# PREGNANCY &CHILDBIRTH

*Other Avon Books by*
**Tracie Hotchner**

CHILDBIRTH & MARRIAGE
*The Transition to Parenthood*

THE PREGNANCY DIARY

# PREGNANCY & CHILDBIRTH

## TRACIE HOTCHNER

Foreword by Karen Blanchard, M.D., OB/GYN

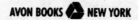

AVON BOOKS ▲ NEW YORK

PREGNANCY & CHILDBIRTH (Second Revised Edition) is an original publication of Avon Books.

AVON BOOKS
A division of
The Hearst Corporation
1350 Avenue of the Americas
New York, New York 10019

Copyright © 1979, 1984 by Tracie Hotchner
Second revised edition copyright © 1990 by Cortona Corp.
Inside cover author photograph by Jonathan Exley
Published by arrangement with Cortona Corp. and the author
Library of Congress Catalog Card Number: 79-63133
ISBN: 0-380-75946-2

Second Avon Books Revised Trade Printing: April 1990
First Avon Books Revised Trade Printing: May 1984
First Avon Books Trade Printing: May 1979

AVON TRADEMARK REG. U.S. PAT. OFF. AND IN OTHER COUNTRIES, MARCA REGISTRADA, HECHO EN U.S.A.

Printed in the U.S.A.

OPM   10   9   8   7   6   5

*Dedicated to the memory
of two Great Women
My beloved mother
Geraldine
and my dear friend
Lisa*

# Contents

vii

# List of Charts, Directories, and Diagrams

# Foreword

## by Karen Blanchard, M.D., OB/GYN

The decade that has passed since *Pregnancy & Childbirth* was first published has borne out Ms. Hotchner's vision that childbearing couples need all the information they can acquire to make decisions for themselves and for their children-to-be. The technology that medical practice makes available grows at an ever-accelerating rate. The appropriateness of its application in any individual situation remains far more than solely a medical decision.

The wise couple and the wise physician recognize that parents-to-be should form a partnership with their physicians, a relationship rich with mutual respect. It is the sole responsibility of the couple themselves to take charge of the care of their unborn child: NO ONE ELSE CAN DO IT.

This book is a first step, a source that can advise and guide you throughout your journey to parenthood. There is no attempt here to tell you the "right way" to go; this book serves as a road map to broaden your choices so that you can find your own way. You will learn a great deal about the natural process of pregnancy and birthing, about the problems that can complicate the process, about the medical interventions that can be applied to better the chances of a good outcome. You will learn how you can enhance your own body's abilities to cope with the changes of pregnancy, birthing, and breast-feeding. Arming yourself with facts and a knowledge of what is normal and what is not will give you the confidence to proceed through all the landmarks of a new territory. Committing yourself to taking charge of your own care will enhance your ability to make advantageous use of your other sources of support, such as your health-care providers, childbirth educators, family and friends.

I feel privileged to have been involved from the beginning in *Pregnancy & Childbirth*. Ms. Hotchner has nurtured it through its first decade with changes when needed. She has listened to criticism and praise, always working toward making it a better instrument of its purpose. I recommend it highly for anyone who is involved in the process of becoming a parent.

KAREN BLANCHARD, M.D., OBSTETRICIAN
Santa Monica, California
October 1989

# Acknowledgments

Karen Blanchard, M.D., has been the medical adviser on this book from Day One—a selfless commitment that has spanned a dozen years and required a great deal of time from a doctor with a large and demanding OB/GYN practice. She nurtured the conception of this book, saw it through a long and complicated gestation, and helped deliver what was originally an 8 lb. 6 oz. manuscript, which has grown even heftier through two revised editions! When I first embarked on this ambitious project, it was meeting Dr. Blanchard that gave me the courage of my conviction to realize a book of such scope. She has been a dear friend and an invaluable professional colleague, without whose experience, insight, and intelligence this book would be less than what it is.

Jeffrey Wasson, M.D., is a special pediatrician who throughout the years has generously answered all the questions I receive from readers about their infants. Dr. Wasson has helped me keep up-to-date on baby-related information and made time to read this revised edition of the book, offering his wise advice, for which I am grateful.

Hal Danzer, M.D., is not only a fine infertility specialist but a kind and gentle man. This edition of the book has a greatly expanded section on infertility, which Dr. Danzer took the time to read and improve upon. I hope those of you with infertility problems find an infertility specialist as downright nice as Hal—and also as successful at helping couples get pregnant!

Thanks to Julie Murrow for helping me organize this totally revised edition.

Nansey Neiman was the original editor on this book, and it still reflects the commitment to its purpose and scope which she shared with me. Judith Riven was my editor on *Childbirth & Marriage,* and I was also fortunate to have her editorial support on the tenth anniversary revision on this book. My thanks to both these special women.

Most of all, thanks to Frank, my life-mate, for his belief in my work and for the quality of love and life that we share.

A special thanks to Baby Gracie, who gave a whole new dimension to what love can be and made me a bigger person. She graced our lives with her admirable capacity for living every day in a state of joy.

And then there are all my delicious godchildren, who have been a continual source of pleasure and information: JESSICA ASTOR, KATE KORSHAK, STEPHANIE KINLOCH, LOGAN LEVANT, MOLLY PENN GERON, MELISSA ROSENBERG, and ETHAN ROSS. I've been privileged to be there as they've grown up, sharing their parents' thrills and chills, vicariously riding the roller-coaster of giving birth and raising children! Thank you all for so generously including me.

I have so many dedicated parents to thank for their contributions to this new edition of the book. I feel close to all those couples I've never met, who call or write with their thanks or suggestions (that's why I always send an inscribed copy of the book with my thanks!) I am grateful to friends who have taken the time to share their frustrations, fears, and joy about pregnancy, birth, and child rearing with me. Then I meet people whose gratitude and enthusiasm about this book reaffirms my dedication to staying abreast of all the news that may affect couples wanting to raise a family. All of them are part of this book—as *you* will be once it becomes part of your childbearing experience.

# Introduction

The tenth anniversary of this book! More than ten years have gone by since this book was first published, and I am honored to know that it has come to be called the "bible" by many couples who have relied upon it. Those of you embarking on the adventure of pregnancy and childbirth in the nineties get the "new and improved" edition: a top-to-bottom overhaul! It is because of the faith of millions of people in the information this book offers that I have undertaken a complete revision to help guide a second decade of expectant couples through the pregnancy experience.

When I first wrote this book, I set out to gather every bit of information that existed about childbearing. In the process I became a consumer advocate in the area of childbirth, a protector of the needs and rights of prospective parents and their babies. Over the years I have continued to read every book and publication relating to birth. I've interviewed many hundreds of expectant couples, veteran parents, childbirth educators, nurses, doctors of every kind, midwives, clinic directors, and hospital administrators. I consider it a privilege that couples continue to involve me in the obstacles as well as the joys of their pregnancies, writing to me from Alaska or calling me from Kentucky.

The staying power of this book proves that expectant

couples are more eager to educate themselves and take responsibility than they're sometimes given credit for by health-care providers and facilities. I am as sure now as I was a decade ago that there is a need for this unique book that offers you the pros and cons of every single aspect of childbearing. By reading this, you can make intelligent, personalized choices on your way to a safe and joyful birth experience.

The nineties are a wonderful time to be having a baby. If you are having your first baby now, you probably don't realize how much different things were for couples giving birth a mere ten years ago. Things you may take for granted, such as the father's being present for cesarean birth, or vaginal birth after cesarean (VBAC), or the choice of whether or not to circumcise a baby boy, or baby foods *without* salt or sugar, or in vitro fertilization, or insurance reimbursement for nurse-midwives, or parent-infant bonding at birth, were practically unheard of then.

If you had a baby years ago and are pregnant again now, you'll be amazed to discover that it's a whole new world out there! Most hospitals are more flexible in their attitudes to the childbearing experience you want, and many obstetricians view the expectant couple as partners in decision making about the pregnancy and delivery. There are new advances in treating infertility, in genetic testing of prospective parents, and in getting prenatal information about the well-being of the fetus. The best news of all is that while the technology of childbirth has continued to improve, so has the awareness of the importance of the human aspects of having a baby.

You'll find the most up-to-date information in this new edition, along with many new charts and directories to give you facts at a glance about such subjects as the protein content of foods, the growth pattern of premature babies, or guidelines for donor sperm. I have tried to make sure that everything and anything you need to know about your pregnancy and childbirth is between these covers.

You might already know that I've written a sequel to this book, called *Childbirth & Marriage: The Transition to Parenthood,* which your bookstore should have right beside this one. Over the years, many couples have written to say, "Thanks, you helped me through my pregnancy. We had the baby. Now what?" I wrote the second book because I saw so many new parents' relationships going through a rough time when the baby arrived. Families must be safeguarded: nurturing the family relationship is vital to the long-term happiness of you and your children. The bonding of parents to each other is as important as parent-infant bonding. I have tried to give you the same kind of thorough, unbiased information in *Childbirth & Marriage* as I hope you will find in this book.

Most of us have no idea the enormous effect that a baby is going to have on our marriage. It can be wonderful if you know how to make it work for you, and it can be miserable if you don't have a support system. I believe the world can be a safer, happier place for mamas, papas, and babies because of these two books. I hope you will take advantage of what they have to offer and let them become good, trusted friends during this exciting, challenging time in your lives. Good luck in the thrilling adventure of childbirth and the new world that parenthood will open up to you.

I'm often asked, "What's the one piece of advice you'd give to pregnant and new parents?" The wisest suggestion I can make is this: give yourself and your mate the same love and patience that you show to your little baby. The three of you have a lot in common: you are vulnerable, learning and growing. To all you new parents out there I send a heartfelt wish: HAVE A GREAT BABY, AND HAVE A GREAT LIFE TOGETHER!

Los Angeles, 1990

# How to use this book

This book is a consumer guide to pregnancy and birth. As such it covers every possible aspect of that experience. I have researched and tried to think of absolutely everything anyone could possibly need or want.

Some people will want to sit down and read straight through the book but others may be interested in one particular issue. For instance if you're already three months pregnant you may want to skip Chapter Two, Difficulties Getting Pregnant. If you are certain you're going to have a baby in a hospital you may have no interest in reading Chapter Eight, Home Birth (or vice versa). My intention in writing the book is to make thorough and unbiased information available so that prospective parents can make intelligent decisions throughout the pregnancy experience.

The more you know about *all* your options, the better you'll be able to get the most out of this time in your life. However, it is possible that your only concern is whether to have a fetal monitor during labor. This book will have served its purpose if you read nothing but that section—because it will equip you with a balanced view of the pros and cons so that once you are in labor you can understand and perhaps share in the decision to use a monitor or not.

The other intention of this book was to organize it so that you don't have the frustration of digging through endless chapters to get at what you want. Just look at the contents pages and go right to the section that covers your area of concern. Don't feel obliged to read the chapters that precede it—the book is intended to be a tool to make things more clear and therefore easier for you. Use the book so that it works for you, not so that you feel that reading carefully through is one more thing you "have" to do while you're pregnant.

Let me explain why I organized the book as I did. I didn't put Taking Care of Your Body before Choosing a Doctor and a Hospital because one is more important than the other. I dealt with the physical changes and demands of pregnancy first because it doesn't mean very much to have a terrific doctor if you aren't nourishing the fetus properly. But if your primary concern is how to choose a doctor or whether to change doctors, then certainly you should go right to that chapter and read about nutrition and other physical aspects of pregnancy another time.

There are going to be people reading this book years before they ever get pregnant and there are going to be people who turn to it in their seventh month. Obviously, what they want from this book will be vastly different. The way they use the book will be different. All I could do was make sure that everything they can possibly need to know is in here. Please use it to suit your individual needs and enhance your pregnancy experience.

# 1
# Taking care of business before pregnancy
## *(Read even if it's "too late"!)*

A friend once asked me rhetorically, "Do you know why most people have babies? Because they get pregnant." That may have been true years ago when women never questioned that they'd (a) get married, (b) have children, and (c) spend their lives being mothers and housewives. Of course there are still many women doing all three of those things, but nowadays they have more choice about when and how to do them. There are women marrying and never having children, there are unmarried women having babies, and there are women choosing between children and a career or making room for both.

Most women don't just blindly accept motherhood—it's a big decision to create another life and help it develop for twenty-odd years. Being a parent involves a lot of time and energy, and there are choices about when, or in some cases if, to become pregnant. The best parents are willing, flexible, loving ones, so listen to yourself, not to other people, when deciding. A baby is going to change your life forever: if you're aware and ready for all that a baby means, that change will be for the better.

This chapter covers some of the things you may want

to think over and talk to your mate about. After you read it you may wonder if I'm trying to talk you *out* of becoming a parent, because it's so overwhelming! But I wouldn't be doing a complete and responsible job if I didn't include these questions. Anyone who tells you not to worry about these things, that everything will "fall into place by itself," is not being a true friend. I have interviewed many couples who split up after their baby was born and lots of women who were confused and miserable about their newborns. They hadn't thought things out beforehand, or maybe it was just the wrong time in their lives for a baby. So please read this chapter, even if you're already pregnant—at least you'll have time to think things through before the baby comes. It's every bit as important as eating well during the pregnancy.

## THE DECISION TO GET PREGNANT

Women often say their pregnancy was unplanned. They insist it was the one time they, or their partner, didn't use contraception. Or they'll say they "got a little high" and took a chance. But if someone always uses contraception and then doesn't "just once," *that is deciding.* Those people should recognize that this was their way of making a decision. Perhaps they feel more comfortable saying the pregnancy was unplanned because the decision is such an enormous one they were afraid to take responsibility for it. We can all learn something from this because even people who are *sure* they want kids can often feel ambivalent. For some people, deciding whether or not to get pregnant may feel like standing on the edge of a diving board. No matter how long you stay on the board you don't get an absolute answer—you see all that you gain by having a child, as well as what you lose. Maybe you finally jump in when you get used to feeling ambivalent and realize it will never be a black-and-white decision.

## DO YOU LIKE KIDS?

This is a logical first question, but you may not know the answer. People live so cut off from others in this country that you may feel uncomfortable around children simply because you're not used to them. One way to learn more about your feelings about children is to go out of your way to be around them—friends' kids, relatives' kids, etc. Your reactions would be different to your own children, but at least you'll get some sense of what you do and don't like about *these* children (and you'll probably have some opinions about how their parents are raising them—which you should keep to yourself if you value their friendship!). It may be that infants make you nervous and bored and that you're more interested in children at the walking-talking stage. Or vice-versa. If you're visiting a two-month-old and are panicked when you see that the baby has to be fed or changed constantly, keep in mind how quickly a child grows. You won't have all that long to put up with—or to enjoy—any one stage in your own child, who will be constantly changing. If you like the idea of having a child or children share your life, that's what really counts.

## OUTSIDE PRESSURES THAT MAY BE INFLUENCING YOUR DECISION

*Friends and relatives* may be urging you to have a baby. Remind them that you're the one who has to live with the child, not they! There is also a lot of general social pressure to reproduce: if you've been married for several years and don't have children you've probably found that even total strangers ask "when" you're going to. There is a group called NON (National Organization for Non-Parents) to give support to couples who choose to be child-free, a word they encourage instead of "childless." They say that people without kids are called materialistic, selfish, and irresponsible—and that some people have children because they can't stand up to that pressure. It's certainly true that you should try to separate your personal desires from what society expects—and if they don't match up, then do what seems right for you.

*Role fulfillment:* You may be having a child because you think you're supposed to find fulfillment as a woman by childbearing and -rearing. You *may* very well find fulfillment in motherhood, but trust your instincts rather than the myth. The women who have formed their identities around the expectation of one day marrying and having kids are the ones who *need* parenthood. They have to fulfill that expectation—even though they may have formed it years ago and things may have changed a lot since then. Some men may feel the need to be fathers to fulfill the age-old idea that masculinity and virility are judged by reproduction (historically, this was gauged by how many *sons* a man could produce). The modern-day measure of a man's power is usually his success in business, but fatherhood is still very important to some men to fulfill their roles.

Even though things have changed a lot because of the women's liberation movement it will probably be at least another generation before we see the real impact of feminism and antisexism in roles. My point here is simply that people should be *aware* of the influence of role-fulfillment—having parenthood as a lifelong expectation isn't "wrong" or "right." But for people who have no real interest in parenthood, it makes no sense to have a baby because they've been taught that it's the way to find meaning for their lives. Those people may wind up feeling emptier than before.

*Having a baby to become an adult:* There are people who feel deep down that they are perpetual adolescents until they become parents, and for them having a baby is a way of entering adulthood. This may be especially true for a woman who does not have a career or who thinks of her work only as something to do until the baby comes. For anyone, the transition from being someone's child to being someone's parent is an important "rite of passage." Many of the emotional flip-flops that people go through during pregnancy are a result of getting used to the idea of themselves as Mommy or Daddy.

There are lots of people who still need to prove their grown-upness, even though they may be 25 or 35. Often this desire is tied up with complicated feelings about their own parents. Having a child may give you a feeling of release, of freedom from your parents—for some of us that may be a relief; for others it may be wistful. Try to be aware of the ways in which your relationship with your parents may be affecting your decision to become a parent yourself. Pregnancy and birth are part of your ongoing personal growth—call it becoming an adult if you like—but beware if a substantial reason for wanting a baby is to prove your adulthood to others.

Everyone is affected by his parents in terms of the kind of parent that he becomes. Some people may overindulge or overrestrict to correct the "mistakes" their parents made with them. Some people may try to make up for lacks in their own childhood by giving a child all the things they didn't get, either materially or emotionally. These are natural human tendencies but if you see them for what they are, they'll be much less of a burden to you and your child(ren).

## Is Your Relationship Ready for a Baby?

**Have you discussed parenting with your partner?** Do you have compatible ideas about the kind of education you'd want for a child? About the part that religion would or wouldn't play in a child's upbringing? Have you talked about discipline and freedom—setting limits while giving space to children? Would either of you be so strict or so lenient that you couldn't modify if your partner disagreed? Many people just *assume* that because they're in a good, loving relationship, their mate shares philosophies about child rearing. That isn't necessarily true, and if you can't iron out any differences ahead of time, raising the child may become a battleground. It may seem unimportant to you now, but if *you* think a baby should be cuddled when it cries and *your partner* thinks that means you're spoiling the child . . . life can get pretty tense.

*Is the relationship stable?* Have you been together long enough to feel you have a good working foundation? Would you be able to share each other with your child without feeling jealous? Your immediate reaction to that question may be indignation—your "conscience" may be telling you that anyone who would even *think* that way, much less admit it, isn't fit to be a parent. You're wrong. There are couples who already feel that their time together is limited by their jobs and it's natural and even healthy for them to feel that the baby is coming between them. You'll probably be a better parent if you toss these ideas around ahead of time and realize that you *are* going to have less time together once there's a baby in the house. By looking ahead you won't take those feelings out on the baby or on each other.

Is your relationship shaky, or do either of you feel it's less good than in the past? People make the mistake of thinking that a baby is a remedy for their problems and will bring them back together. For most people who get pregnant with that hope, the baby usually acts as a Band-Aid that comes unstuck pretty quickly. Childbirth often has the effect of accelerating whatever is going on in a relationship—so if things are on the rocks, it only propels them downhill (and, happily, the reverse also seems to be true for people whose good relationships blossom). Perhaps you're thinking of a baby as someone who will love and appreciate you—to fill in the gaps there may be in your relationship. It just doesn't work that way. You'll be doing yourself and the child a great disservice if you expect him or her to fill an adult's emotional, intellectual, and/or affectional needs.

*If you aren't married* but live together, have you been honest and clear with each other about plans for the future? There are people who hope, often unconsciously, that a pregnancy will propel cohabitation into marriage. Be open and up-front about what you each really want and how a child fits in. If you both truly prefer to stay unmarried, then discuss and perhaps even write up an agreement about child care in the event that you split up. Such an agreement would probably stipulate that whoever did *not* take the major responsibility for the child in the event of separation should contribute in time, money, or both to the child rearing. If you aren't living together or have no long-range plans, then the woman must be realistic: there are financial, logistical, and social burdens in raising a child alone. Don't underestimate them!

*Irreconcilable differences,* as the divorce courts call it. If you had insoluble problems would you stay together just for the kids? Single-parenting: think about it. You may be shocked to learn that one-half of all marriages today wind up in divorce. I'm not trying to throw a pall over things, but *someone* has to ask you how you feel about the prospect of raising kids alone. If you want to think of yourself as part of the American public, then you stand a chance of being a divorced person. Difficult though it may be, many people raise children alone—but does that seem so unthinkable to you that you aren't willing to take the risk?

## CAN EITHER OF YOUR CAREERS AND/OR EDUCATION TAKE THE STRAIN?

A baby may mean postponement of your goals and a temporary or even permanent leave of absence. Are you ready and willing to make adjustments in advancing your career for a totally dependent baby? Does your job involve a lot of traveling? Unless you want to quit working altogether, a baby will place some restrictions on you no matter when you decide to get pregnant. Might there be a different stage in either partner's work when a baby would be less disruptive? Are you willing to restrict your social life and give up certain amounts of leisure time, privacy, and the freedom to do what you want when you want to do it? If you want to breast-feed (or even if you don't), have you explored the possibility of having the baby with you at your job or school? If you plan to return to work full-time after the baby is born do you think you'll feel guilty to the extent that it interferes with your job or your relationship to the child? Even if working full-time doesn't make you feel conflicted, you should prepare yourself for other people's reactions. Most people are conditioned to seeing a mother spend all her time with her child and cannot understand that some women can be mothers and have careers and do both very well. You may have to be the one to educate people, while trying not to let their insinuations make you angry! Finally, can you find ways for both parents to share the tasks of parenting—it doesn't have to be fifty-fifty to work—so that neither you nor the baby is compromised?

## Can You Afford a Child?

It isn't necessary to have a nest egg with the baby's college education already set aside, but if your budget is already tight, then a baby is going to squeeze it even tighter. Before getting pregnant you should take a good look at your financial situation, *especially* if either of you is going to stop working. A hospital birth costs anywhere from $1,200 to $3,500 nationwide for the simplest care. Out-of-hospital births go anywhere from no charge to well over $1,000. And you're going to have to pay for the pediatrician and all the things you *didn't* get at the baby shower! It may be a good idea to wait until you have what *you* consider financial security before adding a baby to your life. Some figures say it can cost over $100,000 to raise a child to the age of 18, not counting the lost income for the parent staying at home. Whether or not that estimate is a little high, the truth is that a baby may mean giving up certain personal indulgences, if nothing else.

A baby may mean you have to move, either because you need more room or because your present neighborhood isn't appropriate for kids. So in calculating whether you're financially ready for a child, you should include the cost of moving and a possible increase in monthly cost.

It may be wise to consider taking out a separate comprehensive major medical policy in advance of your pregnancy. This insurance can be bought through your employer or from an agent. If you purchase it through your employer, be certain you can convert it to an individual policy and continue payments if your employment terminates. Be sure that the policy covers all catastrophic health expenses, with a maximum of $20,000 or more. It should cover all complications of pregnancy, including the care of the unborn child and the newborn baby from birth. There should be no exclusions for laboratory fees, X ray, anesthesiology, equipment, drugs, ambulance, or consultation fees. It will be necessary to have a deductible figure of at least $500— otherwise the policy would cost too much. If you can manage, it is well worth having this insurance "just in case." "It happens to other people" won't pay the astronomical costs of hospitals, so protect yourself with insurance if you can.

While 40 percent of the United States work force enjoy some type of disability coverage, only 40 percent of these benefit plans include pregnancy disability coverage. However, there are twenty-two states that require payment of pregnancy disability benefits. If you live in one of these states be sure to demand the money you have coming to you: Alaska, California, Colorado, Connecticut, Hawaii, Illinois, Indiana, Iowa, Kansas, Maryland, Michigan, Minnesota, Montana, New Hampshire, New Jersey, New York, Oklahoma, Oregon, Pennsylvania, South Dakota, Washington, and Wisconsin. Hawaii is the only state that treats all disability benefits equally: it requires employers to cover pregnancy-related and other disabilities for 26 weeks. Since that mandate, Hawaii's costs for temporary disability insurance have not increased, as might be expected: they have actually decreased.

In order to get benefits, you should contact your state disability office and request the form to apply for disability. You fill out one side of the form and take it to your doctor, who will fill out the rest of the form, stating the date from which you are disabled. The doctor then sends the form to the state, and you tell your employer that you've made this application.

The Pregnancy Disability Act (PDA) applies only to women who work for companies with employee disability policies. The PDA does not help the majority of women who work for smaller companies that are less likely to offer such benefits. If you believe your employer has denied you benefits you're entitled to, you can contact the Equal Employment Opportunity Commission and/or the Department of Human Rights in your state. Under Title 7, Public Law 95555 (insurance coverage for maternity care), you are entitled to benefits for pregnancy the same as for any other disability.

Under most pregnancy disability plans the average leave time is 6 weeks. Two factors contribute to misleading statistics regarding pregnancy leave. First, many employers require a woman to leave work months before she is disabled. Second, many employers impose an arbitrary date for return to work based on the stereotypical notion that women are unable to continue working or do not desire to return to work. However women *do* return to work with impressive regularity: about three-quarters of them return to their jobs after an average of 6 weeks' absence after delivery.

Federal, state, and local governments have programs to ease the cost of pregnancy and the arrival of a baby. Contact the health department of your city *and* state to find out what services may be available. They will probably also have information on free or inexpensive health clinics in your area. The federal government operates the Maternity and Infant Care (MIC) Program for poor pregnant women. There are fifty-six clinics in thirty-four states—in areas that have had high infant and maternal mortality. Chart 1 (page 11) shows the regional office serving your part of the country; all women who live in these areas may receive prenatal care in project clinics.

## CHART 1. MATERNAL AND CHILD HEALTH SERVICE REGIONAL OFFICES

**REGION I**
*(Connecticut, Maine,
Massachusetts, New
Hampshire, Rhode Island,
Vermont)*
Room 1409
John F. Kennedy Bldg.
Government Center
Boston, MA 02203

**REGION II**
*(New Jersey, New York, Puerto
Rico, Virgin Islands)*
Federal Bldg.
26 Federal Plaza
New York, NY 10007

**REGION III**
*Delaware, District of
Columbia, Maryland,
Pennsylvania, Virginia, West
Virginia)*
3531-35 Market St.
P.O. Box 13716
Philadelphia, PA 19101

**REGION IV**
*(Alabama, Florida, Georgia,
Kentucky, Mississippi, North
Carolina, South Carolina,
Tennessee)*
Room 423
50 Seventh St., N.E.
Atlanta, GA 30323

**REGION V**
*(Illinois, Indiana, Michigan,
Minnesota, Ohio, Wisconsin)*
300 South Wacker Dr.
34th Floor
Chicago, IL 60606

**REGION VI**
*(Arkansas, Louisiana, New
Mexico, Oklahoma, Texas)*
1114 Commerce St.
Dallas, TX 75202

**REGION VII**
*(Iowa, Kansas, Missouri,
Nebraska)*
601 East 12th St.
Kansas City, MO 64106

**REGION VIII**
*(Colorado, Montana,
North Dakota, South
Dakota, Utah,
Wyoming)*
9017 Federal Office Bldg.
19th and Stout Sts.
Denver, CO 80202

**REGION IX**
*(American Samoa, Arizona,
California, Guam, Hawaii,
Nevada, Trust Territory)*
Federal Office Bldg.
50 Fulton St.
San Francisco, CA 94102

**REGION X**
*(Alaska, Idaho, Oregon,
Washington)*
Mail Stop 503F
Arcade Bldg.
1321 Second Ave.
Seattle, WA 98101

These clinics offer family planning, special services to adolescent mothers, and patient education. There is medical care that includes vitamin supplements, prescriptions, and other medical supplies (such as elastic support stockings) that are free to any woman in the project who couldn't otherwise afford them. There is dental care—so important during pregnancy—and special attention to women who may have dental problems that keep them from eating properly. There is also a nutrition counseling service that is geared to a patient's limited budget and personal eating habits. The Department of Agriculture also provides nutritional supplements for pregnant and lactating (breast-feeding) mothers. Some project clinics participate in the MIC program through which high-risk pregnant women get milk, orange juice, eggs, and high-iron cereal with special coupons. The Maternity and Infant Care Program also offers social services to help a woman cope with the emotional demands of pregnancy. Once the baby is born, there is free infant care in a well-baby clinic.

## ARE YOU THE RIGHT AGE TO HAVE A BABY?

Most doctors agree that the optimum ages to have a baby are between 20 and 35. Women under 20 are especially likely to have miscarriages, premature deliveries, and still-births. A teenager is still growing herself, which compromises the growing fetus, but the problem is not only a physical one. The complications in teenage pregnancies are usually a combination of social, economic, and emotional pressures—a pregnant 15-year-old is probably unmarried, without much (if any) income, and temperamentally unstable.

There has been a change in the medical community's attitude towards women 35 or older, whose pregnancies until recently were considered risky and who were officially referred to as "elderly" mothers. Medical journals have called this nomenclature archaic, obsolete, and even offensive. It is now agreed that a healthy woman of 35 or older can look forward to a pregnancy as safe, and an infant as healthy, as a 20-year-old mother's. In fact, the statistics show that older women are more likely to progress normally in labor, less apt to require anesthesia, and less likely to deliver an infant that requires care in the neonatal intensive care unit.

However, if you are an older mother, you are at higher risk for having a baby with abnormal chromosomes. About 1.5 percent of the children born to women over age 34 have an unusual chromosome pattern. An older man also has a greater likelihood than a young man of fathering a child with chromosomal abnormality. Like the older mother's ova, an older man's undeveloped sperm have had a longer exposure to environmental hazards which might have damaged genes or chromosomes. In fact, in one-quarter (25 percent) of the children with Down's syndrome (mongolism), the extra chromosome comes from the father, not the mother. On pages 23 and 593 there are some statistics that indicate your chances of having a Down's syndrome baby.

Unfortunately, testing the parents is not usually useful in predicting the disorder. You can protect yourselves by finding a well-informed, supportive doctor and undergoing whatever screening tests are available.

You should have a baby when you are ready. Getting pregnant *primarily* because you've reached a certain age can cause more problems—and longer-lasting ones—than the age factor itself!

If you want more than one child, you should consider that in deciding when to first give birth. A woman's body needs at least one year to replenish itself after a pregnancy. Some studies show that the optimum interval between pregnancies should be not less than two years. There is evidence that if the space between is only one year, low birth weight and prematurity are more likely, both of which may mean complications.

## PREVIOUS CONTRACEPTIVE HISTORY

### THE BIRTH-CONTROL PILL

The many health warnings about the Pill have not been updated to include information about pregnancy. To avoid potential birth defects, there is a warning to discontinue use of the Pill three months before becoming pregnant. A woman's body needs 60 to 90 days to restore its normal metabolic function—perhaps longer if you've been on the Pill for many years (some women who are long-time users wait many months for the return of periods). The safest system is to wait for two spontaneously occurring menstrual cycles before trying to conceive and use other contraception during the wait.

It's been shown that women who get pregnant within 60 days of coming off the Pill stand a 1 to 2 percent chance of babies with abnormalities of bones, heart, eyes, and/or ears. Abnormal nutritional changes take place in women on the Pill that affect the first twelve weeks of pregnancy—when the above-mentioned parts of the fetus are forming. The nutritional change is basically a decrease in the body's absorption, utilization, and availability of the B vitamins: $B_{12}$, $B_6$, folic acid, riboflavin, and thiamine. These are needed for the proper formation of bones, heart, eyes, and ears. The Pill also causes a drop in vitamin E and an increase in cholesterol levels (as much as 35 percent), and vitamin A, niacin, and copper.

*Because of these possible injuries to the fetus, the Pill should never be taken by a pregnant woman.*

## BIRTH-CONTROL INJECTION

Depo Provera is being developed as a 150-milligram injection that will give three months of contraceptive protection. As of now, it is approved only for the treatment of uterine cancer. Ralph Nader's Research Group is trying to block approval of the drug for contraceptive purposes because it has been linked to cancer, birth defects, and sterility. Until studies connected Depo Provera to limb and heart abnormalities in infants, it was given orally to women to prevent miscarriages. Research on dogs has shown that the drug can lead to malignant breast tumors, and there are indications that there may be an increased risk of cervical cancer in users.

## INTRAUTERINE DEVICES

An IUD can cause complications if you become pregnant while you have one in place. A report published by the Cooperative Statistical Program for the Evaluation of Intrauterine Devices (IUDs) analyzed the outcome of pregnancies in which the women conceived while using a Copper T IUD. Many of the women chose to have a legal abortion. Of those who chose to continue the pregnancy, the IUD was removed in about half the cases and left in place in the other half. When the IUD was removed, 20 percent of the pregnancies ended in a spontaneous abortion; when the IUD was left in place, 54 percent ended in a spontaneous abortion. The Copper 7 IUD is similar enough to the Copper T that it is not unreasonable to apply the report's findings to that device also.

It is now being recommended that any intrauterine device be removed as soon as pregnancy is confirmed if you wish to continue the pregnancy. Spontaneous abortion seems to be the main problem of carrying an IUD when you are pregnant. Another possible problem is premature delivery. In the above-mentioned study with the Copper T there were four times as many premature infants when the IUD was left in place as there were when it was removed. However, other studies have not shown a statistical difference between the number of premature infants born when the IUD was left in or taken out; so there is doubt about IUDs and the question of prematurity.

Another concern has been about the effects of the IUD (in particular the Copper 7 and the Copper T) on the development of the baby. The report showed no children born with deformities. Most authorities agree that this is a somewhat reassuring finding about IUDs in general with regard to the safety of the baby. However, this study as well as earlier ones indicate that you should have the IUD removed if you become pregnant while using it.

## SPERMICIDES

Some spermicides—all contraceptive creams, jellies, foams, and suppositories—have been linked with serious birth defects. Research shows that women who get pregnant while using spermicides (or possibly even several weeks after giving them up) may be more likely to bear children with defects. These researchers also found that late miscarriages were almost twice as common in spermicide users as in women who practiced other forms of birth control.

However, this earlier research is disputed by the U.S. Food and Drug Administration's Fertility and Maternal Health Drugs Advisory Committee. This committee concluded that studies have *not* shown an increased risk of birth defects from the use of spermicides immediately prior to or during early pregnancy. The group concluded that the warning labels on spermicides are not warranted.

Because this is one of those controversial issues about which there is ongoing research, you are going to have to decide for yourselves whether to give up using spermicides in the months just before you want to get pregnant.

## THE CRUCIAL FIRST THREE MONTHS

It is during the first twelve weeks of fetal development that most birth defects happen. This is when the body, arms, legs, and internal organs are forming and exposure to damaging substances is most dangerous. Unfortunately, many women aren't even aware that they're pregnant right away so they can't be careful during the time when it matters most. If you are one of those people you must be *very careful* in recalling any X rays, drugs, or chemicals (pesticides, for instance, or materials used where you work) that you have been exposed to since conception.

Any drug used by a man or woman before conceiving a child may have the potential to cause birth defects. This includes topical medicines applied to the skin, which most people would not stop to think about (like Accutane for acne—see page 196). Check with your doctor about whether any medications you use now or have in the recent past may be toxic to the fetus.

## PREGNANCY TESTS

*At-home pregnancy tests* are more accurate than they used to be, if the instructions are followed carefully, but they are still not completely dependable. The advantage is that you can get immediate results in the privacy of your own home. However, these kits can be expensive and many women want to repeat the test because they don't feel confident about the results, thus making the process even more costly. Also, erroneous results have their costs: if you get a false negative reading and are actually pregnant, you may not take appropriate precautions about what you expose yourself to, what you eat or drink, and so forth.

These tests are usually based on the use of monoclonal antibodies to detect HCG (human chorionic gonadotropin), a hormone produced early in pregnancy in the urine of a pregnant woman. HCG can be detected in your urine or blood once the fertilized egg has implanted in the uterus, or as early as six days after conception.

The at-home tests, *if used properly,* are about as accurate as a urine test done in a doctor's office—except that doctors don't use urine for pregnancy testing anymore because it isn't accurate enough! The companies that make these products hope you don't realize that.

*A blood test for pregnancy* is the most accurate way to know if you are expecting. The Beta HCG test is a specific blood test that can pick up pregnancy as early as nine days after implantation. If administered this early (8 to 10 days after conception) the test is 97 to 98 percent accurate. This means you could have this test *one to two days* after a missed period and know whether you were pregnant or not. If you were to wait 4 weeks from your last period, the test could give you 100 percent accuracy. Only a few drops of blood are needed to look for the presence of chorionic gonadotropin. Such fast results mean that you can increase your nutritional intake and avoid potentially dangerous substances right from the beginning of your pregnancy. Unlike the urine test, a blood test can detect the difference between a normal pregnancy and a tubal pregnancy, a potentially fatal condition.

*Progestins (progesterone-like hormones)* are sometimes used as an early pregnancy test. A doctor may inject you if your menstrual period is late, and if the progestin fails to bring on a bleeding phase, the conclusion can be that you're pregnant. The lack of a bleeding phase can indicate conditions other than pregnancy, however, so it is fairly inaccurate. Most importantly, it may cause birth defects. *Allow a doctor to give you a shot of progestin only if you would absolutely abort* if pregnant, because the fetus may be adversely affected by it.

## PSEUDO PREGNANCY

Pseudo pregnancy is a condition brought on by your emotions: pregnancy tests register negative, but your body acts as if it were pregnant. The most common reason for a false pregnancy is that your strong desire to be pregnant may inhibit menstruation. This in turn can set off related changes such as weight gain and enlarged breasts and abdomen. It *is* physiologically possible for thoughts and feelings to stimulate the hypothalamus in your brain, which stimulates the hormones causing the physical changes of pregnancy. Pseudo pregnancy can also be the result of a strong *fear* of being pregnant; that anxiety can suppress menstruation, which in turn increases your anxiety. In cases like these it might be helpful to consult a psychologist or psychiatrist. Once a woman understands why believing in the pregnancy was so important to her, the symptoms usually disappear.

## DETERMINING YOUR DUE DATE

It will be easier if you get in the habit of jotting down on a calendar the day your periods begin. This will eliminate some of the guesswork about when the baby will arrive—the ninth month is nerve-wracking enough as it is! Two hundred sixty-six days is the average time from *conception* to full term, although it may be as long as 300 days or as short as 240 days. In weeks, the gestation period is 40 weeks, give or take 2 weeks. But only 4 percent of babies ever arrive exactly on the day predicted.

The due date is computed, however, as 280 days from the first day of your last period. So take the beginning day of your last period, count back 3 months, and add 7 days. This is the same as saying that the baby takes 9 months and 7 days—280 days—to reach full term. This is called predicting the due day "by dates."

An obstetrician has other ways of determining your due date—for example, by listening for the sound of the fetal heart. The heart sounds can be detected at 18 to 20 weeks with a stethoscope and at about 10 to 12 weeks by listening with a Doppler device. These methods have a two-week leeway, which makes them less accurate than the menstrual data. The same is true of the physician attempting to determine your due date by feeling externally for the height of the fundus (the top of the uterus), which should reach your navel at about the 20th week of pregnancy. Later on in your pregnancy, a doctor can use ultrasound to estimate the age of the fetus by its size.

The duration of your pregnancy will tend to follow your menstrual cycle. If you have periods every 21 days, the baby will probably be early. If you have a 28-day cycle the baby may be late. Women with consistently regular periods are more likely to have their baby on the 280th day than women with irregular periods. A woman's age, race, size, and number of other children have no influence on the length of her pregnancy.

**Ultrasound** is another way to determine due date. Ultrasound works like the radar system of submarines. A quartz crystal is placed on the woman's abdomen and high-frequency sound waves (two million cycles per second) are beamed toward the fetus. Unlike X rays, ultrasound can depict soft tissue in detail, and it prints out a "picture" of the fetus in utero. There are times when a doctor wants to know the exact placement of the fetus, the size of its head, the location of the placenta. Ultrasound is usually done before amniocentesis is performed—see next section—to insure that the needle doesn't touch the fetus or placenta.

Ultrasound can be used to investigate fetal development and measure its growth. It might be used in a case of an anticipated cesarean section in which the due date "by dates" is unsure and the doctor doesn't want to jeopardize the infant by removing it before it has reached full term. Ultrasound can also identify intrauterine growth retardation. Pregnancy can be confirmed from the 4th week and the condition of a blighted ovum—which will lead to abortion—can be identified. This helps prepare a woman for the inevitable.

## PRENATAL TESTING

Each year 150,000 children are born with congenital malformations. The advantages of prenatal testing are many. For a couple who fear a specific anomaly, a negative test will spare them months of anxiety. If the test is positive it is possible to have a therapeutic abortion of an abnormal fetus. And for families who choose not to have therapeutic abortion, the test gives them time to adjust to the fact that their child will have a congenital defect. There is also the school of thought that if you absolutely know you would not abort a fetus regardless of what abnormalities it might have, then you shouldn't have prenatal testing. There is the expense, and, in the case of amniocentesis, the very slight risk of miscarriage as a result of the test.

*A couple should seek genetic counseling* if either of them has a disease with a genetic component, meaning that it can be inherited, or if they have already produced an affected offspring. Some experts say that if the mother is over 35, and therefore more likely to have a child with chromosomal abnormalities, she should have a genetic screening.

*Knowing the health background of your families* is helpful if you are going to have prenatal testing, so both of you will want to review the health history of your relatives.

The March of Dimes offers a free booklet that is helpful in explaining genetic testing and includes a worksheet on which you can note your medical backgrounds before you undergo testing. Send a stamped, self-addressed envelope to March of Dimes Birth Defects Foundation, 1275 Mamaroneck Avenue, White Plains, New York 10605. This gives you a chance to gather information that you'll be asked about in the counseling session—whether your parents, grandparents or other relatives had high blood pressure, paralysis, mental retardation, or other diseases.

*The emotional aspect of testing and treatment* is sometimes overlooked by health professionals. There is usually no real treatment for genetic flaws found in the fetus, other than the option of aborting the fetus. Before you have amniocentesis or other testing, it's important to know this so that you can consider the possible psychological impact of deciding to abort such a fetus. Selective abortion, as this is called, can shake the foundation of your self-worth, if your feelings of self-esteem are closely bound up with your ability to create a normal, healthy child. If you abort a fetus diagnosed as having a serious defect you may experience emotions similar to those of infertile couples, who can be upset when they see pregnant women or couples with infants.

Experts say that some couples can react so negatively to the genetic testing that these feelings can ruin their entire pregnancy experience. Here are some of the pitfalls you may experience during prenatal testing and some practical suggestions about ways to handle your feelings:

- You may feel intense anxiety during the two- to three-week wait for amniocentesis results or even during the shorter wait for results of chorionic villi sampling.
- Try to keep in mind that the odds of a bad result from prenatal testing are very low: amniocentesis and CVS return favorable findings 95 to 99 percent of the time. While the reality of the odds in their favor may not mean much for a couple waiting for these test results, it may help to

remind yourself of these odds when you're feeling particularly vulnerable.

- Some couples wait until after they receive favorable test results to talk about their pregnancy. However, experts say it is not a good idea to avoid talking about the baby while waiting for results, or to stop such pregnancy-related preparations as buying maternity clothing or baby products.
- Denying that you are pregnant is shortsighted and counterproductive. Denial can make it more—rather than less—difficult to cope with a bad genetic testing result, if it should happen.
- You may reason that by telling only a few people you're pregnant, you won't have to endure the emotional drain of explaining the situation to a lot of people if the test results indicate you should terminate the pregnancy.
- You may want to restrict the people who know about the pregnancy to only your closest friends and relatives. You may feel that the pregnancy is less real if fewer people know about it, and that by not discussing it you can protect yourself from possible disappointment.
- Many couples who keep their pregnancy a secret and then have to abort the fetus, however, later come to regret their secrecy. They recommend that you don't try to keep the pregnancy a secret any longer than you would if you were *not* having prenatal diagnosis.
- Try to accept and enjoy the pregnancy right from the start: get excited, buy maternity clothes or baby things, allow yourself to experience all the natural reactions. Couples who thought that by not disclosing the pregnancy they would save themselves pain found that what they actually had done was to deprive themselves of joy.

### AMNIOCENTESIS

Amniocentesis is a test of the amniotic fluid to determine whether the fetus has a chromosomal abnormality. A common use for this test is if a couple has an increased risk for Down's syndrome (mongolism), meaning physical and mental retardation. If parents have a previous child with Down's syndrome, the recurrence risk in other children is 1 to 2 percent. The other high-risk group for Down's is women aged 40 to 44, whose children have a 1 to 2 percent risk. Women over 40 produce a dramatically larger percentage of such babies: 1 in 39 births vs. 1 in 2,300 births for 20-year-old mothers.

A second indication for amniocentesis is in cases of inherited inborn errors of metabolism, which is usually identified by a previous child with a metabolic defect.

A third indication for amniocentesis is when the mother is a known carrier of a serious X-linked disorder. Duchenne's, the most common form of muscular dystrophy, and hemophilia are the diseases that fall into this category. They are not detectable in utero, but amniocentesis can detect the sex of the fetus: a male child has a 50 percent chance of being affected, whereas a female has no risk of being affected by these diseases.

An additional use for amniocentesis is if there are medical reasons to induce labor and there is uncertainty about fetal maturity. Amniocentesis can be used to determine the lecithin/sphingomyelin ratio in the amniotic fluid—this tells the doctor how mature the baby's lungs are. The likelihood of RDS (respiratory distress syndrome), a severe lung disorder in newborns, is greatest for premature babies. The information about lung maturity which amniocentesis offers makes it possible to wait to induce the birth, in most cases, until the fetus is more mature.

The preferred time for obtaining amniotic fluid cells is 14 to 16 weeks after your last menstrual period. A needle is inserted through the abdomen and uterine walls to extract the fluid. Although it usually does not hurt, some women may need a local anesthetic. In any case, the long needle used for the procedure may look frightening. It may be a good idea to turn your eyes away while they are inserting the needle if you are squeamish. Beforehand, ultrasound is used to locate the placenta so that it won't be punctured by the needle. Ultrasound is described on page 19.

---

**CHART 2. INFORMATION THAT CAN BE GATHERED BY AMNIOCENTESIS**

---

*SEX:* Skin cells sloughed off by the fetus accumulate in the amniotic fluid. Under the microscope all male cells are different from all female cells.

*AGE* of the fetus is also indicated by the discarded cells. Measuring the lecithin/sphingomyelin ratio in the fluid tells the maturity of the lungs, which is itself an indication of fetal age.

*CHROMOSOME COUNT* is also determined by discarded cells. Usually any deviation from the normal chromosomal structure means that the child is gravely malformed—mentally retarded, handicapped, etc.

*CHEMICAL COMPOSITION* of the fluid can reveal metabolic disorders caused by missing or defective enzymes.

*BILIRUBIN CONTENT* of the fluid helps determine whether an Rh baby needs an intrauterine transfusion.

*GASES* dissolved in the amniotic fluid can be measured. This reveals the amount of oxygen the baby is getting and whether it is at risk.

*ACIDITY* of the fluid is another indication of fetal distress, often caused by inadequate oxygen flow to the fetus.

---

It takes two to four weeks to get the results of amniocentesis and the cost is around $1,200 because it also includes genetic counseling. However, some state governments will pay the entire cost of the test because the expense to the state of a child with Down's syndrome, for instance, is so much greater.

While the risks are slight—under 1 percent—they must be mentioned. The risks to the mother are basically theoretical: things that *could* happen although it's highly unlikely. They are: intra-abdominal bleeding, blood-group sensitizing (Rh blood incompatibility), or amnionitis (infection, which would induce labor and the abortion of the fetus). The risks to the fetus are abortion and injury by the needle. The fetus instinctively moves away from the needle. In rare cases when the needle has touched, it has left a white line so small as to be minuscule. There is usually no question that the information gained by doing amniocentesis far outweighs the very slim risks.

## BLOOD AND CELL TESTS

Blood and cell tests can detect around sixty-five chromosomal and other disorders. No race or group is immune, although some are more prone to be afflicted than others. Individually these diseases are quite rare, although cystic fibrosis, for example, afflicts an estimated 30,000 Americans and Duchenne's muscular dystrophy appears about once in every 5,000 males born live. Current research is constantly making strides in the detection of the estimated 3,000 different single-gene defects. Fetal tests can now find many more genetic flaws than was previously possible: prenatal detection is now possible for the classic form of hemophilia and is reasonably reliable for muscular dystrophy. The new DNA studies are safer for the fetus than some of the earlier techniques and can find important diseases never before detectable in the womb. However, only a few laboratories are capable of doing the newer testing, which is expensive.

The National Genetics Foundation (555 West 57th Street, New York, New York 10019) has a free service for people seeking information about their personal susceptibility to genetic problems in their offspring. Write to the foundation and they will send you information and a family-health-history form for you to fill out. They will analyze it free of charge and if necessary will refer you to one of 54 genetic counseling centers across the country.

## ALPHA-FETOPROTEIN TESTING

Alpha-fetoprotein testing is a simple blood test done on the mother at approximately 16 weeks into her pregnancy. This test can detect birth defects as well as give doctors an early warning of other possibly dangerous situations, including the presence of twins or triplets, pseudo pregnancy, fetal death, and low birth weight. The test supplies information about development of the fetal central nervous system and can detect such abnormalities as spina bifida, anencephaly, and hydrocephalus.

An analysis of the mother's blood will show the presence of alpha-fetoprotein, or AFP, which is produced by every human fetus throughout prenatal development. The fetus secretes it into the amniotic fluid, where traces of the protein cross the placenta into the mother's bloodstream. The function of AFP is unknown, as is the reason that the baby stops producing it soon after birth.

Small quantities of AFP in the mother's blood are normal, but large quantities (which have been found in about 50 of every 1,000 women tested) are a warning, calling for a repeat of the test.

Those mothers with consistently high levels of AFP in their blood are then given an ultrasound scan. This would immediately show whether there are twins, which would account for the excess AFP in the mother's blood. An ultrasound could also show if there is a single fetus with the abnormally shaped head characteristic of anencephaly. The majority of infants with this brain abnormality are stillborn or die soon after birth.

If ultrasound testing yields no explanation of high AFP levels, the next step is usually to do amniocentesis. A high level of AFP in the amniotic fluid is a strong indication that the baby will be born with spina bifida. In this neural-tube defect, the vertebrae that normally protect the spinal cord fail to form properly, leaving a hole in the backbone where the nerves can be pushed out and damaged. It is through this hole that the AFP apparently pours out into the amniotic fluid. If amniocentesis yields these results then the prospective parents have to decide whether to abort or prepare themselves for the birth of a severely handicapped child. Spina bifida often leaves children paralyzed at birth from below the level of the opening in their spine: this may leave them incapable of controlling their bowels or bladder and highly susceptible to chronic urinary-tract infections. In addition, spina bifida often includes hydrocephalus, or water on the brain, which can lead to mental retardation.

Other benefits of AFP testing are that it can show miscarriages which may have been missed and false pregnancies. Also, doctors are now learning that *low* AFP values, which were ignored until recently, also give them important information. Usually, a very low value means that the fetal age has been grossly overestimated. This is a potentially dangerous situation because if a woman is believed to be overdue, labor may be induced. This can mean a premature baby with all of the attendant complications.

## Chorionic Villi Sampling (CVS)

Chorionic villi sampling (CVS) is one of the newer prenatal tests which may one day replace amniocentesis: CVS can be done earlier in pregnancy and with more rapid results. Amniocentesis is done around the 16th week of pregnancy and it takes 3 to 4 weeks to get the results. Chorionic villi sampling is usually done in the 9th or 10th week, and preliminary findings—including whether Down's syndrome is present—are available in a day or two. It takes two weeks to get a more thorough analysis that is comparable to amniocentesis results.

The obvious advantage of CVS is that it allows a woman to abort a blighted pregnancy much earlier, in the first trimester. If a woman learns through amniocentesis that she is carrying a fetus with Down's syndrome, she is faced with a more complicated, dangerous, and emotionally difficult second-trimester abortion. However, the most recent studies show that there is slightly less accuracy when CVS is used to test for fetal chromosomal abnormalities such as Down's: amniocentesis gives an accurate diagnosis 99.4 percent of the time in comparison to CVS's 97.8 percent accuracy rate.

There is also a slightly higher risk of miscarriage with chorionic villi sampling: the rate is estimated at 0.8 percent higher than that associated with amniocentesis. Other studies show a 1 to 2 percent miscarriage rate for CVS, while amniocentesis is generally thought to be 0.5 to 0.75 percent. It may be worth the slightly increased risk of CVS for women who are at risk for certain conditions such as Tay-

Sachs disease or who are in their forties with a higher risk of Down's and limited time to get pregnant again.

In the relatively painless chorionic villi sampling, a catheter is guided by ultrasound through the cervix and into the uterus. A small amount of chorionic villi tissue is withdrawn; the villi are protrusions on the chorion membrane, which surrounds the fetus and later becomes the placenta. The sample is not part of the fetus but contains fetal tissue which can divulge information about genetic abnormalities, including chromosomal, metabolic, and blood-borne conditions. The only significant conditions that cannot be detected from this sampling are neural-tube defects, including spina bifida and anencephaly, but you can compensate for that with a blood serum taken from the mother in the 16th week.

***Experimental use of early amniocentesis and late CVS*** is being offered at some major medical centers. Obstetricians who perform amniocentesis as early as 10 weeks of pregnancy or chorionic villi sampling as late as 20 weeks of pregnancy stress that because the timing of these tests is still experimental, there are not yet any studies to indicate safety. In doing CVS into the second trimester of pregnancy, doctors take tissue from the placenta, which is made of fetal tissue and nourishes the fetus, rather than from the chorionic villi.

Some physicians are doing this test later because their patients want faster results. For example, a woman might have a routine ultrasound examination in her 20th week of pregnancy that shows something is not quite right with the fetus. She might want immediate results from a prenatal diagnostic procedure because the longer she waits, the more difficult an abortion might be if the fetus has a serious defect. With amniocentesis it can take a week or longer before fetal cells can be grown in the laboratory in sufficient quantities for diagnosis. With CVS, the cells can be analyzed instantly.

## Disorders Detectable with Testing

**Cooley's anemia** is an inherited blood disease. Most carriers trace their ancestry to the Mediterranean region; they are primarily Greeks and Italians. One in 25 is a carrier and 1 in 25,000 has the severe form of the disease: 4,000 young Americans have Cooley's anemia. If both parents are carriers there is a 1 in 4 (25 percent) chance that their child will have the severe form of the disease, a 1 in 4 chance (25 percent) that the child will be perfectly normal, and a 1 in 2 (50 percent) chance that the child will be a carrier like the parents. The odds remain the same with every pregnancy, regardless of the outcome of previous children.

Cooley's anemia cannot be caught from another child who has it, it can't be outgrown, it can't develop later in life, and the carrier state cannot turn into the severe form of the disease. It is not yet possible, however, to detect in utero whether the fetus is affected—but research is under way. Individuals born with the disease are anemic: they can't produce the normal amount of hemoglobin. Carriers are usually healthy, with no anemia at all. The child appears healthy at birth but during the first or second year of life it becomes pale, listless, has a poor appetite and frequent infections. The bones become thin and brittle, which affects the structure of the skull and facial bones; because of this, children with Cooley's anemia often look alike. The spleen often becomes enlarged and must be removed. Children with the severe form of the disease would die of anemia if they didn't get regular transfusions. This can cause a severe iron overload—along with added absorption of iron from the diet—which can lead to fatal heart and liver disease.

There is no cure for Cooley's anemia but the FDA has approved use of a drug called Desferal (deferoxamine) that will remove the excess iron that poisons the hearts and livers of these children.

**Cystic fibrosis** is a genetic disease which affects breathing and digestion. Ten million people, or 1 person in 20, most of them Caucasian, are carriers of the cystic fibrosis gene. It occurs approximately once in every 1,500 births and happens when both parents have the recessive gene. In those couples each child has a 1 in 4 (25 percent) chance of getting the disease, a 1 in 4 (25 percent) chance of escaping both the disease and the carrier gene, and a 1 in 2 (50 percent) chance of being a symptomless carrier. Unfortunately, there is no way of predicting who is a carrier. Research is being done to develop a prenatal diagnostic procedure and a newborn mass-screening system.

If a child has cystic fibrosis, a thick, sticky mucus clogs the lungs and airways, creating breathing difficulties, high susceptibility to infection, and lung damage. The mucus may also interfere with digestion by preventing the flow of enzymes from the pancreas into the smaller intestine. The disease is diagnosed with a "sweat test": a child with CF has sweat with a salt content 3 to 5 times higher than that of a child without the disease. Other lung-damaging diseases don't affect perspiration in this way. For now, the only thing to do is diagnose and treat a child as early as possible until researchers are able to distinguish which parents are carriers.

**DES DAUGHTERS**, women who were exposed to diethylstilbestrol (DES) may have anatomical problems that can cause complications in pregnancy. Prior to pregnancy, these women should have a hysterosalpingogram to determine whether there are abnormalities of the cervix or uterus. This test is done by the injection of dye into the cervix. This dye fills up the uterus and fallopian tubes and will then show any areas where malformations may have occurred. It is characteristic of DES daughters to have a short cervix and T-shaped uterus. This means they have a 20 percent chance of miscarriage in the first 20 weeks of pregnancy.

**DOWN'S SYNDROME**, also known as *mongolism,* means there will be physical and mental retardation of the child. The chances of having a child with Down's syndrome are described on pages 23 and 593. Because the test cannot be done until approximately the fourth month of pregnancy, and the results can take an additional month, there are two ways to terminate the pregnancy if you decide to do that.

Dilation and evacuation (a D&E) can be done under anesthesia. It is similar to a dilation and curettage (a D&C) except that the cervix is widely dilated with *Laminaria japonicum,* a Japanese form of seaweed that is inserted into the cervix and dilates it slowly and safely.

If the fetus is too large for a D&E then it is necessary to perform a saline abortion. This is done by injecting saline solution into the amniotic fluid. This kills the fetus; the uterus expels it. Sometimes prostaglandin suppositories are used in the vagina to help the expulsion process. Since the survival of the fetus is not an issue it is possible to use narcotic agents for pain throughout the process, morphine being a common choice. The risks of a saline abortion are approximately the same as the risks of a term birth. Surprisingly, the risks of a D&E (or D&C) are approximately one-tenth as great as those of a full-term delivery.

HERPES SIMPLEX VIRUS is a common venereal disease in the United States. It is therefore not an unusual complication of pregnancy. It consists of clusters of fluid-filled blisters on any part of the body, although it's usually around the genital area. Herpes is usually noticed 3 to 14 days after sexual contact with someone who has it but who doesn't necessarily have the symptoms. Sometimes there is a fever which may be accompanied by headache and generally not feeling well. Urination can be very painful and there can be severe burning or inability to urinate. The blistery lesions usually open and group together, forming larger open sores which heal within a few weeks.

Once infected, a victim will probably have recurrent outbreaks but the disease can be transmitted (sexually) only during recurrences. Between times, the virus becomes inactive. The drug now used for herpes is called acyclovir (brand name Zovirax). It is not yet known whether it is safe to use this drug during pregnancy; studies are being conducted.

Active vaginal or cervical lesions at the time of birth can pass the virus to the newborn—50 percent of infants that pass through an infected birth canal will get herpes. This means they will die or have severe nerve and/or eye damage. A woman who has had herpes *at any time* must be examined for recurrent infection in the cervix and birth canal as delivery time nears. Infection of the fetus before birth can occur if the membranes are ruptured for a prolonged time. If a woman has herpetic lesions in the genital area at the time of delivery it is essential for the baby's well-being that it be delivered by cesarean section before the membranes rupture or within four hours after they do. Most newborns will be protected by this precaution.

Good health is the best way to prevent recurrences. Mothers with a history of herpes should be sure to eat well regularly, get plenty of sleep, keep clean, and wear loose-fitting undergarments. Mental and physical stress are important factors in whether herpes recurs. Be sure not to have any sexual contact if lesions are present.

*Diet therapy* in the control of herpes is one result of the research being done in the field. Recent studies have shown that certain viruses like herpes, mononucleosis, and chicken pox are affected by the protein composition of their environment. It has been found that one of the protein building blocks, an essential amino acid called L-lysine, inhibits the growth of the herpes virus. At the same time, researchers found that another amino acid, arginine, enhanced this viral growth. Clinical data is not yet conclusive, but it does suggest that manipulating your diet can reduce the chance of infection and the recurrence of the virus, as well as helping to heal any lesions which are already present.

Since this treatment does not involve the use of drugs, it poses no problem for use in pregnancy. Any woman with a history of herpes should take care, especially in the last six weeks of her pregnancy, to avoid arginine-rich foods. She should also supplement her diet with L-lysine supplement. It is available in health-food stores and most drugstores. The usual recommended supplement is 1,500 to 3,000 mg. a day, taken in three doses.

---

**CHART 3. DIETARY GUIDELINES FOR WOMEN
WITH HERPES**

---

| LYSINE-RICH FOODS (FOODS TO EAT) | ARGININE-RICH FOODS (FOODS TO AVOID) |
|---|---|
| fish and chicken | all nuts and seeds |
| beef and lamb | chocolate, cocoa, and carob |
| milk and dairy products | coconut and raisins |
| beans | buckwheat and whole-wheat flour |
| brewer's yeast | brown rice and corn |
| shellfish | oatmeal |
| eggs | gelatin |

---

**NEURAL TUBE DEFECTS (NTDs)** are defects involving the central nervous system and development of the neural tube, anencephaly (absence of the rear half of the brain and skull, which is fatal before birth or soon afterward), or spina bifida (an open or malformed spine—survivors suffer paralysis, deformity, and/or brain damage). These birth defects arise early in pregnancy, at the end of the first month after conception. At that time the neural tube, which later forms the spinal column, starts to close, in a zipperlike fashion, progressing both up and down. If there is no closure near the bottom of the spinal column, the fetus has spina bifida.

NTDs occur in 1 in 1,000 births; if your family has a history of such a defect, you are at increased risk. If you already have had a child with an NTD the recurrence rate after one such child is 4 to 5 percent; if you have had two children with a defect, the risk rises to 10 to 12 percent. Neural tube defects can be detected prenatally because a fetal protein called alpha fetoprotein pours out of the opening of the spinal cord and enters the mother's bloodstream. A blood test is done on the mother to find signs of alpha fetoprotein in her blood. If you have a high level of the protein, you will probably be referred for a sonogram to confirm the findings. If the sonogram results are suspicious, you will be referred for amniocentesis to confirm the existence of high levels of alpha fetoprotein in the amniotic fluid.

Researchers have speculated for years that a pregnant woman's diet might have something to do with NTDs. Spina bifida has been found to be most common to northern Europeans, especially the Irish. NTDs in general are more likely to occur in babies born to women of lower socioeconomic classes and women who have poor diets for other reasons. There was an epidemic of neural tube defects during the Depression, and the incidence has been falling since then.

A recent study showed that women who take multivitamin pills at the time of conception have less than half the risk of having a baby with a serious neurological defect than women who do not take vitamins. Although some authorities are advising all women of childbearing age to take vitamins, other experts are waiting for more data from other studies before officially making this recommendation. However, there is the danger that some women will overreact to this information and take large quantities of vitamins at the time of conception, which can actually *cause* birth defects! *NOTE: It is unsafe to take more than the recommended daily amount of any vitamin.* Please see page 142 for Warnings about Vitamins.

RUBELLA (GERMAN MEASLES): 1 in 7, or 14 percent, of women of childbearing age are susceptible to this disease. Rubella is most dangerous if contracted in the first 3 months of pregnancy but the fetus may also be affected if rubella occurs after that. For example, maternal rubella infection during the first 4 weeks of gestation results in a malformation rate of nearly 50 percent. After the 25th week, malformations occur in less than 1 percent of exposed fetuses.

The disease can cause miscarriage, stillbirth, and defects, although only 1 in 5 fetuses are affected in utero if the mother does get rubella. If you have had German measles (which is NOT the same as ''regular'' measles) then you are immune—but before you get pregnant *have a blood test to find out if you are.* If you're married and if you had to have a blood test, that often indicates whether you've had rubella or not.

If you are not immune, get immunized . . . and do not get pregnant for *3 months* afterward. *Do not get inoculated while pregnant:* the vaccine can harm the fetus. Vaccination against "regular" measles is no protection. If you are pregnant and not immune, stay away from young children you don't know. Children between the ages of 1 and 12 are the main sources of infection; although they are required to be immunized, many are not.

Symptoms are so mild you might not even be aware you have German measles. The signs take 2 to 3 weeks to appear after exposure and include a low-grade temperature, a rash spreading from the face down the body, and swollen lymph glands in the neck. *If you come into contact with rubella, your doctor can give you a gamma globulin shot to prevent you from getting the disease.*

**RH BLOOD INCOMPATIBILITY:** The Rh factor is a genetically determined substance in the red blood cells of most people; those whose cells don't have the factor are Rh negative. A woman without the Rh factor in her blood—who is pregnant with an Rh-positive baby—has a chance of becoming "sensitized." Every year 100,000 to 200,000 women face this hazard. Rh incompatibility exists in a couple in which the woman is Rh negative and the man is Rh positive. The incidence of this Rh incompatibility in marriages occurs in 13 percent of marriages between Caucasians and 5 percent between black Americans.

The danger of sensitization exists only when an Rh-negative woman is pregnant with an Rh-positive child. Sensitization occurs if fetal blood cells mix with maternal cells: the mother's blood then develops antibodies that attack and destroy the baby's red blood cells. Sensitization only very rarely occurs during a first Rh-positive pregnancy: there are raised levels of certain hormones that suppress the mother's immune system until after delivery. However, if the Rh factor from the baby's blood enters the mother's bloodstream at delivery, it acts as an antigen and stimulates the production of anti-Rh antibodies. These destroy, or "hemolyze," the baby's Rh-positive cells.

Not all Rh-negative women with incompatible pregnancies become sensitized but there is no way of predicting which women will, so they all should receive Rh immunoglobulin. The intramuscular injection should be given within 72 hours after the delivery of an Rh-positive baby, or after any miscarriage or abortion (blood cells can mix then too). The vaccine prevents the destructive antibodies from forming and should be given after *every* Rh-positive pregnancy in unsensitized mothers.

Once a woman has become sensitized all her pregnancies must be carefully watched: once the antibodies have developed, the Rh immunoglobulin will not work. Once Rh-positive fetal blood cells enter the mother's bloodstream they may stimulate her immune system to produce the anti-Rh antibodies which can cross the placenta, enter the fetus, and destroy its red blood cells. This causes hemolytic disease of the newborn and infant, with differing degrees of impact from stillbirth to mild jaundice and anemia. Babies who develop the disease in utero can often be saved by intrauterine transfusion.

*Intrauterine transfusions* are high risk, but the procedure must be weighed against the high risk of delivering a baby too early. Since there is considerable risk either way, the most desirable situation for an Rh-sensitive mother is for her to carry an Rh-negative baby. This can be done by artificial insemination using a donor who is Rh negative, or at least by determining if the woman's husband is heterozygous, which gives a 50-50 chance of her carrying an Rh-negative baby.

SICKLE-CELL ANEMIA is a hereditary blood disease that primarily affects blacks: 7 to 13 percent of black Americans, or 1 in 10, are carriers of the disease. Those who have the sickle-cell trait are benign carriers—they don't have the disease but they can pass it on. If both parents have the trait, each child has a 1 in 4 (25 percent) chance of having sickle-cell anemia, a 1 in 4 (25 percent) chance of having neither the trait nor the disease, and a 1 in 2 (50 percent) chance of only carrying the trait, as the parents do. If only one parent has the trait, none of the children will have sickle-cell anemia, but each child has a 1 in 2 (50 percent) chance of carrying the trait. And if one parent has sickle-cell anemia and the other parent has neither the trait nor the disease, all the children will carry the trait but none will have the disease itself.

Sickle-cell anemia is not apparent at birth. It may manifest itself in the first few months but usually surfaces between the second and fourth year of the child's life. The disease is more severe in childhood and the earlier the onset of the symptoms, the poorer the outlook is. Many children who get the disease early succumb to it in childhood. Infections—particularly of the respiratory tract—are a frequent cause of death. However, survival to adulthood is *not* rare; the severity and frequency of crisis periods diminishes in adults.

The symptoms are bizarre: irritability without reason, colic, distension of the abdomen, repeated bouts of fever, poor appetite, vomiting, slow weight gain, pale complexion, and jaundice. Some victims have symmetrical swelling of both hands and/or feet with the fever and irritability. Continuous health care is essential in order to prevent infections. A child with sickle-cell anemia will have to cope with hospitalizations, absences from school, and the inability to take part in strenuous sports. There is no way to prevent or cure this disease, but there are several therapeutic procedures that are being researched with good results: administration of urea and alkalinization of blood pH are among them.

A baby with sickle-cell anemia can be diagnosed in utero, but the technique is hard to perform because it involves taking a blood sample from the fetus. However, the test can be done if both parents are carriers and want the fetus tested because they would abort if the test were positive.

A woman with sickle-cell anemia may have serious complications in pregnancy. Increased maternal mortality is associated with it, and the perinatal mortality rate is also high.

Although there is no cure for sickle-cell anemia at present, there are several simple and inexpensive tests available to find out if you have it or are a carrier. There are sickle-cell clinics funded through the U.S. Department of Health and Human Services and the Bureau of Community Health Services operates clinics in the cities shown on the chart (page 11). Early diagnosis is important in treatment and it's also beneficial to go to a clinic for peace of mind, since 9 out of 10 black Americans have neither the trait nor the disease. By knowing the odds for risk within a couple, and what you and your child will have to face if the odds are against you, it will be easier to make decisions about your pregnancy.

TAY-SACHS DISEASE is carried primarily by people of Ashkenazi Jewish ancestry, whose roots go back to Central and Eastern Europe. Ninety percent of U.S. Jews trace their origins to this region. The disease does occur in the other ethnic groups but people of Jewish descent might especially want to be diagnosed before they conceive; in some cases, people might want to be tested before marrying. If two carriers marry there is a 1 in 4 risk (25 percent) with each pregnancy that the child will have Tay-Sachs disease, a 1 in 4 (25 percent) chance that the child will be totally free of the disease, and a 2 in 4 (50 percent) chance that the child will be a carrier like the parents.

Even if only one of the partners in a couple is of Jewish descent, it's a good idea for that person to have the test done. If he or she tests positive for Tay-Sachs, then the non-Jewish partner should be tested too, although only 1 in 900 non-Jews are Tay-Sachs carriers. Also, this gives you the opportunity to have your children checked to learn whether they are carriers.

The disease can be transmitted only from parent to child and the odds remain the same with each pregnancy, regardless of whether other children in the same family have it. The disease is present at birth and does not develop later in life.

One in 6,000 births of Jews with the Ashkenazi background has this crippling, fatal disorder. Tay-Sachs disease is caused by the lack of a specific enzyme, called Hex A for short, in the blood. Since the afflicted child cannot manufacture Hex A, various fatty substances accumulate in the cells, particularly the brain cells. The baby gradually loses motor abilities: it is increasingly less able to sit up, roll over, etc. It becomes deaf and blind and eventually mentally retarded. Death usually occurs at age 2 or 3; almost no children live as long as four years. There is no cure or treatment for this disease at present.

**TOXOPLASMOSIS AND CYTOMEGALOVIRUS** can both cause serious birth defects. Cytomegalovirus is one of the ancient viral inhabitants of human beings. Toxoplasmosis is described fully on page 212. The importance of prepregnancy testing for these diseases is that if a woman has already had them, there is no danger that they will recur during pregnancy. But if she hasn't, the woman is not immune to them and should be retested in early pregnancy to assure that she has not contracted them while pregnant. Since they can cause fetal brain malformation, a woman who learns she has gotten either disease while pregnant may want to abort the fetus.

**WILSON'S DISEASE** can be identified with prenatal testing. The disease results in defective metabolism of copper in the body which causes excess copper in the brain, liver, and eyes. Unless treated, Wilson's disease leads to mental derangement and cirrhosis of the liver.

## BOY OR GIRL?

Many prospective parents care only that they get a healthy baby but there are others who feel strongly about wanting a healthy *boy* or *girl*. Some people plan on having only one child and would prefer a certain sex; others planning a two-child family may already have a child and want one of the opposite sex; some people have two or even three children of the same sex and want one of the other.

If you feel adamant about what your baby's sex should be, discuss it with your mate. Try to understand why the baby's sex means so much to you, or you're going to have a lot of problems if the child turns out the "wrong" sex. It doesn't matter whether the reasons behind a fervent desire for a certain-sex child make "sense" or not—what's important is to find out what's behind it and hopefully feel a little less rigid about it. This might be a situation in which a professional counselor could be helpful, either for you alone or with your partner.

If you are concerned about what sex your baby will be and you get the "wrong" sex, it is important to acknowledge your disappointment. Do not deny your feelings. Do not judge them inappropriate with thoughts like, "At least the baby's healthy; that's all that matters, and I should be grateful. I'm being ridiculous for even thinking about whether it's a boy or girl." Recognize that your feelings *are valid*—think about them, talk about them. But don't project them on the child. Don't let your disappointment interfere with your experience of the child or your child's experience of life. Realize that your disappointment—which is real—has nothing to do with this individual person who is now part of your life.

There are many reasons in a person's history that might make him/her feel zealous about the baby's sex, although many might be unconscious influences. For instance, a woman who was an only child may have always felt her father wanted a boy: her own feelings of inadequacy may be what makes a boy seem more desirable. And by presenting her father with a male grandchild she can give him what she always thought he wanted (which, in fact, may not have been the case at all). Another example would be a remarried man who had a bad first marriage with two boys; perhaps a girl child means the start of a whole new life for himself with his second wife. A woman who grew up only with sisters might fear she doesn't know enough about boys to be a good mother to one. It doesn't really matter how foolish a reason may seem—once you understand it then you begin to be in control, rather than having it control you.

Because it is possible to determine a baby's sex with amniocentesis, there are people using this test solely for sex selection. Certain statistics show that the majority of fetuses aborted in these cases are female. It is a reminder of presumably less-enlightened ancient times when girl babies were left to die on a hill (along with abnormal newborns) because females were considered undesirable. Abortion is a personal decision and there are many situations in which it can be defended and even recommended. But a couple who *want* a baby and then will kill it because of its sex—well, that is another story. The intention of this book is to be unbiased; therefore, you must draw your own conclusions about people who request (and doctors who perform) amniocentesis solely to determine the sex of a baby. A word of caution to those who are considering the test for this reason alone: amniocentesis sex determination can be wrong, just as any test can be wrong. And in the rare instances when there has been a misdiagnosis, the error is usually that a baby predicted to be a girl is actually a boy.

If you have amniocentesis for medical reasons you will probably also be told your baby's sex. You might want to consider asking that the sex not be revealed. Your curiosity may overpower your self-control, but there are reasons not to know. One of the exciting aspects of being pregnant is the mystery: the total unknown about the person growing inside you, what your labor and delivery will be like, how your life will change. By learning the baby's sex you lose part of that romantic aspect. It's also pretty difficult not to begin putting expectations on the unborn child and developing certain attitudes because of its sex. Another reason is that if you're one of the very few people who are told the fetus's sex incorrectly you are going to have an awfully hard time readjusting to a boy when you've painted the room pink, etc. Why not just guess and wonder for nine months like everyone else? It's worth considering.

# 2

# Difficulties getting pregnant

Infertility is defined as the inability to conceive after a year or more of regular sexual relations without contraception, or the inability to carry pregnancies to a live birth. It may surprise you that 15 percent of the population—1 in 6 couples, or more than 10 million people—is infertile at any given time. However, patience is sometimes the answer. The pregnancy statistics for normal women who aren't using birth control and are sexually active are: 25 percent will be pregnant in the first month, 63 percent will be in 6 months, and 80 percent will be in one year. An additional 5 to 10 percent will become pregnant the following year.

Some people just take longer to get pregnant than others and a year is not too long to wait to conceive. However, if you get anxious after even 6 months there is no reason not to have some basic tests done to put your mind at ease or correct any problem that may be discovered. For instance, any couple in their thirties who want to start tests should not wait; very simply, they have less time than younger people. It may take them longer to conceive and they may want more than one child. In fact, older couples are the most likely ones to have fertility problems. A woman is at her maximum fertility in her mid-twenties, tapering to thirty, and then a more rapid decline. The same is true for a man, except there is a slow decrease to forty, and then a more rapid drop-off. Endometriosis and irregular menstruation are other primary causes of infertility in women, as are undescended testicles and mumps in adulthood for men.

Contrary to some people's beliefs, infertility is very rarely a psychological problem. In 90 percent of all cases there is a physical explanation for infertility. The remaining 10 percent have a problem that cannot be diagnosed with current technology and are known as "normal" infertile. In the cases where the reason for infertility *can* be found, it is the woman's problem 40 percent of the time, the man's problem 40 percent of the time, and in 20 percent of the cases the couple share the problem. So if you have difficulty conceiving, you should seek help together—not only because either of you can be the one with the problem, but also because it is a stressful situation and you need each other's support.

---

### CHART 4. FACTORS THAT CAN CAUSE INFERTILITY IN WOMEN

- Pelvic inflammatory disease
- Use of an IUD
- Using medications that diminish fertility
- Post-abortion infection
- Cervical infection treated by cautery or cryosurgery (burning or freezing of cervix)
- Abdominal surgery (for example, for appendicitis or ovarian cysts) resulting in adhesions or accidental cutting of fallopian tubes
- Exposure to such environmental hazards as lead or radiation in your workplace or heavily polluted water or agricultural pesticides at home
- Cancer treatments: chemotherapy or radiation for a patient and in some cases for the health-care provider
- Being the daughter of a woman who took DES when she was pregnant with you (see page 30)
- Being an older woman: fertility tapers after age 25. Chance of conceiving after 6 months' trying is 75 percent at age 25; down to 25 percent in late thirties.

---

### CHART 5. FACTORS THAT CAN CAUSE
### INFERTILITY IN MEN

---

- Venereal disease or other infection of reproductive organs
- Mumps during puberty
- Abdominal surgery (for example, the repair of a hernia) with accidental cutting of vas deferens
- Exposure to hazardous substances (lead, radioactive materials, anesthetic gas, pesticides, benzene, mercury) in place of employment
- Cancer treatments with chemotherapy or radiation
- Exposure to dangerous environmental substances
- Use of medications (some antibiotics, medicine for high blood pressure or ulcers) that lower sperm count
- Being the son of a woman who took DES when pregnant with you (can cause a testicular cyst which will impede sperm production)
- Being a Vietnam veteran who was exposed to chemical warfare substances (Agent Orange)
- Overheating of testicles from tight underwear, hot baths or saunas, long-distance driving
- Extreme stress, which may lower sperm count
- Being an older man with diminished quality and quantity of sperm

## WAYS TO PREVENT INFERTILITY

*Any infection* of the male or female reproductive tract should be treated immediately. Symptoms include discharge from the penis or vagina, pain when urinating, low-grade fever, sores on the genitals, pelvic tenderness or pain in women, rashes.

*Barrier methods of contraception* (condoms, diaphragms, vaginal sponges or foam) will help prevent the transmission of venereal disease, many of which compromise fertility.

*Chlamydia* is the number one sexually transmitted disease (STD) in our country. The tiny chlamydia bacteria strikes between 3 million and 10 million Americans a year, causing an infection that leaves many of them sterile. It is easily treated but as many as 70 percent of its victims never realize they have it and so fail to seek treatment, which can have dire consequences. Both men and women can contract and transmit chlamydia infections. Men generally have no lasting effects, although some researchers suspect it can cause male sterility. In women, however, if the disease is not treated or is treated improperly, it can spread throughout the reproductive tract, eventually blocking the fallopian tubes with scar tissue.

*Gonorrhea* is asymptomatic in 75 percent of women, meaning they do not know they have it. If you are sexually active with multiple partners you should have a culture done every 6 months and use barrier contraception (a diaphragm or condom) whenever possible.

*Mumps:* All prepubescent boys should be immunized against them. When mumps occur in a postpubescent male it may cause inflammation of the testes and subsequent infertility.

*The Pill* is not recommended for women who do not have established, regular menses (i.e., women whose periods are very heavy or very light). Also, some doctors discourage taking the Pill beyond thirty-five years of age.

*An abortion* in which there is hasty or vigorous dilation of the cervix—especially in a very young woman—may cause permanent damage to the cervix. In all cases of abortion—but particularly when a cervix is very tight and firm—a "laminaria wick" can be inserted before the procedure (as little as an hour before or as much as a day). A laminaria may guard against damage to the cervix and is more likely to insure healthy future pregnancies. Any postabortion symptoms of infection should be reported and treated immediately.

There is another way abortion can create problems in later pregnancies. If a doctor uses sharp instruments to scrape the inside of the uterus, the lining can be damaged. Once the uterine lining is compromised, it can cause problems of implantation of the placenta in future pregnancies. If you have an abortion, it should be performed with suction rather than with sharp curettage.

*IUDs* (intrauterine devices) have been linked to infertility and sterility. An IUD is a small piece of plastic that is inserted into the uterus, with a "tail" extending down through the cervix into the vagina. Although doctors are not certain exactly how an IUD prevents pregnancy, it is believed to irritate the uterine lining so that an embryo cannot grow there. The problem with IUDs is that they can cause infection that often leads to chronic PID (pelvic inflammatory disease), which is a cause of sterility. The body fights this infection by laying down scar tissue both inside and outside the fallopian tubes, ultimately leaving a woman unable to conceive.

Studies have shown that a woman using an IUD runs 2 to 4 times the risk of developing PID (an infection of the uterus, ovaries, or fallopian tubes) as a woman who does not use an IUD. A woman with an IUD who has not had any children may run 7 to 9 times that risk. Although surgery can repair some of the damage some of the time, many women do not experience the extreme pain of PID and therefore do not even have the warning signals. The IUD may cause infection, the body may create scar tissue, but a woman can feel little or no pain and so continues to wear the IUD. When she wants to have a baby and has the IUD removed, it is not uncommon for her to discover that she cannot conceive.

## BASAL TEMPERATURE CHART

As a first step in infertility diagnosis you will want to know whether you are ovulating, when you are ovulating, and, based on that, whether you've been having sexual intercourse at the right time for conception. To set up a basal temperature chart you need special graph paper (which your gynecologist can probably supply you with) and either an oral or a rectal thermometer. To make it easier, you might want to buy a special basal thermometer which measures only between 96° and 100° F. with the tenths of degrees clearly marked. It costs around $5. Throw away the directions that come with the thermometer because they are invariably full of misinformation.

A normal ovulating woman will have a low temperature (98°) from the onset of menstruation to just before ovulation. Not every basal body temperature shows the quick "textbook" rise after ovulation which does occur in many women; in some women the rise may be more gradual, occurring over a few days. At about the time of ovulation there may be a dip of several tenths of a degree and then an immediate rise of 0.4° or more. This higher plateau (above 98°) is maintained until just before the next period. The reason for this is that progesterone—which your body releases as a result of ovulation—has a slight heat-producing effect. Ovulation is thought to occur within 1 to 2 days before the rise in temperature.

To set up a chart you mark the first day of your period as day 1 and then take your temperature each morning before *any* activity (talking, smoking, drinking, etc.). "Basal" means the body is at total rest. Take your temperature at *the same time* every morning. On the chart note any reasons you can think of for temperature change: illness, lack of sleep, a large intake of alcohol the night before, etc. Around the time of ovulation you may notice increased vaginal secretions or pain in your lower abdomen (known as "mittelschmerz")—note that on the chart. It may take 3 to 4 menstrual cycles to establish whether you're ovulating and approximately when. Also mark on the chart the days you have sex.

The basal temperature chart is a crude tool at best and far from accurate about the exact time of ovulation. But even with its failings, using a chart has helped people to pinpoint more or less when ovulation occurs so that they can try to conceive at that time.

***Ovulation predictor kits*** sold in drug stores can catapult you into the modern age, allowing you to scientifically calculate when you are most fertile. In a few simple steps you can determine when you are ovulating. However, some people may prefer the "old-fashioned" temperature-taking method. You may not want to spend the money for the kits, or you or your infertility doctor may be skeptical about the accuracy of these tools.

***The best time to conceive*** is within the 3 days (72 hours) prior to ovulation. Within 24 to 48 hours after ovulation, it is no longer possible to become pregnant.

## CHOOSING A DOCTOR

The first step in finding out why you aren't getting pregnant is to try to find a doctor who specializes in infertility. Infertility is a subspecialty of obstetrics and gynecology which requires specific additional training. Try to pick a subspecialist who has a formal fellowship training in infertility with extensive microsurgical and endocrine training. In order to get board certification a true fertility specialist would have had to have this additional training, so do not settle for an OB/GYN who has only spent a few weeks during his residency seeing a few infertility patients. But finding a team of infertility doctors or a clinic isn't always possible in remote or less populous areas. At least try to find a doctor who is affiliated with a teaching hospital or medical center, and who limits his practice to gynecology and infertility, if possible. If a doctor calls himself a specialist then ask what additional training or experience he has had in infertility.

A couple should go into this process together. Before meeting with a doctor you will feel more confident if you learn as much as you can about the possible tests and terminology: this will minimize the feeling of humiliation or the loss of control over your own body that some people experience during infertility testing. Reading this section should give you the information you need. Then you can meet with the doctor to talk in his office and get an idea of his bedside manner and his expertise. If there is something that makes you uncomfortable about the doctor, try to tell him in a constructive way. If you feel you'll be unable to adapt to each other—or if you feel a lack of confidence in the doctor—you should consider meeting with a second infertility specialist if there are others available.

It is reasonable to expect that a doctor can complete an infertility workup in two to three months. He should give you a well-organized explanation of the procedures he plans to do and should give you a diagnosis at the end of that time. It is important that you not be subjected to a long, drawn-out, one-test-a-time process both because of the emotional drain on you and also because you want to get some answers as soon as possible. If the man must be cared for by another doctor make sure that the two doctors are in close communication about tests and treatments.

Most infertility specialists are members of the American Fertility Society. In order to get the names of members in your area, write to: The American Fertility Society, 1801 Ninth Avenue South, Suite 101, Birmingham, Alabama 35205.

## SUGGESTIONS FOR PICKING AN INFERTILITY SPECIALIST

- If you live near a university medical center that has an infertility clinic, you might consider seeking treatment there instead of with a doctor in private practice. The clinic of a teaching hospital is more likely to be using the most up-to-date techniques for infertility.
- Check a doctor's credentials carefully: do not rely solely on membership in the American Fertility Society (not all of whose 10,000 members are experts in the field). What really counts is whether the physician has *board certification* in a specialty area, like reproductive endocrinology.
- Ask a lot of questions at your first consultation with the fertility specialist. Read this whole chapter before going in. Ask questions concerning topics you know something about so you can evaluate the physician based on the replies he gives you.
- If the doctor recommends surgery, *get a second opinion.* Be especially careful about a doctor who wants to perform surgery before doing a complete infertility workup.

There are doctors who do exploratory surgery on a woman without even checking her husband's sperm count.

· Make sure the doctor has a lot of experience using infertility drugs, in case you should need them to stimulate ovulation—particularly if you need to use Pergonal, which is complicated to administer.

### THE INFERTILITY WORKUP: WHAT TO EXPECT

Undergoing infertility exams can be stressful or embarrassing. It can relieve your anxiety and discomfort if you know ahead of time the kinds of questions the doctor may ask you. The doctor will take a detailed history and then do a physical examination of both of you. Further testing may then be recommended. The tests that you or your partner may have to undergo are discussed in the sections on causes and treatments of infertility that follow.

*You will be asked very personal questions* about your medical, marital, and sexual history. Since an infertility specialist will usually see a husband and wife together, at least in the beginning, you may find some of the questions too probing or embarrassing. However, the doctor needs complete information about your past and present health and sexual habits in order to evaluate your situation. You need to share this sensitive information with your doctor if you want to deal with your infertility as quickly and painlessly as possible. You may be able to tell the doctor something that will eliminate the need for you to have expensive, time-consuming, and sometimes painful tests.

*Some of the questions the doctor will ask* have to do with your sex life as a couple. These questions may seem intrusive, but they must be asked in order to find out why you aren't getting pregnant. Here are examples of some questions and what can be learned from them:

· *"How often do you make love?"* If a man has a low sperm count, having sex too frequently can make the count even lower. On the other hand, some couples think that "saving up" sperm will give them a better chance at getting pregnant. Instead, this practice can cause problems. If you abstain from sex for more than 4 days, it can decrease the motility (ability to swim) of the sperm.

- *"In what position do you usually have intercourse?"* Although imaginative and athletic sex can be fun, you have the greatest chance of getting pregnant when the man is on top and the woman is on her back—what used to be called the missionary position.

- *"Does your lovemaking involve using a lubricant?"* You may be hampering your fertility if you use a lubricant like K-Y jelly or Surgilube, which kills sperm.

- *"Do you get up immediately after lovemaking?"* Many sperm can leak out if the woman gets up right after making love. Lying still for half an hour afterwards increases the chance that a sperm will reach the egg.

- *"Do you douche after intercourse?"* A woman can destroy sperm by douching.

- *"Have you ever been pregnant by another man/made another woman pregnant?"* Facts about your premarital lives can provide crucial information to your doctor. A woman will also need to disclose whether she ever miscarried or had an abortion in the past.

*If you will not feel comfortable with your mate's hearing* your answers to the doctor's questions, you should try to cover some of these topics with your partner before you go into the doctor's office. If you cannot handle exposing yourself to your mate's reaction to information about you, then talk to the doctor alone beforehand. Just call the doctor before your visit and explain the facts that you would like kept confidential.

*The doctor will then do a physical exam of both partners,* though some doctors deal primarily with women's infertility problems and may refer the husband to a urologist. In addition to a physical examination, the doctor will want to do urine and blood tests to see whether there is some general infection or other problem that could be interfering with your fertility. You will also be checked for any current infections in the reproductive system. For instance, a couple may not be getting pregnant because the husband has nonspecific urethritis, which can make him temporarily infertile. It may take only a course of antibiotics to clear up the man's infection in order for you to conceive.

## THE EMOTIONAL IMPACT OF INFERTILITY

Your first reactions to finding out you're infertile may have certain stages; knowing this might help you cope. After the initial surprise there is a period of *denial* during which you don't want to accept or deal with the problem. Then you might *withdraw,* cut off your feelings and isolate yourself, until *anger* follows, and a sense of "why me?" You may then feel *guilty* and diminish the way you think about yourself, lowering your self-image. What often happens to people who discover they're infertile and have to undergo tests is that their self-perception is damaged as they come to think of themselves as defective. Following that, it isn't uncommon for people to feel depressed. All this doesn't sound like much to look forward to, but it's better to be ready to experience some or all of these feelings rather than to be hit between the eyes with no warning.

Outsiders often make the mistake of thinking that a couple's anxiety, depression, and frustration are the *cause*— rather than the reaction to—infertility. People may give you advice like, "Just relax and you'll get pregnant," which can only fray your nerves more. In fact, people are being counterproductive when they imply that you're not getting pregnant because you're uptight. It's also ridiculous for outsiders to say you aren't getting pregnant because deep down you have a subconscious wish not to be parents; there is no proof for such ideas, yet many people walk around thinking them. There is also the often-repeated myth that once a couple adopts, they get pregnant afterward, proving something or other to the people who repeat these stories. The fact is that among those with infertility problems, the pregnancy rate following adoption is the same as for couples who do not adopt. In all cases except absolute sterility there is a 5 percent spontaneous cure rate: pregnancy without treatment. Educate people who are close to you by asking them to read this section.

Sexuality is the area in which people are most threatened by infertility. It calls into question what we think a man and a woman *are*. There is a societal idea that a woman must bear children as a display—or as an extension—of her sexuality. She is considered a failure, incomplete, lacking in sexual identity if she doesn't reproduce. Even though the women's movement has helped many people see that women can find fulfillment, be successful, and make contributions outside the home, we are all affected by role conditioning. Social ideas and ideals about what is male and female, feminine and masculine, have been drummed into us for a lifetime.

There are also social beliefs that a man's sexuality is judged by his ability to impregnate: in many cultures, his ability to impregnate with male children is even more important. If a man doesn't reproduce he is considered impotent and lacking in the provable virility that may be a part of his masculine identity. Of course, these are broad generalizations about social conditioning: there is a much broader base, longer history, and more subtle input to your sexual identity than just whether you can reproduce or not. However, it's still useful to realize some underlying social attitudes about how reproduction is equated with sexuality.

Your sex life may also suffer during the infertility investigation. Keeping a basal temperature chart can be tiresome and the loss of spontaneity in sex can create tension and diminished pleasure. Making love just isn't the same when you "have to do it" on a certain day and then have to mark it with an X on the chart! The chart can become even more of an issue if one partner takes full responsibility for recording on it and the other doesn't participate. Just because the woman is taking *her* temperature doesn't mean it's "her" chart or "her" problem. Try to share the task. Each time you have sexual intercourse on a prescribed day there's the chance that "it could be this time"—which is both exciting and nerve-wracking. It isn't unusual for a couple to experience periods of impotence, loss of sexual desire, and a diminished or lost capacity for orgasm during all this.

The first suggestion is to keep a sense of humor about the whole thing; try to see the ridiculous side of the basal chart and "sex on command." One way to put the pleasure back into your sex life is to agree to take a vacation from sex for a while; when it's mutually agreed not to have sex it relieves a lot of pressure and can even make it seem desirable again! You can also change when and where you make love—if it's usually in bed in the morning why not try it at night in the living room? But if either or both of you feel that the problem has become too complex to work out together, discuss the possibility of a couples therapist or one who specializes in sex therapy. Especially if you were happy with your sex life before, it should take only a short time to regain your equilibrium with professional help. If you try to ignore the problem, hoping it will go away—and it doesn't—it will only get more complicated.

In the event of a final diagnosis that pregnancy is not possible—or if a couple decides to give up the effort to conceive—there is an emotional process of grief. In a sense, they are grieving for the death of an unknown child, for the loss of certain hopes and dreams. After initial shock and disbelief there is the suffering and finally a recovery. During this grieving period the infertile partner may behave erratically, often showing anger. She or he is certain to fear that the fertile partner will want to leave, or at least is concealing dreadful negative feelings. Some of this angry, unpredictable behavior may be an unconscious way of forcing these feelings to the surface. It is best to get it out in the open and deal with it at the time rather than letting the feelings—or the infertile partner's *fear* of the feelings—build up. The fertile partner must also have room to express feelings along with the infertile mate—of sadness, of disappointment, and of grief.

Regardless of the outcome of your infertility problem, you should keep in mind that it is a shared problem. Two people who want to have a baby are a team, just as much during conception as during child rearing. If you can keep that in mind, these experiences may help you grow and learn together rather than putting up a wall between you. Infertility tests can be embarrassing, humiliating, and painful; some people might even find certain aspects disgusting. By sticking together, supporting, and leaning on one another, you may actually come out of this with a deeper respect and affection for each other.

## CAUSES AND TREATMENT OF FEMALE INFERTILITY

*Infection* is the leading cause of female fertility problems because infected tissues often result in scars and adhesions within the uterus or fallopian tubes and around the ovaries. This can destroy the normal anatomic relationship of the ovaries and tubes, making it more difficult for the tube to pick up the egg as it is released from the surface of the ovary.

*Gonorrhea* is the most destructive and is usually without symptoms (see earlier, Ways to Prevent Infertility). *Syphilis* is less destructive than gonorrhea in the beginning and can be diagnosed earlier. *PID* (pelvic inflammatory disease) is caused by bacteria entering from the outside. This can happen during abortion, insertion of an IUD, or from a ruptured appendix. Infections like the common *monilia yeast* infection or trichomoniasis *do not* have any effect on fertility.

The treatment for infection can be a D&C (dilation and curettage) to remove polyps, minor adhesions, and excess uterine lining caused by the infection. Extensive scarring may require general pelvic surgery in order to cut adhesions and elevate the entire uterus by tightening ligaments to prevent recurrence of adhesions. The extent to which major surgery can really help depends on how much scar tissue one is dealing with in the first place. It might be worthwhile to do a laparoscopy first to evaluate whether major surgery would be worthwhile. Whether or not laparoscopy should be immediately followed by surgery is a decision a woman may be able to make ahead of time if she discusses the possible variables with the doctor beforehand.

Since the doctor is doing the laparoscopy because he does not know ahead of time the extent of scarring, a woman may wish to discuss his findings with him after the laparoscopy and before she decides on major surgery.

There are several disadvantages to doing a laparoscopy and surgery separately. A woman will have to have anesthesia twice, will have to go through two recovery periods, will have the anxiety of going into the hospital twice, will have to take more time off from work, and will incur a greater expense. Therefore, she will have to weigh the psychological benefit of consulting with the doctor between the two procedures and the numerous drawbacks to not doing them at the same time.

---

**CHART 6. DANGER SIGNS OF PELVIC INFLAMMATORY DISEASE FOR WOMEN WHO WEAR AN IUD**

---

- ABDOMINAL PAIN OR TENDERNESS when lower abdomen is pressed
- ONE-SIDED PAIN DURING INTERCOURSE
- ABNORMAL OR FOUL-SMELLING VAGINAL DISCHARGE
- FEVER
- BLEEDING BETWEEN MENSTRUAL PERIODS
- INCREASED BLEEDING DURING PERIODS
- INCREASED MENSTRUAL CRAMPS

*Important:* VISIT A DOCTOR IMMEDIATELY if any symptom appears. If a blood test reveals you have an infection it may be stopped before it spreads from the uterus to the ovaries and fallopian tubes.

---

*Endometriosis* is a condition in which the uterine lining (the endometrium) grows in places where it should not be, like on the inner lining of the pelvic cavity. This wayward endometrial tissue makes pregnancy more difficult because it causes biochemical or immunological reactions during subsequent menstrual cycles. It can secondarily cause scar tissue which, in turn, makes pregnancy more difficult. Occasionally endometrial cysts occur on the ovaries, which may produce pain, bleeding, leaking, scarring, and the attendant problems becoming pregnant.

Genetics may play a part in such gynecological disorders as endometriosis and polycystic ovarian disease (see page 63). The exact link between the gene and the problem is unknown, but some doctors believe that if you have endometriosis you should contact your sisters or other close female relatives to warn them that they might also develop endometriosis. Some doctors think that sisters should be advised not to delay childbearing in order to enhance their chance of fertility; female relatives might also be advised that if they use contraception they should use oral contraceptives (the Pill) rather than an IUD.

Endometriosis is most common after age 30 and may cause painful periods of intercourse. The conservative approach to treatment is "wait and see." It's often said that pregnancy is a cure for endometriosis because the high estrogen and progesterone levels of pregnancy—along with the absence of menstruation—have beneficial effects. In mild cases of this disorder doctors advise waiting for spontaneous pregnancy, and if you want more than one child, to have them as close together as possible. This is sensible *if* you're ready to have children . . . but of course one shouldn't have a baby simply to cure endometriosis.

The use of hormones which simulate pregnancy is one treatment for this problem. There is improvement in 85 percent of cases. The drawbacks are that the treatment can last a year, that you can't conceive during that time, and that you may get early pregnancy symptoms.

The drug called danazol (the usual trade name is Danocrine) is now the established treatment for endometriosis. Studies have shown no recurrence of endometriosis for up to a year after treatment, and 55 percent of the women getting pregnant. Danazol suppresses ovulation by blocking the production of FSH and LH, simulating pregnancy or menopause. Since you do not menstruate, the misplaced endometrial tissue has a chance to disappear. The usual course of treatment is for 3 to 6 months. You'll probably have one last period after you start taking the drug, and then you won't menstruate again until 3 to 6 weeks after the treatment ends and you spontaneously begin menstruating again.

If you were having pelvic pain from endometriosis you will probably feel better when you're taking danazol. However, the drug can have an annoying side effect, weight gain from water retention, which usually disappears after the fourth month. If you notice swelling in the beginning of treatment you may find relief by maintaining a low-salt diet and perhaps using diuretics (water pills), which should always be taken along with a potassium supplement to replace the potassium you will lose. There is also a side effect of muscle cramping, which most women can tolerate.

Danocrine is expensive: taking 4 pills a day comes out to about $240 a month. Instead of prescribing danazol, many infertility doctors have their patients take birth control pills without a break; this is much cheaper. These physicians find almost the same success rate, if the endometriosis is not at a severe stage. While some women have fewer side effects on danazol than on the Pill, some individuals have more.

Surgery is used to combat the most severe cases of endometriosis. During a laparoscopy a doctor may be able to cauterize (burn) endometrial tissue or vaporize it with a laser. It is even possible to cut some adhesions that may have formed. Often a woman may need more radical surgery—a laparotomy, an incision in the lower abdomen similar to the "bikini cut" for a cesarean—to cut and burn the endometrial tissue.

The usual course is to follow surgery with a treatment of danazol to make absolutely sure that no misplaced endometrial tissue remains. There is now a controversy about this trend, which began when some members of the American Fertility Society pointed out that the most likely time for a woman with endometriosis to conceive is soon after she recovers from surgery. These specialists oppose using danazol post-surgically because using a drug that stops ovulation for months after surgery may deprive you of your best opportunity to conceive.

Lupron is a new treatment for endometriosis. This drug has had excellent results, even for those women who don't respond to danazol. However, Lupron is very expensive (about $300 per cycle) and also has to be injected daily. This means you need someone to give you the injection every day or you have to learn how to inject yourself. It's hoped that it will one day be available in a less expensive, more convenient form such as a skin patch.

*Cervical factors* may be stopping the sperm from reaching the egg. There may be *chronic cervical infection (cervicitis),* which can be treated with antibiotics or cautery. There may be thick and *impassable cervical mucus;* tests can be done on the mucus at about the time of ovulation, and the use of low-level estrogens may help. *Cervical polyps* may be obstructing the opening to the womb and have to be removed. Overly *acid cervical secretions* may be creating a hostile environment for the sperm. These secretions can be neutralized by using certain douches right before intercourse, some of which have a nutrient base to promote sperm survival. If the cervical barrier persists, *husband insemination* may be tried, in which a freshly masturbated semen specimen is instilled into the woman above the cervical opening or even mid-uterus. This may cause cramping and uterine infection since the cervical mucus normally filters out bacteria.

A woman whose cervical mucus is hostile to her husband's sperm is sometimes helped by a small dose of the hormone estrogen on days 10 to 14 of her menstrual cycle. Some doctors are also finding that *guaifenesin,* an expectorant that is an ingredient in some cough medicines like Robitussin, may help thin abnormally thick cervical mucus.

It can happen that there is an insurmountable problem with the cervical mucus—poor-quality mucus, an infection which has gone untreated, or immunological problems in which a woman is producing antibodies against a man's sperm. If there is a poor postcoital test and no success with attempts at artificial insemination with the husband's sperm, the doctor may try insemination with donor sperm. But if none of that works, in-vitro fertilization (described on page 94) holds promise as one way to bypass these cervical mucus problems.

The whole area concerning antibodies is controversial, with many opinions as to whether it's even worth treating. In some cases where there is a significant antibody level, a man is able to impregnate the woman anyway.

***Ovulation problems*** can mean irregularity or periods of not ovulating. *Blood and urine studies* can show estrogen and progesterone levels as well as the presence of LH—luteinizing hormone, which is secreted by the pituitary and peaks before ovulation—and the presence of FSH—follicular stimulating hormone, which stimulates the ovary to ripen a follicle and mature an ovum. Many doctors use *plasma progesterone* for proof of ovulation, but it is more accurate if they do an *endometrial biopsy,* which can assess the quality of ovulation and the tissue. This test can be done in a doctor's office but it is painful because it involves scraping along the uterine wall to obtain a tissue sample. An oral analgesic and/or a paracervical block to numb your cervix will help. The lining of the uterus is then examined and the tissue will show the influence of progesterone if you have ovulated and will show estrogen influence if you did not. There may be no hormonal influences on the tissue at all.

Ovulation can be stimulated and Clomid is one of the most popular drugs. It is given orally early in the cycle. It stimulates the pituitary to produce increased amounts of FSH and LH, which stimulate the ovaries to ripen and release an ovum. If a woman has patent (open) fallopian tubes and a fertile partner, 70 percent will ovulate and 40 percent will get pregnant with this drug. However, you must be monitored monthly to avoid cysts developing or hyperstimulation of the ovaries from Clomid.

*HCG (human chorionic gonadotropin)* increases the potential for the release of an ovum and is sometimes injected after Clomid is used. HCG is always used in conjunction with Pergonal.

*Pergonal (human menopausal gonadotropin)* is

extracted from the urine of postmenopausal women and is more potent than Clomid. It should be used only on women who do not ovulate with Clomid because ovarian hyperstimulation is a common risk with Pergonal. Twenty percent of pregnancies with this drug are multiple, with the majority of them twins, although low-dose Pergonal may be used in certain cases to avoid this. Without the HCG, ovulation probably won't occur. This treatment is expensive, both for the drug itself and the time involved in administering it.

*Bromocriptine* is a drug used for some ovulatory problems. The usual trade name for bromocriptine is Parlodel. Pregnant or nursing women have a high level of the hormone prolactin in their bodies, which decreases the levels of FSH and LH, the hormones necessary for ovulation. Some infertile women also have high prolactin levels, which bromocryptine can help bring down.

WARNING: *If you are taking bromocriptine (Parlodel), notify your doctor immediately if your period is late.* It is unclear whether this drug is completely safe during pregnancy.

**Structural problems of the uterus** can include large fibroid tumors, congenital malformation, or malposition. The result of these uterine problems is more likely to be miscarriage than inability to conceive. A *hysterosalpingogram* (HSG) (described below under Fallopian Tube Blockage) is an X-ray study which allows the doctor to check the internal structure of the uterus. Sometimes fibroids may grow deep within the uterine wall and distort the uterine cavity, or the fibroids may grow directly in the uterus. This may either make pregnancy more difficult to achieve or make it difficult to carry a baby. A common malformation is a *bicornuate uterus,* which is divided by a central septum. If you have one or two miscarriages because of this, surgery can unite the two halves.

*Hysteroscopy* is a device to permit direct visualization of the uterine cavity for diagnosis and some corrective procedures. This can be done in the doctor's office with an oral analgesic and a local, but some doctors say it is too painful and the patient is better off in the hospital. The cervix is dilated, a small telescope is introduced, and fluid is injected so the uterus distends.

*Fallopian tube blockage* may be preventing conception. For many years the *Rubin test,* or tubal insufflation test, was used to determine whether the tubes were open (patent)—but now the test is outdated. Many specialists find this test inadequate, even though it's easy to do in their office and isn't technically difficult or high-risk. Carbon dioxide gas is blown into the uterus and out through the tubes, if they're open. However, this doesn't tell whether one or both tubes are open, or if the gas escaped through some fault in the procedure. X-ray studies are preferred by most specialists; a doctor still using the Rubin test is a bit behind the times.

A *hysterosalpingogram* (a uterotubogram) is an X-ray study to check tubal patency (whether the tubes are open). A radio-opaque dye is injected into the uterus through the cervix. Uterine cramping may occur, and although a doctor may be able to pace the rate of the injection to your tolerance, this isn't always possible. Be prepared for the possibility of painful cramping; even a doctor sensitive to this likelihood can only *try* to make it easier on you.

Normally, dye will fill the uterus, then spill into the fallopian tubes and out the ends, and then will pool in the peritoneal cavity, where it's eventually absorbed. If the dye doesn't pass into the tubes they may be blocked or may be in temporary spasm. According to some doctors, the test itself may have a therapeutic effect from the dye being flushed through.

*Laparoscopy* is used when other tests are negative and tubal blockage is suspected. The recovery is usually easy since the procedure involves only a few stitches underneath a small bandage, with little discomfort for most women. A short-term anesthetic is used and a one-inch incision is made in the curve of the navel. A long, thin instrument is inserted, through which the doctor can see the reproductive organs. Only a doctor who is skilled in tubal or pelvic surgery should do a laparoscopy since he will use what he sees to guide him if surgery is required. Otherwise you will have additional pain and expense because a specialist will have to do the laparoscopy over again in order to gather the information for himself.

*Culdoscopy* was used before laparoscopy evolved in the 1960s but some conditions require this procedure instead of the more advanced laparoscopy. A local or general anesthetic is used and an incision is made in the upper wall of the vagina. A thin instrument similar to a laparoscope can survey the internal organs.

*Tubal* blockage or scarring around the tubes is called *tuboplasty*. Surgery can be performed to separate adhesions; success depends on where the blockage is located in the tube and whether it affects one or both tubes. After surgery there is an increased risk (5 to 10 percent) of ectopic pregnancy (pregnancy in the tube). If one tube is good and the other is hopelessly blocked and both ovaries are intact, some doctors will remove the diseased tube and the ovary on that side so that the woman will ovulate every month from the good side. This will increase her chances of pregnancy, but other doctors disagree; they won't remove the normal ovary on the side of the blocked tube in case anything should ever happen to the other ovary.

**Polycystic ovaries** (also known as the Stein-Leventhal syndrome) are a cause of infertility. The ovaries usually have multiple small cysts and a thicker covering than is normal. The hormonal imbalance which causes this condition usually means that ovulation is irregular or absent and may also cause obesity and excess hair growth. If Clomid is not successful in treating this syndrome, a surgical procedure called a *wedge resection* can be done. A wedge of tissue is removed from both ovaries, a process which is believed to cause a sudden hormonal change back to normal. There is an 80 percent rate of ovulation afterward and a 63 percent pregnancy rate following wedge resection. This procedure should be done *when* you want to get pregnant, however. The best chance for pregnancy is right after the operation, and then the chances diminish.

*Congenital absence of ovaries* occurs in a rare condition called *Turner's syndrome*. A woman receives only half of her sex-chromosome complement and doesn't menstruate or develop secondary sex characteristics without hormone treatment. Other reasons that ovarian tissue may fail before normal menopause is as a result of extensive ovarian surgery, hyperstimulation with fertility drugs, or because the blood supply to the ovaries was cut off, leading to tissue death.

*Immunological factors* should be considered. It is important to check a woman's cervical mucus and her bloodstream to see if there are antibodies present causing infertility.

*Radiation* can damage the sensitive germ cells of the ovary. The abdominal area should be protected from radiation whenever possible, not just for patients but especially for care-givers. Nurses, technicians, and the like show a higher miscarriage rate than other women, in part because of their exposure to radiation and similar influences.

*Stress* and its effect on fertility is an area about which not much is known. One theory is that stress can inhibit ovulation from a hypothalamic level; another theory is that stress can cause the fallopian tubes to clamp down in spasm. More research is needed to understand the effects of stress. Although psychological factors alone can rarely be blamed for infertility there may be *some* times when such a relationship exists. So far, little is understood about it, however.

*Tubal ligation can sometimes be reversed* if you previously had your fallopian tubes cut or blocked as a method of birth control. Although tubal ligation (also called "tying your tubes") is designed to be a permanent form of sterilization, it can be reversed unless there has been total destruction of the tube. This surgical procedure is called *reanastomosis,* which is a success 90 percent of the time. Obviously, the younger the woman, the better the chance for pregnancy because fertility normally decreases as you age.

Unlike tubal ligation, which is usually a half-hour procedure done on an outpatient basis, the reversal is major abdominal surgery requiring a 2-to-3 hour operation and 3 to 4 days of hospitalization. As with any operation in which the abdominal wall is cut, there is a recovery period of a couple of weeks at home afterwards. Also, whereas the tubal ligation probably cost you about $2,000, the reanastomosis will run about $7,000 for surgical fees and hospitalization.

*If you have suffered repeated miscarriages,* technically known as repeated spontaneous abortions, there are various treatments available for you, depending on what caused the miscarriages. If you have benign tumors in your uterus, surgery to remove them will give you a 50 percent chance of having a viable pregnancy afterwards. If your uterus is abnormally shaped, that can also be corrected with surgery. And if you have what is known as an incompetent cervix, that can be remedied by stitching the cervix closed (see page 521).

## CAUSES AND TREATMENT OF MALE INFERTILITY

There are four basic ways in which a man's fertility may be impaired. There may be a problem in sperm production or maturation, a problem in sperm motility (ability to swim), a blockage in the reproductive tract, or an inability to place seminal fluid normally in the vagina.

*Varicocele* is the most common cause of infertility in men and one of the most easily corrected. Varicocele is a condition in which there are varicose veins, most commonly next to the left testicle, although it can occur in the right or in both testicles. *Varicocelectomy* is a surgical procedure done through an incision in the lower left abdomen which has been very successful in improving sperm count and motility. For men who have varicocele and have a preoperative sperm count of more than 10 million per milliliter, about 70 percent are able to impregnate their wives after the surgery. For those with a count under 10 million before surgery, the rate afterward is 27 percent, although it may be possible to double this percentage with the hormone Clomid.

*Prostatitis* is the second most common cause of male infertility. It is an infection of the prostate gland, often without any symptoms, but it can be discovered upon examination and with lab tests and is often easily treated with antibiotics.

*Hydrocele* is less common than varicocele and is a small bag of fluid within the scrotum that may be surgically removed.

*Adult mumps* cause testicular inflammation in more than half the victims, which can impair or atrophy testicular tissue. It is usually severe in only one testicle but if the disease is bilateral and there is atrophy on both sides, the man will be sterile. If the process of atrophy is halted, however, there will be a gradual recovery with return to normal function within a year.

*Infections* are difficult to diagnose and stubborn to treat. Men with *venereal disease,* especially gonorrhea, exhibit symptoms and have a discharge before permanent damage results. If you have symptoms of infection at any time consult a doctor immediately. *Tuberculosis* can invade the male (or female) reproductive organs and impair fertility.

*Acute febrile disease,* meaning any illness with a persistent high fever, can temporarily depress sperm production. Viral diseases like mononucleosis and hepatitis have the same effect. There is usually full recovery within three months of the illness.

*Undescended testicles* will be permanently impaired if they don't descend into the scrotal sac before puberty. The reason for this is that the testes perform at 2.2°C. lower than body temperature. Surgery is possible, with the best results achieved if it's done before age six, although there may be something abnormal in the testis itself.

*Heat* is an environmental condition that seems harmless and yet is frequently to blame for temporary fertility problems in men. If the testes are at or above the normal body temperature for significant periods of time, the sperm cells may stop maturing properly. All heat-related effects in a man are temporary. A man's sperm should return to normal three months after the exposure to heat is ended—the approximate length of the sperm-producing cycle.

- *Very hot baths or saunas,* if used frequently, can cause problems.
- *Frequent use of an athletic supporter* (or cups, padding, or other sports protection) is a common source of such heat.
- *Workplaces with excessive heat*—bakeries, pizza ovens, or any kind of industrial oven, or even sitting all day in the overheated seat of a vehicle—can interfere with sperm output.

*Radiation* in large amounts may damage testes but the effects are temporary in most cases and there is recovery of some sperm production.

*Stress* can impair sperm production if it is extreme emotional *or* physical stress. This is reversible once the stress element is removed.

*Congenital factors* such as *Kleinfelter's syndrome,* which is like Turner's syndrome in females, can affect fertility. A man with Kleinfelter's has an XXY chromosomal complement instead of the normal XY. This has a slight feminizing effect on his body, resulting in small testicles, slightly enlarged breasts, and absence of sperm in his ejaculate. Therefore, such men cannot reproduce.

*Injury* to the reproductive organs by a serious accident, for example, may cut off testicular blood supply, resulting in tissue atrophy. This can also be a rare aftermath of hernia repair or the surgical release of undescended testicles.

*Autoimmunity* means that a man develops antibodies to his own sperm. A woman can also develop these antibodies. Autoimmunity usually occurs from trauma, vasectomy, or infection: if sperm cells enter the surrounding tissue they cause an antibody reaction. If the underlying problem can be treated, the antibodies may stop being produced.

## IMPOTENCE

Impotence, which means the inability to have an erection, is estimated to affect 10 million men in America, or 1 out of every 8. Clearly, it's going to be difficult to get your wife pregnant if you are unable to have sexual intercourse, or if you're having trouble getting an erection or ejaculating! Experts used to believe that most impotence was caused by psychological inhibition. New knowledge and diagnostic methods show that physical problems, often due to drugs or diseases, are more likely to be the cause. An accurate understanding of why you are impotent requires a thorough interview, often with both partners, and also a physical examination.

PSYCHOLOGICAL PROBLEMS are still recognized as factors in impotence, of course, even though organic factors are now thought to be the more frequent reason for it. Chronic depression, anxiety, and marital discord can cause impotence—and then your anxiety about being impotent can prolong it. If there is a psychological cause for your impotence, the program outlined by Masters and Johnson, which is followed by many sex therapists, can be effective.

NOCTURNAL ERECTIONS are a sign that your penis is physically capable of becoming erect. These nighttime erections are one of the most important ways to distinguish organic from psychological impotence. A normal healthy man has from 2 to 5 erections during sleep, which last from 5 to 30 minutes. In order to determine whether a man has nocturnal erections, an electronic device can be attached to the penis to record changes in its size during the night. This can be done at home or in a sleep lab. If there are insufficient sleep erections, this is a sign of a physical disorder.

CIRCULATORY ABNORMALITIES can cause impotence by obstructing blood flow to the penis. Sickle-cell anemia, for example, causes red blood cells to clump in the small blood vessels and often causes impotence as a result. Men who have some degree of arteriosclerosis (hardening of the arteries) may be impotent because of decreased blood circulation, even though the condition is not enough to cause heart symptoms. Many men with this condition respond to drugs that increase blood flow. However, some men just have a reduced blood supply to the penis, even though they have normal hearts and are in their twenties or thirties.

NEUROLOGIC DISORDERS, PARTICULARLY THOSE CAUSED BY DIABETES, can cause impotence. Half of all diabetic men become impotent, largely because the disease damages nerves involved in erection. Sometimes impotence may be the first sign of a gradual onset of diabetes. Other neurologic causes are pelvic surgery for cancer of the prostate, bladder, or rectum, which can sometimes involve severing key nerves and therefore can lead to impotence. Spinal cord injuries can also cause a loss of erectile capacity.

HORMONE ABNORMALITIES, particularly those involving testosterone, the major male hormone, may have a role in impotence. In some testosterone-deficient men, shots of the hormone may restore potency, but others may not get any help from it.

MEDICATION AND OTHER DRUGS are major contributors to impotence today, particularly drugs used to treat such diseases as hypertension and heart disease. Some drugs may act by lowering blood pressure in the penis, while others may affect the nervous system or hormone levels. If you are on a new medication and become impotent, you should check with your doctor immediately. For many men, simply switching to a different medication may solve the problem.

ALCOHOL has been recognized for years as a cause of impotence. In small amounts, liquor may remove inhibitions. In large amounts, it is a powerful central-nervous-system depressant: up to 80 percent of alcoholics have decreased sexual urges or impotence. Some suffer even after they stop drinking because alcohol has caused permanent nerve damage or hormonal imbalance.

CIGARETTE SMOKING has been linked to temporary impotence. Nicotine constricts blood vessels, sometimes enough to affect blood flow to the penis.

RETROGRADE EJACULATION occurs when sperm are deposited into the man's own bladder instead of out the urethra. This condition may be transient or permanent and may be caused by certain medication, surgical trauma, or nerve damage. A side effect of *diabetes* is that there may be erectile impotence and possible retrograde ejaculation because of progressive nerve damage caused by the disease. The signs of retrograde ejaculation are no visible semen and milky-colored urine after intercourse. This condition can be treated with sympathomimetic drugs. For couples who are highly motivated a possible treatment is to irrigate the man's bladder with a favorable solution before intercourse (drinking baking soda, for example). Then afterward he can urinate the sperm, it can be collected that way, and the woman can be inseminated with the recovered ejaculate.

CHRONIC ILLNESS may debilitate and affect sexual relations.

*Penile implants* are now used by about 30,000 American men. Semi-rigid plastic rods are inserted in the erectile chambers and permit the penis to stiffen enough for intercourse. There are more sophisticated and expensive implants that are inflatable and more closely duplicate an erection. The semi-rigid implants cost around $5,000 as compared to nearly twice that much for the inflatables. If implant wearers are capable of ejaculation, they can father children.

***Impotents Anonymous*** is a self-help group based in Washington, D.C., with chapters around the country. In open discussion, men can often better understand the physical and psychological causes of impotence and seek out effective treatment.

## DRUGS AND ALCOHOL

***Alcohol*** in large amounts may cause impotence. In small amounts it may release inhibitions and stimulate the libido. Heavy drinking over a number of years can also result in liver damage, which alters the metabolism of estrogen in males and may lower sperm production.

***Drugs*** of any kind, particularly in excess, appear to affect a man's fertility as well as potency.

- *Marijuana,* even in small amounts, disrupts sex hormones in men and women. It is advisable to avoid it during your childbearing years. Studies have shown that it causes chromosomal anomalies which can lead to genetic damage. Marijuana can cause infertility in men because it lowers sperm count and motility (movement) and can lower the level of testosterone, the male sex hormone. The most potentially damaging effect of marijuana on sperm is that it increases abnormal forms of the sperm cell. However, since millions of new sperm are constantly produced, a man's sperm probably become normal after he stops smoking pot.
- *Morphine and heroin* cause impotence and lack of interest in sex. *Tranquilizers* in the phenothiazine family and barbiturates may have similar effects.
- *Drugs used for such chronic illness* as rheumatoid arthritis, psoriasis, gout, epilepsy, and other nervous system

disorders have all been shown to have an effect on the quality of sperm produced.

- *Drugs that block the sympathetic nervous system*—such as guanethidine (sold under brand names Ismelin or Esimil), which is used for patients with high blood pressure—may cause infertility by producing an aberration called retrograde ejaculation. The man has all the sensations of ejaculation but the semen goes backward, into the bladder. Another high-blood-pressure drug is Inderal, which has not been linked to ejaculation problems but sometimes produces impotence.
- *Tagamet* is used to treat ulcers and has become the best-selling drug in America, surpassing even Valium. It has been found that Tagamet depresses a man's sperm count by as much as 43 percent, yet most doctors are not aware of this. Fortunately the problem resolves itself when he stops taking the medication, or actually around 3 months later, when the entire cycle of sperm production and release has had a chance to operate without the drugs.
- *Certain urinary tract antibacterial medications,* such as Macrodantin and Furadantin, are among the drugs known to affect a man's sperm.
- *Imuran (a chemotherapy or immunosuppressive agent) and prednisone (prescribed for a wide variety of conditions)* are known to affect sperm count, although the doctors prescribing them may be unaware of this side effect.
- *The use of steroids for sports or bodybuilding* can result in a drastically lowered sperm count or complete sterility. The chance of this infertility reversing itself depends on how heavily you used steroids and over how long a period of time.
- *Cancer chemotherapy drugs* have a seriously deleterious effect on sperm production. But the effect of chemotherapy is not uniform. It differs according to the class and dose of the drug as well as the age of the patient. Some of the drugs produce sterility in men and boys of certain age groups but have no effect at all on other males.
- *Tetracycline* has proved to affect sperm maturation in experiments that have been done on animals.

- *High doses of aspirin* used for prolonged periods can inhibit the production of prostaglandins, important chemicals in seminal fluid.
- *Heavy tobacco smoking* may change the shape of sperm, though the significance of this is as yet unknown.

## SEMEN ANALYSIS

Analysis of the semen checks several important factors about a man's sperm. Once the problem is identified, there are various treatments that may correct it. However, the process of being "scored" in semen analysis can be threatening to even the most secure male ego. The advice under The Emotional Impact of Infertility in this chapter might be helpful to a man going through these tests.

*Infertility* in a man is defined as a low sperm count. *Sterility* refers to a man who has no viable sperm at all. It must be recognized, however, that semen analysis is a difficult and inexact science. The technician must count how many of the 50 million to 750 million sperm found in a normal specimen are moving, and how many are moving rapidly. He or she must also determine how many are malformed or immature. All of these determinations are subjective to some extent: what looks like a moderately active sperm to one qualified technician may be classified as sluggish by another. The normal range of a sperm count is greater than 40 million per milliliter. But a man with an exceedingly low sperm count who has, nevertheless, fathered a child obviously cannot be considered "infertile."

An analysis calculates the total semen volume, counts how many million sperm there are per cubic centimeter, and measures the viscosity (or liquefaction) of the ejaculate. It also tests the motility and morphology (the maturity and normality) of the sperm cells. Collecting the semen correctly is important: a specimen is obtained by masturbation, catching the *entire* ejaculate in a clean jar. Most of the live active sperm are in the first half of the ejaculate, so it's important to get all of it. The specimen must be kept at room temperature (never refrigerated or exposed to excessive heat) and delivered within an hour to the doctor's lab.

Coitus interruptus is a less useful technique than masturbation because you may not get the entire ejaculate.

Some people's religion may prohibit masturbation or
coitus interruptus. They can use a special condom (Milex,
for example, is not spermicidal like many other brands) and
make a tiny pinhole halfway down the side of the condom
to satisfy religious rules against birth control.

As mentioned earlier, do not make the mistake of
thinking you will do better if you "save up sperm" by not
having intercourse for a while before being tested. In fact,
abstaining from intercourse for more than four days can
decrease your sperm's motility, or its ability to swim.

Semen analysis should be repeated at least once a
month later, because the various levels that are measured
may fluctuate.

## TREATMENT FOLLOWING ANALYSIS

*Corticosteroids* (especially cortisone) are used infre-
quently to improve sperm production and motility.

*HCG* (human chorionic gonadotropin) stimulates the production of testosterone, which improves sperm motility in
some men.

*Split ejaculate* is a way of dealing with a man who has a
large semen volume with a borderline sperm count. The
most active, live sperm are usually in the first few drops of
any ejaculate. This treatment involves the man catching the
first half of masturbated specimen in a container so the
woman can be inseminated with it. This can also be done
with careful coitus interruptus in which the man comes out
of the woman after the first few waves of ejaculation.

*Sperm banking* has been successful for those couples who
can't achieve pregnancy in any other way.

Once all the environmental suppressors of sperm, like
drugs and heat, have been removed, there isn't much that
can be done for a man who still has a low sperm count. It

is harder to get a man's body to produce sperm than it is to stimulate a woman's body to ovulate an egg. Hormonal treatments for male infertility have not been researched with the same interest and attention that have been given to the woman's hormonal problems. However, more effort and funds may be directed at male infertility as it continues to be identified as a health problem.

***Beware any doctor who attempts unorthodox treatments*** for male infertility. Some doctors subject their male patients to unnecessary, unproven, expensive, or even harmful procedures. For example, there are doctors who administer thyroid medication to men even in instances where the thyroid has not been clinically shown to be the cause of a man's infertility. Similarly, a doctor may give a man antibiotics when there is no evidence of infection. NOTE: Even when some men do manage to impregnate their wives after such treatments, *there is no proof that these medications had anything to do with achieving the pregnancy.* Some infertile couples spontaneously get pregnant without any treatment, so do not allow yourself to be used as a guinea pig by an unprofessional (or perhaps overenthusiastic) physician.

## CAUSES AND TREATMENT
## OF SHARED INFERTILITY

There are some fertility problems shared by a couple that can be solved with basic information about sexual technique. First of all, *never use any kind of lubricant*—Vaseline, cream, jelly—because they all have a slightly spermicidal effect. The *best position* for conception is the good old missionary style, man above, with the woman's hips raised on a pillow. The man should stay motionless inside her for several minutes after his orgasm; she should keep her hips raised and stay there for half an hour before getting up. The ideal would be to go to sleep like that. The exception to this is if a woman has a flexed or tilted uterus: in that case, entry from behind is preferable. *Frigidity* in a woman—the fact that she doesn't reach orgasm—is not known to have any effect on whether she conceives or not.

*Infrequent sex,* because of health problems, fatigue, different work schedules, or sexual problems, can diminish your chances of conceiving. You must have intercourse at least before and during ovulation. Infrequent sex presents another problem: if a man does not ejaculate for long periods there is an increased chance of an imperfect fetus. The ovum may be fertilized by one of the older sperm that has been stored up, rather than by a newly produced, more healthy sperm.

*Weekend sex* can become the norm if both partners work in high-pressure jobs. Sex becomes reserved for the weekends, which can be counterproductive to efforts to become pregnant. A couple must make a conscious effort to change their schedules and habits so that they can have intercourse evenly distributed throughout the week. Since ovulation may happen on a Wednesday, and the prime time for conception is within twenty-four hours, a couple is not going to get pregnant if they restrict their sex to the weekends!

*Postcoital test* (Huhner or "PK" test) is one way of determining whether a couple are incompatible in terms of fertility. The doctor will request that a couple have sex and come to his office 2 to 8 hours later (depending on the doctor). The woman must not wash or douche after sex; a sample of her cervical mucus is microscoped at the doctor's office. This will show how the sperm interact with the vaginal and cervical secretions. If the environment is hostile, some treatments can be tried to alter it.

*Immunologic reaction* occurs when a woman builds up antibody-based resistance to her mate's sperm. There is a blood test to determine whether such a reaction is taking place, but it is available only at major medical centers. If you don't live near such a facility, samples of male and female blood serum can be sent to a medical center for analysis.

If an immunologic reaction is discovered in the

woman, the usual treatment is for the man to use a condom during any sexual intercourse with his partner for the next 3 to 6 months. This eliminates contact between the sperm and her cervical mucus. The woman's blood is checked periodically to see whether her antibody titer (the level of antibodies in her blood) drops. The couple can then have sex without a condom—but only immediately before ovulation. This maximizes the chance of pregnancy and slows the reformation of antibodies.

If the immunologic problem is discovered to be a male problem, he can be given steroids if he has antibodies to his own sperm. There is also a process called *sperm washing,* a lab technique that separates some of the seminal fluid components which contain the antibodies.

**Artificial insemination by the husband** is known as AIH and can be used when there is an immunologic reaction or other husband-wife incompatibilities in achieving pregnancy. The procedure for AIH is very simple: when the woman is ovulating, her husband ejaculates into a specimen jar and husband and wife then go to the doctor's office. The woman takes the routine position for a pelvic exam in order for the doctor to painlessly inject the semen into her cervical canal. She will remain in this position for about half an hour to give the sperm a chance to reach the egg. Another method is for the semen to be placed in a cervical cap (like a smaller diaphragm that fits over the cervix), which the women leaves in place for about six hours.

## ARTIFICIAL INSEMINATION BY DONOR

### WHEN IS AID USED?

**Artificial insemination by donor (AID) is most often used** when the woman is presumed fertile and the man has a fertility problem. However, there are some cases (for example when the woman has built up an immunologic reaction to her husband's sperm, see page 76), where artificial insemination by husband (AIH) can be used. AIH may also be tried for male factor infertility (even though the success rate is fairly low) in order to give the man some transition time before donor sperm is tried. The use of someone else's sperm to impregnate his wife can be emotionally difficult for a man. The chart on page 79 lists most of the reasons for attempting AID, but several of these factors are inconclusive—that is, they do not necessarily mean that you cannot conceive naturally. About 5 percent of couples who request AID are fertile but are afraid of passing on inherited diseases: your baby could potentially get a genetic defect from a father at risk for the inheritable forms of Down's syndrome, blindness, Huntington's chorea or Tay-Sachs disease.

***Impotence is not a sufficient reason for trying AID.*** Great strides are being made in the treatment of impotence (see page 68), which frequently has a physical cause. It may save you a lot of trouble and heartache if you find out more about the treatment of impotence before seeking AID. Experts are finding that one-third of all impotence is caused by nerve and blood vessel disease or hormonal abnormalities. It's also important to consider the role that medication can play in impotence. Sometimes a prescribed drug can cause impotence and the man can be cured by simply changing medications. Among the latest and sometimes controversial treatments to restore sexual potency are hormonal therapy, surgical implants, and an experimental blood vessel bypass operation.

***A low sperm count may be temporary*** and can often be corrected, so do not start an AID program on the basis of a single sperm count. Many environmental and internal forces can affect a man's sperm count, so you should refuse even to consider AID based solely on one test. Before making a referral for AID, a competent doctor will order additional sperm counts with sufficient time in between, counseling the man about how changes in his activities may help increase his sperm count. For example, if a man had the flu within the last three months or he has increased the temperature of his testicles by wearing tight underwear, by taking hot baths or saunas, or even by driving long distances, his sperm count may register low even if he is actually fertile.

*A sperm count is not a reliable predictor* of a man's ability to impregnate a woman, anyway. This means that even if you have repeated sperm counts which register low, you do not need to rush into AID. You still have a good chance of creating a child naturally, and should do everything possible to enhance that chance. For example, "subfertility" in one partner can often be "treated" by enhancing the fertility of the other partner.

*How low must a man's sperm count be for AID to be recommended?* Generally speaking, AID is recommended for couples in which the man has a sperm count under 20 million per milliliter. However, this does not mean that if your sperm count is at that level or below, you should immediately try AID. There are many cases of men with sperm counts under 20 million cc who have impregnated their wives. AIH will increase the chance of pregnancy in this situation.

---

**CHART 7. REASONS FOR USING AID**

- AIH has been tried and did not work
- The man has had a vasectomy
- The man has no sperm at all or there is a severe problem with the number, quality, or motility of his sperm
- The man is impotent
- The man has been exposed to toxic materials
- There is a history of genetic disease in the man's family
- The couple has RH incompatibilities

## How Is Artificial Insemination Done?

The procedure for AID is quite simple, although each doctor's methods may vary slightly. Some doctors use a drug to stimulate ovulation, while many do not. The timing of insemination, which should take place on the day before you ovulate, is done based on a basal temperature chart (see page 46). If your temperature does not rise the following morning (which would indicate that you have ovulated), the doctor will ask you to return for a second insemination two days after the first attempt—in case the egg was released later than expected.

*There are several methods of insemination.* You need to understand the options so that you can participate in the decision about how you, as a couple, want AID to be performed:

1. **THE SEMEN IS INJECTED INTO THE VAGINA.** In this case, the insemination is quick and painless; it is not an injection in the usual sense of a needle piercing your skin. The woman lies on her back with her feet in the stirrups, in the position she would for a vaginal exam. This form of AID is jokingly referred to as the "turkey baster" method because the doctor squirts the semen up your vagina, near your cervix. After the sperm is injected, you remain lying on your back for up to thirty minutes, giving the sperm an opportunity to travel to your fallopian tubes.

2. **THE SEMEN CAN BE INJECTED DIRECTLY INTO THE UTERUS.** This technique, called intrauterine insemination, is used in special circumstances, as it requires special treatment of the sperm specimen ("washing").

3. **THE SPERM CAN BE PLACED IN A CERVICAL CAP.** This method involves putting the semen into a cervical cap (a small rubber dome like a diaphragm) which the doctor places on your cervix. Some doctors do not use this method, especially when using frozen sperm. If the cap is used, it means that you can get up about ten minutes after the insemination, keeping the cap in place for four to six hours.

4. YOU CAN DO THE INSEMINATION YOURSELVES AT HOME. It is possible for a couple to do AID at home. The couple picks up frozen or fresh sperm from their physician and performs the insemination at home by themselves. Some couples who have been through AID (or AIH) in the doctor's office later find out that they could have done it in the privacy of their home, which they would have preferred. Your doctor may be willing to teach you how to do this: all it involves is using an appropriate syringe to transfer semen from the container into the vagina, just as the doctor does in the office.

This option can eliminate some of the difficulties of coordinating your AID with a busy doctor's schedule and an appropriate donor's availability. More important, it is much less impersonal and allows the husband to be actively involved in impregnating his wife. Psychologically this can be wonderful for a man who is feeling displaced, passive, and/or inadequate because his wife has to undergo AID to get pregnant.

5. MIXING THE HUSBAND'S SEMEN WITH THE DONOR'S IS NOT DESIRABLE. There are couples who want the husband's sperm to be mixed with the donor's before insemination, or they decide to have intercourse immediately before or after AID. The emotional impulse behind this is the couple's desire to keep open the possibility that the child who is conceived might be the husband's. However, many experts recommend against the mixing of sperm; they urge couples to refrain from intercourse prior to insemination. The reason for this is that sperm from different men can sometimes cancel out each other's effectiveness: the success rate for AID appears to be higher when there is no mixing.

## DONOR SELECTION

### WHO ARE THE DONORS?

Your physician will probably tell you that sperm donors are screened and will be matched as closely as possible to the ethnic background, physical build, and complexion of the husband. However, to confirm that this is so, you might want to do a little research on the sperm bank you'll be using.

**Most people do not question how donors are chosen.** You might believe that sperm donors are carefully screened young men in excellent physical and mental health. This is not necessarily true. Infertility specialists depend on larger clinics to do the sperm banking because of the cost of maintaining frozen specimens and the frequent testing of donors for AIDS. However, most sperm banks do not run checks on a potential donor's genetic background, physical health (other than freedom from contagious diseases), or psychological stability.

Who are the donors and why do they do it? The financial rewards of being a sperm donor are the incentive for most men. Receiving $50 each time, a sperm donor can make $5,000 to $10,000 a year. However, the concern is not whether donors are mercenary or unethical: a man may be a carrier of a genetic disease of which he is unaware. The issue is whether sperm banks are rigorous enough in their screening process.

**What are the criteria for sperm donors?** Superficial physical traits and academic performance seem to be the main criteria for accepting sperm donors. Most programs that look for sperm donors look for intelligent men: profiles of donors to the largest sperm bank in the United States (Idant Laboratories in New York) show a grade point average of 3.5 to 4.0. Being a good student may be a desirable quality in a person, but there are other aspects that may be overlooked.

A donor's mental state is not considered. There is only *one* sperm bank in the entire world that does a psychological screening of potential donors—a program in Belgium which turns away "emotionally unstable" candidates.

**Don't kid yourself that** you'll have control over the sperm you receive. You may be given a questionnaire about donor selection, and this list may give you an unrealistic impression about the amount of input you or your doctor

has in choosing the sperm donor. Some infertility specialists give an AID couple a form on which to list the physical
and personality traits they would like in a donor. There
may even be a chance to indicate whether you want the
sperm of a man who is a certain religion, has thick hair, or
has athletic ability or cultural inclinations! If you believe
that your answers are going to result in a baby with made-
to-order genes, you're going to be disappointed. Even if you
were to receive sperm from a donor with all the traits
you desire, there is no evidence that any of the qualities
you value can be passed on genetically.

## THERE ARE WAYS TO SAFEGUARD YOURSELF IN AID

***How can you protect yourself against a donor*** who
might transmit a genetic problem or a venereal disease? Because of the concern about AIDS transmission, all sperm
donors are supposed to be tested for AIDS every 3 months.
All specimens are guaranteed for 6 months (2 negative AIDS
tests) before use. The estimated risk of contracting AIDS
from donor insemination is less than 1 in 100,000.

The chart on page 84, based in part on guidelines
recommended by the American Fertility Society, includes
some of the tests and safeguards you may want to demand.

---

### CHART 8. SPERM BANK GUIDELINES

---

- Gives AIDS blood test every 3 months
- Cultures donor's specimen for gonorrhea before collecting sperm for use in insemination
- Cultures subsequent specimens for presence of white cells, indicating infection, even if initial specimen is free of gonorrhea
- Has doctors take a careful family medical and psychological history from donors
- Rejects any potential donors with a family history of mental retardation, neurologic disorders, unexplained deaths under age 30, or significant congenital defects
- Screens for the Tay-Sachs trait in Jewish donors
- Screens for the sickle-cell trait in black donors
- Performs lab tests to insure that donor and recipient have compatible RH factors
- Orders a complete karyotyping (a test that details the size, number, and shape of chromosomes) or biochemical assay. Or you may want to do this only if there is a reason to suspect that a donor may be the carrier of a defect
- Finds out how many pregnancies have already resulted from the donor's sperm (If he has inseminated many women, the chance increases that your child could later marry a sibling.)
- Chooses donors with a blood type and Rh factor as close as possible to the husband's to avoid medical/legal/emotional problems later on—for instance, if you do not want to tell your child he was conceived with donor sperm
- Does a blood test for hepatitis

*Some people claim that screening all donors is too costly.* However, most couples would probably be willing to pay $35 for a Tay-Sachs test of donor sperm, or even $250 for a complete karyotyping. Since you're already going to pay an average of $750 just for the sperm alone during several months of AID attempts, the extra cost seems negligible in exchange for peace of mind.

*Experts recommend that you question your physician* about the extent to which the sperm bank he uses screens donors. If you are not satisfied with his answers, you can find your own donor. One advantage to making your own arrangements for a sperm donor is that you do not have to leave the decision in the hands of professionals, who might make very different choices than you would about a potential donor. Another reason some couples prefer to choose their own donor is if they want to give their child the option of knowing who the biological father is and having contact with him. There are instances in which known sperm donors do take part in the child's life.

Your doctor may not like the idea of your finding your own donor and would probably object on the grounds that careful safeguards in the screening procedure are essential. As you have seen, however, many times the professionals do not do as thorough a job of screening as one might hope. Furthermore, you yourself can certainly arrange to have a donor screened.

WARNING: A donor who knows the mother may want more involvement with the child than the mother or her husband wishes him to have. There have even been occasions when the mother and the donor wind up in court over issues of visitation and custody. You never know the strange ways that people can behave in these situations; it may help to imagine worst case scenarios before choosing your own donor.

## HOW LONG SHOULD YOU KEEP TRYING AID?

*AID does not promise immediate success, so don't give up* after the first try. Some infertile couples drop out after the first unsuccessful insemination, which is a shame. They may be blaming themselves or seeing themselves as failures, which is one of the traps of being infertile. Remember that even fertile couples have only a 20 percent chance each month of getting pregnant through normal intercourse!

Most physicians recommend that if a couple can afford it, they try artificial insemination for at least six months before considering other options.

*You should calculate whether you can afford AID* before you begin the process, since it can take an average of 6 months, and sometimes longer, to conceive. Although you might get lucky and get pregnant on the first try, you'll be better off if you have realistic expectations about the time involved.

Each time you are inseminated, there is the charge for the doctor's office visit, the fee for the sperm sample, and the possible cost of fertility drugs you may be taking to stimulate ovulation. If you are using intrauterine insemination, the office visit will be even more expensive. Artificial insemination usually runs $100 to $600 a month, depending on medical fees in the area where you live.

*Sit down with your doctor after 6 months of trying to achieve an AID pregnancy* and talk about what you can do to increase your chances of getting pregnant. Often the fault lies in poor timing of the insemination, and you need to have a more accurate means of pinpointing ovulation.

Ask your physician whether blood or urine tests can be used to gauge your time of ovulation. Another option is to use ultrasound to predict when one of your ovarian follicles will rupture and release an egg. You will want to go to a radiologist who is expert at reading ultrasound scans for this purpose. Another possibility is to regulate your ovulation using clomiphene citrate so that inseminations are not being performed in months when you have not released an egg at all.

*If your doctor does not offer these options,* consider finding another infertility specialist who will.

## LEGAL ISSUES ABOUT AID

Even if you don't tell anyone about the AID, you must protect your child's legal rights immediately at birth. There are precautions you can take to ensure that any baby conceived by AID is viewed as the legitimate offspring of your marriage.

You and your spouse with the help of a lawyer should prepare a document that is witnessed by someone, perhaps your infertility doctor. You also both need to prepare a will that specifically grants rights of inheritance to your child, whose full name must appear in the will. It is not sufficient for you to state in your will that you leave money or property to your child, intending that to mean the child born to your wife through artificial insemination. If the full name of your child does not appear in the will, your relatives can challenge it, claiming that the child is not your biological offspring and therefore should not inherit anything. The same is true for life insurance. Adoptive parents face similar problems.

*Do not underestimate* the lengths to which relatives may go to fight your child in court if anything should happen to you. There has already been a case in Scandinavia in which a man's relatives successfully claimed that his child conceived through AID was not legitimate and therefore should not have rights of inheritance. After his death, the relatives proved that he had been sterile and therefore the child wasn't "his." The child received nothing.

It is unclear whether there would be the same outcome under the American legal system, but you can take steps to ensure that your child will not be a victim of such a situation by using the child's full name in any documents.

## SHOULD AID BE KEPT A SECRET?

Artificial insemination is usually conducted in an atmosphere of secrecy. There is almost always secrecy about the identity of the donor, presumably to protect him from later claims of paternity and support payments or other responsibilities resulting from fathering a child. This secrecy also benefits the parents of the AID child, whose biological father could theoretically claim custody rights. Though such possibilities may seem farfetched, people sometimes do behave in bizarre and unpredictable ways.

***Most infertility doctors*** advise couples that whether to tell their offspring about AID is a personal decision, but some physicians do recommend that you keep AID a secret from everyone involved—not just from family members or health-care providers involved in the birth and care of the baby, but from the child as well.

In keeping with this preference for secrecy, many infertility specialists who do not deliver babies may not pass along information about your artificial insemination to the obstetrician you choose. It is then entirely your decision whether to disclose the AID origins of your pregnancy to the obstetrician who delivers your baby. If you do not choose to tell, your husband's name will be automatically put on the birth certificate without any question about paternity.

***Some couples feel strongly that they want to share the truth about their AID pregnancy*** with people close to them. You may feel torn between wanting to keep the information private and needing to share your feelings about the AID with others. You may want the safety that secrecy gives you, but feel you are being deceptive if you don't tell the truth to those to whom you feel closest. If you find it difficult to maintain total secrecy, be selective in choosing sympathetic and discreet family members or friends to tell.

***You may want to meet other AID couples.*** You may feel the need for peer support and want to share your experiences with others who have gone through the same thing. If you contact infertility groups in your area, you're bound to find other AID couples who would be willing to meet you (see Appendix IV, page 786, for a listing of infertility organizations).

***If you want to tell your child about his conception,*** be sure that you are both united in the decision and have a well-thought-out plan concerning how to approach the topic. The way that you impart this information will influence the way the child receives it.

**Whether to tell a child about AID is a personal decision** that each couple must discuss and make for themselves. Some experts claim that a child must know her medical history, in part so that she doesn't assume that she and the man she knows as her father share any genetically influenced medical conditions. However, bear in mind that if you know nothing about the identity of the sperm donor, then you have no concrete information to offer her about her genetic background.

Some psychoanalysts feel that keeping your child's origin a secret can be unhealthy for your family: such a secret can exert a powerful negative influence on family interactions. These experts fear that a child may sense something is being kept from him, and the reality may be less troubling than any of his fantasies about what the secret is.

Bear in mind that many physicians who provide AID tend to recommend silence, while psychologists might encourage openness. The ultimate decision is up to the two of you, after weighing the pros and cons of the issue.

## THE EMOTIONAL ASPECTS OF AID

Early opponents of AID worried that the procedure would create a problem in the marriage. The concern was that the child's biological relationship to only one parent could cause tension and create an imbalance in the marriage. However, AID marriages have proven to be wonderfully strong. In fact, a couple with a child conceived by artificial insemination is statistically more likely to stay together than a set of biological parents. AID couples have a divorce rate substantially lower than the overall divorce rate of almost 50 percent in our country.

## THE COUPLE'S REACTION TO AID

*Guilt is the most common emotion that couples experience* around the issue of infertility. A man may feel he cannot fulfill the role of fathering a child that his wife and society expect him to. A woman can feel guilty too, especially if she gets pregnant by AID: she is caught between feeling sympathetic to her husband's feelings of failure and feeling elated about the pregnancy. She may also feel angry at her husband for his infertility, then feel guilty for her anger, and guilty that she is fertile and her partner is not. There are suggestions further on in this section concerning how to alleviate some of the negative feelings about AID. That does not mean repressing them, but expressing and resolving them. Both partners have feelings of guilt, anger, and shame that need to be acknowledged before embarking on an AID program.

*The stress of repressed feelings* can damage your relationship and even interfere with the woman's ability to conceive. If AID is started without both partners expressing their feelings, this stress can sometimes cause a woman who is usually fertile to stop ovulating. If both of you feel angry or conflicted within yourselves or with each other, it is bound to cause sexual difficulties and other conflicts between you.

*Child-rearing problems can arise later* if feelings aren't resolved. The husband may feel like a fraud when people congratulate him on the birth of his child. This feeling could inhibit him from bonding with the child and, later, from disciplining the child. Also, the power balance in your relationship may change if either of you feels it is really the mother's baby.

Get any negative feelings out in the open and don't be afraid of such emotions. Often just openly confronting the issues together can bring you closer together.

*A couple may fear that their AID baby* will be born with a genetic defect or will be enormously different from them in appearance. These are fears that usually come out when a couple learns that the woman is pregnant. These feelings may surface again right before the baby is due. Talking to your doctor about the process of selecting a donor should lessen your fears.

## THE MAN'S FEELINGS ABOUT AID

***The man must come to terms with his infertility*** before rushing to a decision about AID. Many men are shocked and dismayed when they learn they are infertile and unlikely to be able to father a child biologically. A man may experience this as a blow to his sense of masculinity, and may feel ashamed that he cannot impregnate his wife. If he felt dominant or superior to his wife before, the news of his infertility can be particularly infuriating, frustrating, or humiliating.

***Very often, AID is suggested immediately*** following the lab results showing a man's low sperm count. Sometimes health-care providers, who think only about the medical aspects of fertility, may not be sensitive to the emotional stages each man must go through when he learns of his sterility. Professionals may lose touch with how shattering it can be for a husband to be told he cannot reproduce. It is often important to let some time pass before suggesting that a man agree to have his wife conceive with another man's sperm. It has been found that couples who wait at least a few months after the man is diagnosed as sterile tend to be able to handle the procedure more successfully and have a happier pregnancy.

***A man has to go through a natural mourning period*** for his lost fertility before he can go on and discuss other ways that he and his partner can have a child together. He needs a chance to identify his feelings and talk them out with his wife, a counselor, or an infertility support group before he and his wife decide about artificial insemination. He must come to terms with what infertility actually means, and separate this medical condition from feelings he has about his virility and manliness.

*A man may quickly say yes to AID for the wrong reasons.* Though a man may be ambivalent about AID or even opposed to it, he may agree to it immediately simply because the doctor recommends it. A man might feel that he doesn't have the right to stand in the way of his wife's right to get pregnant, or that he might force her to choose between him and having a baby. He might also choose AID over adoption because adopting a baby would be an admission to outsiders of infertility problems. *If you are influenced to proceed with AID for any of these reasons, you should postpone the AID decision until you've given it more thought.* You may even need to get professional counseling to help both of you decide whether AID is a comfortable solution for both of you.

*A man may feel he is letting his wife sleep with another man* if he agrees to AID. This is a fear that should be expressed to the fertility doctor so that the scientific nature of the process can be described and discussed. A woman might need to reassure her husband of her love for him. She might need to emphasize her desire to have a baby and raise a family with him because of qualities he possesses that will make him a good father as well as a good mate. The husband needs to recognize that being a father is not about contributing the genetic materials for the conception, but about loving and being committed to his wife and his child.

## THE WOMAN'S FEELINGS ABOUT AID

*A woman has to be able to express her own feelings* about infertility even though they may be less intense than her husband's reaction. You may have negative feelings about having to be artificially inseminated in order to have a child.

You may feel sad or selfish that your genetic heritage will live on through your child while your husband's will not. You may feel that you wanted to have *his* baby. It is okay to talk to your husband about this. It is natural to feel nostalgic about certain of your mate's emotional or physical characteristics that cannot be passed on to future generations. Your feelings may help him recognize his own sadness about this issue—and the love and admiration you feel for him.

*You may become temporarily infertile yourself* if you don't allow yourself time to resolve your own feelings about AID, or if you feel your husband is withdrawing from you. The emotions that you feel as a result may cause you to stop ovulating. The insemination will then fail, which will create still more tension.

## HOW TO ENHANCE THE AID PROCESS

*When a man feels left out of the AID,* it can cause feelings of guilt. A man may feel he has let his wife down and is contributing nothing. He may think that all that he's done to assist with the pregnancy is pay the bills. Similarly, a woman may feel awkward that she is getting pregnant without her husband, especially if he says, "This is *her* baby," or just feels that way.

*Involving the husband in the AID process* can overcome many of the emotional stumbling blocks. Guilt feelings can be reduced if the man accompanies his wife on visits to the infertility clinic. It also helps if the man is actively involved in the process of learning about AID and of making the decision whether to use it. Some doctors make the husband an integral part of the process by asking him to keep track of his wife's basal body temperature to pinpoint ovulation, and then to bring her in when she's about to ovulate.

*Some doctors try to involve husbands even more actively* in the process. Just as most obstetricians welcome husbands in the delivery room and often let them cut the umbilical cord, the more progressive infertility doctors are now letting the husband do the insemination. Some specialists feel this helps integrate the husband from conception so that the couple starts the pregnancy as a family unit.

Some physicians even teach the husband to do the inseminations at home, where a couple has more privacy and can have a more personal and emotional experience together. Otherwise it can be done by the husband in the doctor's office or clinic, once he is shown how to insert the syringe and introduce the semen into his wife's vagina. Then while the woman remains lying on her back, the couple have that half hour to be alone together, hoping and praying that a sperm and egg are uniting and the wife can finally be pregnant.

## IN VITRO FERTILIZATION
## (TEST TUBE BABIES)

In vitro fertilization (known as IVF, which is how I'll refer to it throughout this section) is a technique in which human eggs are fertilized in a laboratory dish and then reinserted into the uterus. I am including IVF in this chapter, but I am not going into great detail because it is not relevant for most couples. The enormous costs (about $5,000 for each attempt) make it too expensive for most people—but don't feel too bad if this is true for you. Despite what you may have heard in the press about "test-tube babies," the actual success rates for IVF are about 15 to 20 percent.

It doesn't seem realistic to recommend IVF, since so few people who undertake in vitro fertilization go home with a baby. Nevertheless, those who can afford it seem to feel it's worth trying; they want to buck the odds and be among the lucky few. At the same time, some insurance companies will pay for IVF, so more couples may be able to afford to take the gamble.

*IVF is still not a proven medical therapy.* Most experts will admit that IVF is still an experimental procedure, and a very expensive procedure with a fairly low success rate at that. But IVF clinics are becoming big business, because there is a lot of money to be made—both from patients and from research grants. Couples who are desperate to have a child may talk themselves into believing that they, too, can magically have a "test-tube baby," just like the couples they read about in the press. More often than not, the statistics get distorted so that IVF can seem more successful than it actually is.

***What do the statistics say about IVF?*** All the publicity about IVF clouds the bottom line: there are very few IVF births. If you're thinking of trying IVF, consider these numbers:

- Of the 150 clinics doing IVF in 1987, only 45 had a single birth.
- Half of the clinics using IVF in 1988 had yet to achieve a single live birth, although many of these clinics had small or very new programs.
- Only a very few—perhaps as few as 6—of the nation's IVF centers accounted for two-thirds of the IVF births in the United States.
- Almost all IVF clinics claim a 20 to 40 percent success rate: the actual figures (for large programs of more than 100 IVFs a year) are 15 to 20 percent for IVF.

***The "take-home baby" rate is the best measure of success*** in IVF; however, that kind of success is enjoyed by only about 5 percent of the couples who go through IVF. So how do clinics come up with their figures? Most clinics calculate their "success" based on technical pregnancies, which may even include "chemical pregnancies," meaning the transient rise in a woman's hormone levels following embryo transfer, although this is meaningless to a couple hoping for a baby. Ectopic pregnancies (the egg is fertilized in the fallopian tube) are also often counted, although such a pregnancy almost necessarily means the death of the embryo and is also a risk to the mother's reproductive organs as well as to her life. The miscarriage rate is 25 percent for IVF pregnancies, as compared to 15 to 20 percent for the general population.

*The cost of IVF is about $5,000 per attempt,* but the total cost can be far greater than that because repeated attempts have to be made. In addition to the medical costs, if you don't live near a reputable clinic, you have to calculate the cost of travel and lodging for yourself and your spouse for approximately two weeks, not to mention the loss of income. Remember that many such visits are involved: the initial visit and diagnostic tests, and subsequent ones every time an egg is removed and fertilization and implantation are attempted. Of course the costs are that much more if you go out of state or outside the United States.

*Medical insurance will sometimes pay for IVF.* Many insurance companies claim that in vitro is a nonreimbursable experimental process. However, some states are beginning to require insurers to cover infertility treatments: Maryland, Massachusetts, Hawaii, and Texas are the first four to do so. Check to see if your insurance company will cover part or all of the procedure, sometimes for an extra premium.

*There is no federal regulation of fertility clinics,* or any treatments that they perform. Of the more than 150 clinics existing in 1990, more than one-quarter were privately run. Of course there are voluntary professional guidelines, but there is a wide variance in the quality of care you may find.

If you have a choice between a clinic that is private or one that is academic (attached to a teaching hospital, for example), you should take the latter. IVF is very complicated: academic centers have very high standards and are reviewed by their peers.

*There are three world leaders in IVF:* Bourn Hall in Cambridge, England; Monash University in Melbourne, Australia; and Jones Institute at Eastern Virginia Medical School in Norfolk, Virginia. It is recommended that you seek the programs with the most experience. The clinics that have seen the most patients usually offer the best chance for pregnancy. If you are fortunate enough to be accepted by one of the Three Greats, your chances of success will be higher.

***How is in vitro fertilization actually done?*** IVF was first developed as a way to bypass damaged or blocked fallopian tubes and get at a woman's eggs. Now it is used for various other infertility problems. Eggs are removed from a woman's ovary, usually by a surgical procedure using ultrasound. The eggs are then fertilized with her husband's sperm in a shallow laboratory container called a petri dish (not in a test tube!). After waiting two days for the egg and sperm to join together and the cells to divide, the doctor inserts the fertilized eggs into the woman's uterus, through her vagina.

***There are risks to IVF,*** both for you and your baby; you will probably be told about the risks and asked to sign an informed consent. There are potential complications from the various drugs and hormones, from anesthesia and incidents that occur during the surgical procedure itself, and from infection or disease transmission via donor eggs, sperm, or the fluid in which the embryo is cultured (although the last is very rare). There is also speculation that women who are treated with fertility drugs, especially repeatedly, will be at risk for endometrial, cervical, ovarian, and breast cancer for as long as 20 or 30 years after treatment.

    The statistics about the risk of IVF to the fetus are coming in slowly. Australia—which is the only country that has kept reliable records since 1979—reported there may be an increased risk of congenital malformations in IVF births. A French study confirmed these disturbing findings; however, the number of women studied was too small to be conclusive. Ask your infertility specialist's opinion regarding birth defects.

***Check the success rate of the clinic*** you're thinking of using for IVF. Remember that the *take-home baby rate* is the only real measure of success: what percentage of couples who were accepted in that clinic's IVF program actually went home with a baby? The average take-home rate in U.S. clinics is 15 to 20 percent per egg retrieved.

# 3

# Taking care of your body

## NUTRITION

There is no way to stress enough the importance of nutrition. Eating well is essential to your comfort while you're pregnant, for a better labor and delivery, and for a healthy, intelligent baby. If you think about nothing else while you're pregnant, *please* think about what you're putting in your mouth and what effect it will have.

A pregnant woman's nutritional status is actually the result of her lifetime dietary experience. You have no control over it, but even the lifetime dietary habits of past generations have an influence. Your nutrition during prepregnancy is also important, so once you've decided to become pregnant, eat lots of protein and a well-balanced diet.

There are many benefits to good nutrition, starting with the fact that you will feel better and look better if you eat well. The foremost benefit is that good nutrition helps prevent stillbirth and low birth weight. The danger of prematurity and low-birth-weight babies is covered in the following section on Weight Gain. Another benefit is that there is a direct relationship between prenatal nutrition and a lack of complications during pregnancy, labor, and delivery. A good diet creates a strong uterus, which helps insure a good labor with efficient contractions. Good nutrition has

99

also been shown to prevent infections and anemia in the mother. A well-balanced diet, rich in protein, has also been linked with a lower incidence of toxemia in late pregnancy (see the section on Toxemia in Chapter Ten).

It is simply *not true* that it doesn't matter what you eat or don't eat because the growing fetus simply "takes" what it needs from your body. Yes, if you have a severely deficient diet, nature *does* give the baby's needs priority over yours at crucial developmental stages. The fetus and placenta take nourishment from your bones and muscles if you eat inadequately—but all this means is that both of you are being cheated. *Poor nutrition affects the baby directly.* Starve yourself and you're starving your baby.

There are two periods of rapid growth of the baby's brain cells: at 20 weeks gestation and at 36 weeks gestation, about one month before birth. The human brain develops most rapidly in the last part of the pregnancy: the cell division in the brain is impaired if there is malnutrition at that time. Inadequate food intake can cause an irreversible deficit in the number of brain cells, but it can also mean malformed cells and impaired interconnections between cells. The latter results in learning problems and poor motor coordination.

The message should be very clear: *Do not go even twenty-four hours without food. Do not skip meals.* People who don't know any better are compromising a baby's intelligence and physical coordination. That is a tragedy. But if you know the results of poor nutrition and you don't eat well, that is a crime.

## FETAL DEVELOPMENT

You won't have any doubts about the importance of your day-to-day nutrition when you see how your baby is growing inside you. The fetus is attached to you by the umbilical cord and 25 percent of the maternal blood volume is going directly to the uteroplacental system. The baby receives her nourishment not through the umbilicus but via the placenta. The fetus absorbs food and eliminates waste products through this remarkable organ: the bloodstreams of the mother and fetus are ordinarily separate, but they come into close proximity in the placenta, where materials pass over from one blood system to the next. Intrauterine growth is largely governed by the placenta, which weighs one-fifth to one-sixth as much as the fetus. The placenta completely stops growing between the 34th and 38th weeks; fetal growth slows but continues. Placental insufficiency—poor performance due to causes such as malnutrition—may adversely affect the growth and well-being of the fetus.

The baby is surrounded by amniotic fluid. It helps to understand the stresses of pregnancy and the need for extra nourishment when you learn that this fluid is not stagnant, as you might think: about one-third of it is replenished every hour. This fluid is constantly being reabsorbed back into the mother's blood system and excreted into the amniotic sac by the cells of the amniotic membrane. The fetus swallows about 1 pint a day and presumably voids a similar quantity. By the 12th week the volume of amniotic fluid measures 12 ounces. In mid-pregnancy the volume is 1 pint and at term (the end of 9 months) there is usually a little less than 1 quart, although amounts up to 8 *gallons* have been recorded. The amniotic fluid contains skin cells shed by the fetus (which are examined when amniocentesis is performed), fetal hairs, specks of vernix (the creamy coating on the fetus), various minerals, sugar, and products of fetal urine, such as uric acid and creatinine.

Inside your uterus there is constant loud noise: a rhythmical whooshing sound punctuated by stomach rumbles created by air passing through your stomach. There is a pulsating noise that keeps exact time with your heart, due to the blood flowing through your uterus: one-quarter of the maternal blood is pumped to the uterus. Almost all external noises are muted as they pass through your body and through the amniotic fluid. Only extremely loud noises ever exceed the rhythmical intrauterine sound. It's interesting to note that regardless of whether a woman is left- or right-handed, when the baby is born she instinctively holds it on the left, where it is near to the comforting sound of her heartbeat. Studies have shown that colicky babies can be calmed by hearing a tape-recording of the intrauterine rhythmical sound.

Fetal activity in utero can be violent, including kicks and punches. Some babies seem to get more active at night or when their mother is resting; others get very active when the parents are making love (which can be disconcerting!). It is also common for a fetus to have hiccups—short, quick regular jerks of its trunks and shoulders that can be seen as well as felt. An attack usually lasts about fifteen minutes and can happen several times.

***Prenatal parenting*** is a fairly new concept relating to the influence you can have on your unborn child's development. People have traditionally seen birth as the beginning of a baby's life, and may not think of the baby as even alive until she takes her first breath and cries. However, in the days and weeks before delivery, a baby is not significantly different mentally from how she will be at birth. All of the many tasks that a baby needs to master for life outside the womb—like breathing, sucking, swallowing, touching, smelling, looking, and listening—she has been "practicing" in the womb. The baby's mental apparatus is not suddenly activated at the moment of birth: new studies show that she has been preparing in utero for quite some time.

It is believed that from at least the 6th month after conception, the unborn child feels, senses, and remembers. Extensive studies give credence to the theory that everything that happens to the mother also happens in some sense to her baby. There may well be a connection made between the unborn child and her parents before birth, with important consequences for her personality and development.

The Directory of Fetal Development that begins on page 103 gives you some idea of the stages of your baby's growth in the womb, and suggests that expectant parents should feel encouraged to talk to the unborn baby, play her music, read her stories, and massage her when she acts up. You may find that if your baby is kicking inside the womb and you stroke your abdomen gently, the baby will stop kicking and relax. How much interaction you want to have with your unborn child is up to you, but you certainly shouldn't feel this is something you have to do as a good parent. Your child will not be born mentally deprived if you haven't read her all of *Alice in Wonderland* before she is born! Enjoy this information and use it to enhance your pregnancy experience, not to create a new obligation or source of guilt for you.

---

### CHART 9. DIRECTORY OF FETAL DEVELOPMENT

**FIRST MONTH**

*Around 2nd week:* embryo is attached to the uterine wall and consists of approximately 150 cells, already specialized into what will be their different functions—this is the embryonic shield containing preliminary tissues

*3rd week:* shield transformed into a tubular folded structure with a beating heart, brain, and spinal cord—it is a total of 1/10th inch long

*4th week:* the whole embryo is formed

*26th day:* beginnings of arms

*28th day:* beginnings of legs, which will be slower in development than the arms

**SECOND MONTH**

*End of 5th week:* backbone forming: 5 to 8 vertebrae laid down, nervous system and spinal canal forming; foundation for the brain, spinal cord, and entire nervous system will have been established; tubular, S-shaped heart beginning to beat

CHART 9. DIRECTORY OF FETAL DEVELOPMENT *(continued)*

**SECOND MONTH**
*(cont.):*

| | |
|---|---|
| *Beginning of 6th week:* | head forming; beating heart is visible, located on outside of body, not yet within the chest cavity; intestinal tract forming (starts from the mouth cavity downward); mouth closed; has rudimentary tail (extension of spinal column) |
| *End of 6th week:* | all backbone laid down; spinal canal closed over; brain increasing; tail of the embryo quite long; depressions appear beneath the skin where eyes and ears will appear; germ cells to become either ovaries or testes have appeared; length is $1/4$ inch |
| *6th & 7th weeks:* | nerve and muscle work together for the first time; reflexes; makes spontaneous movements by the 7th week but most mothers won't feel movement until between 16 and 26 weeks |
| *7th week:* | primitive embryo becomes a primitive, well-proportioned small-scale baby, less than one inch long; face is flattening; eyes perceptible through closed lids; shell-like external ears; mouth opens—has a human face with eyes, ears, nose, lips, tongue; chest and abdomen completely formed; heart is internal; lung buds appear; arms, legs, hands, feet are partially formed: the arms are as long as a printed exclamation point and have fingers and thumbs; the toes are all stubby but the big toes have appeared |

CHART 9. DIRECTORY OF FETAL DEVELOPMENT *(continued)*

**SECOND MONTH**
*(cont.):*

*Days 46 to 48:*     first true bone cells replace cartilage; this signals transition from embryo to fetus; ½ inch long; 1/1000 ounce

*End of 2nd month:*     abdominal-wall muscles of the fetus (if removed from the womb) will contract if touched; physical structure is essentially complete; has a complete skeleton of cartilage; face is completely formed; jaws well formed; teeth and facial muscles forming; clitoris or penis begins to appear; ovaries or testicles taking form; weight is 1/30th of an ounce or 1 gram—less than an aspirin

**THIRD MONTH:**     face quite human and "prettier," except for jaws not fully developed; eyes—were at side of head—are moving to the front; physical refinements: nail beds form for eventual nails; vocal chords complete; taste buds and saliva-producing glands appear; buds for the baby teeth are present; kidneys have developed; heart forming 4 chambers; palate to form roof of mouth is closing; major blood vessels assuming final form; muscle wall of intestinal tract forming; fetal heart beating 117 to 157 beats per minute; fetus becomes active but mother rarely feels it unless she's very slender

CHART 9. DIRECTORY OF FETAL DEVELOPMENT *(continued)*

**THIRD MONTH**
*(cont.):*
*End of 3rd month:*    male scrotum has appeared, female external vulva and male penis have gradually molded during second and third months; *at 11 weeks:* cycle of circulation starts as baby is able to swallow: swallows amniotic fluid, urinates it back out; ears completely formed; when brain signals, muscles now respond and fetus kicks, even curling its toes; arms bend at wrist and elbows; fingers close to form tight fist; all movements reflex from the spinal cord; brain not yet sufficiently organized to control them, and won't be until after birth; fetus more than 3 inches long and weighs approximately 1 ounce

**FOURTH MONTH:**    fetus grows so much it reaches one-half the height it will have at birth; increases its weight sixfold; takes in a large amount of food, oxygen, and water from its mother through the placenta; movements more vigorous but most women don't feel them yet; fetus fills the uterine cavity; placenta now fully formed and not only nourishes the baby, gets rid of its waste, and provides it with oxygen, but also secretes hormones into the mother's system; grows to a length of 6½ inches and 4 ounces; tests show that by the end of 4th month, fetus will suck if his lips are stroked; if a bitter substance like iodine is introduced into the amniotic fluid, he will grimace and stop swallowing liquid;

CHART 9. DIRECTORY OF FETAL DEVELOPMENT *(continued)*

**FOURTH MONTH (cont.):**

if a bright light is shined on the mother's abdomen, the baby will gradually move his hands up to shield his eyes; at 16 weeks he begins to suck his thumb: thumb-sucking calms the baby and also helps develop coordination and strengthen jaw and cheek muscles

**FIFTH & SIXTH MONTHS:**

thair begins on eyebrows, eyelashes, head; both sexes develop nipples and underlying mammary glands; hard nails form on nail beds; toes develop a bit later than fingers; muscles are stronger: mother perceives movement (probably for the first time); skin has begun to develop vernix, a protective, cheeselike coating; body is covered by *lanugo,* a fine, downy hair; in 6th month eyelids can open and fetus can look around; if born prematurely now might survive in an incubator but usually the breathing mechanism and lungs are too immature to operate; youngest known to have survived are between 23 and 25 weeks, weighing 1 pound; by end of the 5th month, fetus is 10 inches and 8 ounces; by the end of 6th month, fetus is 12 inches and $1\frac{1}{2}$ pounds; at 5 months if a loud sound is made next to his mother, the unborn child will raise his hands and cover his ears; by the 6th month his hearing system is perfectly developed: because water is a better sound conductor than air, the baby in utero

CHART 9. DIRECTORY OF FETAL DEVELOPMENT *(continued)*

**FIFTH & SIXTH MONTHS** *(cont.)*: can hear very well, although with distortions; at 6 months babies in the womb react to sound with increased pulse rates and by moving in rhythm to the music; recordings of the baby's brain waves at the beginning of the last trimester show that the baby has rapid eye movement (REM) sleep, which in adults is associated with dreaming, so the unborn baby may be dreaming by the 7th month

**SEVENTH MONTH:** may practice sucking thumb, which may have begun as early as the 4th month; at the end of the month boys' testicles descend into scrotum; child born alive during 7th month has just better than a 50 percent chance of survival; puts on more than one pound in this month, for a total of 2½ pounds and 15 inches

**EIGHTH MONTH:** baby likely to settle into a vertex (head down) position and has little room to move; gains at least 2 pounds this month, for a total of 4 pounds and 16½ inches

**NINTH MONTH:** eyes usually slate color; average circumference of head equals the circumference of its shoulders; grows 2½ inches and gains 2 pounds this month; during last 3 months, baby gets antibodies for immunity to whatever disease the mother has had, from measles to the common cold, or has been immunized against (polio, smallpox, etc.)

## CHART 10. CRITICAL PERIODS IN HUMAN DEVELOPMENT

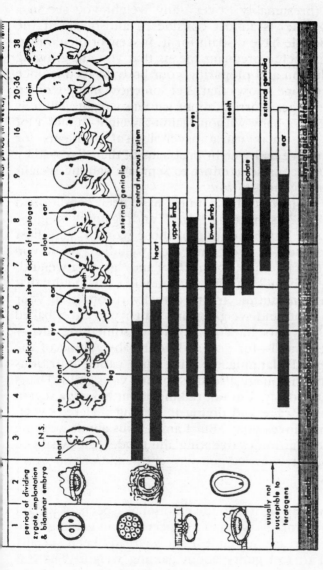

*from Moore, Keith L. The Developing Human, 4th edition, W. B. Saunders Co., Philadelphia, 1988. Reprinted by permission.*

Schematic illustration of the critical period in human development. During the first two weeks of development, the embryo is usually not susceptible to teratogens. During these predifferentiation stages, a substance either damages all or most of the cells of the embryo, resulting in its death, or it damages only a few cells, allowing the embryo to recover without developing defects. Black denotes highly sensitive periods; white indicates stages that are less sensitive to teratogens.

## WEIGHT GAIN

*Emotionally,* weight gain is one of the most sensitive areas of pregnancy. Thinness has a high value in America. Being overweight (presumably "over" any weight you see in a fashion magazine) is almost considered antisocial—at the very least, people have disdain for it. It seems ridiculous to point out that being pregnant means that you are growing a baby inside you and preparing your body to feed it once it's born. Everyone knows that. Yet somehow many women also manage to get worried about gaining weight. There is no way to have a baby without gaining weight—quite a lot of weight. This may cause psychological problems for women who have had weight problems in their lives—they should make a conscious effort to separate gaining weight *then* and gaining weight *now*.

Many women in this country have been conditioned to think of "fat" as meaning "ugly" and "gaining weight" as being "bad." If you are one of those women, you must fight at every meal to overcome your prejudice. While you are pregnant, "fat" equals *protection* and "gaining weight" is *good*. The remainder of this section will explain why that is true. In the meantime try to actually recondition your response to food and weight gain. When you eat a baked potato, praise yourself. You are doing something nice—something essential—for you and your baby. Think of the time you spend planning, cooking, and eating nutritious food as affection you are already showing your child. That's what it is. Obviously, I'm not talking about baking a seven-layer chocolate cake and diving in, saying, "Here, sweetheart, Mommy loves you." But I am serious about working to change your attitudes to eating and food. Otherwise you will be constantly worried/guilty/resentful and/or you won't eat properly.

*Doctors* can play right into the emotional aspects of weight gain. They reinforce a woman's concern about gaining "too much" and increase her guilt if she's already been socially conditioned to feel guilty about gaining weight. There is virtually no nutritional training in medical school and it is rare to find a doctor who knows much about nutrition in pregnancy. Doctors may not be aware of the ways in which good nutrition is preventive medicine—they are trained to deal only with problems that result from inadequate diets. Also, medical thinking about weight gain has changed only in recent times—some doctors are still holding on to the outdated, disproven concept of a rigid weight restriction in pregnancy.

Some doctors are so fierce about imposing a weight gain limit that their patients dread prenatal visits because of the chastisement they get for gaining weight. Some women go so far as to "starve" themselves before a visit to the doctor and then gorge themselves when they leave the office. Some doctors hold these views out of ignorance. Some may have these attitudes because they are raised in the same society that condemns "fat" and they are upholding the social prescription that all women should be thin—whether they've got another person growing inside them or not.

Defy or leave any doctor who puts you on a diet to restrict weight gain during pregnancy, or insists on a low-calorie, low-salt diet. Studies have shown the latter to be dangerous—such a diet can be the *cause* of toxemia (not the cure for it, as was once thought).

**Recommended gain** for pregnancy is a *minimum* of 24 pounds. It wasn't long ago that the medical community battled nature and tried to keep a pregnant woman from gaining more than 15 pounds. The chart on page 112 should show you why that is not only difficult but also compromises the fetus. With a weight gain of 25 to 35 pounds, most women will only have 5 to 10 pounds to lose after the baby is born.

**Underweight women** can gain as much as 40 pounds. If you are underweight at conception—really thin—then you probably already have a nutritional "debt." You should improve your diet as soon as possible or there is a chance that you'll have problems during labor and delivery and perhaps with your baby.

*Overweight women* should not be on a severely restricted diet during pregnancy. It is probably unwise to eat less than 1,800 calories a day. Try to get 6 meals a day, each supplying 20 grams of protein. This will help satisfy your hunger, prevent you from gaining more weight, and build a healthy fetus. For proper utilization of your food, be sure that you drink *whole milk* (not skimmed) between meals and at any meal supplying no fat. Eat frequently if you are cutting down on calories so that you prevent blood sugar loss.

---

### CHART 11. WEIGHT GAIN: "PRODUCTS OF CONCEPTION"

| | |
|---|---|
| Fetus | 7½ to 8½ pounds (average newborn weight) |
| Amniotic fluid | 1 to 2 pounds |
| Placenta | 1 to 2 pounds |
| Mother's blood & body fluid | increases by 4 to 8 pounds |
| Uterine muscles | 2 to 3 pounds |
| Breasts | enlarge by 2 to 3 pounds |
| Fat deposits | 2 to 10 pounds (around internal organs) |

Thus, the absolute minimum you will gain is around 20 pounds, although your gain can be as much as 35 pounds and still be within this range.

---

*Weight loss at birth* is dramatic, which you should keep in mind if you get concerned about your weight gain. If you're a fairly large, big-boned woman, even a 40- to 45-pound gain won't leave you with that much weight to lose after the baby is born. The average weight loss at birth itself is 13 pounds—the baby, amniotic fluid, and placenta. An additional average 3½ pounds is lost between the first postpartum hour and the 12th day, mostly from water in your body tissues. There is an additional weight loss during the first six postpartum weeks—particularly for breast-feeding mothers—so that there are usually only 5 to 10 pounds of weight that you'll have to "work" to lose.

***Rate and cause of weight gain*** are what count during pregnancy. If it's gained from nutritious foods and the weight increases at a steady rate, you're doing fine. However, many doctors and books adhere to fairly rigid ideas about weight gain designating anything but the average weekly weight gain as "abnormal." Of course there *is* an average rate of weight gain—an ideal—but it's unreasonable to expect any one woman's weight gain, or the rate of it, to follow those patterns. *People are individuals*—and each individual's body behaves uniquely (the same woman may even gain weight differently in two pregnancies). Unfortunately, many doctors make women feel there is something "wrong" with them if they don't gain weight according to a certain chart.

For example, you may hear that during the first three months you should gain only 1½ to 3 pounds. You may also be told that that weight gain should average about 1 pound every 9 days, or ¾ pound a week, which would bring you to an ideal total of 24 pounds by the end of your pregnancy. However, the pattern of weight gain will be different for each woman.

Check your weight weekly. A *weight loss* or *no gain* should be checked by the doctor: something may be wrong with the placenta or the baby. A *sudden gain* after the 24th week might mean that you have edema (retention of water in your tissues) related to toxemia; the doctor can test for this.

The greatest gain will take place in the 5th and 6th months. The second trimester of pregnancy is the peak of weight gain for most women. Again, it's important to stress that women rarely gain weight in equal weekly or monthly increments. Usually a woman gains only a few pounds in the last trimester. Even though this is the baby's time of greatest weight gain, a woman can even have a weight loss in the last 2 weeks or so of her pregnancy.

*Appetite increases* substantially by the 4th month of your pregnancy. This is nature's way of stimulating you to eat for yourself and your baby. It is a normal response to the increase in your metabolism. Energy requirements increase about 15 percent during pregnancy. This means you should be getting 300–500 extra daily calories more than before you were pregnant, assuming you were eating a substantial and well-balanced diet then. *Protein* needs increase by about 50 percent because of body-building work in you and the baby and because your systems are putting out added effort.

*Restricting gain to a certain preset weight* can be most harmful. It is during the last 8 weeks of pregnancy that the baby gains 1 ounce a day and its brain develops at the most rapid rate. The catch-22 is that if you've set a certain limit on how many pounds you can gain, you will probably reach your self-imposed limit just as the baby's growth spurt begins. It's at this point that the baby requires more oxygen and nutrients of all types than earlier in the pregnancy. If you restrict calories and salt at this time you compromise the baby's brain-cell growth and reduce the amount of blood that flows through the placenta, carrying oxygen and nutrients.

*Low-calorie, low-salt diet* is prescribed by some doctors. It is not nutritionally adequate—but again, doctors are not trained in nutrition. In the last 3 months of pregnancy a woman needs 2,600 calories a day. During that period she also needs approximately 90 grams of protein a day. This is a generous allotment—some authorities say that 75 grams is sufficient. However, a low-calorie, low-salt diet causes protein to be utilized in such a way that only one-half of the protein eaten is available to build the baby's body and brain. In other words, even if you were taking in 90 grams of protein, if you were also on a low-calorie, low-salt diet that protein would be metabolized in such a way that only 45 grams could be used for fetal growth.

## SOME WARNINGS ABOUT WEIGHT GAIN

Although I've been emphasizing the need to eat well and gain weight, this isn't to say you can go hog wild. Gaining too much weight is a problem too. For one thing, some studies show that there is a correlation between a large weight gain and a higher cesarean section rate. Evidently if there is excessive fatty tissue the uterine muscles don't function as well. It is harder for the baby to descend and for the cervix to dilate. The other problem with gaining too much weight is that you'll have a lot to take off once the baby is born and that can be depressing and arduous.

***Don't overeat in the first trimester.*** Some women overeat out of eagerness when they learn they are pregnant. The baby isn't visible yet and a woman who's really excited about her pregnancy may want to display to the outside world—and have proof for herself—that the baby is there and growing. The only growth you'll have proof of in the first trimester is your expanding thighs! Eat sensibly. The baby probably won't show until after the 16th week. Most women begin to "show" between the 16th and 20th weeks. The pregnant uterus grows upward, reaching the navel at about the 20th week, at which time it will be pretty clear to outsiders that you're pregnant. Eating too much won't hurry it along!

***Avoid or limit sweets,*** which are "empty" calories. Cakes, cookies, soda pop not only have virtually no nutritional value themselves but they fill you up so you haven't got an appetite for foods that *are* good for you. Also, refined sugar products make your blood sugar go way up and then drop way down rapidly—making you hungry again in no time. If you feel you're gaining too much weight, the least complicated and most effective way to control it is simply to cut out sweets. Eat fruit, for example, instead. It is sweet, provides many nutrients, and the fructose (natural fruit sugar) doesn't catapult your blood sugar way up and then drop it down fast the way refined sugar does. A snack of an apple and a piece of cheese can satisfy your hunger, be a mid-afternoon treat, and is good for you and the baby—all without being very fattening. If you find yourself simply craving a sweet, then have it. It makes more sense to have the cookie or piece of cake than to deny yourself because it will just boomerang and you'll go out of control later. Don't make the mistake of thinking that because you're pregnant it's okay to eat things you usually don't allow yourself. Some women begin eating dessert at every meal once they're pregnant, rationalizing that they're "eating for two" and it will all be put to good use. Unless you're an absolute beanpole and are eating well-balanced, nutritious meals along with your sweets—you're going to be very sorry nine months down the road. You're going to be pretty sick of your maternity clothes by the time the baby is born—the sooner you can get back into your prebaby clothes, the better you'll feel.

*Expanding hips and thighs* do not necessarily mean you are gaining too much. In fact, some padding in these areas is essential during pregnancy. One reason for this is that the body has to counterbalance the enormous new weight in front. Another reason for this added fat is nature's way of insuring an "emergency reserve" of fat for the lactation period. Even if you aren't going to breast-feed, your body needs extra energy for the emotional and physical demands of the first weeks of having a new baby in the house.

*Don't eat to cheer yourself up.* It's possible to have periods of feeling low (see Moodiness in Chapter Four) while you're pregnant and some people tend to eat when they're feeling depressed. Do nice things for yourself to feel better but don't start munching. There are many ways to perk up: get into a nice hot bubble bath with a pile of magazines; go to the movies; get your hair done or have a manicure; buy a new set of place mats. Whatever you do instead of eating to cheer yourself up, the most important thing is to recognize that you're feeling blue and deal with it.

*Take a picture of yourself*—don't forget to get a photograph of yourself at your most pregnant. You'll never believe you looked like this, six months postpartum!

## LOW-BIRTH-WEIGHT BABIES

Maternal malnutrition is a major cause of low-birth-weight babies. A low-birth-weight baby is defined as being 2,500 grams (5½ pounds) or less. You do not want to have a low-birth-weight baby. The neonatal mortality rate is anywhere from 17 to 30 times higher for babies weighing under 5½ pounds (depending on which statistics you read). Low-birth-weight babies account for only 8.2 percent of live births but account for 75 percent of neonatal deaths. Low birth weight is the cause of an estimated 53,000 yearly infant deaths within the first year of life.

These babies are ten times more likely to be mentally retarded: the U.S. Department of Health, Education, and Welfare did a study in 1972 that showed a direct relationship between birth weight and IQ. Nearly half of all children who were underweight at birth had an IQ under 70. Oxygen deprivation, birth injuries, and RDS (respiratory distress syndrome) all primarily affect babies under 5½ pounds. Maternal malnutrition also retards the growth of the placenta and low placental weight is related to perinatal mortality.

The most rapid brain development takes place in the last trimester of pregnancy and also the first month of life. As I pointed out before, an undernourished mother can cause irreversible neurological damage and permanent brain underdevelopment in her baby. It is therefore disturbing to learn that in Scandinavian countries the average birth weight of babies is close to 8 pounds, while in the United States the average is almost *a pound less.* Yet studies have shown that with women who gained an average of 35 pounds during pregnancy the result was an average of 8-pound babies. Other studies show that larger babies are easier to care for. The comparison between 8½-pound babies and 5-pound babies showed that the larger ones were more vigorous, active, and mentally alert and suffered less from colic, diarrhea, anemia, and infections.

In a country as rich as ours there is no excuse for low-birth-weight babies as a result of maternal malnutrition. Ignorance is hampering people who can afford protein-rich and well-balanced diets but don't eat them. But if you have financial difficulties there are still ways to get good food for yourself and your baby. Call your local Department of Health and Human Services and find out if you are eligible for food stamps. If you are pregnant and on welfare you may be eligible for an *unborn child allowance*—find out. And contact the Maternal and Child Health Service Office in your region (listed on page 11 of Chapter One) to find out about free nutritional supplements for pregnant and lactating women.

## DIET

There are certain very important guidelines about your diet while you're pregnant, though the "daily food guide" lists (with the required number of servings of each category of food) can be forbidding. Considering the pace of people's lives it's unreasonable to expect them to sit around measuring ounces of this and portions of that. Most daily food guides recommend: 4 servings of *protein,* 4 of *milk and milk products,* 3 of *grains,* 1 *vitamin C–rich fruit or vegetable,* 2 *leafy green vegetables,* 1 *other fruit or vegetable.* Personally, it would drive me crazy trying to remember how many of my grain portions I'd already satisfied by teatime. But for other people keeping a list may help them structure their intake. At any rate, what matters is that you eat balanced, sensible meals. Before I go into detail, here are the *basic guidelines:*

- a 24-pound minimum weight gain which is gradual and steady
- 75–100 grams of protein needed daily
- 500 calories needed over a *normal* diet: i.e., a total of about 2,600. Your calorie needs will be greater if you are: underweight, under severe emotional stress, had a previous miscarriage or stillbirth, are having a baby within

one year of another baby, or any combination of these situations
• no sodium restriction—use iodized salt to taste
• toward the end of the pregnancy, eat 5 or 6 small meals instead of 3 large ones—for your own comfort and easier digestion
• daily vitamin supplements: 30 to 60 mg of elemental iron and 400 to 800 μg (0.2 to 0.4 mg) of folacin
• the nearer foods are to their natural state, the higher their food value—fresh is best, frozen next, canned foods last

CAUTION: If you are thinking of or planning to breast-feed, please read that section in Chapter Eleven. Your diet before and during pregnancy can contaminate your breast milk.

## CHOLESTEROL

There is a widespread misunderstanding about the "danger" of eating too much cholesterol-rich food. The fact is that people's bodies manufacture cholesterol from *any* food source. Limiting the intake of cholesterol-containing food is not the answer. The tendency in some people to over-synthesize and assimilate cholesterol is an inherited problem—if you inherit it from both parents, heart disease can start in childhood, but if you inherit it from one parent the problem manifests itself later in life. The point is not to worry about cholesterol in your diet while you're pregnant unless tests have shown that you have an inherited problem.

## DIGESTION

Many grains and vegetables are composed principally of starch. Cooking renders starch more digestible by breaking down the cell walls.

***Chewing food thoroughly*** is also important. Ptyalin, an enzyme in the saliva, starts breaking starch down into its component sugars. By chewing food completely you help the ptyalin work by mixing it into the food. This is especially important when you're pregnant because your digestive tract is somewhat sluggish and needs all the help it can get.

*Fluids:* You should drink 6 to 8 glasses of fluids a day. There is a 25 percent rise in your blood volume when you're pregnant, and your body has to have additional fluid to meet that need. Liquids aid the circulation of blood and body fluids and help the distribution of mineral salts. Fluids also stimulate digestion, preventing constipation, and aids the assimilation of foods. Protein, for example, requires fluids in order to metabolize. Generous amounts of liquid in the diet also prevent urinary infections, to which one is susceptible when pregnant.

## GRAINS

Grain products supply thiamine, niacin, riboflavin, iron, phosphorus, and zinc. Whole-grain items are preferable because they have higher quantities of magnesium and zinc: brown rice, wheat germ, cold cereals (puffed oats, shredded wheat, wheat flakes, and granola), and hot cereals (oatmeal, rolled or cracked wheat). Whole-grain breads—cracked wheat and whole wheat—are made by many companies. The germ of the grain contains most of the nutrients, yet when grains go through a refining process it is this germ which is removed—so try to eat whole-grain products. Other items considered grain products are: ready-to-eat cereals, although the sugared ones supply empty, expensive calories, cream of wheat or rice, farina, cornmeal, grits, and rice; all breads, including cornbread, corn or flour tortillas, rolls, bagels, muffins, biscuits, dumplings, and crackers. Waffles and pancakes are grain products—add wheat germ to the batter to increase their food value. French and Italian breads are nutritionally inferior even to soft American enriched white bread. They may taste better but French and Italian breads are made with water instead of milk so they are mostly empty calories.

## HONEY

Honey has a number of advantages over sugar. First of all, it contains traces of nutrients, especially the B vitamins. Also, honey is sweeter than sucrose, so only about two-thirds as much is needed to provide the sweetening power of sugar. Honey is immediately absorbed by the system but it doesn't trigger the same cycle as sucrose does: insulin—low blood sugar—more sugar needed—insulin. This explains honey's third advantage: it *satisfies,* so one is less likely to eat it to excess. With sucrose, the more you eat, the more you want, the above-mentioned cycle. So try to substitute honey for sugar whenever you can.

## POTATOES

Potatoes are a vastly underrated food. A potato is only slightly higher in calories than an apple but each potato contains 3 grams of protein vs. only a trace in an apple, and the potato has more calcium, twice as much iron, thiamine, and riboflavin, much more niacin, and 7 times as much vitamin C. Therefore, you should jump at any chance to eat a potato during your pregnancy—especially a baked one, with the skin.

## IRON

Your blood volume doubles when you are pregnant, and iron is essential to the formation of healthy red blood cells. Very few women start their pregnancies with enough iron stored in their bodies to meet the greatly increased need for this trace mineral. It is also hard to eat enough iron-rich foods to keep up with your body's requirements during pregnancy. Even if you do eat a lot of iron-containing foods, only a small percentage of what you eat is actually absorbed, so there is no sure way to know how much iron you're taking in.

The developing fetus will take all the iron he needs from his mother, no matter how low her iron supply may be. A pregnant woman who is iron-deficient may wind up

anemic, exhausted, and susceptible to infection. This is why
iron supplements of 30 to 60 mg a day are recommended
by obstetricians, especially during the second half of pregnancy. Iron pills tend to be constipating, so eating dried
fruits such as raisins, prunes, or apricots can counteract
constipation as well as give you added iron.

Even if you're taking an iron supplement, include
iron-rich foods in your diet. The chart below shows you
the foods highest in iron. It's also good to know that high-
acid foods, including yogurt and those high in vitamin C,
increase your body's ability to absorb iron from pills or
food. Cooking such acidic foods as tomatoes in a cast-iron
pot allows the food to absorb some of the iron from the
pot. Conversely, if you drink tea or coffee with your meal,
it can significantly diminish your body's absorption of the
iron in your diet.

---

### CHART 12. IRON-RICH FOODS

|  | Mg |
|---|---|
| *Cereals* (1 cup) | |
| 40% bran flakes | 11 |
| Raisin bran | 9 |
| Cream of wheat | 8 |
| Oatmeal | 1½ |
| Shredded wheat | 1 |
| Wheat germ (½ cup) | 5 |
| | |
| *Fish and Meat* (4 oz.) | |
| Kidney | 15 |
| Liver (chicken) | 10 |
| Liver (beef) | 9 |
| Clams | 8 |
| Oysters | 7 |
| Turkey | 4½ |
| Beef | 4 |

## CHART 12. IRON-RICH FOODS *(continued)*

| | Mg |
|---|---|
| ***Fish and Meat*** (4 oz.) *(cont.)* | |
| Sardines | 3 |
| Lamb | 2 |
| Pork or chicken | 1 |
| Egg (1) | 1 |
| | |
| ***Fruits and Juices*** (1 cup) | |
| Prune juice | 3 |
| Raisins (½ cup) | 1.7 |
| Tomato juice | 1½ |
| Apple juice | 1 |
| Apricots, dried (½ cup) | 3.8 |
| Figs (2), prunes (10) dried | 1 |
| | |
| ***Vegetables*** (½ cup cooked) | |
| Spinach (1 cup raw) | 3 |
| Beans: Garbanzo, black-eyed peas, kidney, lima, and lentil | 2 |
| Artichoke (1) | 2 |
| Peas, sweet; Brussels sprouts; spinach, cooked | 1½ |
| Swiss chard | 1 |
| Romaine lettuce (1 cup raw); potato (baked or sweet); tomato (raw) | ½ |
| | |
| ***Nuts*** (¼ cup) | |
| Almonds, cashews | 1½ |
| Walnuts | 1 |
| | |
| ***Miscellaneous*** | |
| Blackstrap molasses (1 T.) | 3½ |
| Brewer's yeast (1 T.) | 1½ |
| Soybean curd (tofu, 4 oz.) | 2½ |

## MILK AND CALCIUM

Your body needs a great deal of calcium to build your baby's bones and for many other important body functions. The developing fetus will take the calcium from you even if you don't consume enough in your diet. However, both you and your baby will suffer if your prenatal diet is deficient in calcium: your bones will be weakened when the calcium is forced out of them, and the baby's bone growth will be inadequate.

A 50 percent increase in calcium is recommended during pregnancy, to a total of 1,200 mg a day. Milk and other dairy products are the best sources of calcium: drinking a quart of milk a day will fulfill your calcium requirement, since every cup supplies 300 mg. Do not eat any chocolate at the same time because it reduces your body's ability to absorb calcium.

Your body cannot utilize calcium without vitamin D, so the need for this vitamin doubles during pregnancy from 200 to 400 I.U.s a day. But if you are a young pregnant woman—between the ages of 19 and 22—you need even more vitamin D to support your own and the baby's bone development. The amount of vitamin D in *five* glasses of milk a day will meet this need. Other food sources of vitamin D include fortified margarine, butter, sardines, canned salmon, egg yolk, and liver. Also, spending time outdoors is beneficial because when you're in the sunlight the vitamin is made in your skin. *Do not take a vitamin D supplement without your doctor's orders:* overdoses of vitamin D are toxic and can produce severe abnormalities in the developing fetus.

## MILK AND MILK PRODUCTS

There is general agreement that a pregnant woman needs a quart of milk (4 cups) a day. Whole, skim, buttermilk, evaporated, nonfat dry milk, and yogurt are all equivalent. The important thing to remember is that a quart of fortified vitamin D milk supplies 400 I.U.s of vitamin D—as does an equal amount of nonfat dry milk. If you aren't getting it from milk, you need some source of vitamin D daily (see the Directory of Vitamin Sources and Functions, page 143).

However, you don't want much more than 400 I.U.s. Too much vitamin D can be harmful—unlike other vitamins, A and D are not excreted from the body if taken in excessive amounts.

*Whole milk* meets the needs of pregnancy best—the fat in it promotes the most efficient absorption of the calcium. This is a more important consideration than the slightly higher caloric content of whole milk. However, a quart of whole milk a day does supply a large number of calories, and if this worries you it is possible to take supplements instead. Please refer to the list on page 139 of the daily supplements you would have to take to equal 4 cups of milk.

*Do not be concerned* if you hear that milk has a *high sodium (salt) content*. This is *good* for you. Your body needs more sodium during pregnancy (see Salt in this section) and the excess is efficiently excreted by the kidneys.

*The calcium in milk* and milk products is vital to build strong teeth and bones. The baby's primary teeth begin to form during the 5th month of gestation—and the skeleton begins to change from cartilage to bone early in the sixth month. Do not underestimate the importance of this food group in your prenatal diet.

*Do not take calcium tablets* to satisfy your calcium requirement. It is preferable to get your daily calcium from real foods, since they supply other essential nutrients at the same time. Furthermore, it is not clear how your body absorbs calcium taken in tablet form.

### LACTOSE INTOLERANCE

*You may be "allergic" to milk* and think you have to avoid all dairy products. Some women may not be able to consume milk and other dairy products because their bodies cannot digest lactose, a sugar present in milk. However, very little lactose is found in natural cheeses, with the least amount occurring in fermented cheeses, so you can probably eat those. Also, cultured milk products, like yogurt and buttermilk (brands without added milk solids), have reduced amounts of lactose, and some people with lactose intolerance can consume them without a problem. Another alternative is to drink acidophilus milk, or you can add the enzyme lactase to ordinary milk. The enzyme is marketed as Lact-aid, and you can find it in pharmacies or health-food stores.

*You may just dislike milk,* but that doesn't mean you can't consume it in your diet. You can use milk in preparing soups, custards, or creamed dishes, in baking, or on cereal.

*There are also many milk products* which you can have instead of milk. Two 1-inch cubes of cheddar cheese, for example, are equal to 1 cup of milk. Other replacements are hard or semisoft cheese (but not blue cheese, cream cheese, or Camembert-type cheeses), cottage cheese, yogurt, ice cream, and ice milk. Most other commercial ice creams do not have genuine milk products in them.

*Goat's milk and soybean milk* are acceptable replacements, although they are both low in vitamin $B_{12}$. The chart on page 127 allows you to calculate the nutritional value of soybean curd or milk you might use instead of cow's milk.

| CHART 13. NUTRITIONAL EVALUATION OF SOYBEAN COMPARED TO MILK | | | | | | |
|---|---|---|---|---|---|---|
| (one serving) | | | | | | |
| | Calories | Protein (gm) | Fat (gm) | Carbohy-drates (mg) | Calcium (mg) | Iron (mg) | Vitamin A (I.U.) |
| Soybean curd (tofu) 1 package (4 oz.) | 86 | 9.4 | 5.0 | 2.9 | 154 | 2.3 | 0 |
| Pressed soybean curd (3½ oz.) | 135 | 16.2 | 7.3 | — | 210 | 7.1 | 233 |
| Soybean milk | 75 | 7.7 | 3.4 | — | 47 | 1.8 | 90 |
| Cow's milk, whole (8 oz.) | 159 | 8.5 | 8.5 | 12.0 | 288 | 0.1 | 350 |

## PROTEIN

Protein foods are the building blocks, the basic material from which most cells are formed.

*During pregnancy,* your daily need for protein is a *minimum* of 75 to 80 grams for a 5 foot 2 inch 121-pound woman. Most women feel better if they get more than this; above 100 grams a day.

Some women find that it is virtually impossible for them to comfortably consume 75 grams of protein a day. As with the "recommended requirements" of anything, you have to trust your own instincts and adapt things to your personal needs.

*The most complete protein* foods are meat, fish, milk, cheese, and eggs. *Incomplete* proteins include legumes (dried peas and beans), grains, seeds, and nuts. Most vegetables have small amounts of protein, and fruits have a negligible quantity.

*Proteins are composed of many amino acids,* 8 of which are essential. Another 2 amino acids are essential during the growing period, and the remainder our bodies manufacture. Plant and animal foods contain protein, but the former have incomplete proteins—lacking in one or more of the 8 essential amino acids. Animal proteins contain enough of all the essential amino acids in a proper ratio to meet the body's needs. Incomplete plant proteins can be supplemented by adding animal protein (milk in pea soup or egg and milk powder in bread).

*The protein content of food* is increased when certain foods are eaten in combination: **cornmeal** with beans, cheese, tofu (soybean curd), milk; **beans** with rice, bulgur, cornmeal, noodles (especially wheat noodles), sesame, milk; **peanuts** with sunflower seeds, milk; **whole-wheat bread or noodles** with beans, cheese, peanut butter, milk, tofu. (For a complete list, see the chart under Vegetarian Diet in this section). Therefore, having a glass of milk and a peanut-butter sandwich on wheat bread will increase the protein content of those ingredients. Frances Moore Lappé's *Diet for a Small Planet* and Ellen Ewald's *Recipes for a Small Planet* can give you many such ideas.

| CHART 14. SOURCES OF CALCIUM | | |
| --- | --- | --- |
| | Calcium (mg) | Calories |
| *Milk* (1 cup, 8 oz.) | | |
| Skim (nonfat) | 300 | 85 |
| Lowfat (2%) | 295 | 120 |
| Whole | 290 | 150 |
| Buttermilk | 285 | 100 |
| | | |
| *Yogurt* (1 cup, 8 oz.) | | |
| Nonfat | 452 | 127 |
| Low fat, plain | 415 | 144 |
| Low fat, with fruit | 315 | 200 |

## CHART 14. SOURCES OF CALCIUM *(continued)*

|  | Calcium (mg) | Calories |
|---|---|---|
| *Yogurt* (1 cup, 8 oz.) *(cont.)* | | |
| Whole, plain | 275 | 140 |
| Frozen | 200–250 | 180 |
| | | |
| *Cheese* (1 oz.) | | |
| Cottage cheese, creamed (½ cup) | 115 | 100 |
| Parmesan | 390 | 129 |
| Gruyère | 285 | 117 |
| Swiss | 270 | 106 |
| Provolone | 215 | 100 |
| Cheddar | 210 | 114 |
| Edam, muenster | 205 | 102 |
| Mozzarella | 185 | 72 |
| American | 200 | 100 |
| | | |
| *Fish* (4 oz.) | | |
| Sardines, drained solids with bone | 495 | 233 |
| Salmon, drained solids with bone | 225 | 150 |
| Oysters (1 cup, 8 oz.) | 215 | 160 |
| | | |
| *Vegetables* (1 cup, cooked) | | |
| Collards | 300 | 25 |
| Turnip greens | 265 | 25 |
| Mustard greens | 190 | 25 |
| Kale | 150 | 25 |
| Broccoli | 135 | 50 |
| | | |
| *Miscellaneous* | | |
| Bean curd | 180 | 103 |
| Orange (1 medium) | 55 | 80 |
| Corn muffin | 45 | 125 |

***Note:*** Spinach, Swiss chard, beet greens, and parsley are high in calcium but also contain oxalic acid, which binds to calcium and inhibits the body's absorption of the calcium.

*Animal proteins supply* protein, iron, riboflavin, niacin, vitamins $B_6$ and $B_{12}$, phosphorus, zinc, and iodine. *Vegetable proteins supply* protein, iron, thiamine, folacin, vitamins $B_6$ and E, phosphorus, magnesium, and zinc. People are less aware of which foods are vegetable proteins: garbanzo, lima, and kidney beans; lentils; tofu; any dried beans or peas; and an excellent source: nuts and nut butters (including sunflower seeds).

*Some equivalent amounts* of protein are the following: 1 ounce of meat, poultry, or fish; 1 egg; 1 slice of hard cheese (1 ounce of American or Swiss); 2 tablespoons (1 ounce) of peanut butter; 2 tablespoons (1 ounce) of cottage cheese; ½ cup of dried beans or peas. Eggs are a superb source of protein. The white is 100 percent protein and the yolk is rich in iron. If you don't like the taste of eggs, put them raw in a blender with orange juice and fruit or milk and ice cream—and use them in cooking whenever possible.

*Protein usability* is an important factor to consider when deciding which foods to eat to meet the special protein needs of pregnancy. Our bodies cannot fully utilize the protein in our food. The percentage of protein absorbed by your digestive tract that your body can actually use is called the net protein utilization (NPU). Simply put, the NPU estimates what proportion of the protein we eat is actually available to our bodies.

The protein in eggs most nearly matches the body's own ideal pattern, so egg protein is used as a model for measuring the amino acid patterns in other food. For example, the NPU of cheese is 70 percent, while peanuts are only 40 percent.

The Directory of Protein Foods on page 131 should help you get the most protein value out of the foods you eat so that you can meet the high protein demands of pregnancy.

## CHART 15. DIRECTORY OF PROTEIN FOODS

|  | Total Grams Protein | Usable Grams |
|---|---|---|
| *Flour* (1 cup) |  |  |
| Soybean flour, defatted | 65 | 40 |
| Gluten flour | 85 | 23 |
| Peanut four, defatted | 48 | 21 |
| Soybean flour, full fat | 26 | 16 |
| Whole wheat flour, or cracked wheat cereal | 16 | 10 |
| Rye flour, dark | 16 | 9 |
| Oatmeal, barley flour | 11 | 7 |
| Cornmeal, whole ground | 10 | 5 |
| | | |
| *Meat and Poultry* | | |
| Turkey, roasted, 3 slices | 31 | 22 |
| Pork, loin chop (lean and fat) | 29 | 19 |
| Porterhouse steak (½ lb. raw without fat) | 25 | 17 |
| Hamburger (¼ lb. raw) | 26 | 17 |
| Chicken, breast | 23 | 15 |
| Lamb, rib chop (lean and fat) | 20 | 13 |
| | | |
| *Fish and Shellfish* (Average serving 3½ oz.) | | |
| Halibut | 22 | 17 |
| Sardines, 3 medium, canned in oil | 21 | 14 |
| Swordfish,* striped bass, rockfish, shad, shrimp | 19 | 15 |
| Cod, Pacific herring, haddock | 18 | 14 |
| Crab, Northern lobster | 17 | 14 |
| Squid, sea scallops (3), flounder or sole | 15 | 12 |
| Clams (4 large or 8 small) | 14 | 11 |
| Oysters (2 to 4) | 11 | 9 |

*__Warning:__ Large oceangoing fish such as blue-fin tuna and swordfish, which are at the end of long food chains, have been shown to be heavily contaminated with mercury.

## CHART 15. DIRECTORY OF PROTEIN FOODS *(continued)*

| | Total Grams Protein | Usable Grams |
|---|---|---|
| *Dairy Products* *(1 oz. or 1 square inch, unless otherwise noted)* | | |
| Cottage cheese 6 t. (3½ oz.) | | |
| uncreamed | 17 | 13 |
| creamed | 14 | 11 |
| Milk, nonfat dry solids | 10 | 8 |
| Parmesan cheese | 10 | 7 |
| Milk, 1 cup skim, whole or buttermilk | 9 | 7 |
| Yogurt from skim milk (1 cup) | 8 | 7 |
| Swiss cheese | 8 | 6 |
| Ricotta cheese (¼ cup), cheddar cheese | 7 | 5 |
| Ice cream (⅕ pint) | 5 | 4 |

The following dairy products are not good protein sources because they contain too many calories for the amount of protein you get: cream, sour cream, cream cheese, butter (no protein).

| | Total Grams Protein | Usable Grams |
|---|---|---|
| *Legumes: Dried Beans, Peas,* *and Lentils* *(1 cup cooked)* | | |
| Soybeans or soy grits | 17 | 10 |
| Broad beans | 13 | 6 |
| Peas, lentils, black beans, cowpeas (black-eyed peas), kidney beans | 12 | 5 |
| Tofu (soybean curd) (wet weight 3½ oz.) | 8 | 5 |
| Navy, pea bean or white beans, chick-peas (garbanzos) | 11 | 4 |
| *Grains, Cereals, and Their Products* | | |
| Egg noodles (1 cup) | 7 | 4 |
| Bulgur (parboiled wheat) or cracked wheat cereal (⅓ cup) | 6 | 4 |

## CHART 15. DIRECTORY OF PROTEIN FOODS *(continued)*

|  | Total Grams Protein | Usable Grams |
|---|---|---|
| *Grains, Cereals, and Their Products (cont.)* | | |
| Barley (pot or Scotch), millet (⅓ cup) | 6 | 8 |
| Spaghetti or other pasta (1 cup) | 5 | 3 |
| Oatmeal (⅓ cup) | 4 | 3 |
| Rice (brown, parboiled, or converted) | 5 | 3 |
| Milled, polished | 4 | 2 |
| Wheat germ (2 T.) | 3 | 2 |
| Bread (1 slice), whole wheat or rye | 2 | 1 |
| | | |
| *Nuts and Seeds* | | |
| Pignoli (pine nuts) (2 T.) | 9 | 5 |
| Pumpkin/squash seeds (2 T.) | 8 | 5 |
| Sunflower seeds (3 T.) | 7 | 4 |
| Peanuts or peanut butter (2 T.) | 8 | 3 |
| Cashews (12–16 nuts), sesame seeds (3 T.), pistachio nuts (3 T.), black walnuts (4 T.) | 5 | 3 |

The following nuts are not good protein sources because they contain too many calories for the amount of protein provided: pecans, chestnuts, coconuts, filberts, hazelnuts, macadamia nuts, almonds, English walnuts (black walnuts have about 40 percent more protein than English ones).

| | | |
|---|---|---|
| *Vegetables* *(Cooked weight)* | | |
| Lima beans (½ cup) | 8 | 4 |
| Corn (one medium ear), broccoli (one stalk), Kale, w/stems (¾ cup) | 4 | 2 |
| Collards (½ cup), mushrooms (12 small), asparagus (6 spears) | 3 | 2 |
| Artichoke (1 large) | 6 | 2 |

CHART 15. DIRECTORY OF PROTEIN FOODS *(continued)*

| | Total Grams Protein | Usable Grams |
|---|---|---|
| *Vegetables* *(Cooked weight) (cont.)* | | |
| Cauliflower (1 cup), spinach (½ cup), turnip greens (½ cup) | 3 | 1.5 |
| Potato (medium baking potato) | 4 | 1 |
| *Nutritional Additives* | | |
| Egg white, powdered (½ oz.) | 11 | 9 |
| Tiger's Milk (¼ cup) | 8 | 6 |
| Brewer's yeast, powder (1 T.) | 4 | 2 |
| Wheat germ (2 T.) | 3 | 2 |

## SALT

Salt in a prenatal diet is a controversial subject. It was at one time thought that salt caused water retention, which caused the swelling of toxemia. Therefore, many doctors prescribed low-salt diets for their patients. It is now understood that swelling is normal in pregnancy and by itself is not a sign of toxemia (see Toxemia page 530). However, there may still be doctors who tell women not to use salt—or even to use diuretics (water pills) during pregnancy. They are wrong. Your body needs *more* salt—not less—when you are pregnant.

*A pregnant woman's blood volume and body fluids* must increase by 40 percent and salt is the chief element in maintaining this dramatic expansion. Restricting salt in your diet limits this necessary blood-volume expansion and compromises placental growth and function. Salt is needed to maintain osmotic pressure relationships in the body. Salt in the diet is necessary to maintain the water balance and regulate muscle and nerve irritability.

***Do not eliminate salt from your diet.*** And use *iodized* salt, not the sea salt sold in health-food stores. The iodine is necessary to prevent thyroid problems in pregnancy.

***The best way to determine how much salt*** to use is to salt food to taste throughout your pregnancy—rely on your taste buds, the body's simplest salt-regulating mechanism. The results of limiting your salt intake can be fatigue and loss of appetite.

***You should try to avoid high-salt foods,*** which put more salt into your system than it needs and can cause excessive water retention. The following foods are high in salt: **cured, prepared,** and **processed meat** (ham, sausage, bacon, hot dogs, salt pork, lunch meats, bologna, chipped beef); **seasoning salts** (garlic and celery salts, etc.); **salty snack foods** (salted popcorn, corn curls, pretzels, potato chips, salted crackers and nuts); **prepared meat sauces** (soy sauce, catsup, mustard, barbecue sauce, Worcestershire sauce); **relishes** (pickles, olives); **salted fish; canned** and **packaged soups**. Also, **bicarbonate of soda** (baking soda) is high in salt and should not be used as a digestive during pregnancy. Most dairy products are high in sodium, but they supply important calcium and protein.

## VEGETABLES AND FRUIT

Vegetables and fruits play an important role in the pregnant diet. They not only provide a number of essential vitamins (which the body can assimilate most easily in their natural form, rather than as a pill) but fruits and vegetables are also very important for digestion and elimination (which can be problematic when you're pregnant). Vegetables and fruits are usually divided into two groups: "vitamin-C rich" and "leafy green." Notice the "overlapping" vegetables—watercress, for example, is included in both groups—and do yourself and your baby twice as much good by eating them. Be sure to include fruits and vegetables you like that aren't mentioned—for instance, yellow vegetables have significant amounts of vitamin A.

## VITAMIN C–RICH FRUITS AND VEGETABLES

JUICES (the canned forms have less vitamin C than the fresh): orange, grapefruit, tomato, pineapple

FRUITS: cantaloupe (also high in vitamin A), grapefruit, guava, mango, orange, papaya, strawberries, tangerine

VEGETABLES: bok choy, broccoli, brussels sprouts, cabbage, cauliflower, greens (collard, kale, mustard, Swiss chard, turnip), peppers (sweet red, green, and chili peppers), tomatoes, watercress

## LEAFY GREEN VEGETABLES

Leafy green vegetables supply vitamins A, E, B$_6$, riboflavin, iron, magnesium: asparagus, bok choy, broccoli, brussels sprouts, cabbage, dark leafy lettuce (chicory, endive, escarole, red leaf, romaine) greens (beet, collard, dandelion, kale, mustard, spinach, Swiss chard, turnip), scallions, watercress.

## VEGETARIAN DIET

There is absolutely no reason why a pregnant woman cannot be as healthy or healthier on a vegetarian diet than someone who eats meat.

## PROTEIN NEEDS

*If you are a complete vegetarian* you can get sufficient protein by eating daily, in addition to your vegetables and grains: 1 cup of soybeans plus 12 ounces of soymilk or soy yogurt; *or* ½ pound of tofu and a pint of soymilk or soy yogurt; *or* 1 quart of soymilk or soy yogurt and ½ cup of soybeans; *or* 1 cup of hydrated TVP (texturized vegetable protein) and 1 cup of soymilk or soy yogurt. If you are a *lacto-vegetarian* (you eat dairy products), then in addition to vegetables and grains you could get enough protein by eating daily: 2 cups of cottage cheese, *or* 1 quart of skim milk, low-fat yogurt, or buttermilk plus ½ cup of cottage cheese (whole milk and regular cheese may be too fattening to be your main source of protein).

*It is also wise to keep high-protein snacks around.* Soynuts, peanut butter with wheat crackers or celery, or cottage cheese with corn chips. You can even make soy-milk cottage cheese by mixing crumbled curded soy cheese with soymilk yogurt and a little salt. The chart on page 127 lets you know the food value of soybean products. There is a protein chart on page 131.

*It is essential for you to realize* that if you do not get enough protein, along with certain vitamins and minerals (such as vitamin K, zinc, and copper), you will be more prone to complications in labor such as hemorrhage. Many vegetarian diets are not nutritionally sound. Many do not supply nearly enough protein for general health, much less pregnancy. Please make a constant effort to protect yourself and your baby by taking in as much high-quality protein as you can.

**The main concern** is that a vegetarian receive enough grams of protein daily, but there should be no problem as long as she is aware of this need. Selected combinations of vegetable protein are as good or better in their composition of amino acids than many forms of meat. Even eggs and milk are not absolute requirements for an adequate intake of protein. But the quality and quantity of protein must be the focus of a vegetarian diet.

**Most plant foods,** unlike animal foods, do not contain all the essential amino acids in appropriate amounts. If one of these essential amino acids is missing, the protein is "in-complete" and cannot be utilized to build body tissues (please read the Protein section earlier in this chapter). However, the correct combination of several plant foods eaten at the same meal can transform the foods into com-plete proteins which your body can then fully utilize. If you are on a vegetarian diet, it would be wise to get a copy of Frances Moore Lappé's *Diet for a Small Planet*, which will help you combine foods. On the next page is a chart adapted from that book to give you easy reference. It lists "comple-mentary plant protein sources" for four food groups. If the foods listed are eaten in combination, the missing amino acids will be completed.

---

### CHART 16. COMPLEMENTARY PLANT PROTEIN SOURCES

| FOOD | AMINO ACIDS DEFICIENT | COMPLEMENTARY PROTEIN |
|---|---|---|
| *Grains* | Isoleucine<br>Lysine | rice + legumes<br>corn + legumes<br>wheat + legumes<br>wheat + peanut + milk<br>wheat + sesame + soybean<br>rice + sesame<br>rice + brewer's yeast |
| *Legumes* | Tryptophan<br>Methionine | legumes + rice<br>beans + wheat<br>beans + corn<br>soybeans + rice + wheat<br>soybeans + corn + milk<br>soybeans + wheat + sesame<br>soybeans + peanuts + sesame<br>soybeans + peanuts +<br>  wheat + rice<br>soybeans + sesame + wheat |
| *Nuts & Seeds* | Isoleucine<br>Lysine | peanuts + sesame + soybeans<br>sesame + beans<br>sesame + soybeans + wheat<br>peanuts + sunflower seeds |
| *Vegetables* | Isoleucine<br>Methionine | lima beans<br>green peas<br>brussels sprouts  } + sesame seeds or Brazil nuts or mushrooms<br>cauliflower<br>broccoli<br>greens + millet or<br>  converted rice |

NON-LACTO VEGETARIAN

*If no milk is included in a vegetarian diet* you must have the following daily supplements:

- 12 mg calcium
- 400 I.U. vitamin D
- 4 $\mu$g vitamin $B_{12}$
- 1.5 mg riboflavin

If you consume less than 4 servings of milk products a day, or if you substitute goat's milk or soybean milk, then you must have a partial supplementation. Try to eat as wide a variety of foods as possible and refer to the Complementary Plant Protein Sources chart or Lappé's book *Diet for a Small Planet* so that you are getting complete proteins. Also, please use your iodized salt. Sea salt does not contain iodine, which your thyroid gland needs during the extra stress of pregnancy.

POSSIBLE DEFICIENCIES IN A VEGETARIAN DIET

*Iron* is generally not supplied by a vegetarian diet in the recommended amounts. (See the section on iron on page 121.) Enriched grain products could increase your intake, but a supplement is probably necessary. Depending on your iron-level blood test results you should take 1 to 3 iron pills a day (ferrous sulfate or ferrous gluconate, 5 grains). If your blood is not checked for iron regularly you should take 1 tablet 3 times a day (3 5-grain tablets daily). It will be easier on your stomach if you take the iron with meals; time-release iron is gentler if you find regular pills hard on your stomach. You should take a 100-mg vitamin C tablet (ascorbic acid) with each iron pill because it aids in the absorption of the iron. Do not take one large dose of the iron and vitamin C once a day because you won't absorb as much of the iron and you'll lose most of the vitamin C in your urine. The baby collects most of his iron stores in the last ten weeks of pregnancy so if your iron level is tested only once, do it at about 7 months.

*Calcium* is supplied by cow's and goat's milk. There are plant foods that contain calcium, but its availability (the body's ability to assimilate it) is limited. Pregnant women in the last half of pregnancy and when nursing need to supplement about 1 gram (15 grains) of calcium daily. The baby is calcifying his bones in the last half of pregnancy and if there is no surplus calcium available, the fetus will take it from your bones. The most readily absorbed form of calcium is calcium gluconate; if you take calcium lactate you will need about twice as much. In order to make 1 gram you can take 2 500-mg tablets or 3 5-grain tablets.

*Vitamin D* is supplied by *fortified* cow's milk or soy-milk. If you aren't getting those, be sure to get a vitamin D supplement.

*Riboflavin* is found in limited amounts in whole grain and enriched breads and cereals, in legumes and nuts, and a variety of vegetables. However, meat and milk are the best sources. Non-milk-drinkers may have an insufficient amount and should take a supplement.

*Vitamin $B_{12}$* is supplied by milk. A deficiency of this vitamin causes anemia and eventually spinal cord degeneration, so if you are not drinking milk, be sure to get a supplement.

## VITAMINS

Prenatal care usually includes a multivitamin that you take every day. Most prenatal vitamins contain the following vitamins in approximately the indicated amounts: *calcium* (50 to 600 mg), *vitamin A* (1,500 to 15,000 I.U.) and *vitamin D* (100 to 1,000 mg). Refer to the Directory of Vitamin Sources and Functions on page 143 for complete information so you won't underestimate the importance of all vitamins during your pregnancy. Also, you should recognize the dangers of excess doses on the Warning chart on page 142.

You may not think you need to take a multivitamin supplement as long as you are getting at least the necessary amounts of calcium and vitamins A and D through your diet. Although it is true that the food you eat is the best possible source of vitamins, you can't be certain of the vitamin content of everything you eat, especially if you eat out in restaurants. Also, with a busy schedule and/or the nausea that is so common in pregnancy, you may find it hard to eat carefully balanced meals every day.

Regardless of your eating habits, there are two vitamins essential to your health and the growth of the fetus which cannot be met through the food you eat. You are going to need a daily supplement of *iron* (30 to 60 mg of elemental iron). Iron is discussed on page 121. You are also going to need 0.3 mg of *folic acid* (also called folacin) every day. Folic acid is one of the B vitamins essential to a successful pregnancy. Your body's need for folacin is doubled during pregnancy: folacin deficiencies during pregnancy are common, and can result in spontaneous abortion (miscarriage) or damage to the unborn child. Folic acid deficiency is particularly a problem if you were taking the birth-control pill until shortly before you conceived. Consult the Vitamin Directory on page 143 for more information.

Do not make the mistake of thinking that all vitamins are good for you and that if a little is good, more is better. An excess of any vitamin may be related to birth defects. It should be noted that unlike other vitamins, vitamins A and D are not excreted from the body if taken in excessive amounts. The vitamins listed in the chart on page 142 are definitely dangerous in large dosages (hypervitaminosis).

---

### CHART 17. WARNINGS ABOUT VITAMINS

---

- **VITAMIN A** in excess may be teratogenic (the cause of birth defects) and should be avoided before and during pregnancy. Do not take more than 6,000 to 8,000 international units of vitamin A daily.
- **VITAMIN B₆ (PYRIDOXINE)** can cause a type of neuropathy (nerve problems) in people taking 200 mg a day or more.
- **VITAMIN C** is dangerous in large doses. Do not take more than 1 gram (1,000 mg) a day during pregnancy. Vitamin C is an active metabolic agent; the effects of large doses on the growing fetus are not known.
- **VITAMIN D** in excess can cause mental retardation, heart defects, or bone defects in the baby.
- **VITAMIN E** has a tendency to raise blood pressure in people not accustomed to it. No one should take more than 800 I.U.s a day. Women with hypertension (high blood pressure) or a rheumatic heart condition should restrict their daily intake to 150 I.U.s: larger doses tend to raise blood pressure.
- **VITAMIN K** can cause jaundice, which may damage the baby's nervous system. This vitamin is available only by prescription, anyway.

---

## CONTAMINANTS IN WATER

Sometimes it seems as though there's nothing we can eat safely anymore! I don't want to make you more worried than you may already be about the safety of opening your mouth and inserting any food or drink, but there are some potential hazards you would do best to avoid.

*Is your drinking water safe?* Ordinary tap water all over the United States can contain organic chemicals, mutagens, and/or carcinogens (cause cancer). Several studies have found an association between water quality and the local cancer mortality rates in New York, Louisiana, and the Ohio River Valley. Industrial chemicals discharged into the surface waters are not usually removed by current water treatment facilities. Your community may be one of the rare ones that removes these chemicals by filteration with activated carbon, but if not, you can consider buying an activated carbon filter for your home use.

A study done by the California Department of Health Services showed that tap water may contribute to miscarriages and birth defects. Results released in 1988 indicated that California women who drank bottled water had far fewer complications of pregnancy—fewer even than pregnant women who lived in areas where the tap water was not polluted. The miscarriage rate for women who drank no tap water was about 50 percent lower than for women who drank from the public water supply.

In certain geographic areas the lead pipes have corroded, causing a high level of lead in the drinking water. Boston is one such area. Prenatal exposure to lead can cause birth defects in the fetus. Using bottled water is the most obvious solution to these problems.

---

**CHART 18. DIRECTORY OF VITAMIN SOURCES AND FUNCTIONS**

**VITAMIN A**

*Sources:* fortified whole milk, fortified margarine, butter, egg yolk, fish liver oils, liver, kidney, deep green and yellow vegetables (*cooking* vegetables breaks down the cell walls and releases the vitamin A for absorption—so cooked carrots will supply A more readily than raw ones)

*Daily amount:* 6,000 I.U. during pregnancy, 8,000 I.U. during lactation

CHART 18. DIRECTORY OF VITAMIN SOURCES AND
FUNCTIONS *(continued)*

**VITAMIN A** *(cont.)*

*Function:*  builds resistance to infection; strengthens mucous membranes; functions in vision; is necessary for formation of tooth enamel, hair, and fingernails; is necessary for the proper growth and functioning of the thyroid gland

*Caution:*  in excess may cause birth defects: it is chemically related to 13-cisretinoic acid, a compound in acne medicine that can cause cleft palate, heart defects, and brain abnormalities.

**VITAMINS B** (includes all vitamins listed $B_1$ through $B_{12}$)

*Sources:*  brewer's yeast is an excellent source—some brands have a horrible taste, others have a nutty flavor, so experiment. Start out with a teaspoon in juice, let it stand until lumps dissolve—work up to one tablespoon. Some people take up to 3 tablespoons daily. Brewer's yeast gives a feeling of well-being: rested, energetic, relaxed—for your mate too. Do not use live yeast for baking; get brewer's yeast at the health-food store. Also bread, whole grains, wheat germ, liver

*Function:*  can prevent nervousness, skin problems, lack of energy, constipation

**$B_1$ (THIAMINE)**

*Sources:*  pork and pork products, liver, heart, kidneys, peas and beans, wheat germ

CHART 18. DIRECTORY OF VITAMIN SOURCES AND
FUNCTIONS *(continued)*

**B₁ (THIAMINE)** *(cont.)*

*Daily amount:*  1.2 mg in pregnancy
1.5 mg in lactation

*Function:*  essential for appetite, digestion, muscular tone in the gastrointestinal tract; needed for fertility, growth, lactation, and during illness and infection

*Caution:*  is not stored by the body so your supply can be used up in a few days

**B₂ (RIBOFLAVIN)**

*Source:*  best one is milk—each quart contains 2 mg, approximately the amount needed daily

*Daily amount:*  5 to 10 mg

*Function:*  is necessary for the normal growth and development of the baby from conception

*Deficiency:*  signs are eye problems (burning, itching, dimness of vision, light sensitivity, even cataracts); skin problems (impairment of wound healing, cracking lips, lesions at corners of mouth, dermatitis, inflammation of the tongue tip and edges)

**NIACIN**

*Sources:*  liver, beef, poultry, milk, peanuts, almonds, brown rice, wheat, peas, tuna

*Daily amount:*  20 to 50 mg

*Function:*  aids in building brain cells (as do all B vitamins) and prevents infections and bleeding of gums

CHART 18. DIRECTORY OF VITAMIN SOURCES AND
FUNCTIONS *(continued)*

**NIACIN** *(cont.)*

*Deficiency:*     signs are loss of appetite, nausea, vomiting, abdominal pain, headache, dizziness, burning hands and feet, numbness, and weakness

**B₆ (PYRIDOXINE)**

*Sources:*     yeast, liver, wheat germ, whole grain bread and cereal, green beans, leafy green vegetables, bananas, poultry, fish, meats, nuts, potatoes

*Daily amount:*     2 to 20 mg

*Function:*     essential for the metabolism of fats and fatty acids and for the production of antibodies which fight disease

*Deficiency:*     same as with other B vitamins: sensory disturbances (numbness, tingling, loss of sense of position), anemia

*Caution:*     doses of 200 mg a day or more have caused nerve problems

**PANTOTHENIC ACID**

*Sources:*     organ meats, eggs, peanuts, wheat bran

*Daily amount:*     500 to 100 mg

*Function:*     needed for proper functioning of adrenal glands, digestive tract, skin

*Deficiency:*     signs are constipation, digestive trouble, fatigue, burning feet

**B₁₂ (COBALAMIN)**

*Sources:*     yeast, liver, wheat germ, whole grains, kidney, meat, fish, eggs, milk, oysters

CHART 18. DIRECTORY OF VITAMIN SOURCES AND
FUNCTIONS *(continued)*

**B$_{12}$ (COBALAMIN)** *(cont.)*

*Daily amount:*  8 to 15 mg

*Function:*  essential for the development of
red blood cells

*Deficiency:*  a danger only for true vegetarians
who eat no animal products; can
cause anemia

**VITAMIN C**

*Sources:*  citrus fruits, cantaloupe,
strawberries, green and red bell
peppers, broccoli, kale, tomatoes,
potatoes, cauliflower, parsley; NOTE:
overcooking and cooking in too
much water destroy the vitamin C;
ascorbic acid (synthetic) is identical
to natural vitamin C, but vitamin C
is more completely utilized when
taken with bioflavonoids (i.e., the
white rind of citrus fruits)

*Daily amount:*  varies, but infection, fever, and
other bodily stress factors deplete
the body of vitamin C; alcohol,
smoking, the Pill, aspirin all
interfere with absorption and/or the
levels of ascorbic acid in the body

*Function:*  helps body resist infection; controls
poisons produced by bacteria and
viruses; strengthens capillary and
cell walls; builds a strong placenta;
helps absorb iron from the
intestines and acidifies urine;
detoxifies junk foods and nonfoods
we take in. Smokers require larger
amounts, about 25 mg per
cigarette; important in repair of
fractures and in wound healing

CHART 18. DIRECTORY OF VITAMIN SOURCES AND
FUNCTIONS *(continued)*

**VITAMIN C** *(cont.)*

*Deficiency:* signs that your intake is low are swollen, reddened gums; susceptibility to infection; easy bruising

*Caution:* large doses, over 1 gram, potentially harmful to fetus

**CALCIUM**

*Sources:* milk, stone-ground grain; vitamin C helps in the absorption

*Daily amount:* 1,200 mg; most pregnant women are in a negative calcium balance: they are giving out more calcium to the baby than they're taking in; calcium gluconate or calcium lactate pills should be taken on an empty stomach with sour milk, yogurt, or an acid fruit or juice (vitamin C aids absorption)—if taken after eating, the calcium goes all the way through the digestive tract unassimilated

*Function:* builds baby's bones and teeth

*Deficiency:* signs are sleeplessness; irritability; muscle cramps; uterine ligament pains

**VITAMIN D**

*Sources:* sunshine, vitamin D–fortified milk, fish liver oils, mackerel, salmon, tuna, sardines, herring

*Daily amount:* not easy to determine your supplemental requirement—depends on how much exposure to the sun and your complexion. Dark

CHART 18. DIRECTORY OF VITAMIN SOURCES AND
FUNCTIONS *(continued)*

**VITAMIN D** *(cont.)*

*Daily amount (cont.):* complexions have more melanin in their skin, so dark skin is better protected and dark-complected people need more sun to manufacture vitamin D; 400 I.U. is recommended

*Function:* works with calcium to strengthen bones and tissues by helping calcium be absorbed from the blood into the tissue and bone cells

*Caution:* excessive doses can cause toxicity with a reversal of the effect of normal doses; in excess can cause mental retardation, heart defects, or bone defects in the baby

**VITAMIN E**

*Sources:* whole grains, corn, peanuts, eggs

*Daily amount:* 30 mg in pregnancy and lactation— a breast-fed baby's vitamin E level will rise faster than a bottle-fed baby's, indicating that vitamin E is important both to the unborn and newborn baby

*Function:* a potent antioxidant, governing the amount of oxygen the body uses. If you're low in vitamin E you use more oxygen than necessary; helps to preserve vitamins and unsaturated fatty acids in our bodies and foods; helps metabolize vitamine A; promotes healing; it may be necessary for the development of healthy red blood cells, but its function in the human body has yet to be clearly established

CHART 18. DIRECTORY OF VITAMIN SOURCES AND
FUNCTIONS *(continued)*

**VITAMIN E** *(cont.)*

*Caution:* has tendency to raise blood pressure in people not used to taking it; women with hypertension or rheumatic heart condition should restrict daily intake to 150 I.U. Large doses may raise blood pressure; no one should take more than 800 I.U. a day

**FOLIC ACID**

*Sources:* liver, leafy green vegetables, broccoli, asparagus, peanuts

*Daily amount:* 800 micrograms (0.8 mg); the body does not store folic acid so 800 micrograms (0.8 mg) *must be* taken daily

*Function:* essential for protein synthesis in early pregnancy; also for blood formation and the formation of new cells; prevents "pregnancy cap"

*Deficiency:* signs are anemia and fatigue; a deficiency causes an increase in the chance of premature separation of the placenta, toxemia, premature birth, hemorrhage, even infant birth defects

*Caution:* infection, alcohol, and certain drugs (especially Dilantin used in salt form to treat grand mal epilepsy) all interfere with the body's ability to use folic acid

**IODINE**

*Source:* iodized salt

*Daily amount:* salt food to taste with iodized salt

**CHART 18. DIRECTORY OF VITAMIN SOURCES AND FUNCTIONS *(continued)***

**IODINE *(cont.)***
    *Function:*     helps thyroid gland function properly by manufacturing the hormone thyroxin that regulates your metabolism; the thyroid gland grows half again as large during pregnancy and your metabolism increases accordingly

**IRON**
    *Sources:*     liver (or liver pills if you hate liver), fish, egg yolks, meat, raisins, dark molasses

    *Daily amount:*     many young women are already iron-deficient before pregnancy and even good iron stores are insufficient to meet the requirements of pregnancy. *All* women should get 18 mg daily—with up to a 60 mg supplement in pregnancy

    *Function:*     iron is the main component of blood hemoglobin which carries oxygen to the baby and your cells; especially during labor, your uterus and the baby's brain cells need a lot of oxygen; the baby draws on your supply to store iron in its liver to carry it through its milk diet enough to last through the first 4 to 6 months of independent life

**VITAMIN K**
    *Sources:*     does not come directly from food—is synthesized by stomach bacteria; deficiencies are rare because intestinal bacteria manfacture it

CHART 18. DIRECTORY OF VITAMIN SOURCES AND
FUNCTIONS *(continued)*

**VITAMIN K** *(cont.)*

| | |
|---|---|
| *Daily amount:* | for baby: babies' intestines do not contain the K-producing bacteria at birth—it takes a few days before the bacteria are available to manufacture vitamin K. A vitamin K injection is usually given to babies at birth to guard against hemorrhage |
| *Function:* | is an antihemorrhagic vitamin; necessary to blood clotting |
| *Deficiency:* | the continued use of antibiotics may upset the normal bacterial environment of the intestines and interfere with natural vitamin K production |

**ZINC**

| | |
|---|---|
| *Sources:* | seafood, liver, beets, barley, carrots, cabbage |
| *Daily amount:* | minimum 15 mg |
| *Function:* | healthy function of organs; wound healing |
| *Deficiency:* | loss of sense of taste or smell; unpleasant body odor; white marks on fingernails |

## DANGEROUS INGREDIENTS IN FOOD

*Is your food safe?* Many of the chemicals added to food have not been adequately tested to determine whether they may cause cancer or birth defects. Therefore, while you are pregnant you should try to eat food in as natural a state as possible to avoid such additives. Keep in mind that some natural ingredients such as caffeine can also be dangerous

for the developing fetus. The following substances are particularly risky:

***Fish can be contaminated by the water*** they live in.
Freshwater fish often contain chemical pesticides and other
pollutants that have accumulated in their fatty tissues and
flesh. Swordfish should be avoided when you're pregnant
or breast-feeding because of the high mercury levels in this
fish from polluted waters. Please check the directory on
page 131 for more information about the dangers of fish.

***Artificial colors*** are chemically similar to aspirin and
should be avoided. Red Dye 2, used not only to redden
some food products but also to *whiten* others (like some
frozen fish), is a known carcinogen.

***BHA and BHT*** are preservatives found in almost all snack
chips, in sausage meat, in cake mixes, and even in some
cold cereals and canned foods. These chemicals accumulate
in body fat and the safety of their long-term use has not
been proven. Therefore eat sparingly, if at all, of foods
processed with BHT and BHA.

***Growth hormones and antibiotics*** used in animal feeds
remain in the meat and may have an effect on your unborn
child. DES is a drug given to cattle to fatten them up. It
accumulates in the animals' livers, so the nutritional value
of eating liver may not be worth the risk of chemicals you
might also be ingesting. The law states that cattle cannot be
fed DES for 2 weeks prior to their slaughter, but you might
want to question whether that law is being observed or
enforced. You might also want to consider buying your
meats from a market that has meat supplied by sources that
do not use these additives in their animal feed.

In animal studies ***caffeine*** caused reproductive problems—
miscarriage, fetal death, and stillbirth. It is speculated that
caffeine may have disrupted cell division at a time when
constant splitting of the cells was necessary for the development of the fetus.

*Especially in the first 3 months of pregnancy, eliminate or at least reduce your caffeine consumption.* Here are some suggestions on how to do that:

- Use decaffeinated coffee or tea, but be aware that it still contains a fair amount of caffeine.
- Do not take any of the analgesic medicines containing caffeine (see the chart on page 155).
- Don't let tea steep too long or let it boil, both of which increase its caffeine content.
- Be aware that colas and some other soda pops contain substantial amounts of caffeine.
- After the first trimester continue to keep your coffee intake at a minimum: as few as 4 cups of coffee or the equivalent in caffeine per day may have a serious effect on the developing fetus.

---

**CHART 19. HOW MUCH CAFFEINE DOES IT HAVE?**

|  | *Milligrams of Caffeine* |
|---|---|
| *Coffee* (5 oz.) | |
| Automatic drip | 110–150 |
| Percolated | 64–124 |
| Instant | 40–108 |
| Decaffeinated | 2–5 |
| | |
| *Tea* | |
| Brewed 5 minutes (5 oz.) | 20–50 |
| Iced in can (12 oz.) | 22–36 |
| | |
| *Soft Drinks* (12 oz.) *regular or diet* | |
| Mountain Dew | 54 |
| Coca-Cola, Tab, Diet Coke | 46 |
| Pepsi-Cola, Dr Pepper | 38 |
| Pepsi Light, RC Cola, Diet Rite | 36 |
| ginger ale, 7Up, Orange, Sprite, Fresca, root beer, Canada Dry Diet Cola | 0 |

| CHART 19. HOW MUCH CAFFEINE DOES IT HAVE? *(continued)* | |
|---|---|
| | *Milligrams of Caffeine* |
| *Chocolate* | |
| Milk chocolate (1 oz.) | 6 |
| Baking chocolate (1 oz.) | 35 |
| Cocoa beverage (6 oz.) | 10 |
| | |
| *Nonprescription Drugs* (1 tablet) | |
| Aspirin | 0 |
| Anacin | 32 |
| Midol | 32 |
| Excedrin | 65 |
| No Doz | 100 |
| Dexatrim | 200 |

## BODY CHANGES DURING PREGNANCY

Your entire system is readjusted when you're pregnant. The heart pumps more blood, the lungs work more efficiently, and the digestive system uses all the food it receives more efficiently too. The thyroid gland grows 50 percent bigger during pregnancy to meet the needs of your increased metabolism. Your body stretches in preparation for delivery. Watch a pregnant woman walk and you will see: the pelvis loosens and what was once a firm basket of bone is now equipped with cartilage to "give" with the baby's birth. The soft tissues of the vagina become even softer and more elastic—it is said that the average woman is designed to give birth to a 15-pound baby.

With these enormous changes taking place in your body it is no wonder that you may be experiencing any number of discomforts. Although minor problems can be dealt with, and a listing follows, *do not simply dismiss discomforts.* Pain, extreme fatigue, or distress are signals to check with a doctor. Pregnancy is a normal, healthy state and should be reasonably enjoyable for a healthy woman. On the next page is a chart of signs that something may be wrong—but even if lesser complaints are bothering you, try some of the suggestions here, but also don't hesitate to call a doctor.

---

**CHART 20. DANGER SIGNS DURING PREGNANCY**

(Possible cause for symptoms in parentheses)

- PAIN OR BURNING ON URINATION (urinary tract infection; sexually transmitted disease)
- VAGINAL SPOTTING OR BLEEDING (premature labor; miscarriage; placenta previa or abruptio)
- LEAKING OR GUSHING FLUID FROM VAGINA, less significant near due date (rupture of membranes or bag of waters)
- BLISTER OR SORE IN VAGINAL AREA, itching or irritating discharge (vaginal infection; sexually transmitted disease)
- UTERINE CONTRACTIONS, more than four or five in an hour *not* near your due date (threatened miscarriage)
- SEVERE NAUSEA OR VOMITING, several times in an hour or over several days (hyperemesis gravidarum; infection)
- SEVERE ABDOMINAL PAIN (ectopic pregnancy; placenta abruptio; premature labor)
- CHILLS AND FEVER OVER 100° F. not accompanied by a common cold (infection)
- DIZZINESS OR LIGHT-HEADEDNESS (toxemia)
- SEVERE HEADACHE that doesn't let up, especially in the second half of pregnancy (toxemia)
- SWELLING OF FACE, EYES, FINGERS, OR TOES, especially if the puffiness is sudden (toxemia)
- SUDDEN WEIGHT GAIN (toxemia)
- VISUAL PROBLEMS: dimness, blurring, spots, flashes, blind spots (toxemia)
- NOTICEABLY REDUCED FETAL MOVEMENT (fetal distress)
- ABSENCE OF FETAL MOVEMENT FOR 24 HOURS from 30th week of pregnancy and beyond (fetal death)
- A HOT, REDDENED PAINFUL AREA BEHIND YOUR KNEE or on your calf (phlebitis or blood clot)

## PHYSICAL DISCOMFORTS AND REMEDIES

### BACKACHE

Backache can be the result of the increased weight you are carrying.

***Don't stand in one place or position too long.*** If you cannot move around then you can put one foot forward with all your weight on it and then switch to the other leg.

***Lean forward*** when standing at the kitchen counter, ironing board, drafting table, etc. Bend your knees slightly and support your weight on your hands or elbows. Just taking the weight off your back for short periods can help.

***Pelvic rock*** relieves backache (see a description in this chapter under Exercises). Do the exercise 20 to 30 times before lying down to rest or sleep. It aids free circulation while you're lying down.

***Side-relaxation position:*** Put a small pillow under your side at waist level to keep your shoulders and hips in a proper alignment while you're asleep.

***A footstool*** or a box or block of wood under your feet while you're sitting can relieve backache. To judge how high your feet should be make sure your knees are at a slightly higher level than your hips.

***Lower backache*** can result from walking and sitting improperly. The uterus is moored by two sets of ligaments. The round ligaments insert into the groin on the left and right in front of the birth canal; the uterosacral ligaments attach just below the small of the back to each side of the bony structure of the pelvis. Every time you rise from sitting make sure your buttocks are tucked in and your abdomen is tipped in as far as it will go. Good posture when you walk—also with your hips tucked well in—is insurance against lower backache.

## BRAXTON-HICKS CONTRACTIONS

Braxton-Hicks contractions are periodic uterine contractions which may begin near the end of your second trimester. The contraction begins as a tightening feeling in the top of your uterus and gradually spreads downward until the whole uterus is hard—then it relaxes. If you feel an isolated lump or knob, that is probably just the baby stretching its legs out. To tell if you are having a Braxton-Hicks, feel your entire uterus with your hands. These contractions serve two purposes: they circulate blood to the placental site, but more important, they exercise and strengthen your uterus for labor. Furthermore, these contractions may be responsible for early effacement and even dilation of your cervix before labor actually begins. Another benefit of Braxton-Hicks is that you can practice the breathing from your childbirth education classes on them.

## BREASTS

Your breasts will swell during pregnancy because the milk glands are beginning to develop. They may also tingle, throb, or hurt. The veins often become more prominent because of the increased blood supply to the breasts. The areola—the area around the nipples—may darken and become broader due to hormonal changes. The increased color around the nipples (and the line on your abdomen) usually do not go away after pregnancy.

Lumpy breasts are quite common in pregnancy. If a breast lump feels suspicious in any way—if it is hard or fixed or causes dimpling of the overlying skin—then it may be a good idea to screen for breast cancer. One way that this can be done in pregnancy is diaphanography, which can cause no harm to the fetus. In this method the breast is transilluminated with regular light. A TV camera that will pick up only the infrared spectrum will show areas of dark shadow. This is an indication of new blood-vessel formation and is very specific for cancer detection.

*A biopsy of the breast* during pregnancy may sometimes be necessary if there is a suspicious lump. This is not dangerous for the fetus, although it can be frightening for the mother.

***Wear a support bra*** all through your pregnancy. For women whose breasts get very large it is a good idea to wear a bra even at night. A lack of support *during pregnancy* is what causes sagging—most of the weight gained by the breasts comes in the early months of pregnancy. Breast-feeding is often blamed for sagging bosoms, which actually result from insufficient support in the first and second trimesters. Heredity and poor nutrition also play some part in a loss of tone in the breasts.

***Nipple secretion*** can begin after the first few months of pregnancy. The sticky, yellowish watery fluid is colostrum, which will be the baby's first food, preceding your milk supply. In the later months of pregnancy there may be spontaneous drops of colostrum. As the due date nears it takes on an opaque, whitish look resembling milk. Colostrum may be gently expressed from the nipples if you wish.

### CONSTIPATION

Constipation is a common complaint of pregnancy, when the bowels are more sluggish. The cause is the pressure of the growing uterus on the bowels. Also, the increased amount of progesterone in your system relaxes all smooth muscles, which makes the bowels less efficient. However, being "normal" does not mean a daily bowel movement: every second or third day may be sufficient for many women. At any rate, the proper definition of constipation is the passing of hard stool, not having infrequent bowel movements (unless they happen to be hard).

***Fruit*** has a laxative effect as well as being nourishing. It is especially helpful if eaten at night—fruits with the greatest laxative action are prunes, figs, dates, raisins, and apples.

***Green vegetables*** add roughage to your diet which stimulates the intestines. Raw vegetables are especially good.

*Fluids,* lots of them, are very helpful for constipation. Your body requires more liquids when you get pregnant, so try to get at least 6 to 8 glasses a day.

*A cup of hot water* 3 times a day (with lemon juice if you wish) is helpful to some people.

*Fiber* in your diet from whole-grain breads and cereals and from foods like bran muffins helps stimulate your intestines.

*Exercise,* even if it's only walking, helps constipation.

*Licorice candy* has a mild cathartic action which can give relief.

*There are natural fiber laxatives* that have none of the drawbacks of chemical laxatives. They can be used as often as you want. Some people find these work well if taken before bed; others prefer to take them in the morning. Metamucil and Peridiem are among the brand names for these products.

*Regularity,* establishing a set time to move your bowels, can alleviate constipation. Regular bowel movements also help control gas. Try to train yourself to go to the bathroom right after breakfast, for example. Some people find it easier to move their bowels if their feet are elevated on a footstool or box while they are sitting on the toilet (this releases the anus).

## MUSCLE CRAMPS

Muscle cramps are due to the slowing of your blood circulation. Shooting pains down your legs can be due to pressure of the baby's head on certain nerves, which can be helped by changing your position. Another cause of cramping can be the sudden contraction of one of the two round ligaments that moor the uterus in front. Cold weather seems to set it off in some women.

*A heating pad,* hot-water bottle, and massage all give relief.

*Elevating legs* can prevent cramps.

*Increase intake of calcium and potassium.* Put dried milk powder or bonemeal in a glass of milk before bed. Or have a glass of milk before bed with 10 to 25 mg of vitamin $B_6$ and 2 to 3 tablets of combined calcium and magnesium. To increase your potassium intake, eat half a grapefruit or orange or banana before meals or as a snack. Another possibility is to take *calcium lactate* in 10-grain (650 mg) tablets accompanied by 100 mg of vitamin C as follows: 3 tablets on an empty stomach before breakfast and 2 more later in the day on an empty stomach.

*Relief of leg cramp:* While sitting or lying, *force* your toes back toward your face, and push down on the knee at the same time to straighten your leg.

### DIZZINESS OR FEELING FAINT

Dizziness can have several causes. First of all, your enlarged uterus presses on major blood vessels, causing a blood pressure drop (the size and position of the fetus determine the extent of dizziness or fainting). Second, hormonal changes cause a relaxation of the blood vessels, so blood pools in the legs.

*Move slowly* to avoid creating blood pressure changes.

*Assume new positions gradually.* Faintness is often caused by standing or sitting up quickly. If you're lying down sit up slowly for a moment before standing up all the way.

*Report any dizziness to a doctor* and let him decide whether it is a sign of a problem.

## FOOD CRAVINGS

Food cravings are the perennial joke of pregnancy—ice cream and pickles and all that. Cravings are *not* the body's "natural" way of making up for a nutritional imbalance (almost every pregnancy woman is low in iron yet how many go around craving liver?!). A mineral deficiency may trigger cravings, but the item craved may not be what's missing. Eat balanced meals and get lots of tomato juice and fish, both good sources of trace elements.

**If the food you crave is nutritious,** eat it. Otherwise, beware that pickles, potato chips, and other salty foods that are often the object of these cravings are going to make you retain water. If you find that you are communicating such cravings to your mate in the middle of the night, they're probably an attention-getting device. What you are craving is *not* food. Realize this and find a quiet time to talk about it. The changes that you are going through, both physical and emotional, are already difficult for a man to cope with. It is unfair to both of you to set up a situation whereby he has to prove his devotion to you by midnight forays for jamoca-almond-fudge ice cream!

## GAS PAINS

Gas (flatulence) is a common complaint of pregnancy. The stomach and intestines distend and you get a bloated feeling.

*Milk of magnesia after each meal* increases intestinal activity, which may reduce intestinal gas.

*Avoid gas-producing foods:* in particular, beans, parsnips, corn, onion, cabbage, fried foods, sweet desserts, and candy.

*Pureed vegetables* may give additional relief.

*Regular bowel movements* reduce gas.

## GROIN PAINS

Groin pains, mild, achy sensations in one or both sides of your abdomen, are probably due to the stretching of ligaments that support the uterus. Any of the exercises outlined in this section may help that stretching.

## CHANGES IN YOUR HAIR

Your hair may change when you're pregnant. As with your skin, hair can become more or less oily, in which case you should change shampoos or the frequency with which you wash it. Also, you may find your hair has more or less body. *Do not use hair dye when you're pregnant.* Permanent hair dyes can enter the bloodstream and recent tests are showing these dyes to be cancer-causing.

## HEARTBURN/INDIGESTION

Heartburn is a burning felt in the chest, but it has nothing to do with the heart. There are two main causes for heartburn. The increased progesterone in your system relaxes the smooth muscles, one of which is the cardiac sphincter of the stomach. This allows stomach fluids to reenter the esophagus. These acid stomach secretions are also pushed up into the lower portion of the esophagus when the uterus enlarges and pushes the stomach upward. The esophagus is not protected by the same mucous lining as the stomach so the acid fluids burn. Since the muscular movements are slowed, the stomach secretes less hydrochloric acid and pepsin. These are the substances that start the breakdown of the proteins you eat. Therefore, food remains longer than usual in the stomach, with the muscle between the esophagus and the stomach more relaxed. The *positive* result of this slowing is that food nutrients seem to be absorbed more efficiently (but it can also cause nausea and constipation).

*Avoid greasy, spicy foods.*

*Avoid large meals,* especially right before going to bed.

*Avoid alcohol.*

*Sleep propped up,* with your head elevated. That way stomach acid can't flow back up into your esophagus at night.

*Sip milk,* (warmed, if you like), which coats and soothes the stomach. Buttermilk works better than antacids for some people and provides protein and calcium.

*Don't take bicarbonate of soda* (baking soda), which has a high sodium (salt) content and causes swelling.

*Take an antacid* in liquid form or suck on tablets.

*Milk of magnesia,* a teaspoon or tablet after each meal and whenever heartburn occurs, is soothing.

*Chewing gum after meals* lessens heartburn for some people.

*Engagement* (also called "lightening" or "dropping") will take pressure off your stomach when the baby's head settles into the pelvis.

### HEMORRHOIDS

Hemorrhoids are the result of the increased pressure on the veins in your anus (the equivalent of varicose veins in your legs).

*Kegel exercises* (see section in this chapter on Exercise) stimulate circulation and also help heal hemorrhoids.

*Sit only on hard surfaces* once you have hemorrhoids. Sinking into a soft chair cuts off circulation in the colon. If you have to sit all day or for several hours at a time put a hard board on your chair. The hemorrhoids should clear up soon.

*Yoga position:* Sit tailor-fashion on the floor, let your belly fall forward, taking weight off your pelvis and back. Sit this way whenever possible once you get hemorrhoids—it helps.

*Don't get constipated,* because straining and pushing worsens them—use suppositories if necessary.

*25 mg. vitamin $B_6$* at each meal for several days may clear up the hemorrhoids entirely. Taking 10 mg per meal thereafter will help prevent a recurrence. As with any remedy, check first with your doctor.

*Local treatment:* Cold compresses with witch hazel are comforting. Or put some petroleum jelly on a tissue, lie with your hips on a pillow, and gently push the hemorrhoid back into the rectum with the tissue. Stay with your hips elevated for about 10 minutes, keeping the muscles surrounding the rectum tightly clenched.

## NAUSEA

Nausea is the most common complaint of the first 3 months of pregnancy. One-third of pregnant American women are afflicted with vomiting or digestive disturbance but it usually stops at the end of the first trimester. Nausea is caused by the higher level of estrogen in your system, which influences even the stomach cells and causes irritation as acids accumulate. Another reason for nausea is the rapid expansion of the uterus. Improvement will be gradual: the nausea and vomiting won't clear up dramatically in one day. Good days will gain over bad ones until there are fewer and fewer bad days and the nausea finally disappears.

*Early morning is the worst* because stomach acids have accumulated and blood sugar is low after hours without food. To prevent the blood sugar drop, eat some protein and a little natural starch or natural sugar immediately before going to bed—milk or cheese with fruit or juice.

• A light sweet snack before going to bed (such as milk with toast and jelly) works for some people.

- Set your alarm to go off a little early so you are not rushed and can move more slowly in the morning.
- Keep crackers, popcorn, or dry toast by your bedside, and before you even raise your head, nibble some and then lie back for 20 minutes before you get up.
- At breakfast go easy on food containing fats and eat fruit or fruit juice (which is acidic) at the *end* of the meal.

*Vitamin B$_6$ (pyridoxine) may have antinauseant properties.* Some people have found that vitamin B$_6$, taken along with brewer's yeast, is effective in preventing and controlling nausea. Before pregnancy, your body needs 1.5 mg of B$_6$ a day, which increases about 25 percent to 2 mg a day during pregnancy. However, in order to prevent nausea and vomiting, take 10 mg of B$_6$ a day, or, once nausea has started, take 25 mg with each meal. If you have bad nausea, ask your doctor about taking 10 to 25 mg of B$_6$ frequently throughout the day, trying this for one or two days to see if it gives you any relief. *Under no circumstances should you ever exceed 200 mg in one day.*

*WARNING:* Megadoses of vitamin B$_6$ are not recommended for anyone, pregnant or not. Taking 200 mg or more a day of vitamin B$_6$ has been reported to cause neuropathy (nerve problems) in nonpregnant people. It was once thought that there was no harm in taking large amounts of B vitamins because they are water soluble; but this is not true. As with anything you want to try during pregnancy, always check with your obstetrician first.

*Yogurt,* as a source of B vitamins, is helpful.

*A high-carbohydrate diet* is often recommended, starting with nibbling crackers before rising and staying on a high-carbohydrate diet (starches, etc.) as long as the nausea persists.

*A high-protein diet* works for many people because it keeps the blood sugar high. For instance, it may help to just add an egg to your diet, in the blender with juice and yogurt, or milk and flavoring. Although it is hard to face substantial food when you're nauseated, in order for you to take in a lot of protein you're going to have to force yourself to eat milk, eggs, cheese, fish, and/or meat. See the sections on protein, page 131 and page 138.

*Never let your stomach get empty.* Have 5 or 6 smaller meals instead of 3 large ones. Nibble on nutritious foods between meals. Once you're nauseated it's harder to eat, so get in the habit of keeping some snack you enjoy nearby so your stomach always has something in it.

*Mid-morning snack of a banana* helps many people. Also, you should carry crisp salt crackers, graham crackers, or zwieback so that you are not caught unprepared by a wave of nausea. This is especially important for women who work outside the home: keeping a banana or crackers with you is convenient and may be the only defense you'll have away from home.

*Avoid greasy, spicy foods.*

*Strictly avoid coffee, sweets, and refined foods.*

*Apricot nectar* helps nausea for some people.

*Suck mints or lollipops,* if you must, although if your stomach is empty this could have a reverse effect. The sugar will stimulate your digestive juices and if your stomach is empty it may irritate and make you even more nauseated.

*A baked potato* sprinkled with salt is easily tolerated if you're nauseated and can't face the idea of food. There are many vitamins and minerals in a baked potato, as well as some protein (see Potatoes under the Nutrition section of this chapter).

*Drink very hot or very cold liquids:* The extreme temperatures may make you feel better. Experiment to see which works for you.

*Fluids are more important than solids* over a short period of time if you're having trouble getting anything down. Most women can tolerate iced liquids best. (Ginger ale and *nondiet* colas are valuable because they are rich in carbohydrates and the carbonation often helps too.) A good mid-afternoon supplement is to have some sherbet or water ice.

*Medications:* If you absolutely cannot keep food down, your doctor may prescribe medication, although you should double-check the brand name since many antinausea drugs have been found dangerous. Any risk has to be weighed against the benefit of essential nutrients for your baby.

*Herb teas* are helpful to many women. If you have a health-food store nearby, try peppermint, spearmint, camomile, or peach leaf teas. Red raspberry leaf tea is also said to relieve nausea and vomiting and has the reputation of promoting contractions during labor and helping to prevent hemorrhage. Brew all of these teas with approximately 1 teaspoon of herb to 1 cup of boiling water—or buy them in tea bags.

*Ginger,* an old home remedy for gastrointestinal disturbances, is reported to be a safe and effective remedy for morning sickness. Ginger is now sold in capsule form in many health food stores.

### NOSEBLEEDS

Nosebleeds can happen in pregnancy because of the increased blood volume which puts pressure on the capillaries. There is also increased nasal congestion and the increased hormone levels in your body may be a cause.

*Do not use nosedrops* (see Drugs during Pregnancy, page 196). They have side effects which can be harmful to the baby and the excessive use of nosedrops only makes the condition *worse.*

*Vaseline* will stop the bleeding if you put a little in each nostril.

*Eat citrus fruits* and other sources of vitamin C because a vitamin C deficiency may be the cause of the nosebleeds.

*25 percent solution of menthol in white oil:* Lubricate each nostril with a few drops, using an eye dropper. Tip your head back so the menthol runs into your throat, then spit it out. An application in the morning and evening should stop nosebleeds.

## EXCESS SALIVA

Excessive salivation, also known as ptyalism, can accompany morning sickness (nausea) and usually occurs in the first trimester, as morning sickness does. It is a rare occurrence, but when it does happen it begins 2 to 3 weeks after your first missed period and can persist throughout the pregnancy. What happens is that saliva floods the mouth, more than can be swallowed. You have to spit out constantly and it has a foul taste. Most treatment is unsatisfactory but you can try some of the remedies for Nausea earlier in this section and see if they work.

*Foods containing starch aggravate* this condition, so as a first step eliminate all of the many vegetable foods containing starch.

*Mild sedatives* may help.

*Strong mouthwashes* or sucking peppermint candies may give relief.

## SHORTNESS OF BREATH

Shortness of breath sometimes accompanies dizziness and faintness (covered earlier in this section). A pregnant woman's respiration is deeper—you take in more air than a nonpregnant woman because you are oxygenating the baby's blood as well as your own. Your lungs have more space because the rib cage increases in size. Your total lung capacity doesn't increase—the vital capacity remains the same—but the actual amount of the air going in and out is greater. The increase in the size of your rib cage is permanent, however. You may need a larger bra or blouse size even after you've lost every pound you gained during pregnancy.

*Take three or four deep breaths* before getting up from a sitting or lying position.

*Consciousness of the need to breathe* is a common experience in pregnancy. Move around or take a walk to alleviate the feeling.

*Shortness of breath is worst* in the last weeks of pregnancy. The expanding uterus is largest then and presses on the diaphragm. If it gets too uncomfortable, you can sleep propped with pillows in a semi-sitting position.

## SKIN CHANGES

Your skin is affected by pregnancy. Do not pick at or fuss with any of these skin conditions because they will tend to leave a lasting mark if you do. Be comforted that most of these problems will disappear after the pregnancy—with the exception of stretch marks and darkening of the genitalia in some women.

*Pimples:* If in the past your skin has broken out before periods, you will probably get pimples now (similar hormones are affecting the subcutaneous oil glands). Use an antibacterial soap followed by an astringent. The object is to keep your skin as clean as possible. Around the house use no makeup at all; when and if you must, use a water-based foundation which won't aggravate the oiliness the way heavier makeup will.

*Bumps on your skin* are probably caused by hormonal influences on your blood cells and nerves. They will disappear after the baby is born.

***Tiny red marks*** on your face, shoulders, and arms will also disappear afterward. They are caused by distended blood vessels that rise to the surface of the skin.

***Mask of pregnancy,*** also called "pregnancy cap," is the appearance of brown spots on your face, neck, and abdomen (in black women the spots are white). Like most skin problems in pregnancy they will usually clear in the month following delivery. However, the cause of these spots may be a *folic acid deficiency.* If you take 5 mg of folic acid per meal, it will usually restore normal skin within 2 to 3 weeks. However, you should check this with your OB/GYN and perhaps a skin specialist (dermatologist).

***External genitalia may darken,*** and also you may develop a dark line between your unbilicus and the bottom of your abdomen. In many women the areola (the area around the nipple) darkens near the end of the 3rd month. Also, brown spots may appear on the secondary areola, or the skin surrounding. This darkening is permanent and will not go away after pregnancy.

***Stretch marks*** affect 90 percent of pregnant woman. However, some authorities say this need not be so. They contend that healthy tissues are elastic and that stretch marks are scar tissue formed wherever normal elasticity is lacking. The recommendation is to get adequate protein in your diet and take vitamin C and E supplements to help prevent stretch marks. Stretch marks are most common on the abdomen, which is doing the most stretching, but they affect thighs and sometimes breasts. Keeping your skin supple may help—have oil baths frequently and massage in oil or cream or cocoa butter daily. Lubrication of your stomach, hips, and thighs will not prevent stretch marks, but it will minimize them. Most of these pale, reddish streaks either disappear after delivery or turn a pale, silvery color. They are more pronounced in brunettes, although redheads have the most sensitive skin and should be extra careful of it during pregnancy.

**SLEEP PROBLEMS**

Sleep is affected to some extent in all pregnant women.

***Do not sleep on your back*** because this puts all your weight on your internal organs and can also aggravate hemorrhoids. Sleep on your side with one leg crossed over and a pillow either between your legs or under the cross-over leg to improve circulation.

***Your bed*** should be large; in late pregnancy even a double bed may not be big enough for comfort. Invest in a queen- or king-size bed if at all possible; later on a larger bed will permit you to breast-feed in bed comfortably.

***Try a foam mattress pad*** if you can't get comfortable in bed. A hard bed may be uncomfortable in the later stages of pregnancy: your body may need a surface that has more give. There are "egg carton" and other types of foam pads available from hospital supply stores because they give relief to people confined to bed for long periods. You can get the single bed size and put the pad on only your side of the bed between the mattress and sheet. The softer surface may help you sleep better.

***Sleep apart from your mate*** if you're having trouble sleeping and this is interfering with your mate's sleep. With a larger bed, however (and a reading light aimed just at the page), you will disturb him a lot less.

**FATIGUE** is most pronounced in early pregnancy, when your sleep requirements normally increase by several hours. One reason is that the placenta is not complete until the end of the first 3 months, so you will have less energy in the first trimester while the placenta is being formed. Your body is making the necessary adjustments to pregnancy as it did to your growth during adolescence (when sleep requirements were also high).

*If you feel guilty about sleeping more* (the old American Puritan work ethic), just stop worrying about it. You didn't feel guilty about sleeping a lot when you were an adolescent, so don't now. Your body needs the rest. If your own upbringing makes you worry that you're being "lazy," or anyone tells you that, keep in mind that your body is letting you know what it needs.

*Don't fight the fatigue.* Especially if you're an active, energetic person you might be disconcerted by your diminished capacity. Just accept it; your baby is asserting her needs (you may as well practice getting used to having your life disrupted now!).

*Recognize the side effects* of fatigue because otherwise you may not understand your behavior in the first trimester. Four primary results of fatigue are: impatience, irritability, inability to concentrate, and loss of interest in sex. So you'd better get plenty of rest unless you want to be a complete ogre.

*Remedies: Take naps.* If long naps aren't possible, even 5 or 10 minutes with your eyes closed and feet up can be refreshing. Also, *go to bed earlier.* Simply get as many hours as you need to make you feel rested (and don't think of it as slothful).

SLEEPLESSNESS can occur during any part of your pregnancy, although it's often worst in the last weeks when the baby seems to be more active at night and you are biggest and least comfortable. This sleeplessness may possibly be nature's way of preparing you for the first weeks of the baby's life when the hungry newcomer isn't going to let you sleep through the night.

*Do not fight sleeplessness.* Insomniacs say that resistance only makes it harder to sleep. You can read or do sewing in bed or go in another room and listen to music while doing projects or chores (unless your mate can sleep through noise). Not being able to sleep may be disconcerting if you think of yourself as "needing" a certain number of hours. Give up your previous ideas and think of these months as a time when *everything* is in flux. Fighting these changes instead of accepting them will only aggravate the problem.

*A cup of hot cocoa or malted milk* before bed is good. The calcium in the milk is a relaxant. Also, camomile tea (or herb teas like "Sleepytime," with camomile and other herbs) have relaxing properties. Make the drink as hot as possible for the most benefit.

*A very hot bath* right before bed is so relaxing it can knock you right out. It is so effective at relieving mental and physical tension that you may have to fight falling asleep in the tub.

*Sleeping pills* are not a good idea unless you absolutely cannot rest. Talk to a doctor about it, but under no circumstances take a sleeping pill more often than 2 nights in 3— you will develop a dependence on them.

*Shortness of breath* as a cause of sleeplessness happens at the very end of pregnancy. Take pressure off your rib cage and lungs by propping two pillows behind you, one of them lengthwise to raise your shoulders (see Shortness of Breath, page 169).

### STUFFY NOSE AND ALLERGIES

Sometimes a stuffy nose, watery eyes, and other allergic reactions can occur during pregnancy, even if you have not had those reactions before. Antihistamines are the usual remedy to dry up the watery eyes and a runny nose, but these drugs can be harmful to your unborn child.

*Preventing allergic reactions* is of course the best way to deal with them. If you can determine what it is that you're allergic to, avoid it if possible! But if it's the pollen season or your beloved cat, you can't do much about preventing contact. Whatever your allergies, smoking or being in a smoke-filled room can make the allergic reaction worse.

*Avoid any medicines* designed for decongestion. You should not use nasal sprays or drops except those made with saltwater (called saline). Medicated sprays work by shrinking blood vessels and affect your whole body. Do not take cold or allergy medicines containing antihistamines (for example, Allerest, Dristan, Contac, Coricidin). Antihistamines have caused birth defects in animals and may be harmful to your unborn baby. If you are unsure whether a product contains antihistamines, ask your health-care provider for more information, and read all drug labels carefully.

You can buy saline nasal spray or you can make saltwater nosedrops from ¼ teaspoon salt dissolved in 1 cup of warm water. You should make the solution fresh every day.

*There are some helpful remedies* for a stuffy nose, most of which are age-old:

- Breathing steam in a hot shower or standing above a pot of very hot water with a towel draped over your head can help clear blocked sinuses. You can find eucalyptus oil in most pharmacies: put a few drops in the pot of hot water to help unstuff your nose.
- A vaporizer or cool mist humidifier may bring relief. Use it especially when you are sleeping. If you use either of these machines, be sure to keep them clean, because bacteria and mold can grow in them.
- Placing a hot washcloth on your face may soothe sore sinuses.
- Use finger pressure to massage your sinuses. In firm, gentle circular motions rub on the bony ridge at your eyebrows, under your eyes, and alongside your nose.
- If you have a cold, drink hot liquids, especially chicken soup. Drinking more liquids will make it easier to cough and clear your chest.

## SWEATING

Sweating can increase when you're pregnant. Your thyroid gland is more active so you perspire more. You also manufacture more heat when you're pregnant so the body has to sweat more to maintain your body temperature. Sweat also serves to dispose of additional waste material in your system. If you develop any irritation, powder yourself with cornstarch or a medicated powder. Sweating may be excessive at night; if so, put a towel on your pillow.

## TEETH AND GUMS

Your teeth and gums can be affected by your pregnancy. However, the old saying "For every child a tooth is lost" is not true with today's dental care. First off, once your teeth are formed they are inert and do not undergo remodeling the way bone can. If a mother's diet does not provide the necessary calcium for her baby's development then calcium *will* be taken from her—but from her bones, not her teeth.

However, hormonal changes (estrogen and especially progesterone) can exaggerate the response of periodontal tissues to plaque. These changes can also decrease your body's immune response to bacteria. Bacteria can enter your bloodstream from carious or periodontally afflicted teeth. Some blood-borne infections can cross the placenta, so any infective source should be eliminated.

***There is greater susceptibility to gum problems,*** especially in the upper jaw. The susceptibility increases in severity during pregnancy: it is greatest in the 8th month and then decreases. Bleeding gums may occur because the increased blood volume puts pressure on the capillaries.

***Diet*** helps prevent tooth and gum problems. Sufficient calcium and high-quality protein along with a good supply of vitamins C, B, and D should protect you.

***See the dentist*** at least once during your pregnancy and have your teeth cleaned professionally.

## SWELLING (EDEMA)

Swelling (edema) is a *normal* condition affecting around 40 percent of pregnant women. It may give you some discomfort, but *every pregnant woman will have some swelling.* Any doctor who attempts to tamper with the normal edema of pregnancy by eliminating salt from a pregnant woman's diet or prescribing diuretics is doing harm to her and her baby. The doctor may be acting out of ignorance or the old belief that by eliminating edema you eliminate toxemia. See Salt on page 134 and Toxemia on page 530.

The rise in female hormones during pregnancy—particularly the estrogens manufactured by the placenta—causes a normal fluid retention. These are the same hormones that cause water buildup and swelling in the days preceding a menstrual period and in women on the Pill. In pregnancy this retained fluid is a safeguard for the expanded blood volume: 330 quarts of blood circulate through and nourish the placenta every day. Besides the extra fluid circulating in your bloodstream, the body retains additional fluid to protect you from going into shock during birth when there's an unavoidable blood loss. There is an increase in fluid in all the cells in your body and even in women with *no signs* of edema the total amount of water weight gained can be nearly *15 pounds.* All this is even more true for women carrying twins: a larger placenta means more hormones are manufactured and therefore more fluid is retained. Studies have shown that women with edema have slightly larger babies—and fewer premature babies—than those without edema. Women who are heavier tend to gain more water weight and thin women tend to gain more fat during pregnancy. Please read the section on Salt in the section on Nutrition earlier in this chapter so you fully understand the need for salt and fluid retention.

*Anything more than mild edema*—or if edema persists for more than a day—should be reported immediately to your doctor. Although some swelling is normal in pregnancy, more severe edema can be a sign that you have kidney problems or other complications.

*Diuretics (water pills)* have been shown as useless and harmful during pregnancy yet many doctors still prescribe them. Diuretics cause a potassium deficiency, which in turn causes listlessness, fatigue, mental depression, insomnia, constipation, and harm to the kidneys. Diuretics can produce deficiencies of some thirty-five nutrients—or any body requirement which dissolves in water. Diuretics also can lead to impaired placental function, fetal malformations, neonatal thrombocytopenia, hypoglycemia, and electrolyte imbalance.

*Vitamin C* increases urine production and can be even more effective in removing excess fluids than a diuretic.

*Vitamin B$_6$* is a very effective diuretic, particularly when used with vitamin C. Vitamin B$_6$ can sometimes upset the stomach, so take it with food or milk.

*High-protein diet* should soak the extra fluid out of your system. Carbohydrates encourage fluid retention: by eliminating them from your diet and increasing your protein intake—up at least 150 grams daily—you may be able to decrease swelling.

*Apple cider vinegar* can act as a handy, harmless diuretic. Take a teaspoon or two before each meal and it will rid your body of excess retained fluid if you have a temporary flare-up (due to having eaten salty food, for instance).

*Mild frequent exercise* such as swimming and walking helps edema.

*Avoid high-salt foods:* There is a listing under the Nutrition section earlier in this chapter that will steer you away from foods that contain excessive amounts of salt. However, this does not mean you should cut salt out of your diet entirely. You will profit more from increasing your protein intake and continuing to salt your food to taste.

*Avoid tight clothes* that are constricting at the waist or wrists. Wear loose things that feel comfortable.

*Remove rings* if your fingers get puffy. If your hands have already swollen it may be difficult to get the rings off. Soak your hand in cold water, then hold the finger pointing upward and soap the ring and your finger before attempting to remove.

*Avoid standing* in one position for hours: change positions or move around to help your circulation.

*Tired feet* and swollen ankles can be helped several ways. If your feet feel tight and burn, immerse them in cold water. Rolling or rotating your ankles helps swelling there. Pelvic rock (described on page 191) improves circulation in your legs, which decreases swelling.

*Swelling of the vaginal area* can be uncomfortable. A cold compress on the perineal area helps. An easy way is to take a cold can or bottle from the refrigerator and wrap it in a cloth and hold it against the swollen area.

*Swelling of the breasts* can make them tingle, throb, or just plain hurt. The milk glands are developing and there is an increased blood supply to the breasts (which makes the veins more prominent). Again, a cold compress should help.

### URINARY INFECTIONS

Urinary infections are more common during pregnancy when your body is more susceptible to any kind of bacteria. One way to prevent urinary infections is to drink plenty of fluids. Antibiotics are usually used to treat infections, and you should see the doctor if you suspect you may have a problem. Two types of infection are most common:

*Pyelitis* is a kidney infection. The normal path of urine elimination is blocked and waste material backs up into your body.

*Cystitis* is a bladder infection and is more common. You will feel the urge to urinate every 5 to 10 minutes and then will pass only a few drops, maybe with a burning sensation.

## FREQUENT URINATION

In the first months of pregnancy the hormonal changes in your body send you to the bathroom more often. The hormones affect your adrenals, which change the fluid balance in your body. Also, your kidneys work more effectively during pregnancy. They clear the waste products from the body more rapidly. The amount of urine increases in the first 3 to. 4 months; as the pregnancy advances, the amount of urine diminishes to below what is normal for a nonpregnant woman. Another reason for the need to urinate frequently is that your bladder is pressed by the growing uterus.

*Lightening* (also called "engagement") increases frequent urination. It occurs when the baby's presenting part (usually the head) settles into the pelvic cavity. In a first pregnancy this can happen 2 to 4 weeks before delivery. Although it will give your lungs more room to breathe, it will also put additional pressure on your bladder. In later pregnancies lightening may not occur until labor begins.

*Increased urination* at night is caused by water retained in your ankles which may have been causing swelling during the day. When the pressure is off your legs at night, this fluid moves to your kidneys. One way to cut down midnight trips to the bathroom is not to drink any liquids after 7:00 P.M.

*Do not restrict fluid intake* to lessen the problem of frequent urination. Other sections in this chapter have stressed how much your body needs additional fluids when your body is working for two.

## VAGINAL BLEEDING

Bleeding during pregnancy is a danger signal and you must notify your doctor. However, there is not necessarily any cause for alarm in the first trimester. Some women have scanty, short periods even once they're pregnant. Also, it may be *implantation bleeding*. Approximately seven days after conception the group of cells that will become the embryo attach to the uterine wall, and there may be some bleeding accompanying that.

## VAGINAL CHANGES

The vagina goes through many changes during pregnancy. Most noticeable is an increase in discharge due to the normal excess activity of the mucus-secreting glands of the cervix. There is often an accompanying increase in vaginal odor which can be distasteful to some men during sex. Douching will only give short-lived relief, since it is the secretions themselves that have a strong odor.

*The color* of your vagina may deepen. The tissues at the entrance to the vagina and within it take on a purplish, dusky color instead of the usual pink. This is known as Chadwick's sign. The color deepens as the pregnancy advances and is more striking in women who have had more than one baby.

*Softening of tissues* will be noticeable. The vagina becomes increasingly elastic, readying itself to stretch for the baby. Vitamin C in your diet is important to keep the vaginal tissues elastic.

*Increased blood supply* to the vagina can have the effect of causing uncomfortable swelling (mentioned in the preceding section on Swelling). However, this increased blood supply may also have a positive effect: some women become more rapidly and intensely sexually aroused during pregnancy and either become orgasmic for the first time or may become multiorgasmic. This increased blood supply is one of the physical changes of pregnancy you can be grateful for—because some of this increase remains with you after delivery. Read Chapter Five on Sex for more information.

***Douching*** is all right until the last 4 weeks of pregnancy. There are two exceptions. *You may not douche if:* your membranes have ruptured or if you have had vaginal bleeding at any time during the pregnancy.

Use a douche can or bag, not a bulb syringe, with the source of water kept low (less than 2 feet off the ground). The nozzle must be inserted no more than 2 or 3 inches within the vaginal entrance. Do not hold the lips of the vagina together: the water must flow freely in and out. Douching will not lessen vaginal discharge.

***Vaginal infections:*** In pregnancy the vagina offers a chemically hospitable environment for certain infections, in particular a yeastlike fungus called *Candida albicans.* Sexual partners pass it on to each other and it causes irritation and sometimes burning on urination in the man. Your doctor can do vaginal smears and cultures to determine if you have such an infection, which never causes any systemic illness and is readily curable. Although vaginal infections have a tendency to recur during pregnancy, they subside after delivery.

### VARICOSE VEINS

Varicose veins have two combined causes: the increased fluid in your circulatory system and the pressure on the veins in your legs from your enlarging uterus. Varicose veins are hereditary and will recede dramatically after the baby's birth. Hemorrhoids are a form of varicose veins.

***Do not wear stockings*** with elastic tops or girdles with elastic bands on the legs—they cut off circulation. You may find that wearing support hose is helpful.

***Walk and exercise regularly.***

*Do not sit* with your legs down constantly. Elevate your legs when you are sitting. Try not to stay in any one spot for too long.

*Put wood blocks* or old books under the foot of your bed (or between the mattress and box springs). This elevates your feet 2 to 3 inches above your head and at night gravity will be working in favor of your legs. It may take awhile for you and your mate to get used to this new slant on your sleep!

*The lips of your vagina* can develop varicose veins too. You can buy a special four-buckle adjustable support. It is worn on the hips, over the buttocks, and is fitted with a compression vulvar pad and disposable inserts.

*The vitamin E requirement* is greatly increased during pregnancy: there is disagreement about whether an insufficient store of E in a pregnant woman's body is related to varicose veins. Vitamin E aids in the development of new blood cells; it has been credited with preventing blood clots, which might imply a positive effect on varicose veins.

However, some doctors disagree with vitamin therapy as a solution for varicose veins and prefer elastic stockings. You must discuss this issue with your physician: if he is well versed in nutrition he may want to monitor a dosage of vitamin E that can reduce or eliminate the protruding veins. It is known that the vitamin must be in the form of d-alpha tocopherol acetate. Mixed tocopherols are not believed to have any effect on varicose veins. Read the label carefully.

### VOMITING

Vomiting, like nausea, diminishes as your pregnancy continues. You may have vomiting in the morning, in the evening, or at irregular times. You may also have a stretch with none at all and then it may begin again. As with nausea, however, vomiting will taper off; it won't stop all at once. There is no conclusive evidence that vomiting is influenced by emotional factors (as some people may suggest to you). The hormonal changes your body is going through may be intense and/or you may be more sensitive to them than other women. Do not be concerned by blood flecks or streaks if you have been vomiting fairly often. Repeated vomiting may rupture a tiny blood vessel in the throat or esophagus, which soon clots or heals by itself.

*Vitamin B₆* helps control vomiting. Once vomiting has begun, 250 mg a day or more is necessary, or your doctor could give you a 300-mg or larger injection of vitamin $B_6$ if the vomiting is severe.

*Dehydration* and loss of calories is the danger with repeated vomiting. In some cases women have to be hospitalized for intravenous feeding if they can't keep anything down for a stretch of time.

*Hypermesis gravidarum* is a rare complication of pregnancy. It is severe and unremitting vomiting that can be controlled only with anti-emetic drugs and hospitalization. This rare illness occurs more frequently in women with abnormally high hormone levels during pregnancy, as happens in cases of multiple births or placental abnormalities. While there is reason to believe that the illness results from a hormonal imbalance, it may also have an emotional basis. Some women may also be more sensitive to the natural changes in hormone levels that take place during pregnancy. This illness is seen most frequently in pregnant women who are under emotional stress, which suggests that emotions may play a part in the disorder.

On page 156 is a chart outlining the warning signs that something may be going wrong in your pregnancy. By seeking professional help right away, you can avoid serious problems for yourself and your baby. *Notify your doctor or midwife immediately if you have any of these symptoms.*

## EXERCISE

Keeping active while you are pregnant can be as beneficial psychologically as it is physically. Labor and delivery are stressful and require a lot from your body. Giving birth will be more comfortable for you if you have good muscle tone. Also, you will probably get back into shape faster and more easily if you've kept your body in good condition during your pregnancy. Exercising is also good for your mind. It counteracts the tendency to feel clumsy or "fat" or immobile, particularly in the last trimester. The increased circulation that exercising causes can relax a lot of tension. The increased oxygenation of your system can even make you feel a bit "high."

### SUGGESTIONS ABOUT EXERCISING

*If you aren't an active person,* you probably won't change during pregnancy. At least take up regular walks of a mile or more (in a city that is only twenty blocks). Walking is good for your figure, digestion, and circulation. However, for some women the cartilage in the pelvis softens so much that a walk of any distance is difficult.

*If you have to sit all day* at a job, there are several exercises you can do in a chair. You can do *head and neck circles and neck stretches* for tension; *pelvic rock* and *ankle rotation* can be done while sitting (all described later in this section).

*Exercises* should always be *slow, rhythmic,* and *frequent.* You should try to get in the habit of doing 10 or 15 minutes a day. If you exercise only sporadically, you may strain something.

*Never exercise to the point of fatigue.* A little bit of exercise several times a day is better than a lot all at once and then none. A *pregnant women lacks resiliency.* A non-pregnant woman can restore her energy by lying down for half an hour. It can take a pregnant woman *half a day* to recover from fatigue.

Another reason it's unhealthy to exercise to the point of exhaustion is that your body accumulates lactic acid and syruyic acid and this acidosis is not good for the fetus. Though strenuous exercise does divert blood to the muscles from the internal organs, including the uterus, most studies suggest that as long as you don't exercise to the point of exhaustion, the fetus will get an adequate supply of blood and oxygen.

*Monitor your level of exertion,* the length of time you spend doing the activity, and the temperature at which you're exercising. If you're not accustomed to aerobic exercise, then it's suggested you limit yourself to nothing more vigorous then brisk walking. If you were exercising previously, you can continue at the same *perceived* level of exertion, keeping in mind that the weight of the baby changes your ability and capacity. A good guideline for exertion levels is that you should be able to carry on a conversation comfortably while exercising.

*Beware any activity that raises your body temperature* significantly during pregnancy. Hyperthermia, or overheating, can potentially cause birth defects during the first trimester and can lead to premature birth in the last trimester. The safest advice is to avoid vigorous exercise when it's hot and humid: exercise at cooler times of day and wear light clothing. The other way to keep from getting too hot while exercising is to stay well hydrated: drink plenty of fluids, preferably water!

*Limit aerobic activity to 30 minutes maximum,* as some specialists suggest. There are two reasons for this. During exercise, some blood flow is diverted away from the uterus to the exercising muscles, which could endanger the baby. Second, higher internal temperatures might be implicated in certain types of birth defects—neural tube defects in particular—as noted above.

*A stationary bicycle* is recommended during pregnancy because pregnant women have a dramatic change in their center of gravity as the pregnancy progresses. You're more prone to lose your balance and run the risk of a fall if you're riding a standard bicycle, especially in the last trimester.

*After the 4th month* some physicians advise that you not exercise while flat on your back, since the uterus could compress blood vessels that are nourishing the fetus. Certainly problems can arise with fetal distress during labor if a woman remains flat on her back, compromising the oxygen flow to the fetus.

*"No pain, no gain"* is hogwash during exercise while pregnant. If you feel pain while exercising, your body is telling you to stop. *Other warning signals during pregnancy exercise:* uterine contractions, light-headedness, or bleeding.

*Pregnancy is a kind of aerobic activity* in itself. Your heart generally beats faster, there is about 50 percent more blood plasma circulating, and your body is carrying extra weight. It might take as much effort to run one mile now as it did to run three miles before.

*Don't feel guilty* if you can't or don't want to exercise when you're pregnant. There isn't any scientific proof that exercise during pregnancy gives you anything more than a feeling of well-being. So if you're already feeling fine or simply don't want to do it, don't worry if you don't get around to doing the exercise you think you should.

*Play music* while you are exercising. Music will increase your enjoyment and if you choose music with a comfortable beat it can help you exercise rhythmically.

*Never point your toes* when exercising or stretching. Always flex your foot (keeping it perpendicular to your leg) to prevent leg cramps.

*Don't take up a new sport* during pregnancy. As long as it's a sport you've been doing regularly before pregnancy and as long as you do it with some frequency so your body remains conditioned for it, there is no sport that is strictly forbidden. But, for example, skiing and horseback riding are not a good idea once you get big because your balance is thrown off by the new weight in front. Use common sense.

*Swimming and walking* are perhaps the best all-around sports when you're pregnant. Swimming utilizes many muscles while rarely producing strain or any possibility of physical mishap.

*Weight-bearing sports* like backpacking, etc., are not a good idea when you're pregnant.

*Jogging* is not a great idea either. It is hard on your breasts and is jarring to your back. Your heel hits, then your knee and lower back get clobbered. During pregnancy progesterone relaxes the ligaments in your back. Unlike muscles, which go back to their prior shape after being stretched, ligaments remain stretched out.

## How to Exercise

*Any exercise that pulls on abdominal muscles* is not a good idea. Sit-ups are a prime example: unless you are conditioned to them you should not do sit-ups when pregnant (and even then you should quit as soon as it becomes uncomfortable). The longitudinal (up and down) muscles of the abdomen are designed to part in the middle to allow room for the expanding uterus. Sitting straight up from a lying position encourages them to part even farther. Experts say this may slow recovery of abdominal tone after delivery.

*Here is how to tell* which movements aren't good: once your uterus is big enough that you look definitely pregnant, lie on your back and try to sit straight up. You'll see a longitudinal ridge that forms at the midline . . . avoid any action that raises this ridge.

*Leg raises while lying on your back* are equally harmful.

*To sit up from a lying position,* roll over on your side and use your arms to push you up sideways. This way your abdomen won't be working (and stretching) to get you up.

*For comfort* during exercises you might want to have at least one pillow under your knees when you're lying on your back. Another pillow under your head and a small pillow in the small of your back should take care of any discomfort.

*A deep cleansing breath* before each exercise is a habit you should get into. Inhale deeply through your nose and exhale through your mouth. *Don't forget to breathe deeply throughout the exercises*—breathe in as you relax and exhale during the most difficult part of any exercise. It's easy to forget to breathe deeply or even to hold your breath when exercising. You need that additional oxygen for relaxation and for your muscles.

## SOME EXERCISES

*Relaxation* is the most important exercise you'll learn even though it may not even seem like an exercise. Practice it at least twice a day: before a nap and at bedtime. Once proficient at it you'll probably be asleep before you even finish the routine. One problem of early motherhood is grabbing catnaps: if you've learned to lie down and relax so that you can sleep right away you'll be way ahead of the game.

What follows is the relaxation technique you'll learn in childbirth education classes. It teaches you to prevent the spread of tension during labor from the working muscle (the uterus) to nearby inactive muscles—thus the uterine contractions can have maximum effectiveness with minimum discomfort to you. This exercise enables you to recognize the reactions of your own body so you can interpret sensations of muscle tension, fatigue, and release.

1. First, get as comfortable as possible. Add pillows under your knee and foot so no circulation is cut off.
2. Contract (tighten) your right arm; release it. You should feel all the tightness/tension leave. It should feel good.
3. Contract and then release the left arm. Contract and release the right leg, then the left leg.
4. Now contract the right arm and right leg at the same time; release them. Do the same on the left side. Then contract the opposite arm and leg on both sides.
5. Now contract the right hand and release, contract the left hand and release. Then scrunch up your face and let it go; tighten the pelvic floor; release it.
6. Check yourself for relaxation. Your body should be like a rag doll's. Your hands should be loose and open; neck, shoulders, and face relaxed; your jaw should be loose (a lot of tension accumulates around the mouth—open your mouth very wide, stretching the entire area, then release); your tongue should be loose and resting against your teeth; your eyes should be relaxed; not shut tight, not open.

## THE KEGEL EXERCISE

The Kegel (or pelvic floor) exercise is the most important one of all—and again, not a strenuous one. If you do no other exercise, do this one (when you're pregnant and forever after). The point of this exercise is both to strengthen your pelvic floor muscles and also to give you enough control so that you can relax them totally (very important for delivery). These are the same muscles used to stop the flow of urine, so you can get the feel of the muscles that way. When urinating, practice stopping the urine at will: then do the exercise regularly during the day. If you drive a lot, do a Kegel at every red light or make up a similar often-encountered reminder for yourself. Kegels are easiest to do sitting down, but once you get the hang of it, you can do them standing up or even walking.

*"Elevator" is the easiest way* to conceptualize the exercise. Contract the muscles a small amount at a time, counting up to the tenth "floor." Then release down, floor by floor, slowly. Release fully at one, not before (going down is harder). The point of the exercise is to get precision control like this—not just to be able to tighten and release.

*Another way is to contract* the muscles in a wavelike front-to-back rhythm, including the anus in the exercise. Release in reverse.

*A very pleasant way* to practice Kegels is during intercourse. When your mate's penis is inside you and you're relaxing, suddenly tighten the pelvic floor muscles and hold the tension for a count of anywhere from 5 to 10. The man can tell you how you're progressing in developing those muscles.

### THE PELVIC ROCK

The pelvic rock is a very useful exercise. It relieves backache, strengthens your abdominal muscles, and also brings the baby forward (taking its weight off your back, which improves circulation). Kneel on all fours like a cat. Have your elbows straight, legs slightly apart, and your back straight. Curl your back up like a cat while inhaling and tuck your head under. While exhaling let your back slowly relax. Make sure your arms and upper legs are perpendicular to your body and the floor. Arch your back up using the lower abdominal muscles to push the arch up rather than using your backbone to pull (which might increase lower backache rather than relieving it).

### TENSION-RELEASING EXERCISES

Tension can build up when you're pregnant, and there are some easy exercises you can do anywhere to relax.

*Neck stretch:* Rotate your head slowly in a circle. First stretch to the right, then let your head drop gently to the front, then stretch to the left, then back. After a couple of turns in one direction, reverse and make the circle going the opposite way.

*The shoulder roll* is designed to loosen your shoulders and upper back. First press your shoulders *forward* (as if they would meet in front); then pull them *up* to your ears and then drop them down; then push them *back,* pulling your shoulder blades together in back and lifting your chest.

*Stretch and flop over:* Stand with your feet apart, knees slightly bent, and let your head hang down. Let all your weight hang down with your arms loose; touch the floor if you can.

*The back roll* is a good substitute for a massage. Lie flat on your back with your knees up to your chest (or later in pregnancy, as far as they'll go) and your hands resting on your knees. Now roll from side to side with your hands guiding your legs—you can let your hand pull one leg over, leading the rest of the body. This massages your back muscles, where you may have tension.

## ABDOMINAL EXERCISES

To strengthen abdominal muscles there are several exercises that don't utilize the longitudinal muscles the way sit-ups do (which you want to avoid).

*Opposite arm and leg reach:* Lie on your back, lift your head, and with rounded shoulders reach your right arm toward your left toe. Your leg should be straight and about a foot off the ground, with the foot flexed (remember to never point your toes while exercising or you may get leg cramps). Hold the stretch, then lower and relax. Switch legs. The other way to do this exercise is to lie flat on your back with your knees up and your feet flat on the floor. Your opposite hand reaches to the opposite knee, your head raising each time. Note: Be sure to inhale as you lie back down and exhale as you stretch up and across.

*Leg raise:* Lie on your back with your knees bent. Bring one knee up to your chest and straighten the leg toward the ceiling, flexing your foot. Slowly lower it (exhaling) with your leg straight out. This exercise is good for circulation in your legs as well as your abdominal muscles.

### OTHER EXERCISES

*Tailor-sitting (or knee press)* strengthens your inner thighs and your perineum (which is important for labor and delivery). This exercise is quite easy and you can do it when you're sitting around with friends. Sit on the floor and pull your feet, with the soles together, as near your body as is comfortable. With your back straight press your knees gently to the floor six times (do not *bounce* the knees up and down as you may have done in exercise classes pre-pregnancy).

*The hip roll* helps take the bulk off your thighs. Sitting up with your legs straight out in front of you, shift your weight and roll from side to side, massaging the other thigh on each side as you roll over.

*To strengthen the lower back,* Pelvic Rock is the best exercise. If you want an additional exercise: get on all fours like a cat and pull your knee in and tuck your head under so your knee touches your nose. Then straighten out your head and extend the leg straight out behind you at the same time.

## DRUGS DURING PREGNANCY

It is dangerous to use any drug while you are pregnant. The fetus's growing tissues are extremely sensitive. The growing baby's mechanisms for neutralizing drugs and eliminating them from his body are immature and deficient. These mechanisms remain incomplete for at least 4 weeks following a full-term birth.

When drug treatment is considered necessary during pregnancy, make every attempt to limit the use of the drug to the smallest effective dose for the briefest possible time period. If a doctor says you need drugs for a medical condition, discuss the side effects of the drugs—as well as the effects from *not* taking the medication. Get as much information as you possibly can about any drug prescribed and study it beforehand.

Your baby's greatest risk of injury from drug exposure is during the first 3 months. The critical period of major organ development in the embryo occurs from the 4th to the 8th weeks (see Directory of Fetal Development, page 103). Drugs can cause permanent birth defects if you take them during this crucial stage of growth. The use of any drug during the first trimester must be considered hazardous. In the second and third trimesters drugs may impair the normal development of your baby's brain, nervous system, and external genital organs.

***Cocaine and crack*** are causing an epidemic of damaged infants, some of whom may be impaired for life because their mothers used cocaine even briefly during their pregnancy. Many pregnant women underestimate the dangers of cocaine: they won't take an aspirin for fear it could harm the baby, but think that snorting a few lines of cocaine can't do any harm. In fact, cocaine is brutal on the developing fetus: there is a painful withdrawal at birth, followed by developmental and neurological problems as the child grows up.

Cocaine-exposed babies are more likely to die before birth or be born prematurely, with smaller than normal heads and brains. Lasting damage can include retarded growth; stiff limbs; hyper-irritability; learning disabilities; a tendency to stop breathing, with a risk of Sudden Infant Death Syndrome ten times greater than normal; and in extreme cases, malformed genital and urinary organs, a missing small intestine, and strokes and seizures.

Research shows that a single cocaine "hit" can cause lasting fetal damage. While a single dose of cocaine and its metabolites clear out of an adult body within 48 hours, an unborn baby is exposed for 4 or 5 days. Cocaine is fat soluble, which means it can penetrate the placenta, the source of nourishment for the fetus. The baby's body converts a significant portion of it into norcocaine, a water-soluble substance that does not leave the womb and is even more potent than cocaine. Norcocaine is excreted into the amniotic fluid, which the fetus swallows, exposing himself again to the drug. Researchers believe that no baby exposed to cocaine can escape its damaging effects.

If you used cocaine during the early part of your pregnancy, perhaps before you knew you were pregnant, you should seriously consider discussing this with your doctor. Some doctors may not have an opinion about how to handle the situation, while others believe that any use of cocaine during the first trimester is so detrimental to the developing fetus that they recommend an abortion.

***There is a Pregnancy Risk Hotline*** you can call to get the latest information about the effects on your unborn child of drugs and chemicals which may be teratogens (substances harmful to the fetus). Call 800-532-3749 to reach this service of the California Teratogen Registry at the University of California/San Diego Medical Center. This facility also offers a free follow-up program after birth to pregnant women who have been exposed to suspected teratogens.

The directory beginning on page 196 includes drugs that have proven to be teratogenic (causing malformations) or are suspected of causing abnormalities in the fetus.

**CHART 21. DIRECTORY OF DRUGS TO AVOID DURING PREGNANCY**

*Accutane* (isotretinoin) is an acne drug that can cause severe and often lethal birth defects. The FDA is trying to make it more difficult for young women to obtain this drug, since the very strict rules governing the dispensing of Accutane are not always followed by doctors, pharmacists, or patients. The drug is compared to thalidomide: even one pill can be so dangerous to the fetus that in Britain women taking Accutane actually sign a written agreement that they will abort accidental pregnancies while on the drug. Birth defects include facial malformations (ears missing or below chin), severe mental retardation, and serious heart defects.

*Amphetamines* (cocaine, "speed," etc.) act as stimulants on the fetal nervous system. The effects of cocaine and crack are described above. Dextroamphetamines (see Diet Pills) can cause heart defects and blood malformations. All amphetamines are dangerous to the fetus.

*Anabolic drugs:* Also known as steroids, these male sex-hormone-like drugs to stimulate appetite and weight gain are dangerous during pregnancy.

*Antibiotics:* These cross the placenta, which is why some antibiotics can be used to treat an unborn baby if necessary. If you have a cold, sore throat, or stubborn infection be sure the doctor knows you are pregnant when he prescribes.

- *Chloromycetin (chloramphenicol)* is an antibiotic which is dangerously toxic. It may kill your unborn child.
- *Streptomycin and gentamicin* are associated with deafness in infants.

CHART 21. DIRECTORY OF DRUGS TO AVOID
DURING PREGNANCY *(continued)*

*Antibiotics (cont.):*
• *Tetracycline* may cause permanent discoloration of your baby's permanent teeth. Some brand names of tetracycline are: Achromycin, Achrostatin V, Aureomycin, Azot-rex, Cyclospar, Kesso-Tetra, Mysteclin-F, Panmycin, Robitet, Sumycin, Tetracyn.
• *Macrodantin* is a macrocrystal of nitrofurantoin and is a common treatment for urinary-tract infection in pregnant women. However, this drug is contraindicated in pregnant women at term as well as in infants under 1 month old because of the possibilities of hemolytic anemia due to immature enzyme systems.
• *Antibiotics safe in pregnancy are penicillin,* which is often the treatment of choice for various common infections provided that the woman is not allergic, and *ampicillin. Cephalosporins* (Keflex and Anspor are the most common ones) also do not manifest toxic properties for the expectant woman or her fetus.

*Anticonvulsants* (Dilantin, etc.) can cause cleft lip, cleft palate, and other abnormalities. If withholding the anticonvulsant would be injurious to the mother, folic acid may counteract these possible malformations.

*Antihistamines* can cause possible malformations. However, there are now some that have been designed specifically for safe use by pregnant women. Check with your doctor.

*Antimetabolites* such as aminopterin and other antitumor drugs cause malformations.

*Antinausea drugs:* Malformations have been observed in the offspring of animals exposed during pregnancy. Some brand names are: Bonine, Antivert, Migral, Compazine, and Marezine.

## CHART 21. DIRECTORY OF DRUGS TO AVOID DURING PREGNANCY *(continued)*

*Aspirin:* Large amounts can cause miscarriage. Also, frequent use toward the end of pregnancy may disrupt the baby's blood-clotting mechanism and cause hemorrhage in the newborn. Aspirin taken near the due date, may also affect the mother's blood-clotting during labor and delivery. Please see special section on aspirin, page 203.

*Birth control pills:* These cause malformations of the arms and legs, defects of the internal organ systems and some also cause masculinization of the female fetus. Some brand names: Demulen, Enovid, Loestrin, Micronor, Notinyl, Notlestrin, Nor-Q.D., Oracon, Ortho-Novum, Ovulen.

*Blood-pressure-lowering drugs:* See listing for Reserpine, page 201.

*Cocaine* affects both the course of the pregnancy and the development of the fetus. It can cause early onset of labor as well as miscarriage due to the sudden separation of the placenta. The possible consequences for the baby include fetal addiction with painful withdrawal at birth; high infant mortality; low birth weight; and behavioral, development, and neurological problems. Conclusive new studies show impaired fetal development resulting in lighter, shorter babies with smaller heads who are more likely to suffer health and developmental problems.

*Cortisone* can cause fetal and placental abnormalities. It has been implicated in cleft lip and stillbirth.

*Diet pills* (dextroamphetamines): These can cause heart defects and blood vessel malformations.

*DES:* Used into the 1970s to prevent miscarriage. There were no reports of ill effects on the mothers, but many of their daughters have developed cervical cancer; 90 percent of the female offspring of women treated with DES during pregnancGy have precancerous growths on their cervixes.

**CHART 21. DIRECTORY OF DRUGS TO AVOID
DURING PREGNANCY** *(continued)*

*Diuretics* (water pills): Can possibly cause blood disorders in the newborn. With some brands jaundice may also occur. Some brand names: Diupres, Diuril, Dyazide, Enduron, Esidrix, Hydrodiuril, Hydropes.

*Haldol (haloperidol)* is a major tranquilizer used in treating schizophrenia. It has the same possibility of altering a baby's brain chemistry as does Aldomet. The drug may permanently alter the brain chemistry of the baby by causing a decrease in the number and sensitivity of receptors in its brain for a chemical messenger called dopamine.

However, there is a potential benefit to the use of antipsychotic drugs in schizophrenic women during pregnancy, but *not* while nursing. Such drugs might actually decrease the offspring's risk of developing the disease in adolescence or early adulthood, since schizophrenia runs in families and is thought to have a genetic component. If a baby receives Haloperidol via its mother before birth, it might correct an otherwise faulty dopamine mechanism.

*Herbs* are not really drugs, but some people use them in place of drugs, so it is necessary to mention those herbs that have been implicated in causing miscarriage; blue or black cohosh, pennyroyal, mugwort, tansy, and slippery elm.

*Heroin, morphine* can possibly cause fetal addiction, which can mean that the newborn has to suffer the agonies of withdrawal and may need a blood transfusion at birth.

*Iodides* (expectorants) can cause a goiter in an unborn child.

*LSD, other psychedelics* may cause chromosomal damage and pose an increased risk of miscarriage.

## CHART 21. DIRECTORY OF DRUGS TO AVOID
## DURING PREGNANCY *(continued)*

*Marijuana* was once thought to be harmless, but studies have shown it to have the same dangerous effects on the fetus as cocaine. Even moderate smoking can have serious consequences to your developing baby. Studies were done on monkeys using small amounts of THC, the active chemical in marijuana. Effects included delayed conception, problems during pregnancy, stillbirth, early infant death, and smaller-than-normal babies, who are at risk, like any low birth-weight infant, for health and developmental problems. Marijuana interferes not only with cell division but also with your body's immune system: your white blood cells become less capable of fighting viruses. A marijuana smoker may be more susceptible to viral infections, at least one of which, rubella, also known as German measles, is known to cause birth defects. It is known that THC builds up in the germ cells of the ovaries and testes. It is advisable to stop smoking marijuana long before becoming pregnant, although it isn't known how long before conception you should stop to insure a healthy baby. Though the damage to a man may be temporary because he constantly produces new sperm, the effect on a woman could be lasting. You are born with a certain number of eggs at birth, and if those eggs are injured, there is no way to undo the damage.

*Nosedrops* are used to contract the blood vessels of the nose. They can also be strong enough to contract blood vessels in the placenta, which means reduced oxygen and nutrition are carried to the fetus. The nosedrops shrink the nasal mucosa and can also shrink the placental bed. Also, frequent use of nosedrops does not improve stuffiness: it makes it worse. Try using saline nasal drops for congestion.

*Phenacetin* causes possible damage to fetal kidneys.

*Progestins* (progesterone-like hormones) are all linked to birth defects, particularly genital defects in female babies. Some doctors are still writing prescriptions for progestins to prevent miscarriage despite the fact that the FDA has issued

CHART 21. DIRECTORY OF DRUGS TO AVOID
DURING PREGNANCY *(continued)*

---

### *Progestins (cont.)*

warnings. Not only are they dangerous but progestins (or any other drug) have not been proven effective in blocking threatened miscarriage.

Progestins are also used to bring on late menstruation. If such an injection fails to bring on a period then a doctor can conclude the woman is pregnant. Thus progestins are also used as an early pregnancy test. *But if you are pregnant and receive a progestin shot your baby may be adversely affected.* Allow such an injection only if you would *absolutely* abort if you were pregnant.

*Reserpine* (drugs to lower blood pressure) can cause possible blood disorders in the newborn as well as jaundice. It can also cause nasal congestion leading to breathing difficulties. Decreased appetite may be another side effect. Some brand names: Regroton, Salutensin, Serap-es, Serpasil.

*Sulfa drugs:* When taken in late pregnancy sulfa drugs can disturb a baby's liver function. They can produce kernicterus, a form of jaundice in the newborn often associated with brain damage. Animal studies have indicated that other abnormalities may also occur. Some brand names: Azo Gantanol, Azo Gantrisin, Bactrim, Gantanol, Gantrisin, SK Soxazole.

*Tegison:* (generic name etretinate) is related to the acne drug Accutane (page 196). Tegison is used to treat severe cases of another skin disease, psoriasis. Unlike Accutane, which leaves the body within a few days and poses no risk for women who get pregnant afterward, Tegison stays in a person's body for years. Tegison has been detected in patients' blood 2 years after the drug is discontinued and can cause birth defects in later pregnancies. Birth defects in the babies of Tegison users include facial deformities—ears missing or below the chin—mental retardation, and often lethal heart defects. Tegison also causes flipper-like vestigial arms and legs resembling those produced by the sedative thalidomide in the 1960s.

**CHART 21. DIRECTORY OF DRUGS TO AVOID
DURING PREGNANCY (continued)**

*Thyroid drugs:* The thyroid medication used to treat an overactive thyroid can cause a goiter in the infant.

*Tranquilizers* are still the subject of an ongoing debate because studies have not been conclusive. However, the FDA has told manufacturers that they must warn doctors that tranquilizers may cause deformities in the first 3 months of pregnancy. Malformations are possible, although there are now some tranquilizers designed particularly for safe use by pregnant women but of course check with your obstetrician. Some brand names of those to avoid: Librium, Valium, Haldol, Miltown, or Equanil. New studies show that Valium, the most widely prescribed drug in the United States, may interfere with muscle tissue development in the fetus.

*Vitamins:* Although vitamins are covered thoroughly on pages 140 to 152 in this chapter, they also appear here because they can be dangerous if used in excess and some people use vitamins as a substitute for medication. Beware of the following:

- *Vitamin A:* Can injure the growing baby's eyes; vitamin A is chemically related to 13-cisretinoic acid, a compound in acne medicine that can cause cleft palate, heart defects, and brain abnormalities.
- *Vitamin $B_6$:* Has caused nerve damage in people taking 200 mg a day or more.
- *Vitamin C:* Doses greater than 1 gram (1,000 mg) can cause scurvy in the baby due to the rapid drop of vitamin C levels after delivery. May impair bone development in the fetus.
- *Vitamin D:* May cause dangerously high levels of calcium.
- *Vitamin E:* Can raise maternal blood pressure, a danger for women with high blood pressure or rheumatic heart disease.
- *Vitamin K:* Can produce kernicterus, a form of newborn jaundice associated with brain damage.

## ASPIRIN

Aspirin taken by pregnant women continues to be a serious health problem. Doctors have routinely advised against using it since 1970 when it was first linked to unusual bleeding problems (including newborn brain hemorrhage). However, women continue to take aspirin, sometimes not even aware that the products they are consuming contain it. For example, many topically applied ointments and salves contain aspirin that can be absorbed into body tissues. Please consult the chart beginning on page 205 so that you can avoid dangerous mistakes.

Researchers now say that not only should you avoid aspirin during your pregnancy but if you have taken it within 5 days before delivery, be sure to tell the doctor. He may want to have the baby specially evaluated for aspirin-related bleeding problems.

Aspirin has a significant effect on platelets, microscopic discs in the blood that are essential to clotting. If the function of the platelets is impaired, bleeding can become extremely difficult to stop. In newborns and their mothers, aspirin can lead to uncontrolled bleeding and problems of circulation for the baby.

The 5-day interval after taking aspirin and before birth can be significant in cases like circumcising a baby boy. If the mother had taken aspirin, doctors would want to wait several days longer than normal to avoid bleeding-related complications.

Apparently many people do not know which over-the-counter and prescription medicines contain aspirin. The chart should protect you from unintentionally taking aspirin. It includes common brand-name prescription and over-the-counter drugs containing aspirin; however, there are many generic or store-brand-name preparations that also should be checked.

# MISCELLANY

## BATHING

***Bathing during pregnancy:*** Baths are safe at all times except when your membranes (bag of waters) have broken (there is a risk of infection after that). Otherwise baths can be relaxing and soothing. See warning on hot tubs on page 210.

## CLOTHING

Clothes when you are pregnant should be comfortable. Mexican and Indian tops and dresses are comfortable, pretty, inexpensive, and reusable later. A pair of maternity blue jeans with an expandable front panel will take you through much of your pregnancy with a variety of smock-style tops. It's important to buy or borrow clothes you feel pretty in: even if you have only three or four outfits they should make you feel good.

***Wear a bra.*** Your breasts will gain substantial weight during the first trimester, and if they don't get support they may sag later. Wear a bra as soon as you notice the increase in size. Buy only two bras to begin with because your breasts may continue to expand and you will have to get larger bras as the pregnancy continues.

***Maternity girdles*** don't seem to be very helpful because there is a stretchy pouch in front. The point of wearing a girdle is to have extra support of the baby and you don't get that with the loose, elasticized front pouch. If you want to try a girdle buy a regular girdle one size too large and wear it as soon as you get up in the morning. Especially during the last 3 months it will give you help in carrying that extra weight.

**CHART 22. AN ASPIRIN DIRECTORY**

---

*Advil;* Alka-Seltzer; Alka-Seltzer Plus cold medicine; Anacin (and Anacin Maximum Strength); Anaprox; APC; APC with Butalbital; APC with Codeine; Arthritis Pain Formula (by Anacin); Arthritis Strength Bufferin; Ascodeen-30; Ascriptin; Aspergum; Aspirin suppositories

*Bayer Aspirin;* Bayer Children's Chewable Aspirin; Bayer Children's cold tablets; Bayer Timed-Release aspirin; BC Powders; Buff-A comp; Buffadyne; Bufferin; Butalbital

*Cama Inlay-Tabs;* Cetased, Improved; Cheracol capsules; Clinoril; Congesprin; Cope; Coricidin D decongestant tablets; Coricidin for children; Coricidin Medilets for children; Coricidin

*Darvon with A.S.A.;* Darvon-N with A.S.A.; Dristan decongestant; Duragesic

*Ecotrin;* Empirin; Empirin with Codeine; Emprazil; Emprazil-C; En Tab; Equagesic; Excedrin; Extra-Strength Bufferin

*Feldene;* Fiorinal; Fiorinal with Codeine; 4-Way Cold Tablets

*Gemnisyn;* Goody's Headache Powders

*Indocin*

*Measurin;* Midol; Momentum Muscular Backache Formula; Monacet with Codeine; Motrin

*Naprosyn;* Norgesic; Norgesic Forte; Norwich aspirin; Nuprin

*Pabirin buffered tablets;* Panalgesic; Percodan and Percodan-Demi tablets; Percogesic; Persistin

*Quiet World Analgesic/*Sleeping aid

*Robaxisal tablets*

*SK-65 Compound;* St. Joseph Aspirin for Children; Sine-Aid; Sine-Off Sinus Medicine tablets—aspirin formula; Supac; Stendin; Stero-Darvon with A.S.A.; Synalgos (and Synalgos-DC) capsules

*Tolectin;* Triaminicin tablets

*Vanquish;* Verin; Viro-Med tablets

*Zomax;* Zorpin

### CHART 22. AN ASPIRIN DIRECTORY *(continued)*

#### *ASPIRIN-CONTAINING TOPICAL RUBS*

Absorbent Rub; Absorbine (Arthritic and Jr.); Act-On Rub; Analbalm; Analgesic Balm; Antiphlogistine; Arthralgen; Aspercreme; Banalog; Baumodyne; Ben-Gay (all kinds); Braska; Counterpain Rub; Dencorub; Doan's Rub; Emul-O-Balm; End-Ake; Exocaine (Plus or tube); Heet; Icy Hot; Infra-Rub; Lini-Balm; Mentholatum & Deep Heating; Minit-Rub; Musterole (all kinds); Neurabaum; Oil-O-Sol; Omega Oil; Panalgesic; Rid-A-Pain; Rumarub; Sloan's; Soltice (all kinds); SPD; Stimurub; Surin; Yager's Liniment; Zemo (all kinds)

### CHART 23. DIRECTORY OF HAZARDS TO AVOID DURING PREGNANCY

The Hazard Evaluation System in California is the most useful source for information regarding the suspected hazards to the fetus of any chemical you might encounter in the workplace or elsewhere. They can be reached at 415-540-3014.

*Aerosol Ribavirin* is a drug used to treat severe lung infections in young children. There is controversy about its use because breathing its mist may lead to birth defects in the offspring of health-care workers who handle it. The drug is widely used in intensive-care units and pediatric wards across the U.S., particularly during the winter. Several leading medical centers are now severely restricting its use and the FDA is considering a labeling change to include warnings about its potential risk to health-care workers.

*Aerosol Sprays* have warnings on them: if you inhale the fumes they could be harmful to the developing fetus.

CHART 23. DIRECTORY OF HAZARDS TO AVOID
DURING PREGNANCY *(continued)*

*Alcohol* is a poison. In large amounts it may damage the nerve cells of the baby's brain. Some of the alcohol you drink reaches the fetus: during the critical developmental period you don't want the baby's brain cells exposed. The National Institute on Alcohol Abuse and Alcoholism warns that more than 2 drinks a day (a total of 2 ounces of whiskey) may harm unborn children. If you have more than 2 drinks there is a 10 percent chance your baby will have "fetal alcohol syndrome"—physical and behavioral abnormalities in the offspring of women who consume excessive amounts of alcohol. Six thousand children a year are affected with facial abnormalities, heart defects, abnormal limb development, and lower-than-average-intelligence. Testing done on animals indicates that for humans 6 drinks or more a day—throughout pregnancy or a certain phase of it—means a significant risk for fetal alcohol syndrome. There is less risk with less than 6 drinks but some symptoms are still possible. Therefore they are recommending no more than 2 drinks—which means 1 ounce of hard liquor *or* 2 mixed drinks *or* 2 glasses of wine *or* glasses of beer. Binge drinking can also be harmful: one day or night of excessive consumption and then not drinking at all for the rest of the pregnancy gives you no safety.

There are other reasons to avoid alcohol. It interferes with the absorption and utilization of other nutrients. It actually wastes other nutrients by using them for its own metabolism—the body cannot store alcohol, so it must use it when it's taken in. Also, alcohol has the indirect effect of lowering your appetite. It substitutes the empty calories of alcohol for real nutrition—even social drinking lowers hunger.

If you only drink a little, then why not abstain during pregnancy? If a woman drinks as much as 6 beers, glasses of wine, or mixed drinks in one day, she will risk her baby having the symptoms of the fetal alcohol syndrome.

CHART 23. DIRECTORY OF HAZARDS TO AVOID
DURING PREGNANCY *(continued)*

*Anesthetic gases* are encountered in high amounts by anesthetists, nurses, aides, and surgeons working in operating rooms. All these professionals have abnormally high rates of sterility, miscarriage, and birth deformities. Excess exposure to anesthetic gases seems to be the cause.

*Cadmium* is a component of tobacco smoke; it also occurs in wastes from electroplating plants and is released into the air by tires that are wearing down or burning. It seems to retard growth and increase fetal deformities.

*Caffeine (tannic acid in tea)* stimulates the fetal nervous system. Even decaffeinated coffee and tea contain a fair amount of the substance. Please refer to page 153 for more information on why you should avoid this substance.

*Carbon monoxide* is dangerous when you're pregnant: extended exposure can lower birth weight and increase infant mortality rates. Try to stay out of traffic jams and avoid walking around a lot of traffic. The fumes from car exhaust also contain lead, which is a poisonous gas. Do not stay in a running car in an enclosed space (the garage, heavy traffic in long tunnels, etc.). Leave the tailgate open when you are driving a car that might have a defective muffler.

*Chemotherapy cancer drugs* handled by nurses in their first 3 months of pregnancy cause a high risk of miscarriage: nurses exposed to these drugs are twice as likely to miscarry as other nurses. Fetal loss is linked with on-the-job exposure to these three drugs: cyclophosphamide, doxorubicin, and vincristine, medicines that stop cancer by disrupting cell growth and killing cells that are actively growing.

*Dioxin derivatives* in herbicides used in forests are highly toxic in large amounts; even in amounts deemed safe, they are implicated in high miscarriage rates. Dioxin spraying in Oregon to increase timber production was associated with increased occurrence of spontaneous abortions.

CHART 23. DIRECTORY OF HAZARDS TO AVOID
DURING PREGNANCY *(continued)*

*Freshwater or bottom-feeding fish* may be polluted
with PCBs (see below) or other dangerous chemicals.
Pesticide-tainted sport fish from the Great Lakes area may
pose a far greater health risk to you, and therefore to the
fetus, than is acknowledged by local health departments. The
"acceptable level" of toxic pesticide residue in the region,
especially DDT and dieldrin, may be too lenient: regular
consumption of sport fish like salmon and trout at one-fifth
the amount considered "safe" may increase your cancer risk.
The problem is most severe with fatty fish such as trout, and
with the largest predatory fish, which accumulate the chemicals over years of eating smaller contaminated fish. *Swordfish* should be avoided when you're pregnant or breast-
feeding because of its high mercury levels from polluted
waters.

Since 1970 the Great Lakes states have advised residents to eat only one trout from Lake Huron per week
because of PCB contamination. *Pregnant women, nursing
mothers, and children are advised to avoid the fish altogether.* In Michigan you can get information about the
fishing water in your area by contacting: Large Lakes Research Station, 9311 Groh Road, Grosse Ile, Michigan 48138
(313-675-5000).

*Gasoline, other petroleum products, and their va-
pors* are known to cause cancer, birth defects, and other
reproductive harm. This danger is faced by women other
than those who work in an oil refinery or chemical plant:
in fact, you can come into contact with these materials at
your corner gas station. There may even be warning signs
posted near the gas pumps. The seemingly harmless act of
filling your own car can expose you to gasoline vapors. The
vapor-retrieval nozzles on unleaded gasoline hoses are *supposed* to eliminate most of these vapors, but they can be
defective.

## CHART 23. DIRECTORY OF HAZARDS TO AVOID DURING PREGNANCY *(continued)*

*Hot tubs* can be dangerous during pregnancy. A long soak in a tub heated to 106° F. can raise the mother's body temperature to the point of heatstroke. Drinking alcohol at the same time only increases the chances of this. The rule of thumb for pregnant women is to keep the temperature below 104° and get out after ten minutes and let your body cool off before getting back in. Otherwise you risk brain damage to the fetus.

*Lecithin* may cause damage to the developing fetus. Researchers have found that lecithin, a fat-emulsifying agent often sold in health food stores as a diet aid, may produce defects in the development of unborn children. The studies have not been conclusive, but caution is urged in the use of this product during your childbearing years.

*Mercury* is rarely encountered in a pure form, but as a medical or industrial compound (mercurous chloride); overexposure leads to cerebral palsy, blindness, and brain damage in newborns.

*Ozone* is an oxygen variant occurring in high concentrations of smog, as well as in airliners at high altitudes. Flight attendants have an occupationally high incidence of miscarriages and birth defects, and ozone is believed to be the cause.

*Paints* can contain lead. Use paint without lead or toxic vapors; most latex paints are safe. Do not strip or sand old paint yourself. Do not even be in the vicinity when old paint, old plaster, or putty are sanded because they get in the air. This also applies to refinishing old furniture.

*PCB (polychlorinated biphenyls)* are such dangerous carcinogens that the EPA banned their production in the U.S. in 1979. However, PCB wastes remain where dumped on river bottoms, and PCB-containing products, like the electrical insulation in transformers, will continue to release PCBs into food and water supplies for many years. You can

CHART 23. DIRECTORY OF HAZARDS TO AVOID
DURING PREGNANCY *(continued)*

*PCB (polychlorinated biphenyls) (cont.)*
reduce your chance of ingesting PCBs by not eating fresh-water fish or bottom-feeding fish, like flounder and sole. Women who accidentally ingest high concentrations of PCBs during pregnancy may give birth to babies with such abnormalities as eye and tooth defects.

*Pesticides* should be avoided by women in their child-bearing years. The EPA has limited the use of only a very few of the 1,500 active ingredients registered with the Environmental Protection Agency. Partial evidence strongly suggests that excess exposure to almost any pesticide may permanently harm fetuses.

*Photographic chemicals* should be avoided, particularly during the first trimester of pregnancy. Animal studies suggest that high doses of some organic and metallic chemicals used in the photography darkroom may be injurious to the fetus. If you want to resume darkroom work in the second and third trimester, at the least you should be sure that you have adequate ventilation and impermeable gloves and that you wear goggles.

*Smoking:* Studies have shown that lead in the blood vessels of infants increases in direct proportion to the levels found in their smoking mothers. When a woman smokes, she is cutting down the oxygen supply to her baby. The analogy has been made that it's the same thing as taking a baby and instead of giving it three meals a day, giving it only one and a half. Smoking is linked to low-birth-weight infants, which are less hardy. The toxic substances that are inhaled with cigarette smoke—carbon monoxide, cyanide—retard fetal growth.
Another reason for low-birth-weight babies in smoking mothers is that these women have a lower maternal weight gain. They smoke more and eat less. Also, congenital anomalies are suspected from smoking.

**CHART 23. DIRECTORY OF HAZARDS TO AVOID DURING PREGNANCY** *(continued)*

*Smoking (cont.):*
Stay out of smoke-filled rooms, whether you smoke yourself or not. Work areas or social situations where there is a lot of smoke and not much ventilation means you'll be inhaling other people's smoke. This has been shown to have as many ill effects as if you were smoking yourself.

The chart on page 215 has some suggestions for smokers on how to stop smoking or at least cut down. Each cigarette you smoke affects your baby, so even if you cannot stop cold turkey, you will be doing the baby a favor by reducing the number and strength of cigarettes. The point of these suggestions is to make you more aware of how much and when you smoke, in the hope of changing your habits.

*Solvents (toluene, turpentine)* are hazardous during pregnancy if there is a long exposure to constant high concentrations, either in industrial use or arts and crafts.

*Toxic products* should not be inhaled. *Read the label of any material you use during pregnancy.* Some examples are: cleaning fluids, contact cements, volatile paints, lacquer thinners, some glues, various household cleaning agents (e.g., oven cleaner), etc.

*Toxoplasmosis* is a disease contracted from eating raw meat or contact with a cat that is a carrier. If a pregnant woman gets the disease, it can injure her fetus, causing blindness, fetal brain damage, malformation of the head, or fatal illness. The greatest danger from toxoplasmosis occurs in the last months of pregnancy, when infection has the greatest likelihood of causing retardation and other neurological problems. Estimates indicate that 1 to 3 in every 4,000 newborns show defects due to prenatal infection with toxoplasmosis. One in 1,000 may appear normal at birth but may develop the symptoms later.
• Avoid raw or undercooked meat. Do not eat rare steak: make sure all your meat is cooked to at least 140° at which heat the organism is killed.

CHART 23. DIRECTORY OF HAZARDS TO AVOID
DURING PREGNANCY *(continued)*

*Toxoplasmosis (cont.)*

• *Do not clean the cat litter box: feces carry the disease.* Do not feed raw meat to your cat. A cat has to eat infected meat (mice, birds, etc.) to be a host to toxoplasmosis, so keep your cat indoors and feed it cooked, canned, or dry food. Stay away from other people's cats, especially outdoor cats.

• You may have already had the disease if you've eaten raw meat or always had cats. A blood test will tell you. Toxoplasmosis has struck 25 percent of adults in America, who afterwards carry antibodies and are thus immune from future attacks of the disease.

*Uranium wastes* from mining were used for a long time in Colorado to build roads and house foundations. Radioactive slag was made into cinder blocks to build homes in many other states. Rains draining through uranium mining wastes have made the drinking water in parts of Colorado, New Mexico, Utah, and other states abnormally radioactive. This heightened radiation increases the incidence of birth defects and miscarriages. See page 143 for a recommendation concerning bottled water.

*Vaginal products* such as douches and gels that contain povidone-iodine should be avoided by pregnant women because of possible thyroid defects in the fetus.

*Video display terminals (VDT)* have been implicated in increased miscarriage rates in offices, *but there is no proof.* Many clusters of miscarriages among VDT users have been investigated, but there has been no scientific evidence to establish a cause-and-effect relationship. Some studies showed that women who used VDTs for more than 20 hours each week during the first trimester of pregnancy were statistically twice as likely to miscarry as women doing other types of office work, without concluding that the VDT work was the cause of the problem. There is a suggestion that emissions of ionizing and low-level electromagnetic radiation from the VDTs may alter or disrupt cellular development. New studies will consider other factors such as

**CHART 23. DIRECTORY OF HAZARDS TO AVOID
DURING PREGNANCY (continued)**

*Video display terminals (VDT) (cont.)*
smoking, alcohol use, and job stress. *As it now stands, there
seems to be no effect on women who use VDTs less than 20
hours a week. There is a higher miscarriage rate for women
who work at VDTs more than 20 hours weekly, although
VDT use may not be the explanation.*

*Workplace hazards* can expose women to higher than
normal risks of pregnancy complications or birth defects.
Some examples are: motor vehicle tollbooth or exit booth
for pay parking because of carbon monoxide and lead in
exhaust fumes; dry-cleaning facility—benzene vapors can
cause chromosome breaks; vinyl plastic manufacturing (vinyl chloride leads to chromosome defects and higher fetal
death rates); installation of radio or TV transmitting equipment (intense radio waves may impair health of fetus); nuclear power plant (radiation levels can be high enough to
damage egg cells—lead-lined underpants can help); manufacture of storage batteries, paint, or glass (contain lead).

*X rays,* particularly of the abdominal area, should be
strictly avoided during pregnancy unless absolutely necessary for your own health. However, dental X rays are safe
as long as you wear a lead apron.
The use of *X-ray pelvimetry* (X rays of your pelvic structure) is no longer considered safe. This procedure was once
used to determine whether there would be cephalopelvic
disproportion, but studies showed that X rays could not predict whether the fetal head could mold to pelvic dimensions, nor whether the pelvis had the capacity to widen
during labor. Although X-ray pelvimetry may be useful to
determine the position of the baby's head in a breech presentation, most doctors question the potentially harmful risk
of radiation to the fetus.

---

#### CHART 24. HOW TO STOP SMOKING OR CUT DOWN

---

- Use a low-tar, low-nicotine brand
- Change brands with each pack
- Buy only one pack at a time
- Smoke cigarettes only halfway down: more tar and nicotine are concentrated in the final puffs
- Extinguish each cigarette after the first puff, then relight it
- Never hold the cigarette in your hand: force yourself to put it down after each puff.
- Put your cigarettes out of reach so it's an effort to get one
- Do not accept cigarettes from other people. Say, ''My baby and I don't smoke''
- Wrap a piece of paper around each pack of cigarettes and record the time you smoke each cigarette and the activity associated with it. You'll see a pattern after a few days and can decide which cigarettes are most important to you and which you can give up

---

### WORKING

Working while you are pregnant is the same as working when you aren't pregnant—except that you are prey to the physical changes and discomforts listed in the beginning of this chapter. Whether you continue to work depends entirely on why you were working before you got pregnant. Some women work simply as something to do until they get pregnant; others have to supplement their mate's income or the woman may be the sole source of income; other women have career jobs that they intend to continue once the baby is born after a leave of absence. Whichever is your case, there is no reason not to work when you are pregnant unless your job involves heavy physical labor or is in an industry with potentially harmful materials or fumes.

The psychological benefit of working while you are pregnant is that you reaffirm the normalcy of pregnancy. By continuing to work you maintain an important and stable aspect of your life at a time when you may be disoriented by the changes going on physically and psychologically.

## MOVING

Moving your home is not a great idea when you're pregnant. Moving involves a lot of physical and psychological readjustments and pregnancy itself is presenting you with plenty of those. Moving compounds the changes you have to go through and adjust to. However, people need more room once a baby is born and they often decide to make a move once the pregnancy is confirmed. If moving is unavoidable during pregnancy, at least follow these suggestions:

- *Don't lift* or push heavy objects.
- *Don't exhaust* yourself. Don't try to do everything all at once or you will have a hard time recovering from the fatigue (see the section earlier in this chapter on Fatigue).
- *Stay off* ladders and stepstools. Your balance is off when you're pregnant, particularly as you get bigger.
- *Get help* from wherever and whomever you can. You simply do not have the energy and stamina you did before the pregnancy.

## TRAVEL

The one big argument against traveling while you're pregnant is that abortion (miscarriage) or labor can happen at any time. It would be frightening and inconvenient to be in a strange city were that to happen. However, there is no evidence that travel *causes* labor, abortion, or other complications of pregnancy. You would only need to be cautious if you've had spontaneous abortions before or have a history of premature labor.

*Two rules of thumb for travel:* Ask your doctor to give you the name of an obstetrician (hopefully one he may know) in the area you are traveling to.) During the last 6 weeks of pregnancy limit yourself only to trips within 50 miles of your home base.

***Airplanes are not a good idea*** after your 7th month because you could go into labor. Flying itself has no effect on labor, but the chance of going into labor increases as your due date approaches. Check with the airline about whether they require a doctor's letter to let you on the plane after your 7th month. Do not fly in small private planes that have *unpressurized cabins. Sit over the wings* or toward the front of the plane where you will feel less of the plane's motion. *Eat lightly* when flying because pregnancy makes you more prone to motion sickness. *Go to the bathroom* before boarding. There may be a delay in takeoff, or the seat-belt sign may stay on a long time, and during pregnancy you feel the need to urinate more frequently. *Fasten your seat belt* below your belly, across the bony pelvis.

***Cars*** can be exhausting, so limit your car traveling to 300 miles a day. *Get out* at least every 100 miles and have a short walk to insure good circulation. *Fasten your seat belt:* studies show that it prevents ejection and reduces injuries in a crash. Buckle it low across the bony pelvis and also use a shoulder harness if you have one. *You can do the driving* as long as you fit behind the wheel!

## CHART 25. FETUS IN UTERO AT TERM

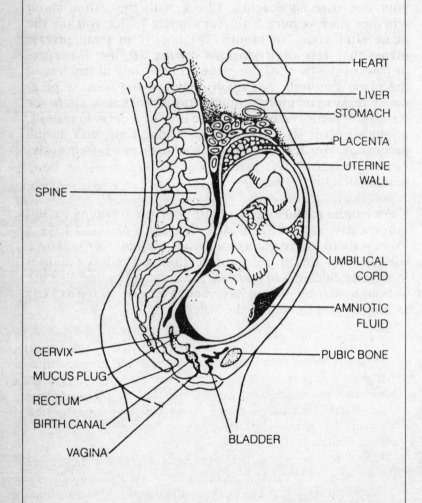

HEART

LIVER

STOMACH

PLACENTA

UTERINE WALL

SPINE

UMBILICAL CORD

AMNIOTIC FLUID

CERVIX

MUCUS PLUG

PUBIC BONE

RECTUM

BIRTH CANAL

VAGINA

BLADDER

# 4

# Taking care of your mind

## *(and your mate's)*

Pregnancy is a life crisis. Everything is changing. Change is disorienting at the least and can be frightening. However, this difficult, pivotal time in your life can also be enriching and thrilling in the new insights and outlooks it gives you.

Pregnancy is a maturational crisis similar to puberty and menopause. Think back on how you felt as an adolescent. It was a time of "becoming," when you were teetering between being a girl and becoming a woman. If you were like most young women you felt anxious, awkward, self-conscious, and like a stranger in your changing body. You might have felt angry and confused by the rapid transformation going on over which you didn't have any control. The rest of the time you probably felt daring, adventuresome, attractive, and on the brink of great things. At times you may have experienced all these feelings at once and your system would get overloaded by so much input. The "circuit-breaker" was a fit of tears or anger or withdrawal. Or simple bewilderment. Pregnancy throws you into a similar state.

The biological and endocrine changes of being pregnant bring an accompanying psychological disequilibrium. You are in limbo; it is a time of Becoming. It is an *identity crisis.* You are going from Woman to Mother; some women may be going from Girl to Mother because they have always associated "really growing up" with having a baby. Either way, all aspects of your life are spotlighted: your personal direction, your relationship with the baby's father, your adequacy as a person (and potential mother), the world condition, and your own mortality. One aspect of reproducing is that you are "replacing" yourself, which forces you to think about how far along the road *you are*.

When you resolve all the confusion caused by pregnancy the result is *emotional growth*. You will probably be more in touch with yourself and have a better understanding of where you have been and where you are headed. There are women, however, who go through the nine months trying to avoid facing the psychological aspect. The issues raised by being pregnant are weighty and thorny; some are hard to wrestle with and others leave you certain that you have no answer at all. It *is* possible to avoid all that, just as it would be possible to have the baby and ignore her. If you sail through your pregnancy as if nothing were different—as if the only change is that your belly is getting bigger and bigger—you will probably get hit with all the feelings somewhere along the way, as if by a boomerang. Instead of denying that pregnancy makes a difference, you'll be better off accepting that pregnancy involves *all* of you: your mind as well as your body.

The maturational crisis that began with pregnancy doesn't just end with the delivery of your baby. The reality of being a parent—and the extent to which it matches your expectations—is going to extend this unsettled period in your life. You will be in a state of psychological disequilibrium during the early weeks and sometimes months of your child's life. One sure thing is that you will never be the same as you were before you had your baby.

You'll want to live through this crucial time in your life with as much understanding as possible—and as much pleasure, too. Knowing what to expect and having some landmarks for the emotional journey you'll be taking will help you accomplish that.

## THE BABY'S MOTHER

*Absentmindedness* often afflicts pregnant women, and it can give you the creepy feeling that you're losing your mind unless you know it is normal. You may find that you forget appointments, mix up information, or can't remember where you put things. It can make you feel like a senile little old lady—or someone whose sanity is slipping! All that has happened is that your attention is focused on yourself and the pregnancy and taken away from other things. Don't get upset by it. Just knowing that it is not a unique phenomenon may help you *accept* the fact that you forgot to take a certain book to your office—three times in a row!

Absentmindedness may even get worse in the last couple of weeks of pregnancy. All your concentration will be on when the baby will arrive and what labor and delivery will be like. You may not only forget things, you may also drop things and generally walk around in a daze.

### ACCEPTING THE PREGNANCY

Accepting the pregnancy is the first and most important psychological task you have. That may sound obvious, but there are women who glide through the early months of pregnancy giving it as little thought as possible (which is especially easy before you begin to "show"). You and the baby's father have to come to terms with the pregnancy and begin to think about the reality. Until now your thoughts about a baby and parenthood have probably all been in soft focus, a pastel picture of the loving threesome (or more, if you already have other children—although *that* picture is probably more realistic, in bright colors, with a good deal of crying heard through the sound of chirping birds!)

*Conflicted feelings* are sure to surface once you begin to really accept the pending realities. Don't be worried that there is something wrong with you for feeling this way: it is good to have conflicted feelings. It means you are coming to terms with the situation. You won't have the horrible shock of parents who wait to face all this until the last possible moment: once the baby is in residence. The very fact of the baby's existence will be plenty to cope with: you'll be glad that you've done some emotional preparation in advance.

*Marriage and finances* are two areas in which you're sure to feel the conflict. Another subject of conflict is housing conditions (closely related to finances). Whether to move or to stay where you are and have less room is a question that can induce a surprising amount of stress.

Many of the questions raised in Chapter One may only come to a head now. Whatever conclusions you came to then may not apply now or may need revising. Don't be too surprised at the discrepancy between then and now, between theory and reality.

*Emotional turmoil* is a positive force in your adjustment to being pregnant and becoming a mother. Don't imagine that having second thoughts or fears (discussed later on in this chapter) means that you've made a mistake. You need to toss pregnancy around in your head the way one wrestles with any big life decision. Social conditioning implies that once a woman is pregnant she should walk around with a Madonna-like expression and attitude. Baloney. Being pregnant isn't all fun. Neither is being a parent. Accepting that reality is the best thing you can do for yourself and your child.

## TALK ABOUT WHAT YOU'RE FEELING

Communicate what you are feeling and thinking during your pregnancy. Talk to your mate. Talk to your friends. Talk to older women (whether your mother is included among them depends on your relationship with her, discussed later in this section under Grandparents and Others).

It is not uncommon for a pregnant woman to feel isolated nowadays. Many women are postponing motherhood until their thirties or even forties, and some are deciding against it altogether. You may find that you're the only pregnant person you know, or the first in your circle to have a baby. Also, most couples live far away or cut off from their extended families. It can be lonely. If that is true for you, find someone to talk to. The baby's father is the logical first choice, and he will also profit from hearing your thoughts and unburdening himself.

***Talk to your mate:*** You are both going through a lot of emotional flip-flops. Keep your channels of communication open. If you don't share your feelings with each other, they can create a distance between you, instead of being a way for you to understand and get closer to one another. Do not make the mistake of thinking, "He's got enough to worry about right now, so I won't bother him with this. It's too silly." What *is* silly is trying to deny or belittle your feelings. Unacknowledged feelings have a way of becoming a problem, which they won't if you communicate them. It is far better to tell your mate you don't think you're spending enough time together and have him explain why he disagrees and thinks you're being unreasonable than to harbor that feeling. Your resentment can accumulate until you feel angry and hurt, and then you explode. He then feels unjustly attacked, which he *has* been, because without any prior discussion, how could he possibly know what you've been feeling? Then you will have created a much more complicated problem. (See Food Craving on page 162 to see how lack of communication can manifest itself.)

***Your childbirth education teacher*** is an excellent person to talk to. You may choose a teacher fairly early in your pregnancy and make plans to start classes in your 7th month. But there is no reason why you can't call her up before that just to discuss something that may be bothering you. Some teachers will even invite you to do that when you first contact them. Childbirth instructors, for the most part, are sensitive, caring women who have dedicated a good part of their lives to helping other women through childbirth. They make fast, intense bonds with many of the women and couples they have trained, precisely because pregnancy is a time in people's lives when they need support. These teachers are aware of and sensitive to the needs and problems you may be encountering. Don't let their expertise and kindness go to waste if there is something bothering you.

*Talk to your friends,* even if they don't have children—in which case they may be interested in what you're going through, but not ideal confidantes. Imagine trying to discuss a difficult love affair, for example, with someone who has never been in love or made love. It may be like talking to a friendly person who nods and looks sympathetic but unfortunately speaks only Tibetan. Still, a friend is a friend, and you need yours now.

Those friends who have opted for a child-free lifestyle are unlikely to be able to give you the kind of support you need. Because of social and family pressures on them to procreate, they may feel defensive about their decision not to. Others may have ambivalent feelings about their decision not to have children (perhaps a mate who refuses—or a career which would not allow them enough time to be the kind of parents they would want to be). These women might feel confused and threatened by your pregnancy—talking intimately with you about it might make it worse. Some friends who have decided against being parents and have resolved their decision may not be terribly interested in helping you deal with your fears and conflicts.

*Early bird classes* are rare, unfortunately, but some communities have them. They are discussion groups designed for prospective parents anywhere from the 4th month of pregnancy on. Some of the group time may be spent discussing pratical issues like breast-feeding and baby care, but usually the primary purpose is as an outlet for the psychological changes of pregnancy. Early bird classes are usually organized by the people who are in charge of childbirth/ education classes; ask around in your community. If you're really energetic you might want to put together such a group yourself.

*Communicate with yourself: start keeping a journal.* Get a notebook and think of it as a place to let go of feelings and ideas that you may not want to share with anyone else. If you make a habit of writing in your journal—even one sentence a day—it will not only serve as an outlet but will help you focus on yourself. Writing in a diary at any time in your life can give you information and insights about yourself that you otherwise wouldn't take the time to recognize. A pregnancy journal is also a very special remembrance of this time in your life. You will no doubt cherish the notebook long after you've forgotten the daily hopes and fears, ups and downs, of pregnancy.

## DREAMS

Dreams can be vivid and sometimes disturbing. Do not be frightened by your dreams. As with dreams at any time, they can seem real—and you can be more impressionable about such things when you're pregnant. Dreams have an important function at this time in your life. Think of them as messages, information about yourself that you have no other way of finding out. Dreams are things to discuss— ideas to recognize. No matter how real they seem, don't get carried away thinking of them as realities.

***Dreams of mistreating the baby*** or not caring for him properly are common. They represent a realistic, legitimate fear: you probably don't know much about baby care and are worried about doing a good job. Try to see these dreams for what they are. If you dream that you haven't fed the baby and he shrivels up, don't start worrying that something is already wrong with your baby before delivery or that you want to harm him. The dream is not an omen—it simply reveals your underlying concern about "doing right" by your child, about your abilities as a parent.

***Dreams of losing the baby*** may have a meaning similar to the preceding kind of dream. The theme of losing the baby, however, may not necessarily be about losing the newborn. It may be your concern about losing the baby from your *uterus*—where you have had him all to yourself, closed and safe.

***Nightmares about the baby dying*** come from an understandable concern for your baby's health and perfection. If you have dreams like this near the end of your pregnancy they may be a defense mechanism. Everybody worries at one time or another that something will be wrong or go wrong with their baby—dreams like these may be a psychological preparation for a possible unwanted outcome.

***Nightmares,*** in general, may be a way of expressing *hostility* toward your unborn child. She is going to overtake your life, disrupt your privacy and comfortable routines. Nightmares can express feelings you may not be able to— or may not be consciously aware of. Again, don't make the mistake of taking dreams and nightmares literally and then feeling guilty or frightened. You may be more superstitious when you're pregnant, so don't let that tendency carry you away.

## THE EIGHTH MONTH

The 8th Month may be the most uncomfortable for you physically. The baby has almost reached maximum size and hasn't yet settled down into your pelvis ("engagement" or "lightening"). Your veins may be swollen; you may be short of breath, have less mobility, or have an embarrassingly leaky bladder. You'll probably feel pretty sick of your maternity clothes and fairly fed up with being pregnant. Impatience and anxiety about when the baby will arrive can start to nag at you.

***You must prepare*** for the physical separation from your baby, as well as the labor and delivery. You may dream about "losing" your baby (see previous page) or of having her delivered in some bizarre, frightening way. It is natural to be anxious about the Great Unknown of what your baby's journey into the world will be like—how childbirth will feel and how you will handle it. Dreams or daydreams are ways to express those concerns. As for losing your baby, ultimately every fetus is lost at the moment a baby is born.

***You need a lot of assurance*** at this time from your mate. You need to be reassured that he will support you through labor and delivery in whatever way you've agreed upon (even if it's in spirit only). Your mate may need some reassurance and comforting for similar concerns he may be having—so don't depend on him for all your assurance. Seek outside supports too. Turn to friends, relatives, your childbirth teacher, your midwife or doctor. This can be a tough time—you're sad that your pregnancy is over but eager to be done with it; you're excited about meeting your baby face-to-face but sad about losing her from inside you. You may be fearful about being a good mother. You need outside support and should make sure you get it.

***Do nice things*** for yourself. Get a pedicure. Go out to a lovely dinner. Take a drive. Go to the movies or to a concert. Do things to lift your spirits (if they need elevating) or just take your mind off yourself. Enjoy these last few weeks of precious time you have to yourself or as a couple.

***Practice breathing exercises*** from childbirth classes *every day* though your motivation may be low. Daily practice is essential to comfort and ease when the real thing happens. You may be getting Braxton-Hicks contractions (see page 158 for more information), which are not only accomplishing effacement of your cervix but are an excellent opportunity to practice your breathing exercises.

## FEARS

Fears of one kind or another have probably bothered you at some time during your pregnancy. You may have worried about some pill you took before you knew you were pregnant. You've probably been afraid of losing your freedom. Fear is nothing to be ashamed of—fear of the unknown is healthy. You dispel fear by getting information, by getting an understanding of what is happening.

*Acknowledge you are scared.* Unacknowledged feelings can assert themselves psychosomatically or through otherwise inexplicable behavior. If you deny your feelings there is a good chance that they will surface as some physical complaint (since you wouldn't pay any attention to them when they were "only" in your head!). Accept whatever you are feeling and do not discount your feelings or your mate's. Never say, for example, "I feel scared but there's no reason to be." Don't place judgment on your feelings— or feelings your mate is having. Listen. Deal with the feelings: get reassurance.

*The baby's normalcy* is a fear you may have at various times during your pregnancy. Everybody worries that her baby won't be perfect: that something has already gone wrong or will during delivery. It doesn't give you much comfort that only a tiny percentage of the babies born in this country have any problems. If you're a true worrier you'll be concerned that *someone* has to be in that small group and it may be *you!* It is more likely, however, that you will be in the majority and have a healthy baby. As with all fears, don't try to deny that you are worried: recognize the fear and then put it out of your mind. Worrying won't change anything. If you are superstitious (which is a trait that can get exaggerated during pregnancy) you may worry that too much worrying can *cause* something to go wrong with the baby. The only documented ill effect so far is loss of sleep for the mother!

*An inability to care for the baby* once he is born is a common and legitimate fear. Most middle-class Americans grow up isolated from childbirth and from early child care. American girls play with dolls and then they do some babysitting. This isn't a culture where there are babies around all the time so that you can learn by watching how to dress, diaper, feed, burp, calm, or amuse a newborn. Many women in this country don't have female relatives around when they're pregnant or after birth, so there is no trusted, experienced person to ease you into child care by leading the way. It is frighteningly overwhelming to be faced with a teeny, fragile newborn who is at the same time capable of raising hell if he doesn't get fed/burped/changed/soothed right this *instant!* As with all fears, the way to lessen them is to get information. So read books (Spock is still the tops), talk to people who have had babies *recently,* and try to spend time around any babies you can, just to get used to them. If you get accustomed to seeing how a little baby's face gets all scrunched up and red when he is having a good cry, it won't be such a shock when *your* little angel starts wailing and looks like he's going to burst!

*Loss of freedom* is another concern for prospective parents. Of the many fears you may have, this is the one to spend the most time thinking about. You *are* going to lose your freedom, it's that simple. One thing you can do is redefine what freedom means. If you cling to previous ideas that freedom means being able to go *wherever* you want exactly *when* you want then you are going to experience frustration and anger—having a child in your life makes that kind of freedom close to impossible. Even if you can afford full-time help, your schedule will still be secondary to breast-feeding, to care for a sick child, etc. Having a child means having to think about her health, education, and welfare a great deal of the time (more or less constantly!). Even when you're away from your baby, your "freedom" is compromised by having had to arrange for someone else to be with the child and to organize all her paraphernalia for the substitute; and then while you're away, you think about whether everything is all right at home.

What you lose when you become a parent is the spontaneity (or impulsiveness) of movement. Once you have a baby it's hard to make a move without considering the child. This is as true when you have a toddler and you want to walk into another room (risking total destruction of the first room if you don't think about the child!) as it is of planning a business trip. The conclusion of all this is not to fear your loss of freedom but to anticipate it. Spend some time now deciding what your priorities are and which activities—to do with business or pleasure—are the important ones for you. Once the baby arrives you will have less time for yourself. If you have decided ahead of time what you are *not* willing to give up, as well as what *is* expendable, you are less likely to experience the baby as "taking away" your freedom.

***Loss of attractiveness*** is something many women worry about. It is not merely a question of vanity, nor does it have only to do with American ideas about Thin Is Beautiful (although that may be part of it). Your body image changes when you are pregnant. It helps to understand how this affects you emotionally. If you once again recall adolescence, you will remember that your body-image changes in puberty had a powerful effect on you. Developing breasts, pubic hair, your first menstrual periods, stronger body odor—you had many things to adjust to. Pregnancy presents you with its own set of physical changes that demand your adaptation. Just as with puberty, pregnancy changes the way you look—the new shape of your body and therefore different clothes. Every woman has some idea about her body image: her stature, coloring, and the makeup and clothes she chooses. The way you look is tied up with the way you feel about yourself, with who you are, with how others perceive you. When you are pregnant, your body image changes, and this can be disconcerting to some women. They have to revise the way they "see" themselves and they have to get used to being "seen" differently by the outside world.

When women are afraid of losing their attractiveness during pregnancy it is usually their *sexual appeal* that they are concerned about. A large part of most people's identity has to do with which sex they are and how the opposite sex reacts to them. The feedback they get from other people reinforces their feelings about themselves—it is "stroking" from the outside world. If that feedback diminishes or is greatly changed, it can be disorienting.

I will exaggerate a little to dramatize what being pregnant can *feel* like to women who are used to getting a response to the way they look. A strikingly attractive woman, wearing a stylish outfit that accentuates her sleek figure and her graceful walk, comes into a restaurant. The captain rushes over and leads her to a table. Heads turn. Conversations undergo a slight pause. Men admire her, women admire her. Cut. The same woman comes to the same restaurant, only now she is six months pregnant. Her maternity dress billows around her as she waddles in, albeit gracefully. The captain takes her to a table; she has to go so slowly that he turns around to see if she's following. His is the only head that turns. To this woman, being ignored in public is like being hit with a wet washcloth. She may experience this change as mass rejection; she is no longer attractive, at least not the way she was before.

If you are feeling any loss of attractiveness, seek out reassurance. The most obvious place to go is to your mate, but start with yourself. Try to view what is happening to your body as a wondrous transformation. If you stop thinking of your bulging belly as fat, you will begin to see it as globelike, shining, and uniquely beautiful. A pregnant belly is a sensual, sensuous object; have you noticed how people want to stroke it? Once you have begun to perceive your changing body more positively, encourage your mate to do the same. If you want to hear nice things about yourself, don't go around saying "Ugh, I'm getting huge": You rob your mate of the chance to say, "You look fabulous," and you will most likely color the way he views your changing body. He has some adjustments to make too, and if you say, "Oooh, come feel how big our baby is getting," your chance of getting a positive response is greatly improved.

**Phobias and obsessions** may overtake you during pregnancy. You may get a car phobia and suddenly be very nervous about driving in a car. You may find that you are suddenly superstitious and obsessed with dreams and symbols. Phobias and obsessions are one way to express some of the fears you may be having (discussed earlier in this chapter). Pregnancy is an intense time in your life and you may experience many things more intensely. Don't worry, you aren't going crazy (no matter what other people say!).

**Questions** about your changing body and psyche, about labor and delivery, and about your baby may nag at you.

Read, ask, listen. That's the whole point of this book. And never precede a question with, "I know this doesn't matter, but . . ." or "This sounds stupid, but . . ." *No question is stupid: It is only stupid not to question.*

## MOOD SWINGS

Moodiness, known also as "emotional lability," affects all pregnant women at one time or another. You may have a wide range of rapidly shifting moods in response to situations that wouldn't generally trigger such extreme reactions. You may have unexplained crying, emotional outbursts, and attacks of anxiety.

*Hormonal changes* have to be considered along with the body-image changes and identity crisis that may be affecting you. Progesterone is produced in large amounts during most of your pregnancy and has a depressant effect on the central nervous system. It can feel as if you're walking around in a fog. Some women are more sensitive to these hormone changes. They are similar to the shift in the estrogen-progesterone balance which makes some women short-tempered and/or weepy before a period. If that has happened to you, be prepared now.

*Ambivalence* about being pregnant and about the baby may be a cause of shifts in your moods. As I've said before in this chapter, acknowledge your feelings, do not try to suppress them. It is *okay* to have mixed feelings about pregnancy and parenthood. Only a fool imagines that once a baby arrives, everything's going to be just as it was before. It's all going to be changed—and in ways that you have no way of knowing yet. Thinking ahead may make you wonder if you've done the right thing—at the right time—with the right mate. It is fine to have those feelings. Do not, however, expect that you can *resolve* your ambivalence and reach a place where you no longer feel any conflict. If parrecogents are honest with themselves, they will probably accept ambivalent feelings at times about their child(ren), regardless of how it goes—right through the twenty-first birthday (if not longer!).

*Depression, anxiety, confusion* are going to occur in even the most positive pregnancies. Try to roll with it and not make a big deal out of it. You will only prolong these periods if you feel the need to figure them out—*"Why* was I depressed on Wednesday? Nothing *seemed* to be wrong." If your instinct is that you *can't* figure out why, then leave it at that. Obviously if there are real problems in your life causing depression, you should deal with them and get help wherever you can. If you expect to have times of feeling low and realize they are a normal part of pregnancy, they will pass more readily.

*If you are 100 percent happy,* with none of these mood swings or other effects, *beware.* Look over your shoulder a lot because there may be a boomerang headed your way, carrying all the feelings you have suppressed or ignored. You may be denying a deep hostility or resentment toward your pregnancy. Many women are ambivalent about having a baby before they get pregnant. Others don't realize their ambivalence until well into the pregnancy when they begin to give it serious thought. These feelings may be so powerful that they are frightening, so you swallow them down and go through your pregnancy on an even keel, without the normal dips and turns. The result can be that these feelings will hit you like a ton of bricks one day, before the baby's birth or after. Unless you recognize these feelings for what they are, you could wind up taking it out on the child. Of course there may be women who genuinely are totally, 100 percent happy during their pregnancy—which is wonderful.

*Motherhood*—the process of "becoming mother"—is an awesome task. You may develop an identity for yourself as a mother that is separate from that of your own mother. You may accept those qualities you respected and valued in your mother and reject those aspects of her mothering that you disagreed with. This is a complex task full of guilt and conflict. You may feel some identity confusion with your own mother and other women until you sort this out. And unless you *do* go out of your way to consciously re-examine how you feel about what kind of mothering you (and your siblings, if any) had, you will unconsciously re-peat it. What you saw around you has become "fact" for you: whether a baby is picked up when she cries, whether a baby is chubby or thin, whether a baby is bundled with three layers in the carriage. You might automatically repeat what you saw and will socialize your child(ren) in the exact same way unless you stop to look at your feelings about mothering.

## THE GRANDPARENTS AND OTHERS

Parents, in-laws, and other people can be a source of com-fort and support during pregnancy and/or a meddlesome aggravation. Whichever the case in your life, you should be aware that whatever relationship is established with these people during pregnancy will probably continue during the early part of the baby's life. If you live far from the baby's grandparents then the only decision you have to make is whether you want your mother or your mate's mother to be there after the baby is born. That decision depends on how well you get along with those women and whether you want them to be the one(s) to help you through the first weeks.

But if you live within visiting distance of your par-ents or in-laws (or other people who have similar roles in your life) then during your pregnancy you must set the stage for how much involvement—or lack of the same—you want them to have later. It is great to have an extra pair of hands around during those first few weeks but your helper should be doing housework and cooking, freeing you to get to know your baby. Some grandparents will shun such "men-ial tasks" and want to take charge of the baby . . . which is not what you need. So try to honestly evaluate how it will be—even discuss it with your parents and in-laws if they are open enough to have a direct talk about it.

If you *know* you don't want any of them closely involved during the first weeks then don't let them get too involved in the day-to-day aspects of your pregnancy—because then they may *assume* they are going to have an active role in the early postpartum period.

## THE TWO OF YOU

Your relationship with your mate may have to weather some difficult times during your pregnancy. Nine months is a short time in which to make the rapid shift from being "just Alec and Cynthia" to being "Cynthia and Alec, parents of Neil." You have to change your entire orientation to the world and in a short time learn the underpinnings of each other. You are about to become Mommy and Daddy.

*A sense of permanency* is one effect that pregnancy has—it is like a seal on your marriage (or whatever other arrangement you may have). Now that there's going to be a baby it's no longer so easy to leave. Regardless of how good a relationship may be, this new bond may feel a little tight at first. Get used to the idea by talking to each other about it—agree ahead of time that neither of you will take the other's comments as a personal affront or rejection. You are discussing the sense of permanence a baby implies—don't let this spill over into the other areas of insecurity that can exist during pregnancy.

*There is a need to depend on someone* during pregnancy. Don't deny that pregnancy makes a difference, just admit it. Let your mate know how you are feeling and the ways in which you especially need him or her right now. The baby is a representation of your union and this may be the first time that you realize the extent to which you and your mate are interdependent psychologically, socially, and economically. This merger may feel like a trap—you may feel stifled by the *idea* of your diminished independence if that has been important to you prior to your pregnancy. The effect on your relationship may be that you fight the need to lean on your mate; you may even pull away from each other. Once you realize what's motivating you, you probably won't feel the need to withdraw.

*Evaluating each other* as prospective parents can be a source of conflict. Although in the past you may each have had daydreams about what kind of Mama and Papa your mate would be, now it is nearly a reality. You are evaluating "the father" in your mate and he is judging "the mother" in you. As mentioned earlier in this chapter *you* are evaluating *yourself* along the same lines, so being judged by your mate only compounds the confusion you may already be feeling.

Don't be surprised if you start criticizing little things about the baby's father—or if he does the same with you. This process of facing the reality of parenthood frequently causes tension in a couple. You may also find that you make unusual demands to test his loyalty and devotion to you. If these sorts of petty grievances do crop up, try to recognize them for what they are . . . and point it out to each other. As with many of the psychological changes you have to work through during pregnancy, if you do not understand why they are occurring—and "call" each other on them—then the friction and conflict can become problems in themselves.

## STRESS FACTORS

When you are pregnant you can be more sensitive to outside stresses. Any sort of problem—your health or that of relatives, your financial situation, marital discord, having to move, changing or ending a job—can be more difficult to cope with now. You should be aware that stress may hit you harder and you may not bounce back from it as easily as you did before you were pregnant.

A baby's activity in utero can also be affected: it increases when the mother is under emotional stress. Studies have shown that maternal emotional upsets lasting for long periods resulted in a prolonged increase in fetal activity: up to ten times the normal level. Some mothers find that when they are really tired their baby's movements increase then, too.

It is speculated that a relationship may exist between emotional stress during pregnancy and general restlessness in the newborn. A mother's anxiety in pregnancy has been linked to a newborn baby who cries more, particularly before feedings. These studies may be the flip side of the traditional saying that a happy pregnancy makes for a happy baby. But please don't think that because you are under considerable emotional pressure you will definitely have a fussy baby. By the same token, an easy pregnancy will in no way guarantee you an easy baby.

Stress during your pregnancy can be an impediment to the natural bonding process that occurs at birth. If you are under stress it may delay your preparation for the infant and retard your formation of a bond with the baby. During pregnancy a foundation is laid for maternal-infant bonding. If you skip any of the following stages in the process of creating that bond it can alter the bonding process, which is particularly likely to happen if you're under a lot of stress. Your subsequent relationship with your child may be affected.

First, you must get medical confirmation that you are pregnant; second, you have to accept the pregnancy. Third, you have to accept the fetus as a separate person even before he is born, a recognition that is often set in motion by the first sensations of fetal movements, which are signs that the baby is asserting himself.

Among the stressful events that may delay this process are:

• moving to a new geographic area
• marital infidelity
• death of a close friend or relative

As a *reaction* to stress you may experience one or more of the following symptoms, which suggest a conscious or unconscious rejection of the pregnancy, expecially if they persist beyond the first trimester:

• preoccupation with your physical appearance or a negative self-perception

- excessive physical complaints
- excessive emotional withdrawal or mood swings
- absence of emotional response to fetal movement
- lack of preparatory behavior in the last trimester (making plans and getting the baby's room and clothes ready)

If you are aware of some of these symptoms in yourself and know you are under stress, try to seek out professional help while you are pregnant. That way you can cope with the problems before the baby is born, and save yourselves heartache later.

## THE BABY'S FATHER

Many books and care-givers virtually ignore the baby's father. Aside from the physical carrying of the child, which of course he cannot experience, (though he may suffer from some of its symptoms; see page 242) a man is as deeply affected as the mother by pregnancy and birth. The health of the family depends partly on a man's successful transition to parenthood, yet there are few support systems to help prepare him. He is often left out of the pregnancy experience yet expected to deal with a woman who may be complaining and demanding, to cope with new financial burdens, and to struggle with his feelings about becoming a father. There is rarely any help for him. All the attention is focused on the baby's mother; the father's needs might as well not exist. This can cause justifiable resentment, followed by anger and withdrawal.

The coming of a child can mobilize a man's personal strengths or highlight his weaknesses. He needs to be encouraged to participate in the new threesome. The traditional concept of male virility did not allow a man to experience the nurturant feelings elicited by expectant parenthood. In the past a man was excluded from almost every aspect of pregnancy, birth, and early child care. That has changed now—or at least men now have the option to get more involved without risking their male identity, which has been redefined in recent years.

A mutual alliance is the essential foundation that al-

lows and encourages a man to take part in the pr
process. It is a difficult and exciting time for parei
you need each other in order for it to bring out the k
both of you.

## FEARS

Fears are as common in men as in woman, but it may not
be as socially acceptable for a man to admit to them. Encourage him. When a woman talks about her fears it can be
a natural extension of the discussion to ask what is worrying him. One fear a man will certainly have in common
with his mate concerns the *baby's normalcy;* the same advice given to mothers (see page 228) applies to fathers.

*Finances,* insurance, and other money issues are often
considered the man's domain. Though the coming of a child
*can* mean a real change in your finances, some men may
focus too heavily on the financial aspect as a defense against
more fundamental worries about competence and security.
A man can share his wife's fears about being able to care
properly for the baby, but he may express this fear by con-
centrating on finances, just as a woman may express her
need for additional attention by having food cravings.

*A loss of independence* is a common fear for men, particularly as a pregnant woman's changing identity becomes
more anchored to him. The woman does need to lean or
depend more heavily on her mate during pregnancy and
this can frighten a man, not just because it threatens his
sense of autonomy or independence but because he may be
unsure of whether he can give her the support she needs.
His anxieties may become more concrete in the third
trimester when the woman needs his help more because she
is less able to do for herself. In addition, the baby's room
is being readied as the due date nears, which can add to his
anxiety.

*Sex* is an area where a man may feel fearful. Some men feel
a drop in sex drive and activity during pregnancy. They are

afraid that they will hurt the fetus during sex regardless of whether medical facts contradict that. Do not be worried about this decrease in sex, which generally comes from positive feelings about the pregnancy. It is part of a man's increased protectiveness and nurturance—and a chance to put the baby's needs before his own. It does not matter whether there is proof that sex cannot hurt the baby; what matters is that his paternal drive is developing. For more information about sex during pregnancy, see Chapter Five.

## ENVY AND JEALOUSY

Envy can affect a man without his knowing it, so it may come out in disguised ways. The unconscious longing to experience pregnancy and birth may manifest itself in a burst of creativity or an increased drive to accomplish, which may be ways of sublimating the desire to be pregnant.

A man may also feel jealous of a woman's new *closeness with her mother* during pregnancy. He may feel shut out, fearful that she doesn't love or trust *him* enough. If your wife does have a renewed closeness with her mother (or other female friend or relative), be aware that this may hurt your feelings. It's natural for you to need reassurance that her attachment to you is not jeopardized by her closeness elsewhere.

## NURTURANT FEELINGS

Her mate's nurturant feelings may not even be noticed by a woman, but many men do feel more protective and gentle during pregnancy. A prospective father's needs are secondary and he has to learn to "mother" a woman—doing additional tasks, taking care of her in new ways. He may even become the prime mothering figure for her if her parents are far away.

*This may be a chance for a man to try out being nurturant* in anticipation of the baby's arrival.

*Nurturance also comes from a need to be more involved* and identified with the woman in order to begin a paternal tie to the coming infant.

*When a man's motherliness is awakened* during pregnancy he is better able to respond to his baby—and he can get great pleasure from his nurturance if the woman, and later the baby, are receptive. Dr. Erik Erikson has said, "Each sex can transcend itself to feel and represent the concerns of the other . . . so real men can partake of motherliness."

*Identification with feminine aspects of themselves* can be frightening to some men, however. Pregnancy precipitates this identification and can be so worrisome as to cause impotence. A man may throw himself into supermasculine (macho) endeavors in order to counteract this fear.

*A man has few socially acceptable ways* of expressing to others and himself that he will soon be a parent. Instead of (or in addition to) increased nurturance a man may take on extra chores or ready the house for the baby's arrival to express this nurturant drive.

*The Paternal role* is something a man has to prepare himself for and may be worried about. If his relationship with his own father has been good, he will probably be more relaxed about developing as a father. If his relationship with his father was bad, however, a man may distrust his own abilities to father.

    *Try to talk* about what you liked or disliked about your father and the way you interrelated. This will help you formulate your own image of what a good father should be. A man is reidentifying himself as a model for his child when he thinks about his own childhood and/or feelings of his possible inadequacy as a father himself. He will need support in thinking this through and asserting the best aspects of his personality.

***Pregnancy syndrome,*** also called the Couvade syndrome, is any symptom developed by a man which disappears after the birth of his child. The symptoms include: nausea, dizziness, heartburn, headache, abdominal cramps, constipation, diarrhea, food cravings, marked changes in appetite or weight during the prenatal period. These symptoms are not a psychiatric disorder but a way for a man to express identification and involvement with the pregnancy. However, they *are* a manifestation of deep psychological stress in anticipation of the birth. *Anxiety, envy,* and *hostility* can be expressed by pregnancy symptoms. A man may be feeling left out; he may be worrying whether his mate and the baby will be okay; he may be concerned that the woman will be even *more* withdrawn from him after the baby arrives.

Couvade syndrome can also be seen as a man's inner psychological reorganization in preparation for fatherhood. It can happen long-distance if the parents are separated. These pregnancy symptoms usually disappear right after the delivery of a healthy baby.

## WITHDRAWING

A man's reluctance to participate during labor and delivery can be detrimental to both partners. By supporting his mate through pregnancy and delivery a man is preparing himself for fatherhood. If he is present at his baby's birth, a man's paternal feelings can be aroused and the "bonding" that takes place then will encourage his later participation in child care. You get out of being a parent what you put in: men don't get much chance to "put in." By asserting his involvement with his mate and then with his baby, a man can claim the place that has been denied all men for too long. Both partners must be aggressive in assuring him that right and responsibility.

A woman should not view a man's disinterest as a personal insult or as a sign of a rift in their relationship. Pregnancy and child-rearing are areas where women are often several steps ahead of men, if only because the sexes are raised with such different attitudes about this. A woman has to be patient for her mate to catch up with her: she can hold out a loving hand and encourage him along the way or she can pout and withdraw and selfishly regard his lack of interest as an attack on her or the baby.

In order to involve a man during pregnancy you might ask him to read this book or others. You should be careful not to project an attitude (which women can do without even realizing it) of superior knowledge or sensitivity. Men feel excluded and uninformed as it is; if you are uppity in any way it can just reinforce his feeling of inadequacy and drive him away. If you want to go to childbirth education classes (see page 302) and your mate does not want to attend, ask him to come to one class. After that, if he is still against it tell him you'll use a friend as coach. Choose a class that is oriented to couples (not just to women) and that has a relaxed atmosphere. You might ask any couples you know who have been through prepared childbirth classes how the men liked the teacher and pick an instructor who gets a good "review" from other men.

If a man feels truly uncomfortable about participating in the labor and delivery, don't push it. Stick to your word and *do* choose a friend or relative to be your labor coach. A man may simply not be very interested in the birth process and it may take him weeks or months to really get turned on to the child. Let it happen at whatever his natural pace is or your enthusiasm or criticism may put him off even more.

However, there are two reasons for a man's adamant refusal to be involved that you may be able to alter:

1. *Fear of hospitals* is a reason some men are reluctant to be there during childbirth. Many people are afraid of hospitals—just on the general principle that they are places of sickness and death (which they are, primarily) or else because they had a bad experience in a hospital. Familiarize yourselves with the hospital you plan to deliver in, if you are having a hospital birth. Take the official tour, more than once, perhaps. Just getting used to the place may help alleviate his fears.

2. *Fear of inadequacy* is another reason some men choose to avoid staying with their mate at this crucial time in her life. Some men are quite squeamish and are afraid they won't handle themselves well during the messy parts of labor and delivery. Other men are more concerned about not being able to meet a woman's emotional/psychological needs during the rigors of childbirth. In both cases all that is needed is some gentle encouragement. Men who imagine that they will "faint seeing the blood" should talk to other men who have stayed by their mates' sides and been so involved that they hardly noticed whether there was blood or not. Men who may not feel equal to the emotional demands should be assured that their simple presence—even if they barely say a word or give more than a gentle pat— may make a woman feel more secure and relaxed.

*Running away,* either figuratively or literally, is a response some men have to pregnancy. They find excuses: longer working hours, sports events they "must" participate in during nonworking time, business trips, and the like. These men feel so overwhelmed by the external and internal demands of pending parenthood that they run away from these responsibilities and personal confrontations.

One danger is that this creates a vicious cycle: the woman feels ignored or abandoned and either makes outright demands on her husband to give her more time and attention or exhibits extravagant emotions to.get his attention. Either tactic simply drives a man like this farther away. His autonomy is threatened (see page 239). He is being called upon to *give:* this makes him feel suffocated or angry or inadequate.

It is not unlikely for a man like this to have an affair as a way of proving his independence to himself and asserting his denial of what is happening at home. Unless either or both partners can recognize his running away for what it is—and get help in the way of professional mediator—*the marriage may break up.* This is not just idle dramatics: marriages *do* break up during pregnancy or soon after a baby is born. In cases like this, such an outcome may be avoidable if the couple seeks help.

**Work** can take on new importance for a man when he is an expectant parent. He may throw himself into work for a variety of reasons. It may be his unconscious desire to procreate (see page 240). It may be his raised consciousness of duties as a provider and the additional income needed to support a child. And it may be a way to avoid facing the pregnancy. Impending fatherhood may so overwhelm him that he puts a great deal of energy into an area where he feels competent, safe, and ultimately rewarded—none of which he may feel about pregnancy and childbirth.

Whatever the reason that a man throws himself into work, do not make the shortsighted and self-centered mistake of regarding this as rejection or neglect of you. A man has to face and resolve his feelings about this crucial time in his life as best he can. Work is one area where a man may express some of these complicated and unfamiliar feelings.

Best of all, concentrate on the *quality* of time you spend together, not the *quantity*. Diminished time together will be a fact of life once the baby is born. Don't forget that *your* time will be more limited then, so don't get hung up now about your mate's long hours at work. Begin to view your time together as special time, to be utilized in ways that give both of you pleasure, relaxation, and stimulation.

# 5
# Sex

## SEX DURING PREGNANCY

Sex is what got you here in the first place, yet ironically sex during pregnancy can be touchy and anxiety-ridden. It doesn't have to be. Your sexual relationship has the potential to be more communicative and rewarding than ever before. In order to take advantage of this special time, you and your mate have to understand the ways in which your sex life may change during pregnancy, and then you have to *talk to each other* about it. If you both can overcome any reticence you may have about discussing or experimenting, pregnancy may give a new breadth to your sex life that can continue after the baby is born.

### ANXIETIES

*The most prevalent fear* is that sex will *harm the fetus.* Some people are afraid they will "infect" the passage. The fact is that intercourse does not introduce infection to the baby, who is safely protected by an intact bag of fluid on the other side of a closed cervix. Another fear is of crushing the baby. Nature has provided excellent cushioning for the fetus: a woman can even fall without harming her baby. If either partner remains fearful about hurting the baby, then talk to your doctor or midwife about it, together if necessary.

*Some people's anxiety comes out as guilt.* They are afraid that their increased sex drive during pregnancy can lead to abnormal sexual behavior later in their child. They are "projecting": the parent feels guilty and perhaps overwhelmed about this new eroticism and projects a judgment onto the baby, imagining that there must be a punishment (a sexually deranged child) to compensate for so much pleasure. Enjoy yourself—you deserve it. Pregnancy has so many *unpleasant* side effects that the very least you deserve is a good time in bed!

*The baby's reaction* to its parents' lovemaking can make some people anxious. A fetus does respond to sound waves and to his mother's movements (some of them sleep when their mother is active, and when she is napping or bathing, they wake up). After lovemaking some babies kick or squirm; this can give the impression that the baby is watching. Some parents are worried by this feeling that a third person is in the room (especially when it is an impressionable child!). Don't worry. The baby cannot see what you are doing. Some men actually have fantasies that the baby not only can see but might bite their penis.

*A fear of miscarriage* may affect either partner. Sex and orgasms have not been shown to have any bad effects on pregnancy, but if a couple is afraid, they are not going to enjoy intercourse. A woman may be so concerned about a possible miscarriage, particularly in the first trimester, that she would rather give her mate oral and/or genital pleasure but abstain herself. A good way to deal with this anxiety is to concentrate on massaging and caressing and especially talking things over. It is important to stay in touch emotionally as well as physically. Eventually the anxiety should subside if you take things slowly. The partner who is fearful needs validation first of all: he or she needs to know that the other person accepts the fear even if it isn't rational. Then you can ease past it.

*The role of sex in bringing on labor* makes some people anxious. Some doctors routinely prohibit sex during the last six weeks of pregnancy (without giving a reason—see page 265), which may reinforce some people's fears. However, labor will *not* start just because of coitus or nipple stimulation. It is true that if conditions are ripe for labor to begin, lovemaking can facilitate the progress of labor. Hormonal activity resulting from sex is the same as that during labor—and the sex hormones seem to enhance labor's progress.

Research hasn't determined what factors or hormonal balance cause labor to begin. Uterine contractions alone—which can be initiated by medical induction—do not cause cervical dilation. Similarly, uterine contractions resulting from orgasm are not linked to dilation. If you are already in labor, however, sexual stimulation can increase your contractions. Stimulation of the nipple has a direct physiological effect on the uterus, causing it to contract. This effect is the same whether it is from lovemaking or from the baby sucking later on—studies show that a breast pump stimulates uterine contractions during labor.

## BLEEDING

If bleeding accompanies intercourse it may not be serious but you should consult your doctor to rule out the possibility of miscarriage or other problems. In the first trimester, bleeding may be caused simply by a deep thrust by the man that brings his penis up against the cervix (the mouth of the uterus). The cervix is softer than usual during pregnancy and there is so much extra blood in the vessels that pressure may cause a small amount of bleeding. This is nothing to worry about; such bruises, which are like a nosebleed, heal quickly. This bleeding can be eliminated by avoiding deep penetration. Shallow penetration may solve the problems of pain or vaginal spotting after intercourse, but it is still worth the peace of mind to have any bleeding checked out by the doctor.

## WOMAN'S BODY IMAGE

This subject was discussed in the preceding chapter, which suggested ways in which the change in your body might be causing changes in your head. Perhaps the most significant way in which a woman's changing body image affects her is in the area of sexuality.

*The strangeness of your new body* shape may make it hard for you to accept this new image of yourself. You may lose confidence in your ability to attract your mate.

*You may recall times* in your life when you were heavy and think of this as the undesirable body you had before. It is important to recognize if "old tapes" are playing in your head, touching on negative feelings about yourself and your body you had in the past.

*Your fear may be that you are becoming fat,* which is a dirty word in America. We are conditioned to believe that if a woman is fat, she is undesirable. And fat (undesirable) women are ignored or abandoned by men. Thus the change in your body image may be making you worried, unconsciously, that your mate is going to leave you. If this anxiety is preying on you, it will certainly affect your ideas, conscious or not, about lovemaking—whether sex will help you "hold on to" your mate or drive him away (since you are unconsciously operating on the assumption that he is so disgusted by your new body that he is going to leave).

*Your mate may have less interest in sex* and you may translate his lack of turned-on-ness as displeasure with you physically. There are many reasons why a man's sex drive diminishes during pregnancy (see the section on Desire, page 252).

*Your mate may find your body ugly,* with the big belly and perhaps stretch marks. What may happen is that *you* will then feel ugly and then be angry at the baby for making you that way. Try instead to focus your attention and your mate's on the positive aspect of your new body.

*In the last trimester* you may get disgusted with your body. You may be sick of being pregnant and your awkward size. However, most men are *not* negatively affected by a woman's body at its most pregnant—and it may be your fear of this (or a projection of *your* disgust onto your mate) that is upsetting you as much as the body change itself.

**Certain body changes may be confusing and anxiety-provoking** for you. Early in pregnancy your breasts will increase in size and in the same way that breasts do when they are sexually stimulated. Then during sex they may become slightly more enlarged. See the section on Increased Desire on page 254, which covers a woman's possible guilt or anxiety about the increased eroticism that is part of her new body image.

**Take positive actions** to counteract your negative feelings about your body-image change. As with any of the irrational worries that may bother you during pregnancy it does not matter whether they "make sense" or not. They are your feelings and they are real. If your body-image change makes you feel insecure, then get reinforcement to bolster your ego. Your need for affection and reassurance increases—so get those needs met.

*Find the beauty* in the fullness of your new shape, because it is there. Share with your mate the changes that your body is going through and marvel at the transformation. Your belly can be a new part of you for both of you to enjoy. A pregnant belly is sensuous. The tight roundness feels good to run your hands over. And it is exciting later in the pregnancy to lie naked together and watch the baby move.

Some woman *like their bodies better* when they are pregnant. They find their new body image more positive than prepregnancy. They enjoy the new roundness and mystery, the feeling of ripening and creating. Try to see it that way yourself.

## COMMUNICATION

Communication about sex can be difficult—because most of us are raised *not* to discuss it—but it is essential during pregnancy. A lack of communication at this time can draw partners apart, when the honesty of shared feelings is so crucial to meeting their own and each other's needs.

***You have to be willing to discuss*** the fact that *your mate may be turned off* to your changing body shape and odor. Unless you can both discuss it as objectively as possible, the man may simply withdraw.

***You may be disgusted*** with your body. It is important to talk this out with your partner in order to resolve some of these feelings so that they don't control your sex life.

***The "dependency period"*** is roughly ten weeks before and after birth: this is a time when a pregnant woman feels the most vulnerable and needs the most support. However, although she may need reassurance during these sensitive weeks, she may often be giving off rejection signals. Unless a man and woman have learned to really talk to one another, the man is not going to realize that this is a "mixed message" and that the woman *really* needs and wants the most is stroking. Sex is especially beneficial during this time because it helps alleviate tension, which can build up as the due date nears. Also, when other kinds of communication fail, sex is a way of talking to each other without words, forming bonds that words might not be able to.

**SEX CAN EXPRESS UNACKNOWLEDGED FEELINGS** (which have been cautioned against in many sections of this book). Withholding and aggression can crop up in the sexual part of your relationship when they aren't acknowledged or resolved by other kinds of communication. The feelings of pregnancy are intense and changeable—the first step in handling them is to consciously acknowledge them. Refusing sex can be a way of expressing unmet needs or fears. Unless you realize that, the needs and fears will remain unresolved, and in addition, you will have a problem with your sexual relationship. Also, having intercourse when you don't want to can produce morning sickness. During pregnancy your mind and body (the psyche and the soma—thus the word *psychosomatic*) are particularly tuned into each other, so you have to pay special attention to your thoughts and feelings.

A MAN MAY WIND UP HAVING AN EXTRAMARITAL FORAY if the two of you have not nurtured an atmosphere of open communication. A prospective father may have an affair if he does not feel free to express *and* listen to the confusing, powerful emotions of this time in your lives.

GENTLE REASSURANCE is what both of you need from each other. You are both faced with a lot of new information and sensations during pregnancy and you need to support one another. If you talk about these personal, frightening feelings, the communication can create a stronger, deeper, more trusting relationship.

## A DECREASE IN THE MAN'S DESIRE FOR SEX

Sexual appetites can go through some dramatic changes during pregnancy—and the partners won't necessarily be feeling their interest increase or diminish at the same time. A decrease in sexual desire affects men and women for different reasons. There are several reasons for a decline in sexual interest for the man:

• FEAR OF HURTING THE FETUS, mentioned at the beginning of this chapter under Anxieties, is a major reason. Although it *is not possible* to hurt the baby during sex, some men will feel better if a doctor reassures them of this. However, the man's weight should never rest entirely on the woman without the support of his arms. Some men will still avoid sex—the rational facts cannot dispel their emotional response.

- **UNWILLINGNESS TO IMPOSE** on the woman, who may be tired or feeling some of the discomforts of pregnancy, is a reason some men back off of sex.
- **THE "MISTRESS/MOTHER CONFLICT"** is behind a decrease in sexual desire in many men, who may not even realize it. A man can have mixed feelings about the growing motherliness of the "girl" he married. His interest in you sexually may decrease as your belly grows because you become associated with his mother in his mind. This throws him into a conflict because there is a sexual taboo against a man sleeping with his mother. A man is usually not even aware that this is what is influencing him.
- **SEE THE SECTION ON THE MAN'S FEELINGS**, later in this chapter, which covers many of the sexual reactions a man may have to a pregnant woman, some of which cause him to withdraw from sexual activity.

## A WOMAN'S DECREASED SEX DRIVE

A decrease in a woman's sexual desire also has a number of causes:

- **FATIGUE, NAUSEA,** and some of the other physical discomforts of pregnancy don't make a woman feel very sexy. However, although there are physical deterrents to sex, it is often emotions—guilt, conflict—that have more effect on a woman's desire for sex or lack of it.
- **A WOMAN MAY FEEL A CONFLICT BETWEEN HER SEXUALITY AND HER DEVELOPING ROLE AS A MOTHER.** In making the transition to "mother" demanded by pregnancy, a woman may have some trouble integrating her sexual self (which she probably associates with her prepregnancy identity: a more self-centered, self-gratifying existence) and her maternal self (which in its purest, least realistic form has to do with being concerned with the child's well-being ahead of, or even instead of, her own). Until a woman has resolved some of this identity crisis in developing her mothering role, her interest in sex may dwindle. Some women have a hard time connecting the image of "mother" with the idea of sexual desire and activity. It

is important to sort this out to restore a healthy sex life, and also to pave the way for breast-feeding. Breast-feeding can stir up some of the same conflicts: sexual pleasure (which many women get from breast-feeding) versus breasts as the means by which to nourish a child.

- **IN THE THIRD TRIMESTER** a woman can lose interest in sex because all of her physical and mental energies are going into fixing up the house for the baby and getting ready for labor and delivery.

- **IF A WOMAN WHO IS UNINTERESTED** in sex makes love just to please her mate it can cause worse problems than abstaining. A man will feel her unspoken reserve and lack of enjoyment and *take it as a rejection of him*. A woman who makes love without wanting to is setting up barriers. If you don't want to make love it is important you tell your partner that your disinterest is caused by the anxieties and pressures of the pregnancy. These are times when both of you are very sensitive, so you must each guard against situations where you can take things the wrong way.

*You can stimulate* your sex drive in a number of ways. Plan a purposely sexy evening of candlelit dinner with wine and romantic music. You can read a sexy book together, or see an X-rated movie. Buy an outrageous negligee and surprise your mate with it. Or he can surprise you by wearing a raincoat with nothing underneath. Sure I'm kidding, but kidding-on-the-square. Enjoy yourselves. Laugh. Play out fantasies. Experiment. Each of you ask the other what his or her secret sexual fantasy is. Tease each other; fulfill each other.

## INCREASED SEX DRIVE

An increased desire for sex can grow. You may feel mentally and physically free because you don't have to worry about birth control. However, a major reason why many women feel an increased desire for sex is because a pregnant woman's body state is the same as a state of sexual arousal. The hormonal changes are the same as during arousal. The breasts and genital tissue are engorged with extra blood; there is increased vaginal lubrication and increased steroid and estrogen production. The vascularization of the pelvic viscera can explain the increased sexual tension a woman may feel in the second trimester. When sexually aroused a pregnant woman feels yet a further increase. She may get *vaginal sensations* in the night which are the equivalent of a man's "wet dream." Breasts are supersensitive to any arousal because the already engorged tissues become even more engorged (although the tenderness that may accompany will pass as the body accommodates to it).

Even women who usually have a low sex drive can feel a new urge. It can be frightening and feel all-consuming. *Talk about it with your mate.* Some women become very erotic and are obsessed with strange sexual fantasies. Some become preoccupied with sex and are then afraid that their increased sexual appetite will frighten their partner. Don't hide these feelings—share them with your mate.

The second trimester is the time when most women feel this increased eroticism. Some women reach orgasm for the first time in this period, and other women experience multiorgasmic capabilities. This is because of the increased blood flow to the pelvis, which means a woman becomes aroused more rapidly and more intensely.

## The Man's Feelings About Sex

Your partner's reactions to your body-image changes, your increased eroticism, and the coming baby all affect him sexually.

*The underlying change* is that a *woman is being transformed* right before his eyes. She can feel the changes going on inside and out, but he can only guess at them. A man has to make a mental and physical adjustment to a "new" woman—a woman who is different in many ways from the lady he has known.

*A man may be overwhelmed* by the "earth mother" aspect of your changing image: your superfeminine body, heavier scent, extra lubrication, and increased engorgement. It may be frightening to him. Give him a chance to adjust slowly.

*A man may become impotent* because of changes in your vagina. Because of your *engorgement* he may feel there's no room for him inside you; because of your *lubrication* he may feel there is too much room. Either feeling can make him lose his erection. This womanliness—this difference in you—may make him feel temporarily pressured and inadequate.

*Similarly, a man may feel inadequate* because you are now having rapid orgasms and he is going at the same rate he always was. Also, if you have become orgasmic—or multiorgasmic—for the first time a man has to adjust to this both physically and mentally. He may worry that he cannot meet your increased sexual needs or capacities.

*A man may turn to a nonpregnant woman* rather than trying to make love to his transformed mate. As with all these changes you will both be best able to cope with them by keeping your lines of communication open.

*Even if a man does not literally leave he may feel kicked out* by the fetus and withdraw emotionally. A man needs to feel that all your attention is not focused inward, that the baby is not getting all your love and energy. If he feels left out now, it will only be worse once the baby is born. Postpartum there will be times you will have *no choice* but to give your attention to the baby, instead of your husband.

*A man may feel guilty* receiving sexual gratification when a woman doesn't want any for herself. There are times when a pregnant woman is not interested in being aroused herself but wants to give pleasure to her mate. One example of this is a woman who is afraid that sex may cause a miscarriage. The man may be picking up signals that the woman does not really want to be giving him oral and/or genital stimulation, that she is doing it out of a sense of "duty." He must talk to her about this so that he doesn't have to feel guilty or in her "debt." Things must be straightened out so that a woman is participating sexually because she *wants* to.

***New forms of sexual behavior*** are not easy to get used to. We are all creatures of habit; change can be disorienting or frightening. Our attitudes toward sex are formed by what we learned in childhood and adolescence. For instance, some people may not be able to enjoy mutual masturbation (discussed on the following pages) because it feels regressive—unclean, something children do (and perhaps should not). Try out new sexual alternatives at your own pace and make an effort to talk together if either of you feels uncomfortable. If you still can't enjoy yourself then try something else. The whole point is to share enjoyment—it's not a test or contest.

*Exotic new postures* may be embarrassing at first. A man may be afraid of failing (consciously or not). He may fear that his penis is not big enough or his erection not hard enough for any positions other than ones he already knows and has tried. Once again, loving, gentle reassurance will get you through these awkward or funny moments.

## ALTERNATIVES TO INTERCOURSE

### MASSAGE

Massage is both an alternative to sexual intercourse and a lovely way to initiate lovemaking. You can say things with your hands, through stroking, that are beyond words. Massage creates a whole new avenue of communication and expression. It is also a wonderful way to rid your body of tension and really relax.

Once you become proficient at erotic massage, you will be giving your mate reassurance, pleasure, and love. If you have never given (or gotten!) a massage before, first get a nice oil. Any vegetable oil (olive, safflower, etc.) is fine, but it is more fun to get a pleasantly scented oil from a drugstore or a health-food store. First of all, the person to be massaged should have a warm shower or bath, to get extra clean and relax the body. Then place towels over the bed—or wherever you've chosen to give the massage—and have your mate lie down, naked. Cover him with two or three towels: they will keep him warm, feeling cozy and protected. Start with his hands. Coat the palms of your hands with some oil and then rub them together so that your hands and the oil are warmed. Then firmly caress his hand, pulling gently on each finger as you massage it. When you feel comfortable with your technique on each of his hands, move to his feet and do the same thing.

If you feel awkward giving a massage, you might want to buy any of the books now available that describe sensual massage with drawings or photographs. Basically you want to firmly and smoothly caress your mate's body, which can be as pleasurable and gratifying to you as it is to him. Using your hands skillfully shows your desire and love for your partner (even if your vagina doesn't want his penis right then, or vice versa).

Obviously all these suggestions apply equally whether the pregnant woman is receiving or giving the massage. The reason that I describe the man receiving a massage is only because so much attention is paid during pregnancy to what the woman wants and needs. I wanted to balance the scales a little and remind both of you that the man deserves loving care, too.

## MASTURBATION

Masturbation has an important place in your sex lives during pregnancy, but either of you may have hang-ups that you need to overcome first. Some women may feel guilty about their increased erotic needs. Once you read the earlier section of this chapter that explains the increased sex drive in a pregnant woman, you should be able to accept and enjoy this heightened eroticism. Masturbation is an excellent way to relieve sexual tension, particularly in the second trimester. Your mate may not be around, he may not be in the mood for sex, or you may have had intercourse with him and still feel aroused. If you have old "tapes" playing that tell you masturbating is evil or dirty, try to recognize them for what they are: the words of a generation of parents who were frightened or disgusted by sexual impulses and expression. Masturbating can be a very pleasant alternative or supplement to sex that you share with your mate.

*Although many women find they have orgasms more easily* during pregnancy, there are some who have a *fear of "letting go" sexually* when they are pregnant. They hold back the experience of orgasm, which in some women evokes the image of letting go or of releasing the fetus. Masturbation may be a way to overcome this feeling because it may give you a feeling of being more fully in control of the sexual situation. If you have difficulty reaching a climax during sexual intercourse, you might try masturbating—by yourself or with your mate—as a way of gradually overcoming the fear of letting go which may be inhibiting you.

*Mutual masturbation* is an excellent alternative to intercourse during pregnancy. It relieves tension and can encourage you to explore new sexual avenues together. Mutual masturbation, and variations on it, is the perfect answer when you want to share a sexual experience but either partner does not want to have coitus because of anxieties or discomfort.

*Using a vibrator* either when you are masturbating alone or together can add a fun and exciting dimension. Remember, pregnancy is a time for change. So if you haven't tried a vibrator before, you can make up for lost time now—and discover what you've been missing! And there's no harm to the baby from the minimal vibration or the noise.

*As with intercourse, if you have spotting, pain, or reasons to suspect you might miscarry,* abstain from orgasm with masturbation. The uterine contractions from an orgasm with masturbation can be even more intense than those from coitus.

## ORGASM

Orgasm is one of the areas of change in sex during pregnancy because there is an increased blood flow to the genitals, which increases sexuality.

***Some women experience orgasm for the first time*** when they are pregnant. Although this is exciting and pleasurable, it also involves some mental readjustments. If you have been anorgasmic you may have resigned yourself to it—discovering the thrill of orgasm for the first time will mean changing your mind-set about yourself sexually.

***If you become multiorgasmic for the first time*** you may feel overwhelmed and perhaps frightened by your new capacities and sexual appetite. Until now you may have always assumed that sex involved a period of arousal in which there was foreplay, then increasing sexual tension and excitement which reached a peak and a climax—and that was it. Then you'd lie in postcoital bliss, feeling drowsy and loving. Now you discover there is more! That first orgasm may go on longer than you've experienced before—or you may have an additional orgasm(s) on the heels of the first one—or you may still feel aroused after the first orgasm and want to continue energetic lovemaking. You have discovered that there is not just *one* peak, but perhaps several. Although some of this heightened sexual capacity may stay with you after pregnancy, much of it is one of the delightful side effects of your condition. If you feel disconcerted by this increased appetite, you should know that after the baby's birth it will return close to what it was prepregnancy. So don't feel worried—*feed* the appetite now while it's there!

## PROBLEMS WITH ORGASM

***Orgasmic problems*** for a pregnant woman are not uncommon. If you read all this and do *not* feel an increased orgasmic capacity you may wonder if there's something wrong with you. You may begin to worry about having orgasms. There is no better way to insure *not* having an orgasm than to be focused on wanting one (it is just the same as when a man is worried about erections—the more he worries, the more likely he is to be impotent). The best treatment is to create a relaxed, nondemanding space in which you feel loved and cared for. Make a conscious decision to have sex *without* orgasms—just for the pleasure of caressing and kissing. Take away the orientation toward a goal—remove the element of "achieving"—and you not only will enjoy sex again but will probably have an orgasm before you know it. Just remember that a strong desire for an orgasm can inhibit it. If you are having trouble reaching orgasm you can get more tense and make it even harder for yourself to relax, enjoy, and climax. Some of the reasons you may be having orgasmic problems are:

- You may generally have trouble relaxing because of anxiety about the impending birth. You may be worried about labor and whether you will be an adequate mother. Try giving each other massages as an introduction to lovemaking. It can relax you and relieve any pressure you might be feeling about your sexuality and orgasmic capabilities.
- When you are pregnant your life is out of control and you know it. The pregnancy and baby have taken over. This fear of a loss of control can lead to generalized tension in some women. For them orgasm may equal "letting go." They are so anxious about this feeling of their life being out of control that sex and orgasm are areas where they can express their fear and "hold on" by not climaxing.

*Some women's genitals remain engorged* even after orgasm in late pregnancy. This may mean that lovemaking leaves them in a state of continued sexual tension; a state of lingering semiarousal. Orgasm occasionally fails to relieve this tension. Some women compulsively seek orgasmic release but don't get it regardless of how many orgasms they have. If you have this feeling of continuing sexual tension, you should know that it is because of the increased blood flow to your genitals, which can take quite a while to subside. The more you are stimulated, the longer this tension will remain.

*Uterine spasms after orgasm* may occur in the third trimester instead of the rhythmic contractions you are accustomed to with orgasm. Near term some women may have regularly recurring contractions for as long as half an hour after orgasm. Pain and abdominal cramping are also possible, although usually in women who are having their first baby. This residual vasocongestion can become chronic. In a woman who is pregnant for the first time, the postorgasm resolution can be 10 to 15 minutes longer than prepregnancy. If this is not your first baby, you may find that it takes your body 30 to 45 minutes longer than before you were pregnant for your body to return to a relaxed state.

*The rate of orgasms often declines* in the last trimester. So if you find you are less orgasmic as your due date nears, be assured it is normal.

*Early labor contractions are similar* in rhythm and intensity to the uterine contractions of an orgasm. People often liken labor contractions to bad menstrual cramps—but labor is a lot more fun to anticipate (and easier to tolerate) if you look at it in this rosier light!

*If you were wondering how the contractions of orgasm affect the fetus*—they do cause a slight change in the fetal heart rate. This change does no harm. Think of it as giving your baby a nice ride in your contracting uterus.

## POSITIONS

Positions for lovemaking have to be adjusted to your pregnant body; as the fetus grows you have to try new ways to be comfortable during intercourse. For conservative people this experimentation with new positions and alternate modes of sex can be threatening. It may make them feel guilty or they may try to avoid sex altogether. Take it a little at a time and go back to positions you are comfortable with if you get uptight. You must protect yourselves from having strain develop in your sex life. These new explorations can give you increased pleasure, both during the pregnancy and in your continuing lives together. If either of you feels really hung-up about new positions or an otherwise expanded sexual relationship, think of it this way: sex is good for you and your baby. Intercourse is good exercise for the pelvic-floor muscles. You need these muscles to be in prime condition for labor and delivery. So the message to these people is: make love as much as you can.

If you continue to feel guilty due to how good it feels, you can rationalize that it's for your own good!

*One position* which will carry you through most of pregnancy is with the *man on top but lying partly sideways* so that most of his weight is off of you.

*The woman-on-top position* is comfortable for many people, especially because the woman can control how deep the penetration is.

*Side positions*—either front-to-back or front-to-front—are excellent during pregnancy. There is no pressure on your belly, which can now be caressed as a new erogenous zone. Side positions can give you both a whole new perspective on lovemaking, freeing your hands for exploration and letting you see each other in a new light. A side position with the man behind so that you can fit together like a "spoon" is good for the end of pregnancy when the woman's belly is largest.

## VAGINAL SECRETIONS

There are increased secretions when you are pregnant. These secretions may also have a strong odor, which can be a turnoff to you or your mate. Douching will not stop the secretions or their smell (see Douching on page 182). The change in the odor or taste of this extra lubrication is caused by the increased blood supply to your genitals during pregnancy. One way to change the scent is to massage the area with a scented oil, perhaps the same one you may be using for massages. Health-food stores and some drugstores sell oils scented with lemon, spices, or other scents.

## THIRD TRIMESTER

This can be the most awkward time sexually. Your belly is big and it may be cumbersome. You get tired more easily; ordinary physical movements can be more difficult. This doesn't leave you with much enthusiasm for sex or much energy once you are making love.

*Certain positions* may be more comfortable, particularly rear-entry positions with the woman standing and bending over or on her side and the man behind.

*You may want to avoid maximum penetration positions* not only because they may be uncomfortable but because they may also cause anxiety.

*Mutual masturbation* can be very satisfying in the last trimester. It can open communication between you and your mate and can lead you into sexual experimentation, which will add new richness to your sexual relationship.

*In the latter part of pregnancy many women feel the need for increased affection.* Hugging and kissing not specifically related to sexual intercourse can meet this need. It can also be lovely just to lie together and cuddle: touching, caressing, massaging, and just looking at each other without talking. These kinds of "nonsexual" (i.e., nonpenetration and perhaps nonorgasmic) times can be intensely romantic and bring you closer together.

## FORCED ABSTINENCE

This can be a big strain on a relationship. Some women do withdraw emotionally during pregnancy, and if this is coupled with a ban on sex by your obstetrician it can drive the man elsewhere to get his emotional and physical needs met. Sex is an important outlet for many feelings (anger, anxiety, insecurity) that you may not be conscious of during pregnancy; sex is also a way to express love and affection. If this avenue of communication is shut off, it can do real damage to a couple who are already riding on the roller coaster of pregnancy.

Some doctors still routinely say to abstain from sex for the last 6 weeks of a pregnancy. Most of these doctors do not give a reason for this decree. Don't just follow these orders without understanding *why* you can't make love. You don't need any more strains on your relationship than are absolutely necessary; and a long, forced abstinence can be damaging. There are many people who make love right up to delivery time. There are many doctors who put no restrictions on a couple's sex life. If your doctor's orders to abstain seem very rigid, then discuss it with him. Consult another doctor if you are not fully convinced of his reasoning. The chart below outlines the accepted reasons for banning sex.

---

**CHART 26. WARNINGS ABOUT SEX DURING PREGNANCY**

---

1. BLOWING AIR INTO THE VAGINA CAN BE DANGEROUS. This is the only sexual activity that has been documented as potentially harmful. (But who does this anyway?!) By doing this you can detach the placenta from the uterine wall and cause an air embolism. *This does not rule out cunnilingus.*
2. THE MAN'S ENTIRE WEIGHT SHOULD NEVER BE ON THE WOMAN. He should support himself at least partially with his arms if he is on top or lie slightly sideways. A corollary warning is that *great pressure should never be put on the uterus.*
3. REASONS FOR NO SEX AT ANY TIME:
    - vaginal or abdominal pain
    - uterine bleeding
    - membranes have ruptured
    - you have been warned or think miscarriage might occur

## THE SEXUAL ASPECT OF BIRTH

It is usually after home birth that women discuss the sexual and/or sensual aspect of their experience. A woman in a hospital may not be aware of the sexual side of childbirth because it is an authoritarian atmosphere with rigid routine procedures. A woman cannot feel emotionally free in that setting, which is controlled by the people in charge. The laboring woman has never even seen most of the people who come in and out of the room and examine her or tend to equipment.

Regardless of whether a woman feels free to experience the sexual aspect of birth, it does exist. It may not be a directly sexual experience for her, but the sexual overtones are there, though they may be unconscious. Childbirth creates an emotional bond which some women do feel despite the hospital environment. This sexual undercurrent may be the reason that women who do not have their mate with them during birth have "fallen in love" with their obstetricians afterward.

A few women experience birth as intensely sexual. Some of them have an orgasm at the moment of birth; it can be a sexual experience for a couple. In a socially permissive atmosphere a woman may masturbate or want to be masturbated to orgasm during the first stage of labor. She may experience the second stage as an orgasm with each contraction. The birth itself may be one huge orgasm. Although this is not a widespread phenomenon, it does happen—and not just to women in out-of-hospital settings. If nothing else, it can be an indicator that there is a sexual aspect to birth even if it is usually suppressed or ignored.

There are certain similarities between intercourse, the birth of a baby, and breast-feeding. Some conservative people may insist that women who have intensely sexual experiences during birth or breast-feeding are "weird" or "are imagining it." The chart on page 267 shows that the links do exist—it is simply a matter of recognizing them. If you are interested in exploring the sexual aspect of your labor and delivery, you will need an environment in which you feel both freedom and support. Once you are aware of the physical ways in which birth is sensual and sexual, you will have to be able to let go emotionally. Even then not every woman will have a dramatically sexual experience, but she may connect with that aspect of the experience.

---

**CHART 27. SIMILARITIES BETWEEN INTERCOURSE, BIRTH, AND BREAST-FEEDING**

---

1. In all cases the uterus contracts rhythmically.
2. The genital area becomes engorged with blood and the vagina lubricates and opens.
3. The genitals go through rhythmic spasms. In orgasm there are 3 to 12 throbs, and in birth there are hours of regular and progressively stronger contractions. Many women have contractions during breast-feeding.
4. The stimulation of the breasts and other erogenous zones releases oxytocin, which makes labor progress more rapidly and in sexual intercourse brings a woman closer to orgasm. Some women have orgasms or come close to them from the stimulation of breast-feeding.
5. The sounds that a woman makes during labor often sound like orgasmic noises.
6. A woman's position for birth and sex is the same: on her back with her legs wide apart and bent.
7. There is a tendency in all three situations to become uninhibited.
8. There is a tendency to be unaware of the world with a sudden return to alertness or awareness after birth or after a sexual climax—with a feeling of joy and well-being afterward. This is also true on a smaller scale for breast-feeding.

---

## POSTPARTUM SEX

Your body has many changes to undergo after birth, all of which can affect your sex life. Your hormones must readjust to prepregnancy levels. Your blood supply and the fluid content in your body must be reduced. Your uterus and vagina have to return to their normal size. Your perineum

has to recover from any tears or bruises or from an episiotomy. And your milk supply has to be either established
or repressed. All that has to take place while you are also
getting accustomed to being a parent and having a new little
person in the house. Recognize what a tremendous upheaval you are going through internally and externally and
give yourself time to cope with it all.

## ANXIETIES MAY INTERFERE WITH POSTPARTUM SEX

*The fear of getting pregnant* may bother some people.
It is something you haven't had to worry about for a while,
and resuming birth control can be worrisome and/or annoying.

*You may be worried* about being "all together again"
internally and be cautious about sex play for this reason.
Generally it is safe to assume that when the lochia has
stopped, the uterus has healed. Lochia is the menstrual-like
flow of the uterine lining that lasts for a week or two after
delivery (see page 274). Some women may still be fearful
after the lochia has stopped, and need to proceed slowly
with resuming sex.

*Your mate may be worried about hurting you.* You
probably will be tender at first and it may upset him to
think he is causing you any pain.

*Fear that the baby will cry* when you are in the middle
of lovemaking is a common concern. It is hard to adjust to
a new presence in the house, and you may not feel as free
as before or as able to be abandoned since you're listening
for the baby.

*Fear that the baby will get infected* from love play is
something you should not worry about unless the father is
genuinely ill—with strep throat, for instance. A child adapts
to the flora of both parents—there is no reason not to make
love and then breast-feed the baby.

## THE BABY'S INFLUENCE ON SEX

***The child can be felt as an intruder,*** ruining your privacy. You may be worried that she will need attention during intimate moments or quiet times with your mate. The baby will undoubtedly intrude on you at awkward moments whether it's right in the middle of passionate lovemaking or when you are playing cards together. *The important thing is to get back to those intimate moments after the interruption.* Learn to be somewhat flexible and not allow the baby's needs to put an end to whatever you were doing—do not let it be more than an interruption. The other solution is to take advantage of other times together with your mate. Just remember: it's your house and your life. Don't let the baby take it away from you by giving up control of your life in deference to the child's needs.

***A woman can get absorbed*** in her baby. You can be so satisfied with your attachment to the baby that you have little need for other emotional ties. However, your mate's emotional needs are the same as—if not greater than—they were before the baby's birth. He is unlikely to be getting the same kind of satisfaction from the baby that you are.

***Physical contact*** with the baby can also be very satisfying to a woman—sometimes to the exclusion of her mate. Your desire to hold, touch, and caress may be met by the baby. The intimacy of this mothering can decrease your interest in lovemaking.

***The baby can demand a woman's energy almost full-time*** if she is home all day. By the time your mate comes home and you have put the baby down for the night you may *need time and space for yourself.* Your mate may want to spend time with you, however. The baby's demands on you have come first and tired you out, which can leave the man feeling uncared for.

## BREAST-FEEDING AND SEX

Lactation alters your estrogen levels and prolongs suppression of ovarian steroid production. Despite this hormone suppression, many women feel a higher sexual interest than prepregnancy. It was thought at one time that this suppression was effective for contraceptive purposes, but it *simply is not reliable:* some women ovulate despite the fact that ovulation is theoretically suppressed.

### INCREASED SEXUAL STIMULATION

*Some women* find that nursing puts them more in touch with themselves and their bodies, which can heighten their sexuality.

*The hormone oxytocin,* which is produced during sucking, is a sexual stimulant. Often the suckling of the baby can also produce sexual stimulation, up to and sometimes including orgasm.

Women who become aroused to this point may feel guilt and have fears about a perverted sexual interest in the baby. Relax. Nursing feels good. It causes hormones that are sexually arousing to be released into your system. That's all there is to it.

Women who find nursing very sexual—to the point of orgasm, for instance—can direct this eroticism toward their mate. You can enjoy this sensuality with your mate rather than regard it as something he is excluded from, even though it was initiated between you and the baby.

Many nursing women experience heightened sexual pleasure and more intense or frequent orgasms. The hormones enlarge your veins and promote growth of new blood vessels in your pelvis. This raises the response potential of your vagina and clitoris.

### DECREASE IN SEXUALITY

*Nursing does inhibit* vaginal lubrication, although it doesn't prevent sexual responsiveness. Use unscented K-Y

Jelly if you have this problem (for more information see page 272).

*The lowered estrogen* levels that lactation prolongs (and which account for decreased lubrication) can also mean a lowered interest in sex. It is quite normal not to want sex or not to be turned on easily. Knowing this can prevent your mate from feeling rejected or confused. Some women who do not choose to breast-feed may be unwilling to experience the possible sexual stimulation from suckling, or the conflict between baby and husband.

*Some breast-feeding women* have painful cramps during intercourse. This might mean you will want to postpone sex until your body has balanced itself.

*Breasts themselves* can be symbolic of a tug-of-war a woman may feel. You may be uptight about your mate sharing the "baby's" breasts—later on you may want your breasts to be for your mate and not for the baby any longer. The larger issue is whether a woman can love both her baby and her mate without feeling a conflict in her devotion to either of them. A man can often feel neglected in favor of the baby—and be sexually jealous when the baby is fed.

## CONFLICT BETWEEN MOTHERING AND SEX

Some women may feel a clash between their self-image as a mother and that of a sexy, abandoned lovemaking partner. This is part of the ongoing identity crisis discussed at length in Chapter Four. It is important that you sit down and discuss this conflict as calmly as possible. If you do not face and resolve this question, it may cause harm to your relationship.

## PHYSICAL CHANGES AND SEX

Even when normal levels of psychic eroticism return, your physiologic responses to sexual stimuli may be delayed and diminished compared to prepregnancy levels. For instance, your vaginal walls are thin and lubrication is sparse for several months postpartum. This means your body will not respond sexually in ways you are accustomed to. You may feel much better after your first period.

*Your diaphragm* has to be refitted after childbirth, when you will probably need a larger size. At first, insertion may be difficult and painful.

*Exhaustion* may leave you too tired for sex. It takes your body a full 6 weeks to recover from childbirth. On top of that you have the new demands of your baby to cope with. Try to explain this to your mate; sometimes men have a hard time really understanding what this exhaustion feels like. Your mate may feel you are using this as an "excuse." If so, let him spend a day alone with the baby. Don't do it in a hostile way, but simply to let him get an idea of how you may be feeling.

*Hormones* play a large part in sexual readjustment. Estrogen levels are low after birth and will remain low if you are breast-feeding. Some women take longer postpartum to return to a hormonal balance. This requires patience on both your parts. A woman may need extra fondling, kissing, and other foreplay to become aroused. Don't worry—you will be functioning normally before long. Low estrogen levels may be one reason for low sexual interest. Hormone imbalance is also the reason for insufficient lubrication, and breast-feeding will prolong this condition. Use unscented K-Y Jelly or have a doctor prescribe estrogen cream until your vaginal lubrication returns to normal.

## PAIN DURING SEX

*Pain* during postpartum intercourse is something many women do not expect. Unless you are prepared for it, you may be shocked by the intensity of pain. Even women who have had cesarean deliveries can have this discomfort. It can occur at the vaginal opening or inside the vagina; there can be irritation, even with the use of jelly.

Do not do too much at first so that you won't get spooked. Take it easy.

It is a good idea to have the woman on top during lovemaking. That way she can control the entrance of her mate's penis. If you are still somewhat dry, you will want to be especially careful and have him come inside gradually.

*Your mate can go in gently and stay inside you without moving much.* Build up your sexual stamina gradually. Be patient with yourself and communicate to your mate what you are feeling and what you do or don't want to do sexually at this point.

*Your perineum* may be sore and stiff after childbirth. There may be tears and bruises that have to heal. If you don't let your mate know and just grit your teeth, you will come to dread even the thought of intercourse. A coldness and touchiness can then build up between you. Your mate may feel rejected. Give yourself a chance to return to normal—attempt sex gradually and with lubricating jelly, if necessary. But let your mate know how you're feeling and why.

*An episiotomy* can make sex especially difficult. (See the section on Episiotomy on page 481 for more information.) A warm bath right before lovemaking may help. Do not use Vaseline or other non-water-soluble lubricants. They can keep the air out and allow bacteria to grow in the episiotomy site. A good position after an episiotomy or with a sore perineum is for both of you to lie on your sides with your mate behind you, "spoon" fashion.

## PHYSICAL INTERRUPTIONS TO SEX

*Leaking milk* can interrupt your sex life. Be prepared for leakage at unpredictable times. Many women lose breast milk in uncontrolled spurts when they are sexually aroused and during orgasm. If the baby cries in another room your breast milk may start to flow, which can elicit the conflicted feelings about mate and baby discussed earlier in this chapter. If the parents are fastidious, this leaking may turn them off. You may feel disgusted with your body and its secretions. There's not much to do about it except take a bath or shower together after making love and clean up the spilt milk without worrying about it too much!

*Lochia,* the postpartum vaginal discharge, may also leak during sex. If you are accustomed to lovemaking when you have your period then this is virtually the same thing. If you have always avoided sex at that time, you may have a negative reaction to lochia, although the flow should not be as great as from a menstrual period if you are taking it easy postpartum. You may feel disgusted by your body and these secretions. It may help you to think of it as your body cleaning itself out after pregnancy and birth—think of it as a *good thing,* as steps on the road to the return of your normal body and its functions.

## RESUMING SEX AFTER BIRTH

Although there are many doctors who suggest a 4- to 6-week wait after delivery, many couples do not wait that long. There are several reasons to start having sex again as soon as possible after the baby is born. Some couples stop having sex 6 weeks before birth and then wait for 6 weeks afterward: that is *3 months* without sex. Even if these couples use alternatives to intercourse, this "celibacy" may not be necessary. The frustration this causes in a relationship can surface in many ways and create needless problems. The six weeks before and after childbirth are a time when sex can be most important and helpful.

### WHEN TO RESUME SEX?

*A 6-week wait* is too conservative for many women. A rapid resumption is better for them—they start having sex 2 to 3 weeks after childbirth and feel great.

*If you had no lacerations* and no episiotomy, there is no reason not to resume within three weeks if you feel the

desire to. Check with your doctor, but if you feel his recommendation is too conservative, then ask another doctor.
However, note the two conditions below before resuming.

*A good way to judge* whether your body is ready for sex
is to wait for it to recover from the delivery. Recovery is
generally complete when the *lochia disappears,* which
means that the placental site has healed and/or *when your
episiotomy incision has healed.* There is a potential risk of
infection until then. Again, check with a doctor if you have
any doubts.

### REASONS FOR RAPID RESUMPTION OF SEX

*Sex reduces tensions.* It is one of the few nonverbal (and
nonhostile!) ways that are available to you and your mate
as an outlet for tension.

*Sex reaffirms your desirability.* Many women come to
doubt their attractiveness while they are pregnant, particularly in the last trimester. By resuming sex you begin to
rebuild a positive self-image in this area.

*The hormonal climate* of sexual activity speeds the uterus
to its prepregnant state in the same way breast-feeding does.
It releases hormones that help return your body to normal—and you to *feeling* normal.

### LOW INTEREST IN SEX POSTPARTUM FOR THE WOMAN

*Lowered estrogen levels,* mentioned earlier in this section, account for some of your possible disinterest in sex.

*A woman's physical and emotional energies* are often
so used up by the baby that there is a delay in the return of
her sexual interest.

*Low sexual interest* may also come from the trauma of
having your life turned upside down, with the arrival of the
newborn and his constant needs. This upheaval may give
you the feeling that your own needs are not being met. *You*

may want to be nurtured for a while without the expectation of sexual intercourse attached to it.

*Sexual activities* short of intercourse seem to be a good solution to this time in your lives. "Pleasuring" is most satisfying to a woman who isn't ready yet for sexual intercourse. Sensual exchanges that include stroking, massaging, and stimulation for the fun of it, rather than as a prelude to intercourse can get you through this transitional time and set the foundation for when your normal sex drive returns.

### DECREASED SEXUAL DRIVE IN THE MAN

*A man may be turned off* sexually from watching the birth. A woman in labor may be frighteningly different from her usual "feminine" self—the noises she makes, her facial contortions, the uninhibited positions she is in may give a man a general impression of an earth goddess. It can be an overwhelming image for a man to integrate into his conception of his partner.

*It may be hard for a man* to believe that his wife's body will ever return to a size that is appropriate for his penis. It can be helpful to a man to try and appreciate the wondrous nature of the vagina—and to realize that it can grow and shrink just as a penis does.

*A man's acceptance* of the changes in a woman's vagina during labor and delivery can help her deal with the fear *she* may be having: "Will I ever be the same again?" It will help you both readjust to sex if you realize that the vagina is designed to make room for the passage of a baby and then to resume its previous size.

*It can take time* for a man to get used to the idea that the lovely, dark, warm place that has always been there just for him has a fantastic and practical function as an exit for the baby! Making love may be difficult until a man gets used to this new concept. Some women may have the same hesitation.

***If a man "knows" ahead of time*** that his sexual attitudes are going to be negatively affected by the birth then it may be better for him not to be there. If he is positive he'll feel this way, then he will create that feeling for himself. And his negative attitude may make it hard for the woman to open up and relax, which is necessary during labor and delivery. Instead of reducing anxiety—which is a main reason for having a mate present—a man with this outlook may increase the tension.

# 6

# Choices in childbirth

You have many options about where you will give birth and who will attend you. In order to decide what is the right setting for you—and what technical aids and attendants you do or do not want—you need to know the pros and cons of the available choices in childbirth. Your community may not offer all the possible options but *you can change that.* This chapter not only describes the choices that exist but it also suggests ways in which you can broaden the opportunities if they are limited where you live.

Time is short. You're about to get pregnant or you already are, so you have to move quickly if you want to bring about change. Consumer pressure and protest are the most effective tools you have. Forming a consumer group, writing letters, and even picketing all bring results. The area in which these tactics are most powerful is *within the hospital.* Because hospitals are profit-making institutions they *need your business:* they have to at least listen to you if they hope to get you or keep you as a customer. However, if you live in a "one hospital town," the monopoly principle applies—if you have no "hospital down the block" to turn to as a threat, then you haven't got as much leverage. The same is true on a lesser scale for doctors. The next chapter, Choosing a Doctor and a Hospital, goes into this in depth.

In terms of out-of-hospital choices (see chart on page

281), you do not have the same kind of consumer power. If these options for where to give birth do not exist you cannot just *create* them. Obviously if you decide to have your baby at home you have the power to make that choice. But if your community has no one who can attend you at home or if the existing medical facilities are so antagonistic that they won't offer you emergency backup care—then your freedom of birth choice has been severely limited by the community. If no doctors in your area offer deliveries in their office your only option is to ask one or two if they would—although you're unlikely to find one who is willing. However, as more couples question and challenge the Establishment—and if that status quo is inflexible in the face of consumer demands—then you will see more out-of-hospital alternatives surfacing.

There are certain rules of thumb you might want to follow in getting what you want in a childbirth experience.

***Ask, don't demand*** is the first suggestion. Simply by asking for anything you are questioning authority. You are calling into question the expertise and years of experience of professionals. Except in the rarest cases this is threatening to them. When people feel threatened they get on the defensive; they become hostile, belligerent, and indignant. Once they feel like that, the *last* thing they're going to do is alter their routine and grant your request.

It doesn't matter whether what you want is "right"—morally, legally, or medically. If you think in those terms you will go in with a chip on your shoulder and a superior attitude . . . and lessen your chances of getting what you want. Keep your objective in mind. Remember that you have limited time and that you want to change what may be a long-standing system. You have to go about getting what you want in the most expedient way. This may be one of the few times in life when the means justify the ends; i.e., it is to your ultimate benefit to adopt whatever attitude will get you results.

***Give reasons*** for what you want. Learn as much as you possibly can ahead of time. The powers-that-be are more likely to listen—to really pay attention—if you make a convincing case for your request. Know the possible arguments in advance so that you'll be prepared to answer them as well. If you know both the pros and cons of what you want and what is currently offered, then you may have some effect. A "reason" need not only be based on facts or figures. Emotional reasons for requesting certain procedures or eliminating certain other ones can be very persuasive.

*Request options ahead of time* even if you're not sure you're going to want them later. In a home-birth situation, for example, arrange for a doctor and/or hospital that will give you emergency backup care—even though you don't anticipate needing them. If you haven't cleared the way ahead of time and you later need to be transferred to a medical setting for either emotional or physical reasons— you may find yourself out in the cold (more on this in Chapter Eight, Home Birth). In a hospital setting you should arrange with your doctor in advance to dismiss certain routine procedures (whether it's an enema or having the baby taken away immediately after birth) or to secure other options (rooming-in, early discharge) even if you haven't yet decided whether that will be what you ultimately want. If these instructions are not written on your chart, you may not have the option when the time comes.

## HOME BIRTH VS. THE HOSPITAL

There are people all over America who have dedicated themselves to making childbirth a safer, more enriching, and more meaningful episode in our individual and collective lives. Many of them disagree about where childbirth should take place and what the priorities are in the situation. Leaders and spokespeople surfaced—as happens in any sociopolitical movement. "Martyrs" have been created: lay midwives have been jailed, a group of feminists was arrested for checking out conditions at their local hospital's labor/delivery area, doctors have been denied hospital privileges because they attend home births. State governments

**CHART 28. CHOICES IN CHILDBIRTH DELIVERIES**

| WITHIN THE HOSPITAL | OUT OF HOSPITAL |
| --- | --- |
| Alternative Birthing Room* | |
| Analgesia | Analgesia (rarely) |
| Anesthesia (general or local) | |
| Cesarean with Mate* | |
| Certified Nurse-Midwife* | Certified Nurse-Midwife |
| Clinic | |
| | Doctor's Office |
| Educated Childbirth | Educated Childbirth |
| Educated Childbirth with Anesthesia | |
| Family-Centered Maternity Care* | |
| Fetal Monitor | |
| Friends Attending* | Friends Attending |
| | Home Birth (unattended) |
| | Home Birth (with doctor) |
| | Home Birth (with midwife) |
| Induced Labor | |
| | Lay Midwife |
| Leboyer Delivery* | Leboyer Delivery |
| | Maternity Center |
| Siblings Present* | Siblings Present |

*Only available in more progressive hospitals
(See Chapter Seven for more information.)

have proposed legislation about childbirth that has touched off heated debates.

Most prospective parents don't even know of the existence of this cross-country revolution and the numerous deeply committed and opinionated people—inside the medical community as well as outside it. Most parents feel only the mild aftershocks of the clashes that go on "behind the scenes." Some pregnant women reap the benefits without even realizing it; others may be equally unaware that they are caught in a conservative backlash.

There may be some couples, however, who get caught right in the middle of the tug-of-war between home-birth and hospital advocates. This may happen because of the community they live in, because of their possible dissatisfaction with the lack of options they find there, or just because they are inquisitive people. If you find yourself in this position try to get out of it! You are on a dead-end street just by accepting *as a premise* that birth should *either* take place at a hospital *or* at home. The intention of this book is to present the pros and cons of *all* options—to illuminate all the gray areas.

There can be many variations and modifications on a home birth, as you will see in Chapter Eight. A hospital birth can run the gamut from nearly-like-a-home-birth to nearly-like-a-prison. In America today childbirth is undergoing an evolution: which means it is thrilling, infuriating, inconsistent, and more complex than it may at first appear to be.

Try to gather as much information as you can and make an evaluation based on physical and emotional considerations.

## CHOICES IN CHILDBIRTH

### ALTERNATIVE BIRTHING ROOM

Called an alternative birth center in some hospitals, the alternative birthing room is a homelike environment within the hospital in which a woman can deliver almost as if she were at home—except that she has the medical facilities down the hall should she or her baby need them. Many people believe this to be the ideal compromise between a technological, depersonalized hospital birth (which cannot offer the emotional experience of a home birth) and a birth at home (which cannot offer the medical backup of a hospital). An ABC, as it is sometimes called, would be the perfect choice for a woman who wants a completely natural childbirth but would not be comfortable having her baby at home.

***Only women who are defined as "low-risk"*** have the option of using an ABC. "Low-risk" means that prior to labor there are no indications of any potential problems. The chart of factors that would put you in the "high-risk" category—thereby excluding you from a birthing room or a home birth—can be found in Chapter Eight, Home Birth (page 415).

***A birthing room approximates a home setting*** as much as possible. Most of them are carpeted, have plants and pictures, a large bed so that the man can lie with his mate during labor if he wants, and facilities for playing tapes or records. There is often a rocking chair, which laboring women can find comfortable, and a beanbag chair, which can be put on top of the bed. It molds to your contours and gives you support during second-stage labor. The beanbag also raises your bottom off the bed so that the baby's shoulders can be delivered more easily. Sometimes there is furniture for other people whom you may have invited to attend.

***An ABC emphasizes the normalcy*** of birth. You labor and deliver in bed, without the usual transfer from one bed to another for birth. Also you are not usually covered in sterile drapes, which is routine in hospitals.

***There are no routine drugs or medical intervention.*** Although it is possible to have an enema, shave, and/or I.V.

in a birthing room they are not required as they are in many normal labor/delivery areas. You can learn more about these routines in the following chapter, Choosing a Doctor and a Hospital. You can then discuss these things with your doctor *beforehand.* They will be options for you when you are in labor but they will not be forced on you in the ABC. The same is true for fetal monitoring. There is no routine use of fetal monitors in a birthing room, but your doctor might possibly need more information about your baby's condition during labor. He then has the option of attaching a monitor until he is satisfied that all is well.

*Eating and/or drinking* are usually optional in a birthing room. You can discuss this with your doctor ahead of time and then see how you feel during labor.

*A couple determines who attends* the birth. Siblings are usually allowed as long as there is an adult whose sole responsibility it is to look after the child. If you want to have friends be with you for your birth, that is your option, although birthing rooms usually aren't very large, so you might be limited in numbers because of that.

*You can choose the position for labor* and delivery that suits you best. You can be on your hands and knees, although many doctors don't feel comfortable with this as a *delivery* position. You can walk around. You can squat. You can deliver from a side-lying position.

*You can wear what you want* in most birthing rooms. This may not sound like much, but to many women it is comforting to be able to wear something familiar rather than a hospital-issue gown. Your own clothes can give you a feeling of being more connected to "real life" or more in control of the situation; you probably aren't going to be wearing much anyway.

*You can leave the hospital within 6 to 24 hours.* This is known as "early discharge," and as long as everything is normal with you and the baby after birth, you can go home.

Among the benefits of early discharge (page 379) are that you save money, you can return to familiar surroundings and begin integrating the new baby into your life right away, and you are not subjected to the hospital routines that can interfere with breast-feeding and your initial relationship with the baby.

*The cost is lower* than for an ordinary hospital delivery and average 3-day stay, which is the routine at most places. You use less (if any) drugs and equipment in a birthing room and usually stay only a short time after delivery: the cost can be one-half to one-third of the average hospital charges for childbirth.

*Alternative birthing rooms (ABCs) are available* in a limited number of hospitals across the country. They have usually been installed because of a trend within the community back to home birth—which often is itself a reaction to inflexible, rigid hospital policies. Prospective parents who are angered and frustrated by a nonresponsive hospital will often completely abandon the system, opting for the "unknowns" of home birth rather than what they know—and do not like—about the hospital. Most medical professionals are frightened by home birth and most hospitals cannot afford to lose customers—thus ABCs are both a philosophic and economic response to people's rejection of hospital birth.

Ironically, however, some hospitals have come so far in their family-centered attitudes that their alternative birthing rooms have become obsolete. What happened was that some hospitals with 4,000 to 5,000 births a year discovered that the birthing room was used for only a handful of deliveries each month. These hospitals, which had been allowing women to labor and deliver in the labor rooms, stopped promoting or enhancing their ABCs. Instead, they concentrated on upgrading the quality of the labor and delivery (L&D) areas, redesigning them as multipurpose birthing rooms. Nowadays ABC is more of a concept, not a specific place.

The new L&D rooms allow a full range of birth experiences, from a totally unmedicated natural birth to the most complex, medically intensive care. This trend is an improvement in health care because it removes the rigid demarcation between high- and low-risk birth. By allowing flexibility for a full range of possibilities in birth, it eliminates the sharp line that was drawn between two kinds of birthing: one that required medical intervention and one that would not permit it. If these revolutionary changes have taken place in the hospital where you are planning to deliver, and you have chosen a doctor willing to help you have the kind of birth experience you want, then you will not need this section on ABCs.

***You can encourage your local hospital to put in an ABC.*** Start an organization and call it "Concerned Citizens." Ask local people to join: psychologists, pediatricians, OB/GYNs, childbirth educators, and anybody else you can contact who has some prestige in your community (bank presidents, clergymen, local government officials). Through childbirth education classes you can contact a lot of prospective parents and get their names. Contact the hospital where you would like to give birth *if* they had an alternative birthing room. Make an appointment with the Director of Obstetrics and Gynecology and go with two or three representatives of your group. Bring documentation of how well ABCs are working elsewhere (you can write to some of the hospitals listed in the appendix and request information about their facility). Bring this book and show them the list of hospitals that have already gone ahead with birthing rooms. Ask if they've read Drs. Klaus and Kennell's book, *Maternal-Infant Bonding,* a medical study which can be viewed as an argument for what a birthing room offers.

If the hospital is at all up-to-date, they will probably tell you that they have already been thinking about putting in an ABC. This is to your benefit because they already know about birthing rooms so you won't have to educate them or have so many prejudices to overcome. However, do not be lulled by the statement that a hospital has been "thinking" about it—talk is cheap. Your effort as a group of "concerned citizens" is what can make the difference between words and action. Follow up your visit with letters restating the importance of going ahead with an ABC as soon as possible. Mention the national trend toward home birth, a trend which causes consternation in medical circles. Point out that valuable public recognition will be paid to their hospital for being the first in the community to adopt such a progressive stand on childbirth. Emphasize that although the ABC may not be the choice of every expectant couple, the hospital will attract couples who would otherwise refuse to deliver there.

There are two major reasons why a hospital may hesitate to open an ABC. The first one is economic. They have to take over floor space that is in the OB/GYN area. This may mean converting an existing labor room or part of a recovery area, which could mean lost revenue. Decorating the birthing room is a minimal cost, but a cost all the same. Then the hospital only gets a patient for an average of 12 hours, usually with no medication costs: yet they have to maintain costly medical/technical options anyway.

The other problem is one of staffing considerations. Some hospitals staff their ABC entirely with certified nurse-midwives, who might also give prenatal care to the hospital's clinic patients. A CNM's training is specifically for attending normal childbirth so one of her strengths is to be able to give constant support, helping insure the normalcy of the labor and delivery. But hospitals that do not employ CNMs may have to reorganize their maternity floor staff so that an obstetric nurse can be assigned full-time to any woman using the alternative birthing room. In most ordinary maternity areas each nurse has several laboring women to look after and she goes from one to another. Therefore the ABC requires more staff to be available—whenever the birthing room is not being used the hospital is "overstaffed." Thus until the ABC is publicized and becomes popular it may be unprofitable.

## ANALGESIA

An analgesic is any drug that relieves pain; this includes tranquilizers, barbiturates, and narcotics. Any woman giving birth in a hospital has the choice to request analgesia. Women giving birth in out-of-hospital settings are almost never given the option of drugs. The emphasis at home is on the naturalness and normalcy of childbirth, and also analgesia during labor can have side effects that are less controllable outside the hospital.

Any drug taken during labor and delivery reaches your baby. *Any drug.* If someone tells you otherwise they are either lying or misinformed. Even a minimal dosage of a painkilling drug has a much greater impact on your baby, whose body is not yet able to rapidly eliminate the drug from his system.

There are many instances in which the benefit of analgesia to the mother is more important than the potential harm to the fetus. A small amount of a tranquilizer may relax a woman who is becoming so anxious that her tension could impede the progress of labor. A small amount of a narcotic might help a woman through a particularly difficult part of labor so that she doesn't need more powerful analgesics or anesthesia. It is also true that the right kind of loving support and encouragement can be at least as effective, if not more so, than drugs. However, there are many instances in which that kind of attention is not available in a hospital.

In Chapter Nine, pages 507 and 510, there are two charts on drugs commonly used during labor and their effects. Be sure that you and your mate have read that section and discussed it with your doctor *beforehand* so that you are all in some kind of agreement about what analgesia should be administered if it becomes necessary. However, you will not know *until you are in labor* just how you will feel and how you will cope with it. Do not hobble yourself by making ironclad decisions that will limit your freedom later. You may think, "I can't get through it without painkillers," or you may think, "I will refuse any drug no matter what!" If you do that you are making a decision based on incomplete information: how you will feel when the time comes. It is fine to have an opinion ahead of time, but for your own sake and your baby's, try to keep an open mind.

## GENERAL ANESTHESIA

General anesthesia is not used very much anymore in childbirth. A general anesthetic is harder for your body and the baby's to recover from. There are times when it is used for cesarean sections, but it is very rarely used for a vaginal delivery.

Besides the physical hazards of general anesthesia, there is also the problem that you do not experience the birth in any way nor do you have any contact with your baby until many hours after her birth. This is a loss for both of you because you miss the "sensitive period" following birth in which maternal-infant bonding most readily takes place.

There are a few cases of women who are so terrified by the idea of childbirth that they do not feel they can handle it at all. They want to be "knocked-out-and-know-nothing," awakening to find a child has been born. Whether it is because of a woman's social conditioning or a personally traumatic experience, it is vital to discover what is causing her such terror. Her fear must be affecting other areas of her life as well—it will certainly have an influence on her relationship with her baby. After investigating why a woman is this afraid, some determination can be made as to whether or not general anesthesia is best for her.

## LOCAL ANESTHESIA

A local anesthetic during childbirth allows a woman to be fully awake for her baby's birth although she is numb in the area that has been anesthetized. Local anesthesia is often used on a woman in labor who has not taken a childbirth education class and therefore does not understand what is happening to her body in labor or how to control it.

A local may also be used on a woman who has had childbirth training but feels the need of additional help for any of a number of reasons: her pain threshold is low, she didn't fully believe the training would work, she didn't practice enough, her labor is very long and she cannot maintain control, etc.

The chart concerning anesthesia during labor (page 510) tells you the various local anesthetics, how they are administered, and what their effects are.

## CESAREAN DELIVERY WITH YOUR MATE PRESENT

This is an option that was once very rare but is now offered across the country. Due to a liberalization of U.S. hospital policies, fathers are frequently present in the delivery room, and prolonged contact between mother and infant is usually delayed only a few hours at most. This constitutes a dramatic and rapid change: in 1979, approximately 35 percent of the hospitals in this country allowed fathers to attend cesarean deliveries; in 1984, 80 percent did. Often hospitals make the change in steps, first allowing father to be present only at repeat C-sections—operations performed on women who have already had a baby by cesarean—and the father is often required to see a film depicting the operation. This insures that a couple is well-informed and therefore prepared for what the procedure entails and looks like. A couple may have many reasons for wanting to be together for a cesarean.

***Probably the most important reason*** is that *you want your mate to support you* through what is a frightening process. No matter how safe cesareans have become and despite the fact that you may have already had an uncomplicated cesarean, it is still major surgery. There are a number of preparatory procedures, then there is the insertion and administration of the local anesthetic that numbs you from the waist down, and then there is the cutting, and afterward the sewing. In the midst of all the attendants with sterile masks and the bright lights your baby is born. You can be more focused on your baby's birth and enjoy that thrill more if your mate is with you for comfort and support during the medical/surgical aspects of a cesarean. Cesareans are described in depth on pages 538 to 565.

***A man wants to see and share*** with his mate the moment of his baby's birth. A cesarean usually denies a man that experience. Paternal-infant bonding is as important as the mother's early attachment to the baby.

*If a couple is together,* it emphasizes the personal, emotional aspect of a cesarean. Often when a woman has a baby by cesarean section she is most aware of the surgical attendants and apparatus. There may be a tense quiet in the operating room or the nurses and doctors may be chatting among themselves. A woman can feel isolated and disconnected from the excitement and joy that are part of a baby's birth. If a couple is together, the birth of their child can have its appropriate emotional importance.

## PREPARING FOR A MAN'S PRESENCE AT A CESAREAN

If you know you are going to have a cesarean and you would like your mate to stay with you there are a number of hurdles to overcome.

*If you are fortunate* enough to live near a hospital that already has allowed couples to stay together for cesareans, then you're in luck. You can reap the benefits of what was undoubtedly a hard-won battle by the couples who preceded you. Simply ask your doctor whether he has admitting privileges at the hospital and whether he is willing to allow your mate to be with you. If not, call the Department of Obstetrics and Gynecology at the hospital and they will give you the names of doctors who have done cesareans with the mate present. Then you can interview them and take your pick.

*If you are going to be breaking new ground,* then most of all you need your doctor's understanding and support. If you cannot convince him of the importance and benefits of your mate being present you might want to interview other doctors.

*Next you must find an anesthesiologist* who will give his or her permission to have your mate present. Your doctor may know of one who is open-minded and flexible. It might be best for your doctor to contact the anesthesiologist so that they can talk about it between themselves as colleagues.

***Once you have found a doctor*** you feel comfortable about, one who respects your desires, then either the doctor or you and your mate have to approach the hospital. If your doctor has a long-standing reputation—i.e., he has some "clout" within the institution—it is possible that they will grant your request. If he does not have that kind of influence, and only a few doctors do, then the Director of the Department of OB/GYN has to be persuaded. It may be an uphill battle. Be prepared for getting the runaround: inconsistent replies and irrational arguments. You have got to be patient and eloquent in order to make this childbirth choice possible. What you have on your side is that several of the most prestigious university hospitals in the country have had successful test programs in which they allowed fathers into cesareans; many have adopted it as official hospital policy. Two examples are Yale University and Harvard University, through its affiliate, Boston Lying-In Hospital.

### ARGUMENTS YOU'LL HEAR

***The first argument*** you will hear is that having the father present increases the chance of infection. Statistics prove that the infection rate was unchanged in the test programs. A father is scrubbed, gowned, and masked just like everyone else in the room. If you are told that each additional person in a sterile area potentially introduces infection, point out that frequently there are students, interns, and residents in an operating room.

***You will be asked,*** with some disdain, why a man would want to watch his mate's abdomen being cut. Explain that the usual procedure is to have the father seated at her head with a screen at the woman's midsection that blocks their view of the actual incision. When the baby is removed either the screen is lowered or the baby is lifted over it for them to see. Restate your positive emotional, interpersonal reasons for wanting to be together.

*You will be told* that it is state law that the father cannot be there. This is misinformation or a lie on the part of the hospital representative. Most state health agencies require only that persons in an operating room be wearing "proper attire."

*You will be told* that the hospital's insurance forbids it. This is also false. Usually one large insurance company covers all of the hospitals in one area. There is almost never a clause which specifically forbids a father, or anyone else, from being in attendance at an operation. Students, interns, and residents are frequently watching and insurance doesn't exclude them any more than it does the woman's mate.

*You may be told* that having the baby's father watch will create a mental strain on the doctor. Restate that your doctor has already agreed to your being together and supports the reasons for your request.

*You will be told* that a cesarean baby has a higher chance of having some trouble breathing at first and if there are any complications that the father would impede resuscitation attempts. Explain that you are aware that being together depends entirely on things going ahead *without complications.* The baby's father knows this—and is prepared to leave the operating room without question if the doctor or anesthesiologist asks him to. Explain that you realize this is for your baby's good and will also insure that other couples after you can have the option of staying together.

*Most hospitals* will consider allowing a father to be present only if the couple is married. If you are not married you have to deal with this in whatever way makes you most comfortable, including lying by omission. You can call yourselves Mr. and Mrs. Abrams or you can use your own names as you do now. If there is any question say that the woman has retained her own name. The best solution is not to raise the issue at all. But at least you are forewarned that if you let them know you aren't married they may reject the entire proposal for you to be together for the cesarean.

## CERTIFIED NURSE-MIDWIVES

CNMs are nurses who have had special training and specialize only in normal pregnancy. They are trained to give prenatal care and attend a normal labor with normal spontaneous delivery with little or no intervention. If any medical problems arise during the pregnancy or labor—a nurse-midwife's training equips her to determine anything that is not normal—then a doctor is called in.

National recognition of certified nurse-midwives has widened only in the last 10 years although the statistics over the past 50 years are impressive. The statistics show an improvement in the outcome of births wherever nurse-midwives have worked, compared to the health status of mothers in other parts of the country who received traditional obstetric care. At this point the majority of CNMs are practicing in hospital clinics. There are few places where a private paying patient can receive care from a nurse-midwife; thus many women who could afford another alternative are becoming clinic patients. The future of nurse-midwifery—where CNMs will practice and the mushrooming demand for them—will be determined by the present and future society at large.

*There are twenty-four schools nationwide* that offer a course in nurse-midwifery. The school training lasts 9 to 12 months, but when she is ready to practice, a nurse-midwife will have had a *minimum* of 6 years' training and experience. She will have had four years in nursing school and one or more years of practical experience and then a year or more of CNM schooling.

If you want to find a midwife, here are three sources that may be of help: St. Luke's-Roosevelt Hospital Center Midwifery Services, Inc., 135 W. 70th Street, New York, New York 10023 (212-877-5556); Downtown Women's

Center, 412 Sixth Avenue, New York, New York 10011 (212-529-7722); and American College of Nurse Midwives, 1522 K Street NW, Suite 1120, Washington, DC 20005 (202-347-5445)

*A nurse-midwife follows your pregnancy* from prenatal exams right through postpartum care, when she teaches infant care and breast-feeding, and does gynecological exams as well.

*Nurse-midwives usually practice through hospital clinics,* so the *total cost for maternity care is lower* than if you were to go to the hospital with a private doctor. Some CNMs also work in doctors' offices (see page 299), others attend home births, and there are a few maternity centers either run by or staffed by nurse-midwives.

*Health insurance reimburses for nurse-midwifery care.* The following states have mandated that private insurance companies in that state must directly reimburse certified nurse-midwives (CNMs): Alaska, Colorado, Connecticut, Florida, Maryland, Massachusetts, Minnesota, Mississippi, Montana, New Hampshire, New Jersey, New Mexico, New York, Nevada, North Dakota, Ohio, Oregon, Pennsylvania, South Dakota, Utah, Washington, West Virginia. In addition, the federal Blue Shield plan, Medicaid, and the Civilian Health and Medical Plan of the Uniformed Services (CHAMPUS) reimburse nurse-midwives directly.

The American College of Nurse-Midwives has compiled the information, along with a list of health insurance companies which provide direct payment to the certified nurse-midwife or reimburse the insured for obstetric services, including labor and delivery, rendered by a CNM. The insurance companies which do this are as follows: Aetna, Allstate, American Hardware, Bankers Life, CNA Insurance, Confederate Life, Connecticut General, Connecticut Mutual, Educators Mutual, Equitable, Fireman's Fund, General American, Hartford, Home Life, Home Security, Interocean, Kemper, Lutheran Brotherhood, Massachusetts Mutual, Metropolitan Life, Monumental Life, Mutual Benefit, Mutual Life of NY (MONY), Mutual of Omaha, Mutual Service Life, National Benefit Life, New England Mutual Life, Pacific Mutual, Penn Mutual, Pilot Life, Provident Mutual, Prudential, Safeco, State Farm Mutual, Union Central, Washington National. The following companies reimburse for midwifery services, although in a slightly more restrictive manner than those listed above: Capitol Holding, John Hancock, Liberty Mutual, Lincoln, New York Life, Peoples Life, Time Insurance, Travelers, Union Mutual.

***Prenatal care from a CNM*** may appeal to women who like the idea of a woman-to-woman relationship. Only 15 percent of the OB-GYNs in this country are female, so that those mothers who would prefer receiving care from another woman are more likely to find a nurse-midwife than a female obstetrician. With a woman care-giver you might feel less inhibited, feeling that another woman can be more empathetic to your physical and emotional experience.

***A nurse-midwife has more time*** than a doctor does to answer your questions about pregnancy and childbirth. With a doctor you might worry about "bothering" him with "petty" questions because he seems rushed. An important part of a CNM's training is parent education: she stresses prepared childbirth and nonintervention in the normal birth process.

***A CNM will be constantly in attendance*** throughout your entire labor. Since she will have given you prenatal care you will have already developed a confident relationship with her. The importance of this trusted, constant-support person (in addition to or instead of your mate) cannot be stressed enough. See pages 496 to 501 for a more detailed discussion of the importance of loving support during labor. If you have a long labor you may not necessarily have the same CNM with you the whole time but you will have met her colleagues during prenatal care so they will all be familiar to you.

*A nurse-midwife usually is flexible* about omitting certain routine hospital procedures during labor and about the positions you choose for labor and delivery. Her training stresses a laboring woman's self-determination in a hospital setting, with medical technology available only in case of need. A nurse-midwife is committed to nonintervention although she is also well versed in medical technology. She will support as natural and personalized a birth experience as you wish—as long as everything remains *normal.* When necessary, she will consult with or call in a doctor.

### THE CASES IN WHICH A DOCTOR INTERVENES FOR A CNM

*Prolonged second stage:* A woman is fully dilated and in good labor, but has pushed for 2 hours and is either unable to continue or the baby isn't descending, at which point a doctor will use forceps or do a cesarean.

*A breech presentation:* If the CNM and consulting doctors deem it safe, a CNM can attend a vaginal delivery of a breech but a doctor is ready and scrubbed in the delivery room to use forceps or do a cesarean if labor doesn't progress or there is fetal distress.

*If the baby is too large* for your pelvis, a doctor takes over surgically.

*In cases of a prolapsed cord,* a doctor intervenes and does surgery.

*If you are carrying twins* a doctor will be present, if only because an extra pair of expert hands will be needed.

*A pediatrician is called in* and will be in attendance for a breech, cesarean, or multiple birth, and when there are signs of fetal distress.

## CLINICS/HOSPITALS

A clinic offers lower-priced maternity care than a private doctor, although you usually receive the same quality of care as private patients in the same hospital. A teaching hospital often has the best clinic.

***The main problem with a clinic*** is that you may see a different doctor at each prenatal visit, so you won't have an opportunity to build a relationship with the person who is going to deliver your baby. In fact, you don't know ahead of time which of these doctors is going to attend the birth; whichever doctor is on duty when you go into labor is the one who will care for you. This makes for a different experience than if you had a private doctor with whom you had developed a relationship. You will not be offered many alternatives during labor and delivery. Nor will you have the backing of your own hand-picked doctor if what you want is not within the hospital's routine. You are somewhat at the mercy of this unfamiliar doctor's philosophy because he will have the final word—for instance, if any medications are used, the choice will be his.

There are two schools of thought about the net result of getting maternity care from a clinic. Some people say that it makes it hard to have control over your own labor because your input doesn't carry the weight it would if you were being attended by a private doctor. Other people point out that since there is no constant "father figure" to depend on, it forces a couple to depend more on themselves. Not having the security of one doctor may motivate a couple to learn more about the birth process and then be more self-reliant and interdependent.

## OUTSIDE-HOSPITAL CLINICS

The outside-hospital clinic is usually a community-oriented facility that offers prenatal care. Many of these are feminist and take a somewhat political stand on health care. The women's movement has raised the issue of the rights of women to have more knowledge about and control over their bodies. These clinics can be the manifestation of the statements made by leaders in the feminist movement that the time has come for women to have control over their own health care. These clinics can be seen as a challenge to the U.S. health care system, which they see as profit-oriented, hierarchical, and expensive.

Expectant women who choose to receive prenatal care from clinics like these are encouraged to learn as much as possible about their pregnancy. You will be encouraged to actively participate in your own prenatal care, often checking your own urine, weight, and blood pressure. The idea behind this is that women have to break away from the traditional attitudes in obstetric care which presume that a pregnant woman has to be "taken care of." Feminist clinics try to stress the normalcy of pregnancy and childbirth and a woman's own capability in these areas.

There is an organization which maintains an up-to-date listing of all the childbirth centers or clinics across the country. There are increasing numbers of these out-of-hospital birth sites so the best way to get a current listing for your area would be to write to: National Association of Childbearing Centers, RD 1, Box 1, Perkiomenville, Pennsylvania 18074. The NACC can also be reached at 48 East 92nd Street, New York, New York 10128 (212-369-7300). The latter is the address of the Maternity Center Association, one of the first and most successful birth centers in the country.

## DOCTOR'S OFFICE

Many doctors refer to their offices as birth centers when they use them for deliveries, although usually all they have is a suite of examining rooms. One or two of them may have been decorated with a homelike style, like an alternative birthing room in a hospital, described earlier in this chapter.

*A doctor's office is an option worth considering* for those who are totally against a hospital birth yet not interested in birth at home. There are no routine procedures in an office birth, little or no intervention, no drugs, and the mother and baby can leave within hours of the birth. A doctor's office is certainly more informal than a hospital but it does not have any of the medical safety advantages, either. At the same time it isn't your own home so you don't get the benefits of familiar, relaxed surroundings in which you feel as if you are in charge. Thus a *doctor's office is neither fish nor fowl,* but it serves a need in communities that have not yet responded to people's changing expectations of childbirth.

***Doctor's offices exist*** as locales for birth for one reason: the *convenience (and economic survival) of the doctor.* In most cities a doctor who is doing out-of-hospital deliveries cannot maintain an OB/GYN practice *and* travel any distance to people's homes to wait during long labors. By having a woman come to his office, a doctor can attend her labor without sacrificing his office patients. Also, there are usually only a very few doctors doing out-of-hospital deliveries and they gain popularity through word-of-mouth. Some of these doctors are delivering over fifty babies a month: it would be impossible for them to attend all those births unless they all come to him rather than the other way around.

***The requirements for being accepted*** for birth in a doctor's office are the same as those for an alternative birthing room in a hospital or for a home birth. See the chart of Factors That Rule Out Home Birth, page 415. If any doctor tells you that he will let you deliver in his office even though you have one of the conditions on that list, *distrust the doctor.* Not only would he be endangering you and your baby, he's just downright stupid. Anyone who would attempt out-of-hospital births for "high risk" pregnancies is eventually going to have fetal deaths or problems.

***If you develop any high-risk indications*** during your pregnancy, a responsible doctor doing office births will refer you to an obstetric subspecialist. Ask the doctor ahead of time under what conditions he would refer you elsewhere and to whom he sends referrals. Some doctors have egos that have grown so large that they like to think they can handle anything and everything themselves. Beware of a doctor like that: once a doctor begins practicing medicine with his ego, he is not using good judgment.

***Even though a doctor may be going against the grain*** of the majority of his colleagues by offering an out-of-hospital birth alternative, his training and orientation are still medical. The next chapter offers more information and insights to doctors, but the relevant point here is that *most doctors coming out of medical school have never seen a natural childbirth.* Modern medicine is oriented toward *controlling* childbirth . . . "improving" on nature. This usually means intervening in the natural progress of labor and delivery. The exceptions are the doctor who is an "old-timer" and has been doing out-of-hospital births for a long time or a doctor who is assisted by lay or nurse-midwives with extensive experience of their own.

***A doctor should have full admitting privileges*** at a hospital close to his office. As with home birth, you are better off if you have paved the way for emergency backup care in the unlikely event that it is necessary. This is even more true with a doctor's-office birth, since a doctor is more likely to seek medical assistance if your labor seems abnormal.

***The chance of infection*** in a doctor's office is open to debate. Some say that there is less chance of infection because fewer personnel are involved in the process than would be at a hospital and there aren't sick, infected people in an office. They point out that a baby has immunity to his parents. Those who do worry about infection possibilities in a doctor's office say that the room isn't sterilized, nor are there sterile gowns, masks, or drapes on the woman, while there have been patients coming through the doctor's office for gynecological exams who *do* have infections. However, most of these doctors contend that their sterile gloves are sufficient protection.

## EDUCATED CHILDBIRTH

Also known as prepared childbirth, educated childbirth is a far better name than "natural childbirth." The latter phrase has come to mean "martyrdom despite suffering," and that is not the desired result from educated childbirth. The point is to *inform* you about what will be happening to your body during labor and delivery and to *train* you to minimize the discomfort. Every expectant woman and/or couple can benefit from these classes. It does not matter whether you intend (or wind up) having analgesia or anesthesia: these classes are not supposed to set up a test of your bravery and fortitude. The intention is for you to have as much information as possible so that you can understand—and therefore be less overwhelmed by—what your body is going to go through. You have nothing to lose and everything to gain by taking classes.

*Pain* results from intense stimuli—noise, heat, cold, light—that are strong enough to cause, or threaten to cause, tissue damage. The *mental state* of an individual may alter the significance of the incoming pain impulses so they are minimized or exaggerated. Childbirth education classes prepare you to *control your mental state for the management of painful stimuli.*

## PAIN AND CHILDBIRTH

There have been important discoveries of substances produced by the body which are changing previous beliefs about pain. These morphine-like substances are called "endorphins," and they have been found in the brain and other areas of the body. They seem to have a special role in pain perception.

Studies have shown that individual differences in pain sensitivity are related to individual differences in endorphin production. Research has shown that treatments such as acupuncture and electrical stimulation which can reduce pain are associated with endorphin production. Each person's endorphin-production system responds differently; as more research is done it may be especially useful in childbirth.

Childbirth preparation varies in its effectiveness for each individual. It is known that a small percentage of women are insensitive to pain during labor and delivery, even in cases where a woman has had no childbirth preparation. It is also known that childbirth education reduces pain for many women. More must be learned about these morphine-like substances and what can be done to stimulate production of endorphins in laboring women.

Keeping this information in mind, expectant mothers and those supporting her in labor must make some allowance for her individual endorphin system. It is not unusual for a woman to take childbirth education classes, consider herself well prepared for labor and delivery, and yet have unexpected difficulties with pain control despite her determination and training. It just may be that certain people's endorphin-producing systems are less responsive.

*"Pain is evil"* is an American belief. Culturally we regard pain and even discomfort as evils to be avoided at all costs. Just look at the aspirin commercials on television to see the intensity of our national warfare on pain, with instant medication the moment there is the slightest discomfort. Medically, the goal is to control and suppress pain. These social attitudes will have an influence on your experience of labor contractions unless you can at least temporarily revise your outlook—for example, "the pain I am experiencing is not evil; it is a natural, normal aspect of expelling a baby from the womb."

*Your expectations may be unrealistic,* which will make it difficult for the childbirth education to be effective. The training methods which advertise "painless childbirth" are guaranteeing their own failure. We have to get away from the myth that if you can just find the right way to breathe during labor, it's going to be pleasant and easy. Childbirth education is *not* a magic tool that makes it all okay. It is going to be hard. It is going to hurt. Classes simply make it easier and less painful. But if you are looking for a way to have "natural childbirth" and feel no discomfort, you are in for a rude shock. Being prepared for the pain and knowing ways to lessen it is a realistic outlook on birth.

*Another theory* that is somewhat contradictory says that *if you are expecting to feel pain* you will find the contractions painful. The point is "negative prophecy": you will create what you expect. The cultural conditioning says that childbirth is painful, and therefore that is how you perceive the sensory input. However, if you liken labor and delivery to a grueling sports event, it can give you a new perspective. A marathon runner is in great pain during the final stretch. The runner's entire body is in pain, but he or she expected it and keeps on going. Personally and socially their pain is not considered "evil" . . . therefore, no one would think to give them an anesthetic to finish the race.

## How Much Will Labor Hurt?

How much pain you will have will be partially determined by whether you have childbirth training and how committed you are to it. There is no doubt that a *belief in the techniques* is part of what makes them effective.

*Studies show* that anywhere from 3 to 14 percent of women naturally experience no pain at all during labor and delivery (without using breathing techniques, etc.). In childbirth education classes 10 to 20 percent of women report having felt no pain.

*People differ greatly* in their anatomy and physiology. This means that there are *individual differences in the number of pain messages* reaching the brain. This is what is referred to as a low or high threshold for pain.

*Your menstrual history* is an indicator of pain during childbirth. Women with irregular periods with acute cramps at the onset tend to have significantly more childbirth pain. There is less pain in women who menstruate regularly with little or no disturbance of their daily activities.

***Do not make the mistake*** of thinking that if you take childbirth classes you are going to have to suffer, and that if you don't, there are drugs which let you be fully awake yet feel no pain. *Every women* (except those 3 to 14 percent) *will feel discomfort; the trained ones are simply better able to deal with it.* Even if you decide absolutely that you want an epidural during labor, for instance, you are not going to be allowed to have it until you are halfway dilated (read the section on drugs, pages 501 to 513). Ordinarily an epidural is not administered until at least 5 centimeters dilation: sooner than that and the anesthetic can slow down or stop the labor altogether, necessitating the use of synthetic hormones to speed things up again. This means that you are going to have to get through the first half of first-stage labor no matter what. The painkilling drugs you can be given during that time are not going to remove the pain entirely—only dull your senses.

If you had taken classes, you would be able to consciously relax and do breathing techniques to ease your way through it. A woman who hasn't gone through any training often can feel as if labor is one continual never-ending contraction—which soon becomes terrifying and overwhelming. With education you know that there is going to be time to relax between contractions and how to prepare for the next one. You learn that the discomfort will stop periodically and you'll have a break.

If you are unsure about whether you want to take the classes *talk to couples* who have used or are planning to take prepared childbirth courses. Talk to ones who have gone through without any drugs and talk to those who had an epidural anesthetic as soon as they could. Regardless of how much they liked their teacher or how their birth went, you are going to have a hard time finding any couple who won't recommend that you take advantage of what the classes have to offer.

***Accepting analgesia or anesthesia*** is not a violation of childbirth education. Some methods of teaching are more adamant about refusing medication: for instance, the Bradley method (which is described on page 310), which can lead you to feel guilt and a sense of failure if you do accept drugs. However, the training is really just a tool. For some women its main benefit is to lessen fear by giving them an understanding of what is happening; for other women the techniques make them able to wait longer before having drugs; for some women the techniques mean they will need less medication; for many women it makes possible a drug-free labor and delivery. The important thing is not to allow a childbirth teacher, your mate, or your next-door neighbor to set up the techniques as a *test of your strength of character*. Don't fall into that trap if someone baits it and do not set it for yourself. The more you rely on the technique, the less you will need drugs; the fewer drugs you take, the better off you and your baby will be. However, childbirth should not be a torture chamber. The psychological harm of extreme pain during labor is greater than the potential harm from drugs. It is better to have a baby slightly groggy from medication than to have a woman so devastated by the pain her baby's birth caused her that it has a negative influence on her mothering.

## How Childbirth Techniques Work

The theoretical explanation of childbirth techniques sounds more complicated than it really is. Laboratory studies on human subjects have defined five major psychological strategies that are effective in reducing pain. All childbirth methods utilize some or all of the following:

1. **Systematic relaxation** is described on page 189. It is based on the repeated tension/relaxation of muscle groups in the body. Childbirth classes train you so that relaxation becomes a built-in response.When your coach says, "Contraction begins," you will have practiced enough so that you can automatically release any tension in your body. After a while during practice sessions you can add distractions like the radio or television and will eventually be able to relax in situations with stress or confusion. In labor itself you must remember to check for tension not only during a

contraction but *between* contractions in order to insure complete systematic relaxation.

The goal is to relax all the body muscles to produce a mental state of *minimal anxiety.* This increases your pain tolerance: you are less fearful of the pain stimulus, therefore your mind decreases its awareness of the painful sensation. Thus you can endure the pain for longer.

2. COGNITIVE CONTROL means involving the mind in mental activities other than the awareness of the incoming pain sensation. There are two types:

DISSOCIATION is concentration on a *non*painful characteristic of the pain stimulus with distracting imagery. For instance, putting your hand in ice water causes pain. The pain is lessened if you imagine yourself on a hot desert island where the water is coolly refreshing. In childbirth training this is applied in teaching you *how* to think about the sensations. If you think of them as muscular contractions of the uterus—not as "labor pains"—it is effective in reducing your pain perception.

INTERFERENCE involves two forms of cognitive control: *distraction* and *attention focusing.* Distraction works only for *slow-onset pain* like labor contractions, which usually build slowly to maximum levels. The breathing techniques you learn are a form of attention focusing: active, intentional mental attentiveness.

3. COGNITIVE REHEARSAL means a clear explanation of what the upcoming experience will involve. You rehearse specific fear images and accommodate them so as to reduce your anxiety. By discussing what you are afraid of and getting a description of what you can realistically expect during birth, your anxiety is lessened and therefore your tolerance for pain is increased. In order for this to be effective, you need to get both objective and subjective information—a factual explanation as well as personal accounts of how the childbirth training works. It is vital that an instructor is careful to provide accurate, verifiable information on a broad range of possible childbirth experiences. A lack of verifiability of subjective information at the time of

exposure to pain will cause you to lose confidence. In plain English, if what you have been told doesn't jibe with what you experience, you will distrust the entire training.

4. HAWTHORNE EFFECT is a finding in psychological research that "more and special attention to a subject increases results in reducing pain." This is scientific proof of what prepared-childbirth advocates (and people who oppose hospital birth because it is depersonalized) have been saying for years: give a laboring woman constant and loving support and she will not need, or will need fewer, drugs. The childbirth instructor—but especially a woman's mate—can contribute immeasurably to her success in controlling her discomfort. The other side of the Hawthorne effect is that *insufficient* attention by a woman's attending doctor may actually be the *cause* of unnecessary requests for drugs. It may be her unconscious attempt to get attention and reassurance.

5. SYSTEMATIC DESENSITIZATION is what a childbirth class does for you, combining the preceding four other strategies in preparing you to manage the pain. This strategy is mostly for high-anxiety cases—women who need more intense and individualized preparation in order to go into labor with less fear and a well-developed ability to relax at will.

An example of systematic desensitization is a technique used in some classes in which the coach pinches your leg very hard to simulate the pain of a contraction. By the end of the course many women find their pain threshold has become higher: they can tolerate harder squeezing for longer. Some women find that even with their coach's hardest pinching, there is no pain (although he should not pinch so hard as to bruise you).

*Studies have shown* that childbirth classes *shorten the length of labor*. The psychosomatic techniques applied in the training have a calming effect that allows labor to progress unimpeded by muscle and mental tension. One study showed a 14-hour duration of labor for the group of women who had taken classes, compared with an average labor of 18½ hours for the control group, who had no training.

*One of the most useful things you learn* in classes is to *take labor one step at a time.* You deal with each contraction as it happens and are taught not to worry about the preceding contraction or about what is coming afterward. There is a misconception many people have about labor, sometimes not corrected even in classes: it is not true that labor gets worse as it goes on and that the contractions get stronger and stronger. Some women don't take childbirth classes because they have this misconception and they figure, "It's going to get unbearable at some point and I'm not going to be able to stand it, so why bother with all the breathing?" Other women who have taken classes may lose heart part of the way through because they figure, "If it's this bad now, I'm not going to be able to handle it when it gets worse."

Labor contractions have an ebb and flow, like waves on a beach. You can have a very strong contraction which will do a lot of dilating and then it may be followed by several light contractions which consolidate the work of the strong one. As you will learn in Chapter Nine, Labor and Delivery, the uterine contractions are stretching and pulling your cervix open. A strong contraction accomplishes a lot of stretching but it doesn't mean that every contraction after that is going to be progressively harder. In fact, if you can stay relaxed and your cervix is fairly cooperative, as labor progresses, the contractions can do more dilating with less pain as your cervix becomes more elastic. It is true that near the end of first-stage labor, when your cervix is close to full dilation, the contractions can last much longer and can have several "peaks" rather than just one. This interlude (known as "transition") is often the most difficult part of labor for a woman but it is usually a great deal shorter than the early part of labor. Therefore, if you can remember to deal with each contraction as a separate event (rather than as "Oh, no, how many more after this?") your childbirth training will give you the greatest success in managing your labor and delivery.

*Childbirth classes* were available in only 10 percent of the nation's 7,000 hospitals 25 years ago but now it would be hard to find a hospital that doesn't offer them. Classes may be less expensive through a hospital than with a private teacher. However, there are two problems with hospital classes: they may be larger than a private class, and teachers of such classes may have less freedom because they are beholden to the institution for which they work. Hospital classes may offer partial information or may give subtle support to hospital procedures. Expectant parents may not know they might have other options (although if they've read this book they'll know!). Childbirth classes should teach about not only the birth process and how to manage labor contractions, but also how to cope with (and if necessary fight against) the hospital.

*To find classes in your area,* ask your doctor or midwife for a recommendation. Ask any couples you know who have had prepared childbirth how they liked their instructor. You can write to the International Childbirth Education Association (P.O. Box 5852, Milwaukee, Wisconsin 53220) or write to ASPO (the American Society for Psychoprophylaxis in Obstetrics, which is the official name of the Lamaze method) (1523 L Street N.W., Washington, DC 20005). You can also try calling the local chapter of the American Red Cross or the YWCA for suggestions.

*All classes are essentially the same:* the exact breathing method they teach does not really matter. People from "rival" methods (Lamaze, Bradley, Dick-Read, etc.) would like you to think there is a difference to debunk other methods in favor of their own. Nowadays most classes have taken the best parts of all the methods and rolled them into one. The Lamaze method is the most well known and widespread—yet originally it did not include the husband as coach. That idea was initiated by Dr. Robert Bradley (whose method is also called Husband-Coached Childbirth). There are slight differences in the type of breathing they teach, but that is not central: it is your intense concentration on breathing patterns which reduces your experience of pain. The other important thing you learn is the ability to relax your body at will; it is the key to pain reduction. All classes are aimed at avoiding the vicious cycle of fear/tension/pain: the more afraid you are the more tense you become and the more you experience pain. The main difference between Bradley and Lamaze is that Bradley teachers tend to be quite adamant about their students having drug-free births. Bradley teachers are recertified each year and sign a policy to strive for at least a 90 percent unmedicated rate. This is fine for expectant couples who have no doubts about having a drugless birth. It can be an extra incentive for those who are eager to deliver without any drugs. It can, however, be felt as a pressure by couples who may have anxiety about "disappointing" their instructor or may feel like failures themselves if they wind up wanting or needing medication.

*A class can be a substitute for your extended family,* which you may not have nearby.

*An important added benefit* of classes is that they are a support system for a couple. The camaraderie with other expectant couples is something you may not have during your pregnancy if your peers are postponing or deciding against childbearing. It is a great help to be able to share feelings and experiences with other people who are in the same situation. Discussing common problems and knowing that the things you feel are normal can help relieve tension and anxiety.

*The class dynamic* depends on the individuals in your group. First you have to trust yourself, then you have to trust your coach, then the teacher, and finally the class. If the class dynamic is good, with shared participation and support, the personal bonds you make in these classes can be strong and the friendships can continue after your babies are born.

*Classes usually start in your 7th month* and meet once weekly for anywhere from 6 to 10 weeks. If you have not delivered by the time the class has finished many instructors will arrange for you to have "refresher" sessions to keep up your practicing until the baby is born. Most classes meet in the evening and last two to three hours. The cost is usually around $125, although it may be more or less depending on the part of the country you live in. A good class size is 8 to 10 couples. Any larger than that and you aren't going to get enough personalized attention or the kind of group interaction which can give you so much support. Some teachers get a bit greedy and take 15 or more couples at a time: it really isn't fair to any of them. The only time to consider a large class is if the teacher lectures to all of you and then for the practical application of the techniques splits the group up and meets with you in a smaller section.

***Choosing a class*** is mostly a matter of finding a *teacher* you feel good about. Trust in the instructor is essential in order for the method to work for you. Most teachers will give you a class outline, their credentials, and let you sit in on one of their classes before signing up.

FIND OUT WHETHER FILMS are shown, and whether the teacher has free discussion, formal lectures, or a combination of the two.

IS THE TEACHER ENTHUSIASTIC? Does she have a sense of humor? This can be nice because it reduces tension and puts things in perspective. A superserious and determined teacher can be intimidating and make the classes a chore rather than fun and interesting. A good way to judge this is whether the couples seem relaxed yet enthusiastic.

IF NONMEDICATION IS VERY IMPORTANT to you, then you might ask the teacher approximately what percentage of her pupils go "drugless." At the least, make sure that the teaching in her class is not aimed at "breathing until you're ready for your epidural." That kind of class is a farce for any couple who is interested in natural childbirth with commitment to prepared techniques. Instead it is just lip service, with the *assumption* of anesthetic completely undermining any possible success with the training.

ASK WHETHER "CONDITIONED RESPONSE" is the basis of the techniques that are taught. In Lamaze-type training the emphasis is on definite, repeated instructions by the coach to which you will eventually have an automatic relaxation response.

## THE MAN'S INVOLVEMENT

*The inclusion of the father* is one of the important benefits of childbirth classes.

*It gives you a unique opportunity as a couple* to work as a team toward a common goal. The technique requires that you have total trust in each other. It elicits an intense nonverbal communication between you in which the coach is attuned to respond to your facial and body signals. When a couple is working well with childbirth techniques they block out everything else that is going on and focus completely on each other. Some observers have noted that seeing a couple like this is almost like watching them "make love," they become so private and intense.

*Most men feel somewhat reluctant* about starting the classes. Don't let that upset or stop you. All couples feel nervous at the first class but as the man begins to see what his role is going to be during labor he usually relaxes and becomes more confident.

*Just how central a role your mate plays* during labor itself depends entirely on his personality, his attitudes toward childbirth, and how well you have been able to work as a team in practice sessions.

*Some men are energetic* and determined to learn as much as they can about labor and delivery. This kind of man is probably eager to be fully involved in the birth and it is important to him that he be your primary and sole support person during labor.

*Some men remain baffled* and overwhelmed by the prospect of labor despite childbirth training (as do some women). A man like this will probably feel uptight and inadequate if he feels he has to be fully responsible for supporting you through the birth. Women who have mates like this often find that if there is someone additional to depend on, their mate can relax and enjoy the experience more and they still benefit from his emotional support. Their doctor, midwife, or an obstetric nurse experienced in prepared childbirth can all be useful for information and reassurance during labor.

*Having your childbirth teacher as an additional coach* can either give you a wonderful feeling of security and support or it may be an extra burden. You may feel you have to do the technique perfectly and live up to your teacher's high standards. This really depends on how gung-ho your teacher is and your relationship with her.

### KEEP PRACTICING

*Practice* is absolutely essential. The techniques cannot work unless you practice them so that they become second nature.

*Do not skip practicing*—or going to class—because your coach is not available. You are the one having the baby. You are the one who needs the conditioning. Practice by yourself. There are going to be times during labor when your coach may leave the room and you'll have to handle a contraction alone. Practice now; don't use his absence as an excuse to be lazy.

*If your coach is unable to practice* with you routinely—because he has to be away during that time, for instance—tape-record his voice giving you instructions during a practice session. This will help condition your reflexes specifically to his voice.

*Do not let anything interrupt* a practice contraction. Let the phone ring, the pot boil, or people ask you questions. There will be interruptions in labor too, and this is good practice for your concentration. If you want to you can even *add* distractions once you've got the technique—turn on the radio or TV—and develop your concentration.

*Practice your breathing* with a Braxton-Hicks contraction. Try it with a headache or to control the pain of bumping your shin. Test how well the techniques work and whether your use of them is improving.

*If you do not have a coach,* prepared childbirth techniques can be done alone. Some mates flatly refuse to get involved. Trying to convert a man who feels this way may be a hopeless battle that causes a problem rather than solves one. If a man can't be gently swayed you may be better off without him because you'd be worried about how *he* was feeling during labor and delivery instead of the other way around. You may not have anyone else in your life that you want to ask to be your coach. Don't worry; much of a coach's tasks are busywork anyway. The main importance of a coach is for emotional support—and to call out contractions and time them. To do it alone you have to have a strong will and motivation. You will be forced to depend more on yourself, knowing there's no one to lean on. It may be a rewarding experience.

*Your anxiety level is high during pregnancy,* particularly as your due date nears. This may not be something you are consciously aware of but it is certainly there. The effect of this anxiety level on your childbirth training is that you only hear about one-third of what you are taught and retain perhaps one-eighth of it. Try to remember that *you are not absorbing information normally* and that if you don't make a special effort to make things sink in, they may go in one ear and out the other. Ask the same question(s) of your teacher as often as you want to. Read and reread anything you want to be able to know during labor and delivery. It is common for an intelligent, seemingly calm woman who has had classes to ask questions during labor that sound as if she just awakened from a nine-month sleep and knows nothing about childbirth! There's nothing wrong

with this except that you may not want to leave it to chance
that there will be someone around at the time who can
refresh your memory with accurate, reliable information.

## FAMILY-CENTERED MATERNITY CARE

Offered by the more progressive hospitals nationwide, it
means just what it says: that the hospital respects the importance of the family unit during labor and delivery and
after the baby is born. Such hospitals usually have nurses in
labor and delivery who are familiar with prepared childbirth techniques and can help you with them. However, the
problem with the phrase Family-Centered Maternity Care is
that *any* hospital can advertise it. Some institutions are using it as a catchphrase to attract patients but the administration and staff are not genuinely committed—either in
theory or practice—to what *should* be included or excluded
from hospital routines and policies.

In order to determine just how family-centered a
hospital is, you are going to have to take a tour and ask
questions. Chapter Seven, Choosing a Doctor and a Hospital, describes the various family-centered options, including
optional routine procedures on admittance, breast-feeding
on the delivery table, Leboyer delivery, nonseparation of
mother and baby after birth, rooming-in, early discharge,
etc. If you decide that you want any or all of these options
available to you, you will choose a hospital accordingly.
Chapter Seven also discusses how to *change* a hospital so
that it meets your needs.

## THE FETAL HEART MONITOR (FHM)

Perhaps the single most controversial subject in childbirth
today, this machine is hailed by some as the greatest advance in the history of maternity care. Others attack it as
inaccurate, dehumanizing, and the cause of physical harm.
In order to make a fully informed, balanced decision for
yourself about fetal monitoring it is necessary to learn how
it works and then to look at it from three perspectives:
philosophical, medical, and legal. Only then will you be

able to formulate an opinion . . . as you will see, this is easier said than done. There is no absolute Right or Wrong about monitoring, but the issue *is* complicated by controversy about when it should be used, how it is used, and what medical action should be taken on the basis of results.

## HOW THE FETAL HEART MONITOR WORKS

***The monitor is a boxlike machine*** that looks like a large receiver for a stereo system. It is usually on a wheeled table that is approximately the height of your hospital bed.

***Two wide plastic straps*** (connected by wires to the FHM) are placed around your abdomen. The nurse will probably squeeze some electroconductor jelly onto your skin to improve transmission of signals. The upper strap has a pressure gauge to record your uterine contractions. The lower strap holds an ultrasonic transducer to pick up the fetal heart rate. The straps must be fairly snug to get readings, but if they are too tight for comfort, tell the nurse.

***You must lie quite still*** because the monitor produces indiscriminate *tracings* (called "artifacts") from your movements, the baby's movements, and other vibrations—the artifacts interfere with an accurate tracing of the fetal heart rate. These tracings come out of the machine on a narrow strip of paper and are two parallel squiggly lines with big dips in them indicating contractions. There is a microphone that picks up the baby's heartbeat, although the volume can be turned off in case you don't want to hear the steady, fast beat-beat-beating. A small light on the machine also flashes with each heartbeat and a digital number flashes (sometimes on a separate TV screen) a reading every second—153, 139, 146—which is a computation of the baby's heartbeats per minute.

***An internal monitor*** is more accurate and more artifact-free (and allows you to move around more freely in bed without disturbing the tracings). The internal monitor can ascertain variables in the fetal heart rate which are impossible to detect with the external monitor. The lower strap is replaced by an internal monitor. The internal monitor is either a clip or screw electrode—a small metal ending on a long wire. Your cervix must be dilated at least 1 to 2 centimeters in order for the electrode to be inserted, which can be painful for some women. The metal end is passed up inside you and clipped onto your baby's scalp or inserted just under the skin. There are as yet no studies determining whether this increases the risk of infection to the baby. The issue is rarely even raised as to whether this electrode causes the baby pain. Some hospitals use an internal monitor whenever a woman's membranes have already broken. Other hospitals only use it when fetal distress has been detected with external monitoring (in such a case the membranes would be artificially ruptured if necessary). A second catheter is sometimes inserted that measures the intensity of your contractions with more accuracy than the external monitor—and replaces the upper strap.

***The purpose of an FHM*** is to supply information about how your baby is responding to the stress of labor. With each uterine contraction the baby's blood supply is temporarily cut off. It seems a bit dramatic to make the comparison that it is like strangling the baby each time, but the baby does receive his oxygen via the blood and that flow is cut off each time you have a labor contraction. Some babies can withstand labor less well than others—depending on their size, the strength of the contractions, the length of labor, and other considerations. The FHM measures each of your uterine contractions and the baby's heart rate simultaneously. It is normal for his heart rate to drop with each contraction; it is also normal for the baby's heart rate to come right back up to where it was before the contraction. If the fetal heart rate is slow in returning to normal it is known as "late deceleration": if the monitor continues to indicate this is the baby's response to your contractions it is called fetal distress. A safe fetal heart rate is considered to be between 120 and 160 beats per minute. Distress is indicated when the rate goes above 160 or below about 110. This introduces an area of controversy about the

FHM—in this section I am only *describing*. Pages 321 to 330 discuss the pros and cons of the fetal monitor.

## FHM AND INACCURACIES

The monitor's only dependable ability at this point is in telling you that everything is okay. The monitor's prediction of a normal outcome is more accurate than any other technique. When the FHM tracing is normal, you can be certain that everything is, in fact, normal. The problem is that the incidence of "false abnormal" tracings is high.

*Monitoring patterns* may sometimes be indecipherable, because of artifacts or a malfunctioning machine.

*The external monitor* can give an inaccurate recording of data.

*Even with the more accurate,* sensitive internal monitor, the data is subject to varying interpretations. The interpretation of distress patterns is not uniform: all tracings are subject to a wide difference in the way they are evaluated by doctors. Even the champions of the monitor agree that a refinement is necessary in the diagnosis of these patterns.

*The maternal heart rate* may be counted by mistake or the fetal heart rate half—or double—counted.

*There is a tendency to "overdiagnose"* when there is fetal distress. Some experts believe that an accurate interpretation of an abnormal tracing cannot be made on the basis of fetal monitoring alone: it is necessary to also do fetal scalp sampling (page 320).

## WHAT HAPPENS IF THERE'S FETAL DISTRESS?

*If there is a distress pattern* the staff first tries conservative measures to restore a normal pattern.

*They reposition you,* usually turning you on your side. A problem with monitoring is that you have to lie on your back, which invites *supine hypotension.* This means that the weight of the baby and your position press on the main vein returning blood to your heart: this can cause a drop in maternal blood pressure and ominous fetal-heart-rate patterns.

***The staff will increase your blood pressure,*** giving you intravenous fluids if you aren't already hooked up to an I.V. and administering oxygen with a face mask.

***The attendants will reduce or cancel any oxytocin*** you are receiving (a synthetic hormone that increases your contractions) or will give you medication to inhibit contractions.

***Fetal scalp sampling*** is performed to determine whether the fetal distress suggested by the FHM is accurate. True fetal distress is almost always caused by a reduced flow of oxygen-rich blood to the fetus. When the oxygen supply is depleted, the pH of the baby's blood is lowered. The pH is a measure of the acidity or alkalinity of the blood; too low a pH level means that the baby is in jeopardy and must be delivered immediately, perhaps by cesarean. A low pH in the fetus is usually from a reduced blood supply, but it may also be the result of maternal disease like diabetic acidosis.

Scalp sampling is done by inserting a cone-shaped speculum into the vagina, which is moved up against the baby's presenting part (which is usually the head) and a tiny prick is made. A drop or two of blood is taken and examined for its concentration of oxygen, carbon dioxide and its pH. The results of these findings help a doctor determine what course of action to take. Although the fetal heart monitor can be inaccurate, when used in conjunction with fetal scalp sampling the monitor becomes a much more reliable tool.

***The rule of thumb*** is that if an ominous fetal-heart-rate pattern in a previously healthy fetus cannot be restored to normal within half an hour, a cesarean section is performed.

*The newest internal monitors* are hoped to be so accurate that fetal blood analysis will not be as frequently needed to verify the baby's condition.

## THE PHILOSOPHICAL POSITION IN FAVOR OF MONITORING

*The mother's condition does not necessarily determine the baby's condition.* You may be in perfect health and have had a trouble-free pregnancy and therefore be considered "low-risk." However, various studies show that the problems that develop during labor and delivery are not confined to women designated "high-risk" (who gave prior indications that there might be complications). High-risk patients only account for one-half of the bad outcomes (newborns with problems). One study which eliminated all high-risk women, by every possible definition of high-risk factors, showed that one-third of all low-risk patients become high-risk during labor. Another study showed that 50 percent of newborns with problems resulted from low-risk pregnancies.

The argument has been made—and rightly so—that many of the routine practices in the hospital can cause physical problems. A woman's emotional reaction to these routines—even to being in the hospital—can also cause complications. However, the larger issue rests on the fundamental position that *labor itself is what generates the problems.* Although the vast majority of births will be normal there is no way of knowing which babies will have trouble coping with the stress of labor and delivery. Thus if you accept the premise that the mother and baby are independent of each other—that information you have about the mother's condition does not guarantee the baby's condition—then you accept the need to monitor. At the very least you accept that the designation "low-risk" is limited in its usefulness as a prediction of how a baby will withstand labor.

*The greatest benefit of the monitor is the confident prediction of a nondistressed fetus* regardless of its mother's condition. If properly administered and read (fairly large "ifs") the monitor removes the guesswork about whether a baby is all right. The pitfalls in its prediction of an *abnormal* fetal condition have already been mentioned. Advocates of the monitor agree that the machine is in its infancy as a diagnostic tool and may be error-prone because the methods of its use and the terminology have not been universally agreed upon and authoritative texts are not available.

*If your number-one priority in childbirth is the kind of safety* the monitor offers (i.e., the certainty of knowing everything is all right) then you will want the monitor. However, you have to decide whether you are willing to pay the personal price for the technology. Monitoring will necessarily inhibit other aspects of the birth experience that have their own importance; you have to be willing to forfeit those. You don't get something for nothing. There are many instances in modern American life where human personal qualities and experience are bartered for what machines have to offer.

At times our technology has outstripped our ability to know when, where, and how to use it. It may be true that the "right" way to use the fetal heart monitor has not yet been discovered. But if this sense of absolute certainty is your foremost concern (there is no way of knowing which baby has the cord tangled around his neck) then you may opt for a machine that can at least assure you that *your baby does not have a problem.* The warning must be added once again that you should not depend totally on the FHM: *normalcy* is the only absolutely reliable information it can give you.

*A doctor cannot make these decisions for you.* If you are considered a low-risk patient then you have to weigh the benefits and disadvantages of the monitor. There is no way of knowing ahead of time who the small number of women will be whose babies will become distressed during labor. Whether *all* women should be routinely monitored to determine if they are in the normal majority is a decision that should not be made by doctors and hospitals. If you are going to have a machine monitor your labor, you must know what you are gaining and what you may be giving up—each individual has to decide that for herself.

## ARGUMENTS AGAINST THE FETAL MONITOR (AND SOME REBUTTALS)

***Inaccuracy in diagnosing distress*** has already been mentioned. The rebuttal to this is that as it is improved, the monitor will become more reliable in predicting problems as well as normalcy.

***The monitors must be monitored.*** Just like the question of whether a falling tree makes a sound if no one sees it, a monitor is useless unless it is being watched. The machine varies from useless to dangerous unless it is being watched by someone who knows the subtleties of what to look for in yards and yards of tracings. This close surveillance which is required is not always available. When there *is* someone reading the tracing—whether it is a nurse or doctor—they may not be properly trained in interpreting the information. The good thing that can be said about the need to monitor monitors is that this increased surveillance may be helping to lower perinatal mortality, irrespective of the machine. There has been a lower death rate for infants at the large teaching hospitals that use monitors routinely on all women. This reduced rate can also be attributed to factors associated with monitoring: closer surveillance, enhanced alertness and education of the staff, changes in routines and procedures, etc.

***All the attention is paid to the machine, not the woman.*** The staff and even your coach can become absorbed in watching the strip that is continuously advancing from the machine. It is not uncommon for a doctor or nurse to walk into a labor room and the first thing they look at is the machine. They may not even make eye contact with you as they say, "How are you doing?" They pick up the long chart of paper that the machine has produced. It's almost as if they're asking the machine how things are going.

The piece of paper has become the laboring woman. Even *you* may come to think of the machine as the controlling influence on your labor.

It is said in praise of the monitor that it can *alert you to an upcoming contraction*. It *is* true that you or your coach can see that a contraction is beginning by watching the needle making a tracing on the graph. But it is somewhat illogical to compliment the machine: after all, it is your body and if you were focused on your uterus (instead of a monitor tracing) you could *feel* a contraction beginning! Very often the coach and staff will watch a contraction from start to finish on the tracing and exclaim afterward, "Boy, that was a big one." It becomes absurd; *they* are telling *you* about the contraction. Similarly you may have a hard time breathing your way through a particularly tough contraction and complain afterward how difficult it was. Your coach or the nurse may make light of it, saying, "No, that wasn't much of a contraction." They were watching the monitor tracing and it didn't look like much *there*. Nonetheless a contraction doesn't have to look huge on a tracing to do a lot of dilation, which may cause you discomfort. If there weren't a monitor to "disprove" your subjective reaction you might get some sympathetic support.

If you feel the monitor is getting all the attention, tell people. There is no use in having a coach and a well-trained obstetric nurse or a carefully chosen doctor or nurse-midwife if you aren't getting the attention and support from them that you want. Even the best-intentioned attendants can unwittingly fall into the trap of focusing on the monitor. There are serious pitfalls in it for you if the emphasis is on a machine.

***We do not yet know the psychological harms to laboring women, their doctors, and nurses*** who take care of machines instead of people. The problem is not just for the woman in labor; the people who care for her may also be suffering psychic damage. They have devoted their training and careers to caring for people; high-risk, technologically oriented maternity care has become a maze of machines, medications, and computer printout. This dehumanization affects the caretakers as well as the recipients.

***The machine may take up so much room*** or be positioned in such a way that the labor room is cramped and the monitor separates a woman and her coach. If this happens, simply tell the staff and move the bed, monitor, or your coach! If the room and machine are arranged so that there is no place for your coach to sit, take it upon yourselves to rearrange things for your comfort and convenience.

***The monitor invites supine hypotension*** (page 320) because a woman must lie flat on her back while it is in place. It is undeniable that lying on your back for long periods cuts off the vena cava (the vein that returns blood to your heart) and thereby shuts off the baby's oxygen supply. There are *alternative ways* of using the monitor that guard against this hypotension occurring. However, you cannot count on your doctor or the staff to suggest them. *You* can suggest them to your doctor ahead of time and then do what you have agreed upon once you are in labor.

1. LIE ON YOUR SIDE. The monitor tracing may not be quite as good when you lie on your side and it takes more skill to interpret the results but it does eliminate the problem of supine hypotension. You might want to shift to your side periodically.

2. THE EXTERNAL MONITOR CAN BE REMOVED and you can walk around or go to the bathroom. The monitor can then be attached periodically to assure that all is going well. One way is to monitor only 15 minutes out of every hour. In between you can take any position you want to, in bed or out. Physically and psychologically it is good for you to walk around during labor. Walking stimulates contractions, allows gravity to help the baby descend, and gives you a feeling of being normal, not a bedridden invalid. Another solution is to monitor once every two hours: leave the monitor on for 20 minutes and if you get a good tracing then you don't need another for an hour and 40 minutes.

Discuss these options with your doctor ahead of time because even the strongest advocates of the monitor believe that these are viable alternatives.

*A doppler or fetoscope* can be used, some critics say, instead of a fetal heart monitor. Unfortunately this is *not true*. These hand-held instruments amplify the sound of the fetal heartbeat, which tells you only that the heart is beating and how fast. The Doppler *cannot* tell you how well the baby recovers after a contraction, which is the whole point of the FHM. It is said that human auscultation (listening to the baby's heart rate with the human ear) is a viable substitute for the monitor. Even if you had enough staff so that someone could stay glued to a woman's abdomen for hours and hours, however, it is *not possible to detect* the kind of late deceleration that indicates fetal distress and can result in problems for the newborn.

*The fetal heart monitor has caused a rise in the cesarean rate.* It is true that there are babies with abnormal FHR patterns who are delivered by cesarean without appearing to have had any signs of problems of birth, for the FHM is not fully reliable at this point in its diagnosis of abnormality. Furthermore, the monitor's accuracy is only as good as the people reading its tracings. For example, a monitor can show a variable deceleration, which to an inadequately trained eye may look like a late deceleration, but is *not* the same and does not indicate distress.

*However, at Yale,* which is the birthplace of the FHM, after a period of increased C-sections when staff and physicians were still learning the intricacies of the monitor, their cesarean section rate has now leveled off to what it was in premonitor days—10 percent. It is hoped that they are now doing cesareans on all the women who do need them, and avoiding them on those who do not, particularly those high-risk patients whose babies register as normal on the monitor.

*The higher cesarean rate* at some institutions may be high because they are just getting accustomed to the monitor, but there are other related reasons. Until now the monitor has been reserved for high-risk pregnancies. And although there is now routine monitoring of all women in relatively few well-endowed institutions, in most hospitals the $6,000-per-machine cost (not counting maintenance, etc.) means that the monitor is still reserved for high risk. *But the high-risk group has grown.*

THERE ARE COUPLES WITH GENETIC OR FERTILITY PROBLEMS (for instance) who might have adopted in the past. Because of improved prenatal testing and fertility cures, they are now able to get pregnant but remain at risk.

NEW TESTS THAT DETERMINE FETAL MATURITY can indicate when an insufficient placenta begins to jeopardize the fetus. This alerts doctors to a potentially complicated labor and delivery, so they elect to do a cesarean instead.

THERE IS A RELATIVELY HIGHER PROPORTION OF FIRST-TIME MOTHERS because parents are electing to have only one or two children, and there are relatively more older first-time mothers because women are waiting longer to conceive. Both these groups are at higher risk.

THERE ARE ALSO LEGAL REASONS for doing a cesarean, which are discussed in the following section and also in Chapter Ten, Complications in Pregnancy and Birth.

*A drop in the FHR pattern may cause a woman or her mate to panic.* A coach may see something that doesn't look right to him on the tracing. He may get upset and perhaps interfere with your breathing techniques. To avoid this potential problem, ask to be shown a monitor tracing ahead of time—either on your hospital tour or in early labor—so that you know which drops are normal (i.e., variable deceleration) and which are late deceleration.

There have also been cases of an internal monitor dislodging from the baby's scalp. This means the fetal-heart-rate light on the monitor stops blinking and the beat-beat-

beating sound stops. You might think your baby has died inside you, although it is only the electrode that has detached. This can be a terrifying and traumatic experience; it can disrupt your relaxation and concentration during labor, and it may be a long time before you recover from it. The only solution if this happens is to supplement the alarming information given by the monitor with what can be learned by the human ear. Ask a nurse or the doctor to listen to the baby through your abdomen to assure you that the baby is still alive.

***What do you do on the day the monitor is broken?*** A FHM is only a machine, and like any machine, it is far from perfect. They malfunction or stop working altogether. We are in the process of turning out an entire generation of doctors and nurses who *know how to assess labor only with a monitor*. They are lost without it. Medicine is fast becoming dominated by machines: that is where all the attention is focused and all decisions are based on machine data. This is a true "1984" situation and one that must be looked at seriously before there is no room left to reverse our steps. Women have babies; machines don't. Women are going to continue to have babies whether or not the machines are ready for them on any given day. The staff of every hospital maternity unit needs training and practice in relying on their own personal experience and intelligence to assess a woman in labor, rather than on what a tracing on a piece of paper tells them.

***Official medical policy on FHMs has changed*** dramatically. In 1988 the American College of Obstetricians and Gynecologists (ACOG) overturned its long-standing policy favoring the use of electronic fetal monitors. The ACOG now states that electronic fetal monitoring will no longer be part of the standard of care for maternity patients. Under the existing standard of care, monitoring is called for only with high-risk patients; however, it is commonly used on all women in labor.

    The ACOG based its decision in part on the results of research which does not show monitors to have any benefit over a nurse listening to the fetal heartbeat every 15 minutes in the first stage of labor, and every 5 minutes in the second stage. Before anyone gets too excited about this, let's stop and do a reality check: where would you find enough nurses to listen to the belly of every laboring woman throughout her entire labor?

The bottom line is that there will probably be no difference in how often electronic monitors are used, despite the data which shows that using FHMs does not produce healthier babies. Obstetricians point to a combination of legal and economic pressures which make it almost impossible to stop using them. Because of the serious nursing shortage nationwide, hospitals could never hire enough nurses to take the place of the monitors.

## THE LEGAL SIDE OF MONITORING

*"Established practice."* Once a medical technique has become standard practice, a doctor can be judged on whether he has followed that standard or not. When a number of doctors state that a technique is necessary, it becomes so. Monitoring has become established practice. This means that if there is a bad outcome in childbirth and monitoring was available but not used, a doctor can be held responsible for the problem that resulted.

*It could be grounds for a malpractice lawsuit not to monitor* once it has become a standard procedure. Theoretically, any doctor who disregards standard procedure is liable for the decision. It wouldn't even matter if a couple were to sign a release form ahead of time. For example, it would be malpractice for a cardiologist not to use an electrocardiograph—a machine which tells whether or not a patient has a heart problem. Even though it can be argued that childbirth is not a sickness or abnormality and therefore should not be treated as one, birth is becoming a high-risk, technologized field.

*In the case of a lawsuit a fetal-monitor tracing can be used as evidence* by a doctor that a patient received thorough attention. The tracing on the strip chart (almost regardless of what is on it) becomes the doctor's defense in the event there is legal trouble later. In a day and age when people *are* litigious and *do* sue doctors, it is understandable that a physician would want every protection possible. A lot depends on the kind of relationship formed by a doctor and an expectant couple: one would imagine that if the relationship was good, then a lawsuit would never result. Not all patient-doctor relationships are optimal—and even those that are take unpredictable twists and turns.

## FRIENDS ATTENDING YOUR CHILD'S BIRTH

This is a choice that either appeals to you or seems distasteful. In home births there are often friends present, both to help with practical matters and to share in the experience. In maternity center births and alternative birthing rooms in hospitals there is usually the option of having guests.

*Your reaction* to having friends attend may be that birth is a private matter, and anyway, "who would even *want* to come?" However, in a hospital there can be a dozen people who see you during labor and delivery—it is hardly a private event. If you think of it this way you may feel differently about the possibility of *choosing* who is with you. As for "who would want to come," there are numerous people who would jump at the chance to see a baby born—it is a fascinating and awesome experience which is denied to most people. However, people with *unresolved feelings* toward births are not going to make good guests.

*Emotional support* is most important during childbirth and being surrounded by friends can give you that feeling.

*Guests are there to focus energy toward the birth.* Although people playing musical instruments or socializing with each other is fine, their activity should always be subject to how it affects you. If you get the feeling that there's a "party" going and you're left out of it (lying there doing hard work!) it can be counterproductive to your labor. Be sure to discuss this ahead of time with anyone you invite. Consider your friends' personalities. If you think they might be so caught up in themselves that they cannot take a back seat to the main event then they may not be an asset to the birth.

***Guests should not arrive too early in labor.*** If people start coming before you are well-established in labor it may make you feel tense, which will slow your labor. See pages 496–501 for more on how your emotions can affect your contractions.

***Curiosity-seekers*** do not make good guests. They are voyeurs rather than participants—both physically and in an emotional sense.

***If there are going to be children present,*** be firm that there must be one adult per child to supervise and entertain them (see pages 345–350 on siblings attending for more on children at births).

***Self-invited guests*** may be tricky to uninvite if they are close friends. If you do not want them there for some reason, it may be awkward to tell them you do not want them there. You can ease out of it by telling a ''white lie'' and saying that your doctor or midwife has been very firm about how many people can be present and you already have invited as many as you can.

## Home Birth

Chapter Eight is devoted entirely to home birth, and includes a discussion of your various options with home birth: without any attendants except your mate; with a lay midwife; with a certified nurse-midwife; or with a doctor (who usually has midwives to ''labor-sit'' for him).

## INDUCED BIRTH

This is a choice in childbirth but it is a dangerous one. Fifteen percent of births in America are by elective induction: a woman and her doctor decide when to have her baby and then they start labor with synthetic hormones. There are only a very small number of births that should be induced, and these should always be for medical reasons.

*Some of the reasons given for elective induction* are for a mother's convenience (so she can arrange care for any other children, so she can be rested, etc.) and/or for the doctor's convenience (to fit in with his office schedule, so he can be rested and alert, so he can choose when the hospital is most heavily staffed—and therefore theoretically can offer better care). None of these reasons is valid when measured against the possible harm. Another frequent use of synthetic oxytocin (the hormone that stimulates contractions) is when you are admitted to a hospital but labor hasn't truly started. More often than not they will keep you in the hospital and administer pitocin, the most commonly used oxytocin, or they may artificially rupture your membranes. This kind of medical interference with natural processes is not even called "elective induction," although that is what it is. The rationale behind inducing a woman in this situation is that she's tired out from being up all night with early labor contractions, that she's nervous and anxious to have her baby, etc. If that is the case, go home and go to sleep. Or stay in the hospital if there's room and sleep there. *Do not allow anyone to tamper with the natural forces regulating your labor unless there are medical reasons* (outlined later in this section). The use of pitocin or artificial rupture of membranes with *no evidence of cervical change* after hospital admission (i.e., you aren't dilating naturally) must be considered elective induction with all its risks. Many women would have stopped contracting naturally and at a future time delivered a mature fetus without the health problems of a baby whose birth was induced before it was ready for extrauterine life.

## THERE ARE SEVERAL METHODS OF INDUCTION

1. *An artificial membrane rupture* is done routinely by some doctors near your due date without your consent. Other doctors may "strip" the membranes: during an internal exam (in the office or the hospital) a doctor can use his fingers to separate the amnion (bag of waters) from the uterine wall. One possible hazard of this is that you could have an undetected placenta previa: the placenta is nearer to the cervix than the baby is. Stripping the membranes could strip the placenta instead of the amnion away from the uterus, causing a critical hemorrhage. However, in an appropriate situation, stripping the membranes is not dangerous and can have a beneficial effect.

THE AMNIOTIC FLUID IS NATURE'S PROTECTION of the baby, especially during contractions. Nature usually keeps the bag of waters intact until the last phase of labor. Most often the membranes rupture with the onset of second-stage labor, when you are fully dilated and the baby is nearing the end of her journey into the world.

INTACT MEMBRANES ARE AN EXCELLENT DILATOR: They maintain equal pressure on the cervix according to the laws of hydrodynamics. If force is applied to an enclosed liquid the force will be transmitted equally everywhere throughout the liquid. Therefore an intact bag of waters makes a better dilator of the cervix than the contour of the baby's head and protects the head at the same time.

However, there are times when intact membranes can hold the baby's head up off the cervix and can therefore slow down the labor. At such times an amniotomy is beneficial.

ARTIFICIAL RUPTURE CAN START LABOR but it often also *accelerates labor,* shortening it by 30 to 40 minutes. This is simply not worthwhile at the expense of possible damage to the baby's head and other complications. When used to speed up labor some of the possible ill effects are: cerebral birth trauma and episodes of cerebral ischemia with permanent CNS depression. In simple terms this means that there may be a temporary deformation in your baby's head and even permanent damage. Although it is known that 95 percent of membranes will rupture in very late labor if left to themselves, there is a common obstetric practice of artificially rupturing membranes midway through first-stage labor, or at 4 to 5 centimeters dilation. *There is no good reason to do this except impatience.* Doctors and even women seem to have lost touch with the concept of normalcy—they have no faith in the body's ability to do the best job in a normal birth. Birth is a normal body function and a woman's body is built for it. In a low-risk, normal situation, Hands Off is the best policy (and this goes for any kind of obstetric intervention). The birth attendant—doctor, midwife, nurse—is there to watch, as a lifeguard, not to interfere.

RUPTURING THE MEMBRANES CAN CAUSE THE UMBILICAL CORD TO BE COMPRESSED and in many cases occluded during contractions. This affects the baby's oxygen supply.

2. *Pitocin,* the synthetic oxytocin, can be used in a variety of ways:

INJECTION of pitocin is less controllable than the other methods—it is hard to predict how a woman's uterus will respond and there is no way to reduce the amount in your system once you've been given the shot.

THE HORMONE CAN BE PUT INTO INTRAVENOUS SOLUTION and the flow into the I.V. can be adjusted. This is called a "pit drip": but there is a measure of error in this method because the hormone is diluted in a large bottle of fluid so the doctor doesn't know exactly how much you are getting.

IVAC OR IMED INFUSION PUMP is a small box mounted on the I.V. Pole. The glucose solution contains the pitocin which flows through the IVAC box, which regulates the amount you receive. This eliminates the hazards of a regular "pit drip."

3. *Prostaglandin* is a synthetic hormone commonly used to stimulate labor. It is applied to the cervix in a gel which is directly absorbed into the cervix and softens it. Prostaglandin stimulates the production of your own natural prostaglandin, which readies your body to give birth. When softened, the cervix will be less resistant and will open more easily and naturally.

One of the problems with using pitocin has been that while it can create uterine contractions, they do not necessarily accomplish any dilation of the cervix. This has meant that some induced births have ended as cesareans because the contractions were not effective. However, if prostaglandins are used first when you are induced, there won't be so much resistance when the oxytocin-induced contractions apply force against your cervix.

## PROBLEMS WITH INDUCTION

1. *The more intense contractions* can make it *harder for a woman to stay in control* and use her breathing techniques. The net result may be that she will require analgesia—or *more* of it. There is almost always an increased need for painkillers with induction, which stay in the baby's system longer than they do in yours.

2. *An effect on the newborn,* shown by some studies, is a slightly higher risk of jaundice when labor is induced. One side effect of jaundice is that the baby spends more time sleeping and less time alert which will interfere with "bonding" (pages 489–493). A groggy baby will interact less with you and create a cycle, influencing the way you respond to her and she reacts to you.

3. *Overdose of the oxytocic substance* is rare. The fetal heart monitor (FHM) has taken most of the danger out of induction because you can get direct information from the FHM about the baby's condition. But problems do still occur when using oxytocic drugs to stimulate labors:

THE DRUG CAN OVERSTIMULATE THE UTERUS and make the contractions so long and intense that not enough oxygen gets through to the baby.

THE DRUG CAN CAUSE THE PLACENTA TO SEPARATE from the uterine wall before the baby is born, disrupting his oxygen supply. Unless a vaginal delivery is possible immediately this will necessitate a cesarean section.

4. *Your due date can be miscalculated* and the baby may be born *prematurely*. RDS, respiratory distress syndrome, also known as hyaline membrane disease, is a severe disorder of the lungs found in newborns, especially those who are premature (less than 28 weeks). Prematurity and RDS can be a problem in elective repeat cesareans and in inductions. RDS claims the lives of 20,000 newborns each year; many of those deaths could be prevented with fewer and more judicious induced labors.

It is now believed that when a baby's brain reaches a certain state of maturity, it releases a substance that begins a chain of reactions leading to delivery. This is the reason that the *spontaneous onset of labor should be awaited* whenever possible.

5. *However, respiratory distress syndrome is preventable.* If an induction is necessary then *maturity studies should be done first* and delivery postponed if the infant's lungs are not mature enough. The tests can be either a pulmonary maturity study (a study of the L/S ratio in the amniotic fluid) or a mature biparietal diameter (measuring the baby's head) demonstrated by ultrasound. It is a good idea to have both studies done for greatest accuracy.

## MEDICAL REASONS FOR INDUCTION

There are medical reasons to induce labor in approximately 3 percent of births. Basically, an acceptable reason is for the *safety of the mother and baby.*.

*If, through testing of the amniotic fluid,* it is determined that *a mature baby is at least 3 weeks overdue,* then it is wiser to deliver than to wait any longer (see Post-Term Babies, pages 576–577). However, many doctors induce routinely after 42 weeks. The problem can be that your due date has been calculated from the last period and not conception, leaving a 2-week margin of error. There are many healthy 8-pound babies born 2 weeks after their "due" date.

***If there is a medical problem in the mother*** such as diabetes or toxemia, it is often mandatory to induce labor. Other medical problems might be severe Rh sensitization or a previous history of severe hemorrhage.

### PREMATURE RUPTURE OF MEMBRANES (PROM):

If the membranes have ruptured spontaneously and labor doesn't begin within a reasonable amount of time, it is standard procedure to induce labor. Medical studies show that if a woman has not *delivered* her baby (not just gone into labor) within 12 to 24 hours after her membranes have ruptured there is an increased risk of amnionitis (infection of the amniotic sac). However, there are some birth attendants, both medical and lay, who point out that the decreased infection rate with a delivery within 24 hours was coupled with a policy of avoiding vaginal exams during that time. That may have contributed to the decline in the infection rate. Some less conservative doctors allow a woman to stay at home after ruptured membranes because the environment there is less pathological bacterially than the hospital. Many lay midwives allow a woman to go 48 to 72 hours after ruptured membranes.

***If dilation begins and then stops*** some doctors advise induction. For example, it is possible to be dilated 3 centimeters for a week or two but the only reason to induce is for your "comfort." Labor may progress quickly once it begins and you may be in the car on the way to the hospital when you're in transition, which may not be the ideal place to go through the toughest part of labor. However, you have to compare it to the possible dangers of induction.

***If an epidural anesthetic (or other drug) stops your labor cold***—if it knocks out the contractions altogether—pitocin may be necessary to get things going again.

*If your uterus is atonic*—contractions are weak and ineffective in accomplishing any dilation—artificial stimulation by pitocin may be necessary.

*In the case of fetal death in utero,* it is sometimes necessary to induce labor if it does not begin spontaneously after a reasonable amount of time.

## LAY MIDWIVES

(Described in Chapter Eight, Home Birth.)

## LEBOYER DELIVERY

Developed by a French doctor, Leboyer delivery has been misunderstood by some followers. It is not intended to be a blueprint of exactly how to manage a delivery: Leboyer's work is best applied if it is seen as an attempt to *sensitize people to understand that the newborn sees, hears, and feels*. The main concern is *the baby's experience of labor and delivery*.

## THE PSYCHOLOGICAL MOTIVATION
### FOR LEBOYER'S TECHNIQUES

Leboyer was influenced by a group of psychiatrists who share the belief that later problems in life stem from birth trauma.

*Otto Rank* viewed the birth trauma as the "primal separation," which profoundly influences our later life. He believed that "neuroses in all their manifold forms [are] reproductions of, and reactions to, the birth trauma."

*Arthur Janov* claims that the primal trauma is at the root of all human problems. He claims that "primal therapy" is the cure of neurosis. This therapy attempts to enable a person to fully experience the blocked-out pain that he felt both inside and outside the uterus at birth. Janov contends that the infant cannot intellectualize that "birth hurts"—the only choice is to feel the pain or repress it and usually it is repressed, which surfaces in adult life as neurosis.

*Leboyer* wants to reduce birth trauma. He says that we carry throughout life the imprint of our birth. He says that a baby is taken from the uterus and bombarded with thundering sounds, the cold openness of the delivery room, and the first breath of burning air. (Personally I find his book *Birth Without Violence* a bit fanatical and overblown. I think his methods are marvelous but his rhetoric off-putting.)

Leboyer agrees with the previously mentioned psychiatrists that birth is a prototypic psychological experience of separation and loss. He believes that the process of birth involves deep pain, hurt, and fatigue for the baby. There are basic defense mechanisms which aid the newborn by blocking out these negative feelings—and it is these defenses which allow a child to become neurotic or preneurotic. The goal, therefore, is to reduce the trauma. Whether or not you agree with Leboyer's reasoning you can still be interested in the net result of gentler, more loving birth.

## LEBOYER'S RECOMMENDATIONS FOR BIRTH PROCEDURES

*Dim, indirect lighting.* This is more comfortable for the newborn's sensitive eyes. There is no doubt that a newborn will keep her eyes tightly shut beneath a bright light and open them and look around if there is reduced light. This can have an important effect in bonding, where eye-to-eye contact is so important.

*A delivery-room temperature is adjusted to the comfort of the baby* rather than the delivery-room personnel. It can be quite chilly in a delivery room; the main reason for this is to reduce chances of infection since bacteria grow where it is warm. The other reason is so the staff can stay cool. One solution is to have portable radiant heaters under which the baby can be placed. The heater can also be positioned over the delivery table so you can hold the baby and have the heat source over you.

***Immediate postnatal positioning of the newborn on the mother's abdomen.*** Leboyer also suggests massaging the baby while she is on your stomach. This accomplishes skin-to-skin contact and lessens the shock of being in the open air because the baby can hear your heart and feel you. It can also hasten third-stage labor, the expulsion of the placenta.

***A minimum of noise and talk throughout.*** Leboyer is concerned that a newborn is shocked by noise outside the uterus, where all sounds have been muffled through the amniotic fluid. However, a newborn's ears are probably still filled with fluid at birth so the sound is naturally softened anyway.

***A minimum of hard, jerky movements.*** Leboyer is concerned about the somewhat rough way that babies are usually handled at birth and the trauma this must cause after the envelopment of the uterus. It is true that delivery-room personnel can be brusque in handing the baby to each other and rubbing her off; a Leboyer delivery focuses everyone's attention on the baby, thereby causing them to be more conscious about their treatment of her.

***A delay in severing the umbilical cord until pulsation has ceased.*** In many hospitals they routinely give an injection of oxytocin to hasten the delivery of the placenta. If you are going to wait for the cord to stop pulsating and delay cutting it, make sure you aren't given that shot of oxytocin at the time of birth because it can cause hemorrhaging. Also, be aware that cutting the cord is a medical procedure and is the doctor's ''territory.'' Discuss it with him but recognize that this is an area in which he may get defensive about being ''dictated to.'' (See page 484 for a full discussion of late cord clamping.)

***Placing the newborn in a tub of warm water*** with gentle, firm support is perhaps the best-known aspect of Leboyer's recommendations. His reasoning is that birth trauma is lessened if a baby is returned to the weightless wet environment he just came from. Some doctors and hospitals encourage the baby's father to give the bath. Some offer practice classes before birth; in any case a nurse or the doctor will assist your mate because a newborn is slippery. It is a wonderful way for paternal-infant bonding to begin and if you are interested you should clear the way ahead of time. It is important that the hospital staff is alerted so that they can have a plastic tub and warmed sterile water ready at delivery time.

Some doctors object to the bath for the following reasons:

1. A BABY HAS A POOR ABILITY TO MAINTAIN BODY TEMPERATURE, so one of the main concerns with any newborn is for her temperature to stabilize. A bath introduces *cold stress*—the water on her skin makes her feel cold when you remove her from the bath, just as it does to you after you step out of the shower and before you dry off. However, since the baby's temperature regulator is not very efficient, even drying her off quickly may not take the chill off. One solution: have a radiant heater placed over the tub of water and wrap the baby in warmed towels and blankets when you take her out.

2. A BABY NEEDS THE SHOCK of the extrauterine environment in order to stimulate her lungs to breathe for the first time. Some experts say that placing her back in a warm liquid environment may not stimulate her enough to insure that she continues breathing. This objection seems a bit too conservative: even with a bath there are still many stimuli unfamiliar to the baby's system that stimulate her to breathe on her own.

***Minimal blanketing of the newborn.*** This recommendation of Leboyer's may be hard to apply if you do give the bath because coverings are necessary to keep the baby warm. However, it is possible to put the baby back on your stomach after the bath and put the covers over her, while maintaining skin-to-skin contact underneath. This way the baby has the additional benefit of your body heat while maternal-infant bonding is taking place.

## OBJECTIONS TO LEBOYER TECHNIQUES

*In many cases an obstetrician or pediatrician may not even know* Leboyer's recommendations for birth. He may be resistant to the mention of Leboyer because of the enormous amount of publicity this French doctor has received. It is not considered "professional" for a doctor to go out soliciting public attention, particularly when his concepts have not first been presented through the "proper" medical channels (carefully controlled studies, published papers, etc.).

*The argument often heard from American doctors* is that there is no "proof" for Leboyer's claims, and *this is absolutely true*. Leboyer's suggestions for childbirth sound kind and loving, but he makes unproven statements about the ways in which his techniques will improve children. He has nothing to back up his claims except his personal beliefs.

*In 1977 the American press* widely circulated a report from the French National Center for Scientific Research. It was the work of one psychologist, Daniele Rapoport. If you read the report carefully it was clear that the results were the *subjective analysis of one woman* who had worked closely with Leboyer. There was apparently no control group, which is absolutely necessary in any kind of controlled "scientific research." The study stated that the 120 Leboyer-delivered babies were better off physically and psychologically than traditionally delivered babies, although there was no *direct comparison*. The study claimed that the Leboyer babies: (1) walked sooner than average; (2) were unusually adept with their hands; (3) had minimal trouble with toilet training; (4) learned to feed themselves more easily.

The problem with this study is that it did not take

into account the possibility—or the probability—that these children did so much better than the average *because of their parents*. The kind of parents who choose a Leboyer delivery are demonstrating a concern for their child's sensibility from the moment of birth: they are bound to be sensitive, attentive, involved, interactive parents.

Rapaport's "study" contends that it was the way these children's births were handled that accounts for their behavior. That may be true—but this study does not prove that. In order for a study to really be conclusive it would have to take parents all of whom *want* a Leboyer delivery and divide the group, allowing only one half to have Leboyer techniques and the other half a traditional hospital delivery. The study could then compare children of these two groups—with parents who all showed an interest in their babies' sensitivity before birth. This would rule out the possibility that the children were well-adjusted and advanced because of the quality of their parenting, not just their birth.

*If your doctor is opposed to Leboyer techniques* ask him to read the book *Birth Without Violence*. If he refuses to read it, then you know exactly where you stand and you have the option of changing doctors. If he reads or has read the book and disagrees with Leboyer's ideas he may be willing to arrange for *some* of Leboyer's recommendations. He might agree not to use the bright overhead spotlight, he might agree to hand you the baby gently and immediately, etc. Again, what counts about a Leboyer delivery is to focus the awareness of all attendants on the newborn's sensitivity to sights, sounds, and smells.

*A Leboyer delivery may be redundant in a home birth* because it was originally intended to humanize hospital birth. The important benefit of Leboyer techniques in the hospital is that it allows a couple to identify themselves as wanting this kind of experience. It jolts care-givers out of their routines and makes them more aware of what they are doing to the baby and the way they're doing it. Obviously there is no problem about this sensitivity at home. In fact, applying Leboyer techniques at home might *decrease* intimacy rather than increase it. Spontaneity would be sacrificed while you were trying to carry out procedures that were designed for a different birth setting. Having a Leboyer bath at home is like carrying the proverbial coals to Newcastle.

***The bath may interfere with bonding.*** Some women find that if they hold the baby immediately after birth and begin breast-feeding on the delivery table that it seems artificial and disruptive to hand the baby over for a bath. Try to be flexible and see how you feel at the time and *do not feel tied* to any of these techniques. Spontaneity—a natural, instinctive response—is more important than anything. If you feel like holding on to the baby, whether she is sucking or not, then do that. Of course your mate may be eager to give the bath, so you'll have your first negotiation over the baby!

## MATERNITY CENTERS

Maternity centers are prevalent in many parts of the world, but there are pitifully few in America. A maternity center is a facility designed to meet the needs of low-risk women during a normal birth. (See page 415 for the chart of Factors That Rule Out Home Birth to determine whether you are eligible). If there are any complications during labor or delivery, in most cases you will be transferred to a nearby hospital. A maternity center is usually staffed by certified nurse and/or lay midwives with a doctor on call, with whom they consult if anything is abnormal. Affiliation with a doctor also enables them to prescribe medication during prenatal care or birth, and to admit a laboring woman into a hospital, if necessary.

Maternity centers emphasize the normalcy of birth. They require that a woman has had childbirth classes; they rarely have any analgesia available for labor, although they may have oxytocins and other drugs in case of complications with delivery. Some maternity centers have cooking facilities and room enough so that a couple can spend the night after birth.

Unfortunately you are unlikely to see more maternity centers developing. The ones that do exist are an anachronism in a day and age when maternity care in the United States is moving toward centralization. It is called "regionalization" and people in favor of out-of-hospital alternatives are concerned about it. The medical establishment is trying to phase out the maternity departments of smaller hospitals, which traditionally have been the more flexible and humanistic for the very reason that they *are* small. The trend is to have all births take place at the largest, most technologically equipped institutions. This not only limits your choices in where the birth takes place but it imposes high-risk obstetric management on all births, including normal, low-risk ones. The large, fully equipped hospital may be medically necessary for some women or it may be the choice for others who will feel more protected knowing the technology is present. However, each woman should have the right to decide where her baby will be born. There is uncertainty about risks in the hospital as well as outside of it. A maternity center offers a middle-of-the-road compromise.

## SIBLINGS ATTENDING BIRTH

This practice is often part of a birth at home. However, parents choosing an alternative birthing room, a doctor's office, or a maternity center may also have that choice. In deciding whether your other child(ren) will be able to cope with and benefit from seeing their sister or brother born, there are several factors to consider.

*Ask the child* whether he or she *wants* to be there. Explain a little of what it will be like. If the child does not want to participate or observe, respect that. Pressure on a child can be harmful.

*Many people believe that ages 1 to 5 are too young to attend.* Some psychologists say that birth and death are trying experiences for any age, requiring maturity to handle them appropriately.

*A child's negative fantasies cannot be predicted.* A child conceptualizes events differently than an adult does and if the child perceives the birth in a frightening way there is *no way to alter that negative fantasy.*

A CHILD MAY IMAGINE THAT HIS MOTHER IS GOING TO DIE or be horribly changed. This is especially true if the labor is long and difficult and you make noises of discomfort and physical exertion.

IN A CHILD'S LIMITED EXPERIENCE, a strained expression means anger or pain; blood means injury. The child may therefore have a frightening impression of what is happening to you—even if it is explained.

A CHILD MAY BE FRIGHTENED seeing you in such a vulnerable state. Children perceive their parents as somewhat omnipotent. Although they must gradually develop refined opinions it may be a shock to a child to see you in the physical and emotional vulnerability of birth.

*What does your child know about sexuality?* The child's age will have some bearing on this, but a child's sexual knowledge and development should be considered.

*What is a child's cognitive development?* This is related to the issue of negative fantasies and how a child perceives a situation. A younger child may have a harder time understanding explanations of what is happening and reassurances that you will be fine.

*Birth is bloody.* How will the child handle that? (On page 347 there are suggestions on preparing a child.)

*Sibling rivalry may be lessened* if a child watches his baby brother or sister born. Some people who have included a sibling in childbirth found that it enhanced family closeness and attachment. There was little sibling rivalry because the older child saw the birth happen rather than being introduced to a wrapped bundle several days later.

It has been suggested that there is a critical attachment period for siblings and the newborn comparable to the maternal-infant bonding period right after birth. Only recently has the bond between the father and the newborn been considered; we can assume that the paternal-infant bond is similar to the feelings a sibling might have if allowed to get involved immediately with the new member of the family. This bond can result in permanently enduring and beneficial effects on the sibling relationship.

*Small children are probably more influenced* by the reactions of adults around them than by the birth itself. A small child's sense of the world and expectations of it are not fully formed. If adults are happy with what is happening, the child probably will be. Of course a child would be distressed if his mother were to scream or cry. This is a rare occurrence but it could cause the child to fear for her safety.

Practice your breathing and pushing exercises when your child is around. Simulate sounds of grunting, groaning, and moaning before birth. Tell the child what hard work labor is and how hot and sweaty and tired it can make you. If the child *does* get anxious during delivery it may be better to encourage him to stay so there will be evidence of a happy outcome to all your hard work. This way the child can see that reality did not bear out the anxiety.

### SUGGESTIONS FOR SIBLINGS ATTENDING BIRTH

*Tell the child* as soon as possible that a baby brother or sister is going to be born.

*Educate and expose* the child to everything you can about the birth process. If you can relate the discussions to what happened when the child was born, it may make it easier to grasp and relate to.

*Take the child* to at least one prenatal visit so that the child can meet the provider of care and listen to the fetal heartbeat.

*Show the child* diagrams, drawings, photos, and, if possible, a color movie or videotape about childbirth. Just as with adults, if a child is prepared and knows what to expect, the experience will be enhanced. It is important that at the child's level of understanding he learns about the physical process of labor and birth, including what uterine contractions are, dilation of the cervix, the stages of labor, etc. There are certain topics that should be discussed ahead of time with any child:

- There will be *blood and amniotic fluid* on the mother and baby. The child must be reassured that it's okay, that it's normal, that it happened when he was born, too.
- The *sounds of work and/or pain* made by the mother can be frightening to a child. It is advisable to demonstrate to children the sounds that are common during labor and delivery.

  The fact that *labor is hard work* and an intense experience is something that should be thoroughly discussed ahead of time. This is an area that can be especially difficult for children: just when they feel they need their mother, she is unavailable to them. They have to understand that it is important that they let their mother work during contractions and not disturb her during them.

  *Their mother's pain* during labor and the facial contortions that may accompany it should be talked about ahead of time. You must explain to the child that this pain is okay, that it's not like when you fall down and get cut. The pain of labor is good—the mother's body is doing the work it was made to do. However, stretching inside and opening to let the baby out can hurt.

- Discuss the *appearance of the newborn,* with special attention to the umbilical cord and placenta. The child should realize that the cord will be cut, which will not be painful to the mother or the baby. Explain that the baby may cry loudly in the beginning, which doesn't mean there's anything wrong; it's a sign of a strong baby. Describe, or show pictures beforehand, of the placenta, explaining what its function was for the baby in the womb.

- *Episiotomy (or tear) repair* should at least be discussed as a possibility. However, some of the people who favor siblings at birth feel that this may be too disturbing to watch. The decision should be up to individual parents, of course. You should see color photos or, better yet, moving pictures of an episiotomy before you subject a child to watching it. You might also ask yourself what can be gained by a child being present, and what the harm might be.

If the child has never or rarely seen his mother naked, or the mother is uncomfortable about being naked in front of the child, that must be sorted out before the birth. Perhaps taking a bath together, if they've never done that, is a natural and easy way to feel comfortable.

***There should be an adult provided especially*** for the child—or for each child if there is more than one attending the birth. It should be the sole responsibility of that person to see to the child's needs. Obviously it should be someone who can answer questions and give emotional support, who is comfortable with the child and vice versa. If the child needs entertaining, needs to go for a walk, needs to eat, and so on, make sure that the support person you pick will be willing to do all that.

Be sure you ask yourself an important question: Who does the child usually turn to if he or she needs someone? If it is always to the mother, *will the child be satisfied with a substitute?* If you don't answer this question honestly—or discuss it with the child if he's old enough—then you may be asking for trouble.

***You might give the child a specific task during labor*** to include him more actively in the experience. Depending on the child's age, you may want to give him the job of supplying ice chips or cool washcloths, for example.

*Allow the child to come and go at will,* both in the birth room and in the house. Some children may be disinterested or may get bored with waiting. There's no use trying to encourage them to be more attentive, some just don't get very involved.

*Wake up a sleeping child to see the birth* only if there is a familiar person to be with him. It can be disorienting to be awakened in the middle of the night and be confronted with the intensity of childbirth.

*Reassure the child after the birth* that everything is all right. Both parents should do this, but the child may need particular reassurance from the mother.

### ALTERNATIVES TO HAVING A SIBLING PRESENT

*Include the child* as much as possible before birth. Bring the child with you to prenatal exams and share any information you have about pregnancy that a child can understand.

*If you are having a birth at home,* you can *send the child to a neighbor's house* for the labor and delivery and have the child return immediately after birth.

*Introduce the sibling to the new baby as soon as possible;* while you are breast-feeding is a good time. Just bringing a baby home with no preparation can create hostility. It can be compared to a man bringing home a beautiful woman and just announcing that she is going to be "co-wife."

## UNDERWATER BIRTH

Underwater birth may be something you'll hear about; therefore it is included as a "choice in childbirth." Fortunately, it is only being done by fringe elements in the birth movement.

The justification for underwater birth is that it allows

the baby to go from one liquid environment to another, thereby lessening birth trauma. There is no mammal on earth that goes into the water to deliver its young, other than whales . . . but then they live in the water, of course.

The fact about birth is that the baby is *supposed* to make the critical adjustment from intrauterine existence to the outside world. The baby's survival depends upon his making the many adjustments that are required for life outside the womb. The moment the placenta separates, the baby is on his own and his lungs must supply oxygen. If the baby is born underwater there is no way to tell when the placenta has separated; the baby may take water into his lungs rather than air. The baby will drown. This has happened to some of the people practicing this new fad in birthing.

The first few minutes of a baby's life are critical in assessing how he is adjusting to the extrauterine environment. This is the point of the Apgar test. If the baby is underwater there is no way to monitor his responses, and therefore no way of helping a baby that may be having difficulty. Why anybody would be willing to take this life-threatening risk is hard to fathom.

# 7
# Choosing a doctor and a hospital

## CHOOSING A DOCTOR

There is some debate about whether your choice of doctor or hospital should come first but choosing a doctor seems to be the first and more essential task. If you can find a doctor who shares your ideology you will have a decent chance of fighting any hospital rules and routines which might stand in the way of your wishes.

### HOW TO FIND A DOCTOR

*Ask women you know* who have had a baby recently whether they would recommend their doctor. However, it is not enough to simply accept a vague endorsement like "Dr. Stevens was really nice." Be aware that most women may not have had the benefit of the information you have gotten from this book and they may not know, to this day, what options they could have had. If a woman you know recommends her obstetrician, ask her specific questions about areas that are important to you: "How much time did he give you in prenatal visits and how did he answer your questions?" "Was he with you during your entire labor in the hospital?" "Was she genuinely supportive of prepared-childbirth techniques or did she suggest drugs at the first sign of your discomfort?"

Perhaps in addition to asking women, you could ask their mates how they liked the doctor. Find out if they found the doctor straightforward, open-minded, and interested in the needs of the baby's father.

*Write to the ICEA* (International Childbirth Education Association) P.O. Box 20852, Milwaukee, Wisconsin 53220. They can send you a list of CEA member groups and individuals in your area who are supportive of Lamaze and other childbirth techniques. This is a particularly good way to find a doctor if you're moving to a new town.

*The La Leche League* and other childbirth groups can make recommendations of doctors that their members have been pleased with. Although these recommendations will be coming from people you don't personally know, the doctors they endorse are probably progressive, flexible, and responsive to consumer demands.

*Female doctors in obstetrics* used to be rare, but they now account for 15 percent of the OB/GYNs in America. Even more encouraging is that 50 percent of the new doctors coming out of medical school to specialize in obstetrics and gynecology are women. However, just because a doctor is female does not necessarily mean that she will be more sympathetic or supportive. If you go out of your way to find a female doctor because you assume her attitude will be very different from a male physician's, you may be disappointed. Medicine has been predominantly a male field and women who have entered that arena have had to sustain a lot of chauvinism and pressure. Some women obstetricians say that in order to finally gain acceptance by their male colleagues they "had to become more male than the men, like being hazed for a fraternity." This is not to say that many of the female doctors around are not excellent physicians—and they *may* be very understanding and warm as well. However, just because they are women does not give you any guarantee of this and may let you in for an unpleasant shock. If you are intent on receiving care from a woman you might want to consider a certified nurse-midwife.

## QUESTIONS TO ASK A DOCTOR

*Asking questions* is the best way of choosing a doctor. In order to have the best possible birth experience you have to make your needs clear to the doctor from the beginning and ascertain whether he is able or willing to meet your needs. This means that you have to inform yourself and *decide* what your needs are before you approach a doctor; otherwise you'll just be stumbling around in the dark.

*Time is limited* so you should choose questions that reflect the aspects of birth that are most important to you. You don't want to bombard a prospective doctor with too many questions.

*The way that you ask* questions is of utmost importance as it can influence the doctor's response. Coming on strong with firm demands is not advisable. It can make a doctor feel threatened or angry. Saying, "I want . . ." is not always a good way to introduce a subject. A doctor has spent a great deal of time and effort reaching his level of accomplishment and a lay person who defiantly says, "I want . . ." is diminishing the importance of the doctor's expertise. The least threatening way to begin a sentence is, "How do you feel about . . . ?" (or "What do you think about . . . ?"). This allows you to bring up an issue while acknowledging the doctor's intelligence and training.

Do not use a strong style of questioning. You'll only be harming yourself and your chances of getting what you want. Many of the controversial issues about birth require negotiation and temperance between doctor and patient—if you assume a greater-than-thou (or even, depending on the doctor, an equal-to-thou) position you will be raising the hackles on the backs of some physicians. Keep in mind your final objective: to assure yourself the kind of birth you want. If getting that requires some self-control or even role-playing on your part, the sacrifice is small compared to the frustration and rage of not being able to make an understanding arrangement with a doctor.

***Try to get direct, specific answers*** to your questions. Some doctors may be unaccustomed to questioning and feel they are being put on the spot. They may qualify their replies with statements like "Depending on the situation. . . ." In this case it is to your benefit to pin the doctor down to a more concrete answer. Tell him that his vagueness makes you anxious. Ask him under what conditions could the father *not* be in the delivery room, for instance, or would the Leboyer technique be abandoned. Although doctors cannot give you absolute promises (because labor is so unpredictable), you can get an idea of how the doctor's mind works.

***Trust has to go both ways.*** While it is important for you to find out as much as possible about the doctor's ideology, it is equally important for him to believe that you respect and trust him. This is why you have to sit down *at the beginning* of your relationship with a doctor and clarify things. If a woman second-guesses a doctor constantly, all through the pregnancy, then she needs another doctor—she obviously doesn't trust him. Of course there will be questions which crop up about information you learn along the way, but it's best to settle important basics at the outset. No doctor can work effectively if he believes he is going to get the third degree every time you walk in.

***Some doctors are going to react badly*** no matter how you phrase your questions. Some MDs have grown so accustomed to having complete control that they consider any question an impertinent attack on their capabilities. Although I have refrained from anecdotes until now I want to share just one with you to let you see how downright nasty a doctor can become. I had given a few questions to a pregnant friend of mine who was trying to decide whether to stay with her longtime OB/GYN when she got pregnant. Until she asked these questions he had been a charming, nurturant man. She asked the question, "Can I keep the baby with me for half an hour after it's born if everything's okay?'' "What do you want to do that for?" he snapped back at her. She was stunned but went on meekly, "To get to know each other; for bonding." "Bonding, shmonding," he said in disgust, "You want to keep the kid between your legs for twenty-one years?! You've got to cut the cord sometime." The woman was so shocked and hurt by his reaction that she said nothing. And found another doctor immediately. This is just a warning that you may see a very different side of your doctor if you ask him questions: you will have to cope accordingly.

***There are several revealing questions*** you can ask a doctor on the telephone before meeting her. This gives you a chance to feel her out and perhaps save you both the time of meeting if you discover you aren't on the same wavelength. Please don't misunderstand: the intention of these questions is not to trick or trap a doctor. It is simply a way of discovering whether you share the same ideas about pregnancy and birth. After that you can make an appointment for a preliminary visit.

### Some Questions to Ask on the Phone

***"What percentage of your patients do you refer to childbirth education?"*** A doctor may not know off the top of his head the exact percentage, so if he hesitates you might add, "One-half? One-quarter? None?" A doctor's reply will let you know his views about prepared childbirth and his attitude toward prepared women. A doctor whose patients usually take classes is going to be more accustomed to expectant couples who want to be together, who ask questions and rebel against certain routine procedures in the hospital, and who generally want to be assertively involved in the process. A doctor who isn't accustomed to this kind of influence on a patient is going to be more resistant to your requests.

***"Would you consider eliminating some routine procedures in the hospital?"*** A doctor's answer to this lets you know where he stands in relationship to the hospital. A doctor may ask you to tell him which procedures you're referring to—he may do this because he's never had a patient make this request before *or* because he wants to get an idea of where you are "coming from." In the following section about choosing a hospital you can decide which of the routines (if any) you would want eliminated and why. Once you are specific with the doctor—for instance you would like the enema to be at your option—you can judge how flexible he is. Do not assume a doctor is *in*flexible, however, simply because he questions *you* after you bring up the issue. A doctor has just as much right—and need—as you do to discover if you're on the same wavelength. If you can give a doctor a valid reason for wanting a change from the routine he may be much more open to it than if you become defensive.

A doctor who is open-minded about eliminating some routines is not cowed by the institution of the hospital. A willingness to forgo routines suggests that he considers your (and his) desires more important than the rules made for the efficiency of the system. For that reason, this question can tell you a great deal.

*"Do you support breast-feeding on the delivery table and nonseparation for about 45 minutes after birth?"* A doctor who is enthusiastic to this question is one who is aware of the work that has been done by Drs. Klaus and Kennell about maternal-infant bonding and its importance. A doctor might add the stipulation that he would allow this if there are no complications with the baby. With all these nonroutine requests, there is the underlying presumption that they take place only if there are no complications with the mother or the baby.

A positive reply to this question can also show a doctor's awareness of the importance of keeping the family unit intact after birth so that both parents can bond with each other and the baby. To give you an idea of how vital I personally believe the reaction to this question is, I made my initial choice of medical adviser for this book based on that. I said to Dr. Karen Blanchard: "Would you think it was irresponsible of me if this book suggested to parents that they refuse to allow a delivery room nurse to take their baby away to the nursery if it is healthy?" "I think it would be irresponsible *not* to suggest that," came her immediate reply.

## SOME QUESTIONS YOU MIGHT ASK IN THE OFFICE

*"What time will you get to the hospital?"* Many of the busier doctors cannot afford to arrive at the hospital when you do and stay there throughout your labor—they have a heavy schedule of office visits and perhaps other women who may be delivering around the same time you do. There are doctors, however, who want to be with a woman throughout her entire labor and they will state that. If you feel that the physical presence of your doctor will make you feel more secure and supported then you should let him know that. If he does *not* usually sit with a woman throughout her whole labor he might be willing to try his best to do that for you.

A doctor may check in on you in early labor to assure himself that you are in true labor and then go back to his office. If his office is near the hospital, he may tell the nursing staff to call him when you are "complete and on the perineum" (meaning that your cervix is completely dilated and the baby's head is bulging on your perineum). Some women have felt abandoned and disappointed by doctors who arrive just in time to "catch the baby." Other women, depending on their relationship with their mate and the doctor, don't mind this at all.

You should discuss the issue of when the doctor arrives with your mate and decide for yourselves how important the doctor's early arrival and/or constant presence will be for you. It can be comforting and reassuring just to have him there; other women may feel a certain pressure in having the doctor hovering around. It depends on your attitude toward labor: how confident you feel about any childbirth training you'll have, what your relationship is to the doctor, how interdependent you and your mate have become, how supportive the hospital appears to be, and so on.

*"What kind of analgesia or anesthesia do you prefer?"* A doctor who says that it depends on what is happening with your labor is giving a fair answer—maybe none will be required. This will tell you that the doctor is familiar with natural, nonmedicated childbirth and does not automatically assume that drugs will be used. You could then add, "If needed, which ones to you commonly use?" A doctor may be somewhat limited in his reply because of the hospital he's affiliated with. However, it is safe to say that a doctor who says he does "routine spinals" (saddle blocks) is not going to leave a lot of room for nature to take its course. In the chart  Drugs During Childbirth (pages 507 to 508) you can see the pros and cons of spinals for yourself. You should be wary of a doctor who routinely uses an anesthetic that can only be administered at the very end of labor, when you need it least, and that can give you a terrible headache for months after delivery.

*"What percentage of your patients are induced?"* For medical reasons there should only be 5 to 10 percent at the very most (the section on induction in Chapter Six explains this). A doctor who has a 20 percent induction rate is a doctor who is unaware of or ignores the dangers of induction. He is also a doctor who is aggressive about interfering with the natural progress of labor. Depending on what sort of answer you get you might want to ask the doctor how many of his patients' labors are *started* with synthetic hormones and what percentage are *stimulated* by them in early labor. A doctor may not know exactly what percentage of his patients receive synthetic hormones at any time during labor but his reply will tell you whether or not he favors the use of it. Doctors who are more conservative about medical intervention in labor will let you know that; those who see no harm in it will give you a reply that reflects that.

*"When do you use forceps?"* The answer to this question may also tell you something about the extent to which a doctor intervenes in the natural labor process. The standard, conservative answer would be, "When a woman has been pushing adequately for 2 hours and the baby is not coming down." A doctor might qualify that answer by adding that, depending on how high up the baby is "stuck," he might elect to do a cesarean instead of a high forceps (a common practice nowadays because the outcome is better for babies). You could also ask, "Do you use vacuum extractors and when?" Although fairly popular in Europe, vacuum extractors have not caught on much in America, and, perhaps because of lack of practice, in the United States there is a high number of cerebral hematomas associated with the use of extractors. By asking, you can find out when and how the doctor favors helping the baby descend. Some women have strong feelings against forceps deliveries (because of bruising the baby) so by asking this question you can find out whether a doctor uses forceps routinely or is more conservative.

*"Do you have any recommendations about diet or drugs?"* A doctor should, optimally, volunteer information about nutrition and medications during pregnancy, but we don't live in an optimal world. Doctors are busy; doctors aren't taught nutrition in medical school; even worse, some doctors hang on to outdated ideas on the subject. Therefore, raise the subject but don't get your hopes up too high. However, there are several replies that you should know the significance of. If a doctor says she likes to restrict weight gain to under 20 pounds, *beware*. There was at one time a belief that toxemia of pregnancy was caused by weight gain . . . it is now known that is not true. It is also known that a *minimum* gain of 20 to 24 pounds will result in a healthier baby. Doctors who try to limit weight gain to below that amount may also prescribe diuretics (water pills) and restrict salt in your diet. These practices are unhealthy for you and the baby and are discussed in more depth in the nutrition section of Chapter Three. If for some reason you wish to stay with a doctor who holds these

ideas you had better be prepared to withstand the pressure she may put on you for disregarding her advice. If a doctor simply says, "Eat a well-balanced diet," and gives you no specifics, it means she does not know the specifics. There is no particular harm in this as long as you *inform yourself* and eat accordingly.

## A DOCTOR SHOULD ANSWER YOUR QUESTIONS WITHOUT RUSHING YOU

Find out from the receptionist when you call for an appointment how many patients are scheduled per hour: appointments 15 to 20 minutes apart is generally good. Then you can see for yourself how crowded the waiting room is—keep in mind that your doctor may share his practice with several other OB/GYNs, so a crowded waiting room doesn't necessarily mean you will be rushed. However, it *can* mean that the doctor is overbooked, rushed, or may be coming to the office straight from a delivery which has held him up. A wait of up to an hour is not uncommon. If you are compatible with a doctor then you may have to make this sacrifice of your time—bring a book or something else to occupy you so that you aren't climbing the walls by the time you are called in. The realities of an OB/GYN practice usually necessitate a fairly long wait but the essential point is whether *once you are with the doctor* he answers your questions without giving you the feeling that you are annoying him and holding him up.

## WAYS TO CHOOSE A DOCTOR

*A doctor should be supportive of your mate.* The fundamental support you should get is for your mate to take childbirth education classes with you and for you to be together in labor and delivery. Your mate should come with you to a prenatal visit at least once, even if you do not plan to have prepared childbirth. The baby's father should have a chance to meet the doctor and ask some questions of his own. One way to get a sense of whether a doctor is supportive of fathers is to say on the phone that your mate wants to come to the first appointment; you may be able to tell just from the doctor's (or receptionist's) attitude whether the office is accustomed to mates participating.

*If a doctor has a group practice,* ask to see the other doctors in rotation at subsequent prenatal visits. Some doctors already have their practice set up that way, but if not you should say you'd like to meet his colleagues. Just because doctors share a practice does not mean that they share views about every aspect of pregnancy and birth. You can find that although your doctor is a firm supporter of prepared childbirth, his colleague seems to give it only grudging lip service. You can also discover that while your doctor's bedside manner is comfortable for you, you feel ill at ease with his partner. If you have this problem try to decide what is bothering you, whether you can talk about it and clear it up or whether you can overcome the feeling.

Realistically, there is a fairly good chance that you will not be attended by your primary doctor if you don't go into labor during the hours that he is "on duty." The only way most obstetricians can keep their offices running fairly smoothly—and get some sleep once in a while!—is to work with another doctor or doctors. If you have a long-standing relationship with a doctor he might be willing to make an exception and promise you, within reason, that he will attend your birth. But do not fail to meet his colleagues even if you get such an assurance. For example, your doctor may have been up with another delivery for twenty hours when you go into labor.

### IMPORTANCE OF THE DOCTOR'S ATTITUDE

*A doctor's attitude to your pregnancy will affect your attitude.* Even once you've chosen a doctor you feel good about you should be aware of how his outlook can affect yours. If he says, "I've examined your blood and urine and everything's fine" ands says nothing about the *feelings* of pregnancy, the underlying message is "Be a good girl and go home; I don't want to hear about your feelings." If you've been aware of the emotional changes of pregnancy you may feel they are petty and unimportant if your doctor doesn't encourage you to talk about them. A doctor who treats you as an intelligent, rational adult is supporting you during a time of personal growth. By encouraging you to participate in childbearing decisions, a doctor helps you to build confidence in your own abilities. That feeling of autonomy is important during pregnancy, and even more vital for motherhood and all the decisions you will be facing.

Your attitude toward your pregnancy—as a time of growth—will affect your attitude toward your child from birth. If a doctor discusses your expectations about parenthood, he is approving and setting into motion your exploration in this new world you are entering. If your feelings are denied during pregnancy and birth, it can influence your parenting, perhaps pushing you toward trying to toilet-train and socialize your child as fast as possible.

*A doctor in his thirties or forties* may be in the best age range, if you have a choice. Doctors in this age group have experience but still have resiliency and stamina. Older doctors can be more set in their ways, inflexible, and may not follow the newer developments in the field. This is a gross generalization, however, and there are many exceptions. There are thirty-year-old doctors who hold rigid, chauvinistic ideas about women (even if they themselves are women), and there are buoyant sixty-year-old doctors doing Leboyer births.

An advantage of an older doctor is that he may be more attuned to natural childbirth because there was not as much technology when he began to deliver babies, so he may have more patience and trust in natural processes. A doctor graduating from medical school in the last 5 to 10 years *probably has never seen a natural birth*. Anything less than a cesarean delivery is considered "natural." Doctors are trained nowadays to view birth as a medical emergency and intervening—with machines, drugs, and procedures—is normal for them. This is not to say that there aren't doctors who are aware of this problem and compensate for it in their practice. Some doctors do trust nature to take its course and have patience before intervening.

*Flexibility from you and the doctor* is essential. Right from the start it is vital for you to make your needs clear to your doctor if you want to have the best possible experience. At the same time you have to leave room for any of the unforeseen developments that can arise in pregnancy and birth. There is no sense in having a doctor if you don't trust and listen to him. The thing to remember is that no doctor can honestly give you a guarantee about labor procedures. You can discuss what you'd like optimally but until labor is in progress no absolute decisions can be made. If you try to demand absolute promises it can make a doctor feel boxed in. If your inflexibility makes a doctor feel helpless or powerless he may become hostile. If your prejudices tie his hands (for example, if you refuse medication suggested by the doctor during labor), it leaves a doctor no room to exercise his best judgment.

*A doctor has his own point of view,* which is based on medical tradition, his training, and personal experience. This does not mean that you may not be able to change his point of view. Give *feedback* to your doctor—educate him. Let him know what you've read and heard and let him know how you feel about his style of doing things. Otherwise, a doctor will think that what he is doing is what people want. Be sensitive to the fact that some doctors may have trouble learning from patients but they can overcome that if you approach them with an unthreatening attitude. If you take the position that you are in this together and you want to share what you've learned, many doctors will make an effort to meet you halfway.

*The doctor as god* is a social attitude that hinders doctors as much as it does their patients. Pregnant women have been partially responsible in the past for putting an obstetrician up on a pedestal and leaving all decisions up to her. In addition, we treat doctors as social dieties. It may massage a doctor's ego every time she goes into a restaurant and gets a better table but in the long run it is an awesome burden that people expect doctors to be all-knowing and all-capable. Pregnant women can gain pride and strength as they exercise their intelligence and free will in birth choices: the doctors benefit also. As prospective parents take more responsibility it reduces the pressure on doctors. When a couple is involved in the decision-making it can reduce the tendency toward malpractice suits. Most of us are raised to believe that doctors are omniscient and omnipotent. The people who say they have *no* faith in doctors are simply rebelling against that social belief. Somewhere in between is the truth—that doctors are people like everyone else. They have training and experience but the human body (particularly that of a woman in labor) is full of mystery and they cannot have all the answers.

Whether or not to call a doctor by his *first name* is tied up with this problem of social reverence. Would you call your lawyer "Mr.———"? If your doctor addresses you by your first name you have the option to do the same. If he calls you "Mrs." (or "Ms." or "Miss") you can certainly suggest being less formal and call each other by your first names. It is only semantics but words carry a great deal of weight—it helps to equalize and demythologize if you call a doctor by his name rather than by his title. It may take a bit of getting used to for both of you but you may find it eliminates some of the role-playing that unconsciously goes along with his calling you "Sally" and your calling him "Dr. Abrams."

## LEAVING A DOCTOR

***Don't stay with a doctor if you feel uncomfortable.*** First try to identify what it is you don't feel right about. Then decide whether it is something you can talk to the doctor about and resolve. Often just by pointing something out you can clear the air and get on a better footing. You also have to determine whether your discomfort is a feeling you can overcome without confronting the doctor.

***If you decide not to choose a doctor***—or if you decide to leave a doctor you have been seeing—you owe it to yourself, to the doctor, and to his present and future patients to tell him why you aren't staying with him. Some women may feel comfortable talking to a doctor about this in person or on the phone, or you may prefer to write a letter. Unless you take the time to explain why you aren't staying with a doctor he will not know it is because you were not satisfied with his attitudes or procedures. In order for improvements to come about in the pregnant woman–obstetrician relationship, each woman has to make at least as much effort as each doctor. A doctor can only respond to consumer demands if he knows what they are.

If you have seen a doctor several times, then you have to write a letter in order to retrieve part of any lump-sum payment you've made, or to release yourself from any future obligation. For example, here's a letter to a doctor whose ideas on natural birth don't agree with yours:

## Sample Letter to a Doctor You're Leaving

Dear Dr. X:
This is to inform you that I will no longer require your services for prenatal care and delivery.

My desire is to have as natural a childbirth as possible. I want to avoid medication and other intervention in the natural process of birth and I feel very strongly about maternal-infant bonding—breast-feeding on the delivery table and nonseparation from my baby at birth. I did not feel that you (and your colleagues) shared my beliefs sufficiently for my pregnancy and birth to be the kind of experience I want.

I do not underestimate the medical aspects of birth or your expertise in that area. The problem is really an ideological one of commitment to safeguarding the personal side of birth with childbirth classes, a Leboyer delivery, and nonseparation of parents and child after birth.

Thank you for the care you have already given me. Please send me a bill for the _____ visits I have made to your office. Would you please send my medical records to Dr. _____.

Sincerely yours,

## PAYMENT

Payment of your obstetrician's bill is often required in full by the 7th month or 6 weeks prior to delivery. It is an unusual financial arrangement to be paying fully in advance, for services *to be rendered*, but that is how many doctors run their offices. There are some doctors, however, who send a bill after the baby is born.

*Preliminary interviews are free* with some doctors, or they may charge a nominal fee. This can be a reflection of a doctor's awareness that it is best for both you and him to discover ahead of time whether you are going to be compatible.

*Do not pay until absolutely necessary.* This gives you the freedom to change to another doctor if you develop problems with your doctor or her associate(s). It also gives you time to learn about ideological differences between you which may not be noticeable immediately.

*Paying in installments* may spare you a lump sum at the end of your pregnancy but it also reduces your freedom to leave. If you have been paying portions of the total bill during the early months of your pregnancy, it makes you feel wedded to a doctor, denying you the leeway to change your mind about him.

*Ask what the fee includes.* Will there be extra charges if there are complications in delivery? Are the prenatal lab fees for blood and urine included? Will the doctor see you more than the routine number of visits if necessary as part of the fee?

### RETRIEVING PRE-PAYMENT

*If you want to change doctors* and you have already paid the full amount for prenatal care and delivery, send a letter asking for "an immediate refund for the 'future services' paid for but no longer desired." State that you wish to pay only for the office visits you have already had up to that time. There is a time problem here: you have given $1,000 (let's say) to a doctor and you need that money back right away in order to give it to the doctor you have chosen as a replacement. You may have only a few weeks in which to do that. Therefore, here are the steps you can take to assure yourself a speedy refund:

- **FOLLOW UP YOUR LETTER** with a phone call to the bookkeeper in your doctor's office. Ask when you can expect a check. If she doesn't know anything about it, explain your situation and say you will call her back the following day. If you are told you cannot get your money back—or you do not feel assured that an honest effort is being made to get a check to you quickly—inform the doctor's office that their lack of cooperation forces you to write to the County Medical Association. This may improve their cooperation; if not:

- **WRITE A LETTER TO THE MEDICAL ETHICS COMMITTEE** of the County Medical Association. Simply state that you have decided not to have Dr. X deliver your baby but that you have paid him in full, in advance, for those future services. He is not refunding your payment (excluding prenatal visits you have already had). Explain that you must have the money back right away to pay Dr. Y, whom you have now chosen as your obstetrician. Follow this letter up with a phone call and ask what action has been taken. If the Medical Association's intervention is either too slow or ineffective, as a last (and surefire) resort you can:

- **PICKET THE DOCTOR'S OFFICE.** If all else fails, this will not! Doctors are not accustomed to being picketed; it is not good for their image. All you need is two or three friends (pregnant ones are preferable) and a few signs that say "Dr. X Unfair to Pregnant Women," or "Dr. X Stole My Money." If the street where you are picketing is not visible from the doctor's office have someone make a call informing him that his office is being picketed. Estimates are that you will be invited into the doctor's office within five minutes and that things will be straightened out. These may sound like hilarious, strong-arm tactics to you now, but if you were to get trapped in a situation like this you would be grateful to have recourse. Courts of law are expensive and can take years—which won't help you when you need it.

## IMPORTANCE OF SEEING A DOCTOR

Visits to the doctor are vitally important. A pregnant woman is not sick, but regular checks to spot potential problems are essential. It may seem boring or unnecessary to you, but many of the complications of pregnancy and birth give advance warning. Regular doctor visits make it possible to clear up problems before they get more serious or to make preparations for a potentially complicated delivery. Routine prenatal visits are scheduled once monthly until 28 weeks, twice monthly until 34–36 weeks, and then weekly until delivery. The exam consists of checking your weight, blood pressure, and fundal height.

### BLOOD PRESSURE

Blood pressure is checked to make sure that you are not hypertensive (suffering from high blood pressure) and to learn what "normal" is for you so that your pressure during labor can be evaluated. A woman who is 130/80 to 140/90 during pregnancy can have slightly higher blood pressure during the late stage of active labor or during pushing without any significance. But a woman who was 100/60 in prenatal exams may be having a problem in labor at the same 130/80 to 140/90 rate. Your pressure is a baseline learned during prenatal care.

The *rule of thumb* is that a 20-point rise in the systolic (top) number or in the diastolic (bottom) number is significant. However, the diastolic rise is more significant. It is the "resting" pressure. Your system is under maximum pressure when your heart is working hardest, which is the systolic (or "pumping") measurement. Thus, when the diastolic is high it may be a sign of problems. For example a 110/60 rise to 130/75 might be normal in labor where a 110/65 to 120/90 might indicate problems.

CAUTION:

A blood pressure of 140/90 is high for a pregnant woman, especially if this is your first baby. At the very least you should question your doctor about it. If he is nonchalant you should have another doctor (or clinic) do a second blood pressure exam on you. Some doctors feel that if a pregnant woman's blood pressure goes to 140/90 that she should be put in the hospital for observation and bed rest.

## FUNDAL HEIGHT

Fundal height is the distance from your pubic bone to the fundus, which is the upper, rounded end of your uterus. The measurement of fundal height is taken externally with a tape measure and can tell the growth of both the uterus and the fetus in relation to the gestational age.

**NORMAL, FULL GROWTH** is 38 to 40 centimeters, although some very petite women will never reach that because their 5- or 6-pound babies won't force the uterus up that far. A large or unengaged (it hasn't settled into the pelvis) fetus can measure as much as 40 to 43 centimeters at term.

**AN EXTREME MEASUREMENT AT ANY TIME MUST BE DIAGNOSED.**

**NO FUNDAL GROWTH** means you are in nonpregnant state (in which case another pregnancy test should be done) or you've had a missed abortion. In the latter case an examination by the doctor is very important because there can be complications.

**SLOW FUNDAL GROWTH** has a variety of reasons. There can be an error in the due date. There can be placental deficiency—the placenta is not nourishing the fetus properly (some doctors will induce labor before 40 weeks because as this condition worsens the baby can die in utero). You may have a small-for-gestational-age baby. Or the fetus may be in a transverse lie position, meaning that you get wider but your uterus does not grow upward.

**RAPID FUNDAL GROWTH** can indicate multiple fetuses, a large baby, a miscalculation on your due date, uterine tumors, or hydramnios (excess amniotic fluid).

***Ask to know the results of any prenatal tests.*** Ask to see your chart. It is your right. It informs you more fully so that you are better equipped to participate with decisions about your pregnancy and labor. Ask the doctor to explain anything you do not understand or are concerned about. It is your body and your baby: if you don't know your blood pressure during pregnancy then you won't know the significance of your pressure during labor. If you know and understand these processes you will better understand what your body is doing in labor.

***Coordinate your obstetrician and internist (general practitioner).*** Any medication that your internist prescribes for any illness or allergy you may have should be double-checked with your obstetrician despite the fact that your internist knows you are pregnant. Similarly, any medication which your obstetrician prescribes for pregnancy-related drugs should be checked with your internist. It is a measure of safety well worth the trouble—why not have the benefit of two expert opinions rather than one?

## SOME THOUGHTS ABOUT DOCTORS

A young doctor graduates from medical school equipped with technical skills and knowledge relating almost exclusively to diaster—to treating patients who are seriously ill. Yet pregnancy and birth are not a sickness: they are a normal, healthy biological process. In only a very small number of cases does anything go wrong. This can make an obstetrician feel useless: he has gone through many years of effort and expense to prepare for complications which rarely occur. It is no wonder that obstetricians so frequently intervene in the natural process of birth: that is what they are trained to do.

People complain that doctors view labor as a purely physical process. It is true that doctors often behave as if they do not understand that birth is a dramatic, socially important event. Perhaps we are asking too much. Some doctors view birth solely as a bodily process in which many things can go wrong and they are there to correct them. Perhaps we should accept the fact that (outside of a few rare obstetricians) doctors develop a viewpoint during medical training. Their viewpoint comes from seeing dire emergencies: women hemorrhaging, babies in distress, blood, death, deformities. In large medical centers where doctors are trained they see a good deal of that: it leaves its mark.

Doctors see a lot of births. Many times women without childbirth education may yell and scream during labor, as much from their fear about the unknown forces taking over their bodies as from the pain. It is understandable that a doctor may see his role as a white knight, who will rescue you from this ordeal.

Patients put unrealistic demands on doctors, who are expected to have all the answers, know everything, and be totally responsible. As women start taking more responsibility for their own bodies it's going to be easier on everyone, but in the meantime doctors are still expected to know and do it all. Giving up traditional procedures in obstetrics may be frightening to doctors because it leaves them hanging—the tradition is taken away as a bulwark and there is nothing to replace it.

Doctors did not design the dangers in being alive . . . they want to minimize them. This is one reason they fall back on traditional thinking. No two labors are alike. The physical and emotional intensity of labor and delivery is awesome. It is *still* not understood what triggers labor; often all the machines and medications cannot control it. Yet doctors are nevertheless expected to know what is going on; to be in charge; to be responsible for the outcome of a perfect baby.

We should keep in mind that doctors may also feel frustration, pressure, guilt, depression, and strain. Being a doctor is a complex and difficult task, perhaps even harder than some doctors recognize. Do not be angry with a doctor who may be rigid—be compassionate toward a person who has been channeled into playing God by his fellow men and women.

The one danger is a doctor who practices medicine with his ego. There are doctors who have gotten so caught up in the role and people's expectations that they actually come to believe that they *do* have all the answers. Beware of any doctor, in or out of the hospital, who does not separate his ego and his medicine. An example would be any doctor who will not listen to any point of view that differs from his own, who refuses to consider any procedure he is not familiar with.

Doctors are not bad people, although some of them may be. Nor are they great people, although some of them may be. Mostly, doctors are decent people under a lot of pressure trying to do the best job they can.

A major facet of American medicine is its ever-growing technology. New machines and tests are seen as progress. Thus a doctor who uses the newest equipment and procedures may believe he is offering you the best (newest, most advanced) care available. Doctors are also acutely aware of malpractice suits. By using the latest technique a doctor can "prove" that he gave the best possible care. In a society that worships technology that makes sense.

The soaring price of malpractice insurance is driving a lot of obstetricians out of their field, in what may become a health-care crisis. Obstetricians are facing more lawsuits, and higher losses from lawsuits, because there is an inherent risk of "bad outcomes" in the course of delivering babies. Mother Nature doesn't guarantee that every baby will be 100 percent perfect: she only cares that the species as a whole is perpetuated. Yet we demand a guarantee of a perfect baby every time from our obstetricians—and sue them when anything goes awry. Many doctors can no longer afford the skyrocketing cost of malpractice insurance—or perhaps they can't tolerate a medical-legal atmosphere in which they have to look over their shoulders and make decisions based *not* on the health and welfare of the baby and the new family, but on what could happen later in a courtroom.

The facts are sobering: close to 25 percent of American OB/GYNs have given up obstetrics. Half of rural Nevada's family physicians no longer deliver babies. Doctors in Brunswick, Georgia, stopped accepting pregnant lawyers, law clerks, or lawyers' wives as patients. By 1985 there were already 17 counties in Alabama with no obstetrical care.

## CHOOSING A HOSPITAL

The only way to find out what a hospital can offer you is to go there and *ask questions*. At the end of this chapter there is a questionnaire you can take with you.

*Take a tour of the hospital,* with your mate if possible. If there is no scheduled maternity tour then ask for a personal tour. If a hospital will not allow you to see their facilities and ask questions, *be suspicious:* they are likely to be equally rigid in their maternity care.

*Find out the night entrance* to the hospital. Many hospitals lock their front doors at 10 P.M. and many women go into labor at night. Trying to search for the night entry during labor can be upsetting. Be sure your mate knows exactly where the night entrance is if he doesn't go on the tour with you.

### TYPES OF HOSPITALS

#### CATHOLIC HOSPITALS

Catholic hospitals are the most restrictive in certain policies but they account for 29 percent of hospital beds in the United States. There are certain procedures which are banned in Catholic hospitals: for instance, if you want to save time and money and have a tubal ligation right after delivery, *do not go to a Catholic hospital.* They will not permit contraceptive procedures.

## Teaching Hospitals

*A teaching hospital has the best medical facilities.* Residents are always on duty, so if you were to run into complications and your doctor was not there, you would be attended by a doctor until yours could arrive.

*Doctors see more births* and more complicated births, which may be transferred there from lesser-equipped hospitals, so they are better equipped to handle problems.

*If a cesarean became necessary* it could be done in a matter of minutes in a teaching hospital, where they have facilities and staff at the ready, unlike smaller hospitals.

*Drawback:* There is resident/intern traffic walking through your labor room in a teaching hospital. The trade-off is that you get better facilities and equipment in case anything goes wrong with you or the baby.

## A Smaller, Community Hospital

This type of hospital is more flexible. A large medical center has more red tape than a local hospital which has a smaller staff and fewer patients. If there are certain procedures you wish or don't wish during labor and delivery you can go to the hospital administrator's office in a community hospital and discuss it ahead of time. It is like the difference between going to the corner store and talking directly with the owner or going to a huge shopping complex. Thus while you may be able to arrange for a more individualized childbirth at a smaller hospital you will probably be forfeiting the costly equipment and facilities of a teaching hospital.

## Family-Centered Maternity Care

This special type of care is offered by some of the more progressive hospitals, both large medical centers and community hospitals. Family-centered care usually involves the optional elimination of certain routine procedures and the optional addition of other procedures, but this varies from hospital to hospital. Just because a hospital says that it has family-centered care *does not guarantee you anything.* You may have to use the questionnaire to find out just how committed a hospital really is to the concept behind the words.

Above all, family-centered care has to do with a philosophy about childbirth: individualized care aimed at nurturing the family unit during labor, delivery, and postpartum. A hospital that has adopted this kind of maternity care is showing its respect for the social importance—both personal and for the society at large—of childbirth. There are certain choices that are associated with family-centered care—including eliminating routine procedures, Leboyer delivery, breast-feeding on the delivery table, nonseparation of parents and baby during labor, delivery, and recovery, rooming-in, early discharge, etc. All of them are discussed in the following section but few hospitals offer all of them. You have to find out what is available at the hospital you've chosen and then see if you can arrange for further options if you wish them. If you are not able to make arrangements you're comfortable with then you may have to go to a more flexible hospital.

## HOSPITAL POLICIES

### ANESTHESIA POLICY

This varies, depending on whether a hospital has an obstetric anesthesiologist on duty full-time. Some hospitals that do keep an anesthesiologist on the premises *will charge you whether you use him/her or not.* Some hospitals give a laboring woman an anesthesia release form to sign when she's in transition (the toughest part of labor), when her resolve is low. Find out whether there is an anesthesiologist "on call" and how long it would take him to reach the hospital and administer anesthetic if you needed or wanted it. Perhaps you might prefer waiting twenty minutes for him to arrive so that you don't have to sign a form obliging you to pay whether you use his services or not.

**BREAST-FEEDING**

Breast-feeding can be overtly or subtly supported or discouraged by hospital policy and attitudes.

*Ask whether babies are encouraged to nurse immediately* after birth on the delivery table. The reason this is desirable is because it reinforces the baby's natural sucking instinct while giving her the colostrum (which precedes the milk and is full of antibodies) in your breasts. The baby's suckling releases hormones into your system that help contract your uterus and stimulate your milk supply. Some doctors prefer nursing in the recovery room instead of on the delivery table; it may be more relaxed because there is less going on around you to interfere.

*Find out whether breast-feeding is supported by the hospital* by asking whether they distribute breast-feeding literature to new mothers and if so, from what source: the La Leche League, a formula company, or other sources.

*Ask whether a test feeding* of glucose and water is given routinely in the nursery. Some doctors believe that such a feeding cleans out mucus from the baby's system although breast milk has the same effect. Giving a rubber nipple to a newborn you want to breast-feed can sabotage your efforts. A baby won't suck properly at your breast if she has been satisfied by the sugar water that was so much easier to suck from a rubber nipple. A baby who does not suck energetically won't stimulate your milk supply to come in, which in turn will not stimulate the baby to suck. Your confidence is undermined and so is your new relationship with the baby. If you do not wish your baby to have these supplementary bottles (which can wind up replacing your breast rather than supplementing it) then discuss this ahead of delivery with your pediatrician and have him note on your chart: *"No artificial nipples"* or *"No supplementary bottles."*

*Ask whether babies are allowed to breast-feed* on demand. This means that your baby is brought in to you (if she isn't rooming-in) when she cries, rather than on an every-4-hours schedule imposed by the hospital. It is extremely hard to establish successful breast-feeding if a baby is not allowed to nurse on demand when she is hungry. When your baby is hungry she will nurse with the enthusiasm necessary to stimulate your milk supply to come in. If a baby awakens in the central nursery (assuming rooming-in is not available or you have not chosen it) she may be given a bottle of glucose and water or formula to quiet her. When the baby is brought in to you on the 4-hour schedule she will be full and sleepy and won't suck properly. She will also have been spoiled by the easy-to-suck rubber nipple and will be less likely to extend the vigorous effort needed for breast-feeding. Breast-feeding babies get hungry sooner than formula-fed babies because breast milk digests more easily and quickly. The 4-hour feeding schedule was instituted for the convenience and smooth running of the nursery staff; if you want to breast-feed it will frustrate both you and your baby.

*Do not assume* that just because a hospital *does* have demand feeding that every person on the staff understands or is supportive of breast-feeding. When you read the section on breast-feeding in Chapter Eleven you will see that there is a substantial emotional component to successful breast-feeding and that if you do not get early encouragement and advice your milk supply may not come in quickly. *Ask for help.* If you don't get it from the nurse(s) assigned to you then ask for the nurse supervisor and tell her you need help: breast-feeding is something you have to learn, it isn't just instinctive. If you feel discouraged and as if you want to give up, don't. The beginning is always the hardest. Nurses who say, "Your baby doesn't seem to want to breast-feed," or, "Your baby isn't gaining much weight," can undermine your efforts. If you can't get support in the hospital, call up your pediatrician, if you've found one who is highly supportive of breast-feeding. Or call up the La Leche League in the phone book; they will have a member talk to you or even visit you in the hospital to show you the ropes.

### EARLY DISCHARGE

This means that you can be released from the hospital within 6 to 24 hours after your baby is born. This option is most attractive to couples who prefer spending the first postpartum days at home and have come to the hospital primarily for the medical care available "just in case." You might consider early discharge in the following cases:

*If you had childbirth education* and went through labor and delivery without analgesia or anesthesia, except a local for the episiotomy if there was one. The main worry about early discharge is that you can have postpartum bleeding if your uterus does not continue to contract—drugs used during birth would increase the chances of hemorrhage.

*If labor, delivery, and a 2-hour postpartum* period are all normal.

*If you get infant-care training* if this is your first baby; otherwise the jolt and sense of helplessness with a newborn at home can be overwhelming. You should take American Red Cross (or other) baby-care classes before delivery or have a trained baby nurse or relative/friend at home who is experienced with newborns.

*If you know that you can force yourself to take it very easy* at home: the tendency is to try and do everything right away and this can be exhausting and even dangerous. Some women regret not having stayed in the hospital where everything was done for them. *Wait to see how you feel* once the baby is born: you may feel terrific and eager to get out of the sterile environment of the hospital and back to your own surroundings or you may be exhausted and not want to move.

*If the hospital has some arrangement for postpartum care.* Some hospitals send a specially trained nurse to your home on the first day postpartum and then once or twice after that; others have a twenty-four-hour hot line you can call for questions or problems. Early discharge works best if there is some ongoing contact with professionals who can assist you and the baby if necessary.

### REASONS FOR EARLY DISCHARGE

*You save a great deal* of money because you do not have the 3- to 5-day hospital stay, which can be around $150 to $300 per day. You can easily hire a registered infant nurse to come to the house for that length of time and *still* save money.

*In a hospital you have no privacy* because there are people constantly coming in and out of your room. If you don't have a private room you have to contend with a roommate at a time when you might prefer being alone with your baby.

*A hospital is a place of sickness* and there will be patients around who are not well. You may be treated as a sick person: your temperature will be taken, your "bathroom performance" questioned and so on. If you walk around in your bathrobe for 3 days and you are treated as if you aren't well, it is apt to influence your attitude.

*Most hospitals don't provide rooming-in,* so you will be separated from your baby at the time when you most need each other. When a baby is kept in a central nursery and brought out for brief visits every 4 hours it can make you feel as if the baby "belongs" to the nursery staff and they are "allowing" you to see him. Many women report that they only begin to think of their baby as their own once they are out of the hospital. Also, as mentioned earlier, separation from your baby makes breast-feeding very difficult.

*Most hospitals don't provide facilities for the baby's father,* siblings, or close relatives to bond with the baby, whereas at home they have natural access to him.

*Breast-feeding is enhanced* by early discharge; you are together at home in relaxed, familiar surroundings. One study showed that women who chose early discharge developed their milk supply in 36 to 72 hours. Mothers who breast-feed but who stay in the hospital usually have milk within 72 to 120 hours. This difference is party because demand feeding is unavailable in most hospitals.

## FATHER PARTICIPATION IN CHILDBIRTH

A father's presence is fairly widely accepted nowadays, but some hospitals attach certain conditions.

*The first thing to ask* is whether fathers are allowed to be with their wives in labor rooms; then ask whether they are allowed in the delivery room at birth. Then ask under what conditions a father must leave his wife. Although there is no medical justification for it, some hospitals require a man to leave if regional anesthesia is used (others ask only that he leave while the anesthesia is first administered). There are hospitals with double labor rooms which allow a man to stay only if there is no one sharing the labor room. If you find that there are any stipulations like this on your staying together, discuss it *ahead of time* with your doctor. Find out whether he can intervene and arrange for some sort of exception so that you can be assured of staying together. If that doesn't work, have your mate contact the hospital administrator and explain how important it is for you both to stay together and ask whether you can be guaranteed that option unless there is a medical emergency necessitating his departure.

*Once you are in labor* and the father is told to leave, *ask for a definite reason* for his exclusion from the labor room. Say that the doctor promised you could be together (assuming that the doctor is not there to protect your agreement). Do not just meekly have the father leave: don't back down unless the staff can convince you that it is an emergency situation. Try to stay calm and reasonable but do not leave unless you are convinced it is in the best interest of the mother and baby.

*Several recent court cases* have upheld the right of local hospital administrators and doctors to make the final decision about whether fathers will be allowed in the delivery room at individual hospitals. *All lawsuits by fathers demanding entry have been unsuccessful so far*—so if you were considering that challenge to the system before birth, forget it.

*Do it anyway* is radical advice, but the only choice you have as a last resort. Legally the hospital *could* call the sheriff on the grounds that you are trespassing, but it's highly unlikely that the hospital will do that as a baby is being born; it's more trouble than it's worth to them. Besides, it is illegal—considered a tort—for anyone to seize you. They will undoubtedly figure it's a one-time problem and they'll let you go in the delivery room. They may be nasty, say you're crazy, and even threaten you—but if you're willing to go through that, you can get anything you want in a hospital. It is cheaper and quicker than suing and you've got a better chance of satisfaction.

*Some hospitals require that the father take the hospital's own prenatal classes.* Ask whether this is true at the hospital you are considering.

*Some hospitals require that a couple be married* in order for them to stay together during labor and delivery. If you are not married, call and find out hospital policy without saying who you are. If they do have that rule, when the time comes and anyone asks, just say you are married. Being together for the birth of your child is more important than honesty. There is no reason, however, not to use your own names since more and more married couples do that. If anyone questions why you have different names say that the woman uses her own name. If they say, "Oh, you've kept your maiden name?" you can say, "Yes, and my husband decided to keep his maiden name also."

***Be sure that the father goes on a tour*** of the hospital so that he knows where to change into hospital clothes for the delivery room. There can be a rush to the delivery room and if there isn't anyone free at that moment to show a man where to change he may wind up missing the birth.

***Ask whether fathers have unlimited visitation*** hours or at least can be with the mother and baby at times in addition to visiting hours. Find out whether fathers may hold their babies. Yes, there actually are hospitals that do not allow fathers to touch their own babies.

***Find out whether the father is allowed into the recovery room.*** Most hospitals do *not* allow the father in, but it can be lonely for you if you feel great and are separated from both your baby and your mate at a time when you most want to be with them. It can be even more unpleasant if you are alone and lying next to a drugged woman or one who had a difficult labor and is upset.

## FETAL MONITORS

Monitoring is discussed at length in pages 316 to 330. You should find out whether fetal monitors are used in the hospital you are considering and whether they are mandatory or optional. You can then discuss the pros and cons with your doctor.

## FOOD AND DRINK POLICY

Whether you can eat or drink often depends on what your doctor has noted on your chart. Most hospitals allow a woman to have *nothing by mouth* once she is admitted in labor. This is to guard against vomiting in case general anesthesia is used). Some hospitals allow a woman to have ice chips during labor; others will allow her to suck on candy. *However,* it is really not a good idea to eat candy while you are in labor: it stimulates stomach acids which can be uncomfortable and are more dangerous than a stomach full of food if you *were* to have general anesthesia, vomit, and aspirate it back into your lungs. You might ask whether you would be allowed to have spoonfuls of honey for energy but, as with all these options, you should discuss them ahead of time with your doctor.

Some people assert that the effect on the mother and fetus of food and drink deprivation over many hours is unknown and that it adds to the "pathologic environment" of the hospital. In countries other than America, light food and drink are permitted during labor; even in the United States they tell you to stay at home during very early labor because you can have liquids and other nourishment there which will be denied you as soon as you enter the hospital. Eliminating nourishment by mouth can cause carbohydrate deprivation, which has been implicated in the precipitation of metabolic acidosis of the mother, which occurs in approximately 20 percent of births. The consequence of metabolic acidosis is that fetuses whose mothers develop it are more prone to become acidotic themselves during labor.

Some hospitals will not allow a man to eat in the labor room. Some couples feel it is inconvenient and also disruptive for him to have to leave. Often it is nice for the man to have a break and go to the cafeteria but that should be his choice, not the hospital's.

## LABOR ROOMS

Labor rooms are an important part of your childbirth because you'll probably be in one for many hours.

*The most important question* is whether the rooms are single or double. If you have taken childbirth training and cannot be assured a private labor room then ask to be paired up with a woman who has also had classes. It is hard enough to maintain your concentration, relaxation, and control during labor: if you have an unprepared woman in the next bed it may be difficult for you to be successful. She will probably be frightened, ignorant of what is happening to her body, and in pain—it can be upsetting to listen to a woman who hasn't had the benefit of classes to prepare her.

If it is not possible for you to be alone with another prepared mother and your roommate is voicing a lot of pain and fear, then do your best to tune her out. Bring a radio or cassette machine and play music. Ask for cotton and stuff it in your ears. This is not a joke—if you do not have a suitable atmosphere it is very difficult to concentrate, relax, and breathe. Ask if there's anywhere you can be moved to—find out if another room has opened up since you were admitted, which happens just as soon as another woman is ready to give birth and is moved to the delivery room. Ask if there is another room you could share, preferably with a quieter woman, if not a prepared one. *But don't ask to have the other woman moved* . . . she's got enough problems as it is.

**Ask whether you will be confined to bed** in the labor room. Many hospitals require a woman to stay in the bed. If you have also been given some sort of tranquilizer, the combination will slow your labor, compromise uterine circulation, create muscle weakness and less effective contractions. Walking during labor can stimulate your contractions, help your pelvis open, and take advantage of gravitational force to bring the baby down. If you know this and are in a hospital with a stay-in-bed policy at least get up to go to the bathroom frequently. You can also walk around and let your mate deal with any nurse who orders you back to bed.

## LEBOYER DELIVERY

Leboyer delivery can be done even in hospitals that are not set up for it but it is easier if the staff is familiar with the technique. Of course first you have to discuss and agree on it with your obstetrician. If you are told that a hospital does do Leboyer deliveries ask whether this also includes facilities for the Leboyer bath.

All that is needed for the bath is (1) a plastic baby tub, (2) warm sterile water, and (3) a radiant heater. If a hospital has never done Leboyer deliveries but your doctor agrees to it you need only bring a plastic baby bathtub. Arrange ahead of time for the hospital to have bottled sterile water ready or bring 3 or 4 bottles yourself. These can be set unopened in hot tap water to warm and poured into the bath after the baby is born. Since the main concern about the Leboyer bath is the possibility of the baby getting chilled, it is important to have a heating element over the bath. However, no special equipment is required. There is a radiant heater over the wiping/warming tray that the baby is put in after birth. Either that heater can be moved away from the tray and positioned over the baby tub or the bathtub can be placed inside the warming tray.

This means that you can have a Leboyer delivery even if the hospital is not familiar with the procedures, as long as your doctor is in favor and will encourage the staff's assistance.

## PHOTOGRAPHS AND TAPE RECORDING

Both photographing and recording are forbidden in many large medical centers. The hospitals' main worry is that photographs could be used later in a malpractice suit. Hospitals that do allow photographing and recording may require you to sign a photography release form when you preregister; sometimes hospitals won't allow flash equipment to be used. If there is no rule against photos you still must have the consent of the hospital and your doctor. Many people have found, however, that although the hospital may have a policy forbidding picture-taking, their doctor is not against it: so they simply take pictures but keep a low profile. One way to do it without a flash is to use the fastest 35mm film (Tri-X) and push the ASA to 800. Be sure to tell the lab that you have done this—there may be an extra charge for development.

## PRENATAL EDUCATION CLASSES

Offered by some hospitals, classes are sometimes free of charge; other times there is a fee but it is lower than for outside classes. The problem with in-house childbirth training is that the teacher is an employee of the hospital and therefore cannot comfortably criticize hospital policies. However, as long as you get the training in breathing, relaxation, and working as a team, it really isn't important whether the teacher challenges the hospital's policies or not: you can do that yourself.

If the hospital does have classes ask whether they also include exercise sessions, a benefit you don't get in most private classes.

The most important question is what percentage of the women who deliver at the hospital have had childbirth preparation. This will give you a good idea of whether the staff is familiar with and supportive of the techniques: nurses can help coach with your breathing if necessary or can just boost your morale at low points. There is a world of difference between that and a hospital where little is known about prepared childbirth and nurses ask you questions during contractions, refer to them as "labor pains," offer medication, perhaps unintentionally sabotaging your training.

## PREREGISTRATION

Offered by some hospitals, it can save you a lot of time and aggravation to be already registered when you arrive in labor. Preregistration allows you to fill out all the many required forms ahead of time so that you can go right in when you're in labor. Be sure to also find out how much money is required on admittance and discharge so that you can come prepared. If you can keep your hospital suitcase in a safe place at home you could put the money or money order in an envelope so you don't forget it in the rush to the hospital.

If a hospital does not offer preregistration you still are not obliged to fill out all the forms when you arrive. It is not legally necessary to have the paperwork done before the birth takes place. You will have to sign a few things, but if you don't want to be separated from your mate and you're having some difficulty coping with contractions, *go to the labor room.* Your mate can complete the forms later.

## ROOMING-IN

This is one of the fundamental features of family-centered maternity care which provides for your baby to stay in your room with you.

***Find out whether the hospital offers the choice*** of rooming-in and then ask whether it is an all-or-nothing option. Some hospitals provide only 24-hour rooming-in, meaning that the baby is always in your room and you don't have the choice of sending her back to the central nursery at night. This system is most convenient for the staff; the logistics are more complicated if they have to bring a baby back and forth. Some cynics suggest that a hospital may offer only full-time rooming-in as a way of discouraging mothers from choosing it because it is easier for the staff to keep all the babies in the central nursery, bringing them all out at the routine 4-hour intervals. This seems an unfair accusation, although it is true that rooming-in means that the nurses have to keep track of which babies are with which mothers, as well as going to their rooms to give them help.

***Some hospitals offer the choice of having the baby with you during the day*** but sending him back to the nursery at night. This can give you more rest, especially if you are tired out from a long labor; but then you have the shock of reality when you go home a day or two later and there is no central nursery at night!

***A few hospitals have an innovative circular layout*** with the central nursery in the middle and the mothers' rooms encircling it like pieces of a pie. There are "drawers"—the same plastic bassinets used in most hospitals to hold the baby that pull out so you can return your baby to the central nursery if you want to sleep or go out of your room. You can retrieve your baby instantly whenever you want him. This way you can choose how much the baby will be with you and the nurses can keep an eye on him when you don't want to.

*An important advantage of rooming-in* is that you can learn your baby's needs and begin adjusting to her habits. The average American woman doesn't have previous experience with newborns and probably won't even know what normal color, breathing, and bowel movements are like. With rooming-in you get exposure to your new baby before you take her home. It also gives you a chance to discover the realities of newborn care while you are still in the hospital and can ask for advice from the staff. Many women's ideas of what is good mothering come from magazines and television ads—rooming-in gives them a chance to test out what it's *really* like so that they don't go home and make themselves miserable trying to be Supermom. A woman who hasn't had a chance to get used to her baby may have little tolerance for even small problems which arise once she's home—she may have unrealistic, idealized expectations of herself and the child.

*Rooming-in does not mean that you're totally on your own,* helpless and isolated in your hospital room with a newborn baby. Nursing care and teaching go with rooming-in. This is even better if there are unlimited visiting hours for the baby's father because he can also benefit from baby-care demonstrations. This can help you and your mate feel more confident about caring for and sharing the baby once you're home.

*If you don't choose rooming-in* or if the hospital doesn't offer it, the father may not even be allowed to touch his baby. Needless to say this is detrimental to his bonding with the infant. If rooming-in is the only way you can be assured that father and baby can spend time together then it is one more advantage to consider.

*The baby's adjustment to life outside the womb is affected* positively by rooming-in. Studies show that a rooming-in baby more readily organizes his cycles of sleeping, waking, and crying if he is exposed to a single caregiver in the first 10 days of life. The studies also showed that the baby cries distinctly less and establishes a day-night rhythm more quickly than in a traditional nursery with multiple care-givers and 4-hour feeding schedules. Thus, the baby you take home after rooming-in may be different than he would be if you had left him in the central nursery. You will probably be more adjusted to the baby's cycles and the baby will already be settling into patterns of sleeping and waking that will make it easier to fit the newborn into your life at home.

## ROUTINE HOSPITAL PROCEDURES

This is the catchphrase for the procedures that most hospitals perform on all woman who are in labor. There is nothing wrong with any of these procedures per se: the problem is that they are carried out *routinely* without any regard for individual circumstances or preferences. Hospitals are large institutions and function most efficiently when there are rules and tasks that are performed across the board. However, this disregards what may be your personal wishes in some areas. The more subtle harm of routine procedures is that they can make a woman feel as if the hospital is in charge of her body; it may undermine her feeling of strength and capability. A hospital and its staff are authoritarian by nature; the automatic imposition of routine procedures simple magnifies this quality. The question to ask the hospital is whether any of the routine procedures can be eliminated if your doctor agrees to it and notes it on your chart ahead of time.

*Enemas* are given routinely to women in early labor. One reason is so that your lower bowel is emptied to give the baby as much room as possible. Another reason is so that during the pushing stage you will feel free to push. The fear (embarrassment) of pushing out fecal matter may make some women tense and they push with inhibition. Also, if fecal matter is pushed out with the baby it can contaminate the sterile area into which he is born. These are all legitimate reasons for an enema.

However, there is a natural cleaning-out process in many women prior to labor or in early labor. In fact, one sign that labor has begun is that you may have several bowel movements or diarrhea. Also, you may not have eaten very much prior to the onset of labor and may have had a bowel movement fairly recently. In those cases you might want to forgo an enema and you should discuss this possibility with your doctor ahead of time so that he can note on your chart that the enema can be eliminated at your discretion.

An enema can bring on stronger contractions. It can also cause you considerable discomfort and anxiety, rushing to the toilet and then having to sit there while you are coping with intensified contractions. In addition, your mate or other labor coach has probably been asked to leave, so you have to deal with this alone. If you choose to have an enema or are given no choice, at least be prepared for this temporary difficulty.

Another word of caution: the nurse may administer the enema, see you to the toilet, and then leave, telling you to stay there for 15 minutes. You do *not* have to stay there exactly 15 minutes nor do you have to wait for the nurse to return—nurses get busy in other rooms and may not be able to get back right away. Many women feel they must "do as they are told" and they get trapped on the toilet much longer than necessary! Once you feel your bowel has emptied you can go back to the bed or to a chair—the worse that can happen is that you feel the need to go back to the toilet or else you mess up the bed a little. It's better to have to clean up the bed than it is for you to feel alone and uncomfortable and have your prepared childbirth techniques disrupted.

*I.V.* is the abbreviation used for "intravenous solution," a bottle of liquid which is fed into your system through tubing which is inserted into a vein, often in the back of your hand. An I.V. of glucose and water is routinely hooked up to women in labor for a variety of reasons. It gives the body energy and fluids when food and liquid by mouth are prohibited. Also, synthetic oxytocin like pitocin can be administered through the I.V. solution (although it is an inaccurate method—see the section on Induced Birth, pages 332–338).

If a woman objects to an I.V. for those reasons she

is often told a third and more dramatic reason: that an I.V. has to be inserted "just in case" she should hemorrhage or "just in case" they have to do an emergency cesarean. This raises the issue of "just-in-case" obstetrical science which advocates the use of "preventive" measures which pervert the normal into the abnormal and deviate from the natural process. The nurse or doctor may tell you that an I.V. is "preventive" but it doesn't prevent anything: this alarmist view of childbirth is a philosophy that can create problems which then demand more interference. This is not to say that an I.V. is *never* necessary—it is of great benefit in a situation in which a woman has had a long hard labor and can become dehydrated because she hasn't had any nourishment by mouth. But that can be determined at the time and an I.V. can then be inserted. The same would be true if pitocin were necessary and the hospital did not have an infusion pump to administer it: putting it in the I.V. solution would be the next best way to stimulate contractions.

Having an I.V. hooked up contributes to making you feel like a sick patient instead of a well person going through the normal bodily process of giving birth. It is often difficult for the nurse or doctor to insert the I.V. needle and catheter so they may have to "stick" you more than once. An injection to numb the area on your hand or forearm precedes the insertion. This process can be painful; it is also disruptive . . . it can interfere with your relaxation and concentration if you are using prepared childbirth techniques. The I.V. limits your movement—it immobilizes your hand, or you may feel it does, and going to the bathroom, which you should do every couple of hours during labor, involves the I.V. hookup and tubing having to follow you into the bathroom. Veins can be aggravated for weeks afterward.

Some doctors feel strongly about having the I.V. hooked up. It makes them feel more secure to have that safeguard against the slight possibility of an emergency. As discussed in the earlier section of this chapter (Some Thoughts About Doctors), they have seen many frightening situations in maternity care. If your doctor won't dispense with an I.V. he may be willing to wait until delivery to insert it, giving you hours beforehand without it. Or you may want to have it right from the beginning. The intention of this section is simply to let you know that the reasoning is weak for *everyone* to have an I.V.

**Shaving** your pubic hair is still done in some hospitals. It is not necessary. The reason given for it is that pubic hair harbors bacteria, although there has never been any proof that removing it reduces the incidence of infection. In fact, just the opposite was proven in one study, where *infection increased* with shaving. The actual reason for the shave is to facilitate the episiotomy repair for the doctor. If an episiotomy is done the alternative is to push the hair aside or clip it with scissors.

One option is to request of your doctor and have noted on your chart that you want only a "mini-prep," which means that rather than your entire pubic area being shaved only the lips of your vagina will be. The other possibility is to arrange with your doctor ahead of time to clip yourself with scissors around the lips of your vagina. This way there is no itching when the hair grows back from being shaved.

Your pubic area is washed down with antiseptic or iodine solution before the baby's head is delivered, anyway, so the chance of infection is eliminated by that.

**Straps and stirrups** are part of the routine procedures in the delivery room. Some hospitals still require your hands to be strapped down to keep them clear of the sterile field where the baby is going to be born. This harks back to the days when women were so heavily drugged that they were not in control of themselves. Having your hands strapped down is undignified and degrading. If someone tries to strap your hands, do not allow them to; say that you understand why they want to do it and that you will respect the necessity of keeping your hands under the sterile sheets.

Stirrups are used on most delivery tables. They are not just the foot stirrups you've seen in the doctor's office: they are usually a metal and/or plastic molded form into which your entire leg is strapped. When your feet are elevated and your legs stretched apart it puts tension on the vaginal membranes during delivery and increases the chance of tearing and injury to your tissues. Also, if you are made to lie flat with your feet high in the air the position you are in defies the gravitational force which could be aiding in the descent and exit of the baby.

One option is to have the stirrups adjusted lower. You may have agreed upon this with your doctor who, for whatever reason, may not be there. You are entitled to a reasonable voice in the matter: tell the nurse you are uncomfortable and cannot push well unless the stirrups are lowered.

***Transfer for delivery*** is done in most hospitals. Right when the baby's head is crowning (is showing at the lips of your vagina) you are wheeled, often in a hurry, to the delivery room. You are then made to shift from the labor bed onto the narrower delivery table, which has stirrups. This transfer is awkward and disruptive of the natural process. Just as the baby's head is ready to be born you are whisked down hallways, often instructed to pant so that you don't push the baby out any farther, and then you have to get onto a different surface for delivery. It is more convenient for the doctor to deliver the baby with your feet in stirrups, at the edge of a hard surface, and with a stool for him to sit on.

Talk to your doctor and the hospital about the possibility of laboring and delivering in the same bed. If they'll agree to that then ask if you can deliver in the labor room if everything is normal. It will be more peaceful for you and won't put you through that last-minute rush and move. One reason hospitals may not agree to it is that you save a good deal of money if you don't use the delivery room— for which they charge a hefty fee. The drawbacks of staying in the labor room are that you don't have the mirror overhead to watch the birth in and you cannot give the baby a Leboyer bath in the labor room. It must also be mentioned that in the rare situation where something goes wrong (the baby cannot exit or it has difficulty breathing or you begin to bleed) you won't have the delivery-room facilities right at hand. You will have to be rushed into the delivery room at that point.

## SEPARATION OF MOTHER AND BABY

This is considered by many experts to be the most harmful routine procedure in a hospital. *Avoiding* this separation is often the primary reason that some couples decide against a hospital birth. Even those hospitals that have family-centered maternity care—which is theoretically intended to keep a family together—nevertheless routinely separate mothers and their babies at birth and for many hours afterward. This procedure is cruel because it violates a mother's and baby's emotional and physical needs: the damaging effects can be far-reaching. Studies have shown that a large percentage of battered children in the United States were premature infants, for whom separation was a medical necessity. It is not unreasonable to predict from this that the separation of normal, healthy children from their mothers also has its consequences in their relationship. Separation is a routine procedure which must be questioned.

Maternal-infant bonding begins with the "sensitive period" for the 30 to 45 minutes immediately after birth. However, it does not stop there. It is contradictory to give parents this protected time with their newborn and then remove the infant to a stabilization nursery. Birth *creates* a mother and a father and redefines them as a family with their new baby. The family is a unit, and its unity should not be broken, least of all in the earliest hours, at this crucial juncture in their lives.

In most hospitals a baby is taken at birth to the stabilization nursery for anywhere from 2 to 24 hours after birth. The medical rationale is that a baby's body temperature has to stabilize. Since delivery rooms are chilly, and a small baby's system is not yet efficient at maintaining his temperature, it can take quite a while for him to reach a temperature of 98.6° F. But opponents of routine separation point out that the best "baby warmer" is a mother's arms. A baby can be wrapped up and held close to his mother's body and he will warm up *at least as well* as he would in a plastic bassinet.

The other reason given by the hospital for removing the baby is that a newborn needs constant observation. It is unrealistic, however, to think that in a busy hospital a baby is actually being watched constantly or that his needs for holding and feeding are met. The stabilization nursery staff is busy cleaning, weighing, and swaddling other newborns. If you were to keep your baby in your arms while you were spending the obligatory postpartum hour(s) in the recovery area, the nurse checking on you could observe the baby as well. Babies are routinely taken to a stabilization nursery because they always have been; it is more convenient for the staff.

Another possible way to circumvent routine separation is to go to the hospital administrators ahead of time with a plan for positive action. The parents should make an appointment and go in together. Do not put the hospital official on the defensive—on the contrary, make it clear that you understand his position. "We accept the hospital position that parents cannot observe a newborn as well as professionally trained personnel. We know that the first twelve hours after birth are a crucial time to a baby and we'd want our baby to have full benefit of observation by nurses. However, we cannot accept being separated from our baby at birth because of the damage we feel this creates in parent-infant bonding. Therefore, we have a compromise we'd like to implement. We are willing to hire a special-duty nurse at our expense to replace the routine observation period in the nursery. This way we can stay together with our baby without sacrificing the safety measure of close observation by a professional."

Birth—compared to your womb—is rough for a baby. She has to make many physical adjustments to her new environment. Your baby needs every assurance that all is well and will continue to be. A hospital tends to dehumanize the mother-child relationship and disturbs its continuity. The necessarily rigid schedule of a nursery does not have the proper regard for the needs of the baby and mother. The first infantile needs are prompt satisfaction of hunger and the urge to nuzzle and suck. A baby needs the feeling of warmth and support from a nurturing mother and peaceful, undisturbed rest in between. You need only go into a stabilization nursery and see the babies less than an hour old, looking around and trying to suck on their hands or the blanket, to know that they belong with their mothers.

Nursing and what happens around it influence a child's later feelings about herself and other people: whether cries for help are met, whether one is worthy of attention, whether others are to be counted upon. An important milestone for a baby is learning that crying results in being fed. This is a baby's first experience of trust and communication. When separated from her mother in the nursery she is kept from forming this close relationship based on love and need. Hunger is a terrifying experience for a new baby: not only is it painful but the child has no way of knowing that the pain will stop. In the nursery a baby may cry herself to sleep and then be too tired to nurse well when feeding time arrives. This can discourage you and create a cycle of rejection and disappointment.

It may seem as though this section on the separation of babies and mothers is not objective enough. I accept that criticism. I feel a moral responsibility to encourage new mothers to protect themselves and their babies from the sometimes unthinking, unfeeling routines of the hospital. The issue here is about normal, healthy babies. Certainly a baby with any kind of problem must be cared for in the stabilization or intensive care nursery. Obviously a heavily medicated mother will not be sufficiently awake and aware to keep her baby with her. However, the overwhelming majority of mothers and babies have no complications. Many doctors, nurses, and midwives are aware of the possible damage being done by hospitals that whisk babies away from their mothers for many hours following birth. One doctor put it eloquently: "Eventually . . . twenty years down the road . . . the public is going to sue for the psychosocial malpractice of the hospital. Natural bonding processes are impeded: the routines interfere with the development of the family and the male-female relationship. The birth process affects the individual and collective lives of the family. A man not allowed to be present at his child's birth—or not allowed to stay with the baby and his mother during recovery—is being denied important rights. We're worried now about medical malpractice—just wait until people realize the irreversible harm of separation at birth.''

### SIBLING VISITING

This is another important aspect of maintaining family unity during childbirth. Your other children can feel frightened, angry, and rejected by your sudden, even if explained, absence from home. The first thing to find out is whether children are allowed to visit you in the hospital. Some maternity floors have visiting rooms for this purpose and it gives your other child(ren) a chance to be reassured that you are fine and still love them.

Ask whether the hospital allows siblings to see the baby. A very few hospitals that permit viewing also allow the children to touch their newborn brother or sister. Some contact is better than none at all. It is hard for children to accept a new baby that will be taking the major portion of their mother's attention in the first weeks. If you bring a new baby home without some ''icebreaker,'' it can increase the older child's jealousy and feeling of displacement. As noted earlier, it can be compared to how you might feel if your mate were to disappear for several days and then come home with his arms wrapped around another woman, stating that she was to become ''co-wife.''

## HOW TO COPE WITH THE HOSPITAL

Although you should know what you do and don't want from a hospital birth experience *you have to be realistic in your expectations.* Administrative and physical needs are going to get priority. Emotional needs and individual requests and personalities impede efficiency. This is not to say that you should not make every reasonable effort to get what you want and refuse what you don't want, but don't set yourself up for confrontations and disappointment. For example, don't *expect* support and aid with breast-feeding—

it will be wonderful if the hospital staff is able to help you, but in many cases assistance is not available. If you seek advice elsewhere you can avoid being discouraged by an unsuccessful start to breast-feeding.

## HOSPITALS ARE INTIMIDATING

Once you enter a hospital it is easy to feel overpowered by the authoritarian atmosphere, as if it's your first day of school. Is is natural to feel "they" are in control and that you have to follow orders. There are some personnel in a hospital who are bound to be particularly intimidating—don't let anyone push you around or make you do anything you don't want, but keep in mind that *everybody in a hospital is following rules.* There is a chain of command that affects everyone—what can often happen is that when people are ordered around from above they try to exert a similar kind of control over other people. Nurses' aides and orderlies are at the bottom of the ladder and have to take orders from everyone else on the staff. Nurses are controlled both by hospital regulations and by any doctor, including interns and residents who often know less than an experienced obstetric nurse. You may notice that many doctors treat nurses with a callous arrogance showing little respect for a nurse's opinion or expertise. Nurse supervisors have to enforce hospital policies, criticize their nurses as well as defend them, *and* answer to any doctor. You should not be surprised that hospital personnel can be bossy with you when they work in a system structured on authority.

The very atmosphere of a hospital can create anxiety—and its side effects—for you. As discussed earlier, your emotional state has a considerable effect on the physical progress of labor. If you are aware of the possible negative influence of the hospital atmosphere you can attempt to minimize that aspect.

*A wheelchair* will probably be used to transport you from the hospital entrance or the admitting office to the labor area. If you are in hard labor you may welcome a wheelchair but if you are able to walk comfortably, a wheelchair can make you feel like an invalid. It can undermine your feeling that you are well, not sick, and coping well with your labor. If you'd prefer not to be wheeled to the labor room, state your preference.

***Personal effects*** are usually removed when you get to the labor room. Often any hairpins, jewelry, and eyeglasses are removed. This can be *depersonalizing*. It may seem like a petty issue, but taking away your personal belongings does have a way of undermining your sense of being in charge— the implication of putting on ''their'' clothes is that you are in their control. The army, prisons, and other institutions can exert control by removing personal belongings and imposing institutional apparel. You can make your own decision about how you want to handle this in the hospital—just understanding it may make it unnecessary to challenge it. Insofar as glasses are concerned, if you are nearsighted, you should demand to keep them, so you can see the birth. Some hospitals do not allow contact lenses; find this out ahead of time, so you can bring glasses instead.

***Confinement to bed*** can make you feel powerless, particularly if the bedrails are raised, which can make the narrow bed seem like a crib. It can make you feel as if you're a sick child. Again, this is subtle intimidation, but it may affect you subconsciously unless you recognize it. You cannot help but be affected by being confined to a labor bed, hemmed in by metal rails on either side, with nurses and doctors (Mommy and Daddy figures) asking, ''How are we doing?'' It can be important during labor for a woman to feel she is capable, self-sufficient, and has a say in what takes place. If the bedrails bother you, for instance, then ask to have them lowered. They were intended to keep medicated mothers from falling out of bed, but some hospitals raise them routinely.

***Questions, examinations, lights, equipment, needles*** can all create anxiety. A hospital and its procedures make most people edgy and nervous—in addition, you have labor to cope with, and you may be anxious about how well you're going to be able to do that.

*If you or your mate are frightened by hospitals*—if you have always felt queasy about visiting people in the hospital, for instance—then make a point of visiting the hospital several times before labor. The more chance you have to walk around in a hospital, the more accustomed you will become. If either of you knows beforehand that you dread hospitals, it is well worth the trouble of making a few trips there. To make it more fun you can find out what the hours are for viewing the babies in the nursery and make that your destination: you can look at all the newborns and decide which one yours is going to look like.

 I personally know that this system of getting your feet wet works: my mother was hospitalized several times before she died and I could never go into a hospital (then or afterward) without getting a migraine headache. To research this book I had no choice but to spend many hours in many hospitals. After the first few times the headaches disappeared; then I was jumpy for a while, afraid of seeing sick people on stretchers in the halls. Before long I could march into a hospital and feel right at home. Many people share my ex-phobia about hospitals; these feelings can interfere with both the personal and physical aspects of birth if you don't deal with them ahead of time.

*Act at the time* if you aren't happy with a staff member or some procedure. Don't cave in to intimidation—you are only going to have this baby once. If you can't face standing up to bullying or negativism, have your mate go to bat for you. Confrontations are never pleasant, least of all when you have the work of labor to cope with—but if you don't stick up for what you want you only have yourselves to blame for a less-than-optimum experience. If you realize what a hospital can do to you, you're okay. A lack of freedom of choice and individual privacy and an assembly-line attitude deny your personal experience. *Fight against every indication of it.*

## AVOIDING ROUTINE PROCEDURES

Routine procedures can be avoided in a number of ways. It is important to find out hospital policies ahead of time so that you know what you are going to have to deal with. You should be aware that in side-stepping routines *you take on the responsibility for anything that goes wrong* as a result. Of course one of the purposes of having a say in what happens during your labor is so that you are more involved and responsible. If you have read the section on routine procedures in this chapter, then you know that there is not much that can go wrong by avoiding certain routines in a normal labor and delivery . . . on the contrary, the routines themselves can cause physical and emotional problems. Also, just because you decide against a routine doesn't mean you can't change your mind. If you want to skip an enema you can always have it later in labor—or if you have decided against having an I.V. inserted in early labor your doctor can ask to hook one up if he feels it is necessary at any point. Here are some ways to avoid routine procedures:

*Get a note from your obstetrician* stating that certain routines can be eliminated: this is a good tool to protect your wishes. Some doctors will not sign anything, however. The only assurance you may be able to get is an exact understanding and agreement ahead of time. If there is any argument in the hospital, you, your mate, or the nurse can call your doctor.

*Get a note from your pediatrician* stating that certain routines should not be employed with your baby. This is especially helpful in a hospital that does not have family-centered maternity care. If there is a note attached to your chart that says, "Baby rooming-in. No supplementary bottles," it will protect your wishes. When the order comes from a doctor—rather than just being your individual request—it carries more weight with a hospital staff accustomed to certain routines.

***Admission forms can be a protection against routines.*** There are forms you must sign when you preregister or when you are admitted in labor. Before you sign the form write in: *All procedures subject to my complete understanding of need.* This makes it clear right up front that you question routine procedures in principle and will need to be shown justification for the application of them in your individual labor.

## How to Get What You Want

***Dealing effectively with the staff*** will get you what you want with a minimum of hassle.

***Labor room nurses need information*** about your labor prior to admittance. If you come well prepared it simplifies their job and can gain you their respect. You will probably be asked when your contractions began, how strong and frequent they have been, whether there's been any discharge of bloody show, if/when your membranes ruptured, whether you've felt nauseous, when you last ate, and any allergies you have to medication.

***Be sure to tell them you've taken childbirth preparation,*** whether they ask or not. Be sure to tell every new staff member with whom you come into contact. You might also add that you'd appreciate being kept informed of your progress during labor so that you can cope with it most effectively and cooperate with the staff. If hospital personnel know you will be using prepared childbirth techniques and want to be involved in the labor and delivery they will deal with you differently than they would an untrained mother.

***Refuse to answer anything during a contraction.*** Some staff members may forget or not understand that you cannot be interrupted when you are in the middle of a contraction. Explain afterward about the need to answer any questions *between* contractions.

### Some diplomatic ways to ask for nonroutine treatment or to complain:

"WE KNOW THIS ISN'T ROUTINE, but we have our doctor's permission and he said you'd all be helpful . . ."

"WE KNOW YOU'RE HERE TO HELP US and we'll cooperate if you will please . . ."

"YOU PROBABLY DIDN'T INTEND TO UPSET NANCY but your comments about 'pain' and 'suffering' make it harder for her . . ." (from your mate to a staff member who doesn't understand prepared childbirth and keeps offering medication or making negative comments about contractions).

"I KNOW YOU'RE TRYING TO HELP and we appreciate that, but . . ."

"WE KNOW YOU'RE VERY RUSHED and we appreciate the help you're giving us . . ." (when even a flexible hospital becomes less so when the staff gets very busy).

*Tactful stubbornness* in the face of opposition is the best stance. Let the staff know you are knowledgeable, calm, and confident. In some cases it is probably best for the baby's father to speak up—judge for yourselves.

### Ask to speak to the director of nursing or the obstetrical supervisor if you have a problem you cannot resolve comfortably with the staff. Don't let a staff member's personal attitude aggravate you so much that you or your mate get into a heated argument. If you cannot calmly come to an understanding in a reasonable way then go above the person you are dealing with—not as a way of threatening but to get your needs met as expediently as possible. Getting upset is going to interfere with your labor. A supervisor is usually interested in helping make sure that customers are satisfied—the hospital may be very rigid or it may be that you are the first person to make a certain request.

***Write a letter as soon as possible after the birth*** if you were unable to get satisfaction in some aspect of your hospital stay. It may be more effective coming from the baby's father—we are still a male-dominated society and the truth is that a letter from a man, especially on business stationery, carries more weight. Address the letter to the nursing supervisor or the hospital administrator—call the hospital and find out their names. If your problem concerns a doctor, intern, or resident, address it to the Chief of Obstetrics. Whichever official you write to, send copies of your letter to the other two and note at the bottom, for example, cc: Dr. William Brown and Mrs. Judy McDevitt so that the person who receives your letter knows that the other officials in the hospital are now also aware of the problem. Be specific about dates, room number, names of people involved, and *exactly* what displeased you. By writing a letter you are not just finding an outlet for your disappointment and anger but, even more important, you are helping pave the way for future couples to get what they desire in a birth experience.

***Write a letter as soon as you have time*** if you were *pleased* with the overall or individual care you received. It is just as important to support positive childbirth practices in the hospital as it is to change those that are detrimental. Every person who praises a flexible, humanitarian hospital helps insure the survival of these qualities which are so vital to making hospital birth a good experience for everyone.

## HOW TO CHANGE THE HOSPITAL

The intention of giving you information about routine practices in hospitals is *not* to drive you away from hospital birth. For some couples the hospital management of childbirth may be one of their reasons for deciding against it but the hospital setting is still where most people will go to have their babies. The point is *you can change the hospital.* You don't have to abandon the system; you can help improve it.

A hospital is there to serve you; health care is a consumer issue; hospitals *must* change if they are going to attract or hold on to their "customers." What is happening in maternity care is a consumer rebellion against medical practices applied indiscriminately to all pregnant women.

The first thing to know is that *you can legally refuse any medical procedure*. You cannot *dictate* medical practice, however, and tell a professional how to do procedures on you. Thus what you have is *reactive control:* you can refuse certain things but you cannot demand that things happen in a certain way. Hospitals can establish and enforce their own procedures within their walls—but you have the option of refusing anything you choose to.

Courts and lawsuits are ineffective in bringing about change. The law supports "standard medical procedure" in every case. It doesn't matter whether it is the parent or the doctor who is suing for a change in policies. The status quo is protected by law—the courts go by the way things have been done in the past. There are avenues for change that work, however. State legislatures, health regulatory agencies, and especially consumer pressure and protest can affect the way that childbirth care is delivered.

If you are sufficiently motivated—either by a bad hospital maternity-care experience or by your desire to insure a good one—form a *local council on maternal and child health*. It is much easier than it sounds.

## FORMING A LOCAL COUNCIL ON MATERNAL AND CHILD HEALTH

*First seek out people to be members* of the council. Speak to women you know who are interested in childbirth, whether they are simply knowledgeable consumers or members of a group like the La Leche League. Call up—and ask the other members to contact—clergy or other religious leaders. Call the college, university, or even the high school in your area and speak to the heads of the psychology and sociology departments whose studies will have made them aware of the importance of childbirth. Contact teachers of disabled children, who work every day with the results of complications or mismanagement of birth.

Health professionals of any kind may be interested. Call obstetricians you know or have heard are committed to natural childbirth. Call the local childbirth education organization or write to some of the national organizations listed in the appendix and learn what related organizations exist in your community. When you have a meeting it can be decided who will be the officers of the council; this nucleus can then represent the council in meetings.

***Contact the chief administrative officer*** and/or the chairman of the obstetrics department of all hospitals in your area and request permission for your group to tour the obstetric department, including the labor and delivery area. You can take the questionnaire (see page 408) with you and find out in detail about each hospital's facilities.

Hold public hearings and "speak-outs" on obstetric care. This can have impact on state and local obstetric practices. Invite the people from the state and/or local Maternal and Child Health Department to attend and participate.

***You can issue press releases*** to alert the media to the present state of obstetric care in your area. Once you have gained enough information you can hold a press conference to highlight the issues.

## CHART 29. QUESTIONNAIRE FOR HOSPITALS

### I. ANESTHESIA
1. Do you have an anesthetist on duty full-time?
2. If so, do you charge whether I use the anesthetist or not?
3. Do your anesthetists mostly use general or local anesthesia?

### II. BREAST-FEEDING
1. Is breast-feeding encouraged here?
2. Do you encourage or allow breast-feeding on the delivery table?
3. Do you allow babies to be breast-fed on demand?
4. Do you give mothers breast-feeding literature? If so, from what source?
5. Do you routinely give a test feeding of glucose and water in the nursery? If so, can it be eliminated if my pediatrician requests it?

### III. EARLY DISCHARGE
1. Do you offer early discharge?
2. If so, do you offer infant-care classes—or require them—ahead of delivery?
3. Do you have follow-up visits made by nurses or other professionals?
4. Do you have a way I can contact the hospital, postpartum, if I have questions or problems at home?

### IV. FATHER PARTICIPATION
1. Are fathers allowed in the labor room? Are there any exceptions (shared labor room, for example)?
2. Are they allowed in the delivery room? If so, under what circumstances are they asked to leave?
3. May a friend or relative substitute if the father cannot come? If so, must that person have taken the childbirth training with me?
4. Are fathers allowed to stay with wives in the recovery area?
5. Are there unlimited visiting privileges for the father? If not, can he be with me at times in addition to the regular visiting hours?
6. Are fathers allowed to hold their babies?

**CHART 29. QUESTIONNAIRE FOR HOSPITALS** *(continued)*

## V. FACILITIES

1. Do you have an alternative birthing room? If so, under what circumstances would I not be permitted to use it or be transferred to a regular labor room?

2. Do you allow women to labor and deliver in the same bed, either in the labor room or in the delivery room (so that there isn't the awkward transfer of beds when the baby's head is crowning)?

3. Are labor rooms double or single? If I can't have a private labor room, can you assure me that I'll be placed with a woman who has also had childbirth-preparation classes? Am I permitted to walk around in labor?

4. Are fetal monitors used? If so, are they mandatory? Can an exception be made if my doctor were to agree to it?

5. Do you sponsor prenatal classes for parents? If so, do they include exercise sessions? Is there a fee charged?

6. What is your policy on food and drink in labor? Are ice chips provided? Is there any rule against fathers eating in the labor rooms? If so, do you have a cafeteria in the hospital?

7. Do you do many Leboyer deliveries? If so, do you provide a bathtub, sterile water, and a radiant heater? If not, to whom do I speak about bringing or arranging for these?

8. Do you have preregistration facilities? If not, would it at least be possible for me to fill out most of the forms and bring them with me when I arrive in labor? How much do you require as a cash deposit on admittance?

9. Do you allow cameras and/or tape recorders? Would you allow me to use them if I were to sign a release form of some kind?

CHART 29. QUESTIONNAIRE FOR HOSPITALS *(continued)*

## VI. THE NEWBORN

1. Are babies and mothers allowed to be together from birth?
   - If not, what is your separation policy? Are all babies automatically taken to the stabilization nursery?
   - If so, what is the *least* amount of time my baby would have to stay there, assuming it is normal and healthy?
2. What is the average length of stay in stabilization: the first two hours after birth? the first 12 hours? the first 24 hours?
3. If my pediatrician agrees, would I be allowed to keep my baby with me in the recovery area?
4. If not, would the baby's father be allowed to stay with the baby in the stabilization nursery?
5. Do you have rooming-in?
   - If so, is it available to all mothers or only those with private rooms?
   - Must a mother commit herself to full-time rooming-in or is it flexible (so that she can have the baby or return it to the nursery as she wishes)?
   - Are babies all returned to the central nursery at night?
   - Do you have nurses available for questions and help in the room?
6. Does the hospital offer infant-care classes to new mothers? If so, are fathers encouraged to attend?

## VII. ROUTINE PROCEDURES

1. Do you administer enemas, I.V.s and/or shaves routinely?
2. If so, could any procedures be eliminated if my doctor agrees?
3. Are women's wrists ever strapped during labor or delivery? Are there cases in which they are routinely strapped down?
4. Are stirrups optional during delivery and if so, is that my doctor's decision or hospital policy?

CHART 29. QUESTIONNAIRE FOR HOSPITALS *(continued)*

## VII. ROUTINE PROCEDURES *(cont.)*
5. Do you routinely transfer from labor room and bed to delivery room and table?
   - If so, with my doctor's agreement could I labor and deliver in the same bed?
   - Could I labor and deliver in the labor room in that case?

## VIII. SIBLING VISITATION
1. Are children allowed to visit their mothers?
2. If so, are they allowed in her room or is there a visiting room?
3. Are children allowed to see the newborn?
4. Are children allowed to touch the newborn?

# 8

# Home birth

Contrary to what some people in the medical profession believe, home birth is not a fad and cannot be ignored. Medical care-givers usually characterize home-birthers as ignorant antiestablishmentarians who either have to be punished or enlightened. In states such as California where home birth flourishes, just the opposite has been found: many of those choosing birth at home are middle- to upper-middle-class, well-educated couples. They are dissatisfied with the hospital system of birth and are not willing to make compromises; and many of them would choose home birth even if hospitals were to suddenly make sweeping changes.

There is a basic philosophical position behind the choice for giving birth at home. There is a strong and growing home-birth "movement" in this country comprised of individuals and organizations dedicated to informing the public, to improving the legal status of home-birth attendants, and to securing decent medical backup care. The home-birth movement reflects not just attitudes about birth but about life as a whole: to simplify one's life and to get back to real human values in a technologized society.

Home birth is a matter of conviction—not of monetary need, ignorance, or rebellion. The revolutionary aspect of the home-birth movement is that it has redefined birth as a normal physiological process rather than an illness requiring hospitalization and aggressive medical intervention. The question is not simply home birth on its physical and emotional merits: it is home birth believed to be a necessary

412

way of life for some, just as hospital birth is believed to be a necessity of life for others.

The out-of-hospital movement began at the same time, in the same communities, in which the principle of obstetric intensive care began to be applied to all women in childbirth. The trend toward home birth has been in direct proportion to the trend within the hospital to treat every birth as a potential high-risk situation. In a technologized society there are constant trade-offs between technical advances and human values: people who choose home birth are not willing to pay the price tag of birth in a hospital where the individual and emotional aspect of birth has been compromised.

Home-birthers believe they are doing the best thing for their children and themselves. These are parents who judge the risks of the hospital greater than the risk in giving birth outside it. They are concerned about the routine administration of often unnecessary treatments which themselves have not been proven risk-free. Some members of the medical community have made ugly, unwarranted public statements that those who choose home birth are endangering the lives of their children and are guilty of child abuse. These professionals are angry and frightened by the home-birth movement: it threatens them at the core of their belief system. But let it be said up front, *no sane parents would willingly choose to increase the risk to their babies*. Most people choosing home birth do so in the belief that for them it is as safe or safer than a hospital.

## SAFETY OF HOME BIRTH

The question invariably raised about home birth is whether it is safe. Those who choose home birth do not ignore the fact that things can go wrong but they are also aware that *life* is fraught with danger (the odds are greater of harm coming to you and/or your child in a car than in giving birth outside a hospital). Those opposed to home birth might say this is foolhardy reasoning—why "flirt with danger" rather than take advantage of the hospital which has machines and expertise *in case* the unlikely complications arise? Home-birth advocates could reply that the same people making that argument are inconsistent and foolish themselves because they'll give birth in a hospital, then drive home with the baby in their lap in "the death seat" next to the driver.

For people who are considering or have chosen home birth, giving birth is not an event to be measured in terms of statistics or to be decided on the basis of other people's lists of possible problems. Birth is a personal and interpersonal experience—one of life's great events—and it belongs at home where this aspect is foremost. Home-birthers understand that there are no guarantees in life and that in birth there is no such thing as "absolute safety"—many people who give birth in a hospital go on the misguided *assumption* that the medical setting assures them absolute safety, which no one can provide. Those who have babies at home must know what to do and where to go if problems should arise; they also have to be able to accept that in nature there is a measure of unpredictability and cruelty.

There are two main factors to be considered in the safety of birth at home. One is that candidates must be carefully screened and receive excellent prenatal care. The other factor is the availability of emergency backup personnel and equipment. If these two elements are carefully taken into account then home birth is relatively safe.

A study comparing the outcomes of a group of home births vs. hospital births in California matched two sizable groups of women so that those giving birth were as similar as possible except in the location of their babies' births. The result of this study was that the home-birth outcomes were better than the California state average, with fewer complications than might have been expected. The conclusion of the study was that home birth is a safe alternative for women who have been medically screened as healthy. There was no increase in risk at home: in fact, with avoidance of medication in the home births there were higher Apgar scores and less fetal hypoxia.

In order to have the greatest margin of safety, those attending home births as well as those choosing to have them should employ very careful screening of candidates.

The chart beginning below lists those factors which contra-indicate a birth at home.

---

### CHART 30. DIRECTORY OF FACTORS THAT RULE OUT HOME BIRTH

**Abnormal Presentation** . . . a baby in a breech, transverse, or other abnormal position might require last-minute obstetric procedures not possible at home.

**Active Herpes Simplex Virus** . . . can be transmitted to your baby if you have lesions at the time of delivery. If you have a history of herpes, have a doctor examine you right up until your due date; if there are lesions, your baby should be delivered by cesarean section.

**Bleeding** . . . with or without pain before labor can indicate placenta previa. In this case the placenta is covering the cervix, in front of the baby, who must be delivered by cesarean).

**Cephalopelvic Disproportion** . . . if it is suspected that the baby's head is too large to fit through your pelvis, a sonogram can confirm whether this disproportion does exist. If cephalopelvic disproportion is not detected prelabor, labor will not progress after a certain point and you will have to be transferred to a hospital.

**Complications in Previous Pregnancies** . . . includes anything on this list as well as previous cesarean or history of small-for-date babies, who have a higher risk of respiratory distress, low blood sugar levels, greater heat loss, and cerebral edema) . . . complications have a tendency to recur in subsequent pregnancies.

**Diabetes** . . . involves high risks for the baby and is a dangerous situation even in the hospital.

**Grand Multiparity** . . . there is a higher incident of uterine inertia in women who have had 6 or more previous pregnancies.

**Hydramnios** . . . too much amniotic fluid.

CHART 30. DIRECTORY OF FACTORS
THAT RULE OUT HOME BIRTH *(continued)*

**Hypertension** . . . also known as high blood pressure, is one of the unpredictable complications of birth. Some women develop hypertension during labor with no previous history of the problem. It gives no warning signals until you go into convulsions. *At least* have prenatal exams every week near your due date and abandon plans for home birth if your blood pressure rises.

**Malnutrition** . . . involves risks to the mother in labor and may mean a small-for-date or otherwise compromised infant.

**Maternal Anemia** . . . is determined by blood tests. It can result in low birth weight and prematurity; it also predisposes you to postpartum hemorrhage.

**Multiple Pregnancy** . . . increases the possibility of: (1) small-for-date babies who require special care; (2) abnormal presentation of both babies or the second baby; (3) separation of the placenta before the second baby is born.

**Postmaturity** . . . is best determined by a 24-hour urine test which indicates whether there is placental dysfunction (the fetus is no longer being properly nourished); determining postmaturity by dates (42–44 weeks gestation) can be incorrect because there may have been an error in calculation of dates.

**Preeclampsia or Eclampsia** . . . can be detected in your prenatal exams.

**Prematurity** . . . is any baby that goes into labor at less than 36 weeks gestation: he may be low birth weight or have other problems.

**Primipara over 35** . . . if this is your first baby and you're over 35, more complications are possible. This factor is something you can discuss with a doctor sympathetic to home birth.

---

**CHART 30. DIRECTORY OF FACTORS
THAT RULE OUT HOME BIRTH (continued)**

---

**Rh Blood Incompatibility** . . . is a problem *only* if a blood test shows a rise in titre (maternal antibody production) before delivery. Otherwise, an umbilical-cord blood sample is sent to a lab, and if positive you must get a rhogram injection within 72 hours of the baby's birth.

**Those who are not ideologically committed to home birth** . . . will depend heavily on the attendant(s) instead of themselves and may not be able to handle the physical or emotional demands of home birth. The wrong reasons for choosing home birth are religious (to avoid drugs, transfusions), financial (too poor to afford the hospital, not poor enough for government assistance programs), peer pressure (your friends have all had home births or your mate feels more strongly about it than you), or you just don't like doctors or hospitals.

---

## REGISTERING HOME BIRTHS

This is essential in demonstrating the safety of home births. Many people giving birth at home do not file birth certificates. However, the law requires that deaths must be reported. Therefore the statistics showing the fetal death rate in home births are accurate, *but* neonatal mortality is computed by *comparing* the number of births with the number of deaths. Obviously this makes the infant mortality figure for home births look much worse than it is.

The medical community, in particular the American College of Obstetricians and Gynecologists (ACOG), is convinced the neonatal mortality is greater at home than in the hospital. The current statistics are grossly inaccurate and make it appear that this is true—this gives the medical establishment ammunition with which to bring greater pressure against home birth. What is at stake here is maintaining the *choice* of home birth for those who want it. Those who are considering home birth deserve accurate information on which to base their decision. Home-birthers who do not register births are creating a false impression of lack of safety as well as a smaller number of home births than actually take place. Adequate medical backup for home birth will not be available until the statistics show that a sufficient number of people are giving birth at home to justify the expenditure of public or private funds for emergency facilities if they become necessary. One reason that couples do not register home births is because of the harassment they get from health officials who are opposed to home birth. But the long-term consequences for a child are worse than the temporary abuse her parents may have to withstand. A birth certificate is necessary for getting into school, getting a driver's license, a passport, proving majority, voting, establishing citizenship, claiming inheritances, qualifying for old-age pensions, Social Security, and Medicaid. A couple should take the responsibility of reporting a birth for their child's sake and also so a more accurate picture of home births is available.

In order to register a birth, look in the telephone book under County Health Department, Department of Public Health, or Registrar (or Bureau) of Vital Statistics. It does not require a doctor's signature, only that of a witness to the birth. Anyone can register a birth if he or she was present; it can be the mother herself. Depending on the state there is a time limit on registering that is anywhere from a few days to a year. After that time late registration can be considered a misdemeanor—which may be a hassle but is still worth the advantages of registering.

## EMERGENCY PRECAUTIONS

Taking emergency precautions and planning ahead what to do in case of an emergency increases the safety of home birth. It is all very well to maintain a positive attitude toward birth as a normal physiological process but you must also consider the "what if . . ." when you are planning a home birth.

***Tape the paramedic's telephone number*** on your phone. Find out who you should ask for in case of complications in childbirth.

***Find out the closest hospital*** with emergency facilities, or preferably with obstetric facilities. Find out whether it is necessary to have a doctor who has admitting privileges there in order to be cared for. It is morally damnable—but a grim reality—that many hospitals may reject a woman in labor who has chosen home birth. Hospitals are ideologically opposed to home birth and may turn you away if complications arise. They also may not want the responsibility of a situation that has already become serious—and the courts will uphold a doctor's refusal to assist you; however, your moral indignation and anger at a hospital, which is presumably there for the good of society, won't do you any good if you're in need of medical care during childbirth. So find a hospital that will accept you.

***Take a run-through of the hospital beforehand*** so you know your way around if necessary. It also can't do any harm to preregister, just in case—this way if you do need the hospital's facilities there will be less hassle. Pack a bag with some nighties, other necessities, and baby clothes in case you do have to be hospitalized. This may seem overcautious but it will smooth the way in the unlikely case that you have to leave home.

***Make sure that your car is in good condition.*** This is more than a precaution; it is a necessity. As your due date is nearing be sure that you always try to have a full or close-to-full tank of gas. Sometime during your labor have your mate or someone he chooses start up the car just to be sure it's ready to go. A station wagon or van is preferable because there is room for you to lie down in the back. If you have complications in your labor the last thing you need is the anxiety of a car that isn't working.

***Do not be more than 30 minutes from a hospital.*** If your house is too isolated, then choose a friend or relative's home that is nearer to a hospital.

***Try to make a relationship*** with a family practitioner or an obstetrician beforehand. You might even consider getting your prenatal care from a doctor so that you know each other. If you have no experienced birth attendant or if you have a lay midwife you must know ahead of time who will take over in an emergency.

It may be hard to find a sympathetic doctor, although it is not hard to understand why most of them have such a negative attitude toward home birth. Doctors spend years of their lives and a great deal of money on medical training—by choosing to give birth at home you are questioning the value of that. By asking a doctor to give backup care you are asking him to violate what he believes to be the only right way and place to have a baby. A doctor's reaction may be fear, outrage and indignation—you are threatening the foundation on which he has built his life's work. You should also realize the pressure put on doctors by hospitals. Some institutions threaten that any doctor who participates in a home birth will have his admitting privileges revoked at the hospital.

It may not be a good idea to have a doctor as your primary *attendant* at home birth. A doctor is medically oriented, trained to intervene, and has had no training for home delivery. Hospital deliveries are very different because labor is affected by drugs and other routine interventions. Many doctors with extensive hospital experience don't know what to expect at home. For example, they may never have seen a natural-length wait in the third stage of labor and they might expect the placenta to come out right away as it does in the hospital where synthetic hormones are routinely administered to speed things along. Therefore a doctor might pull on the umbilical cord in third stage, a dangerous practice which could cause hemorrhage.

Generally, a midwife (either certified nurse- or lay) is a better choice for a home-birth attendant for these reasons. If a couple feels strongly about having a doctor attend them they should consider that they may not be 100 percent committed to home birth and may be choosing a doctor as a psychological crutch. There are two instances in which it might be advisable to have a doctor at home. In many states delivering a child is considered the "practice of medicine," and only licensed physicians are legally permitted to attend births. The other reason is that a doctor has hospital admitting privileges in case complications arise.

***Contact the Visiting Nurses Association,*** which will probably be listed in your phone book, and find out if they have a nurse who specializes in maternity care if you are not going to have a medically trained attendant at the birth. Find out whether she will make a postpartum visit *as soon as possible* after the baby is born. The nurse can examine your perineum to see if there are any tears and whether any stitches are needed. She can also check the baby.

***Contact a pediatrician*** ahead of time, particularly if there is not going to be a medical attendant at your birth and/or no visiting nurse is available. Find a pediatrician who is not opposed to home birth because many of them will refuse to see babies who have been born at home. Then get the baby to the pediatrician (or to a clinic) for newborn checkup. Even though the baby may seem fine, *confirm that*—do not neglect that early checkup just because everything seems fine. There are some birth defects, like cleft palate, which need medical attention.

***Stay very quiet*** for the first few hours postpartum. No matter how good you feel, you must stay still and rest quietly for the hours after birth. This is the time when hemorrhage can happen. Make sure that your uterus is hard and have someone massage it with a gentle downward pressure within the limits of your comfort so that it stays firm.

## THE LEGAL ASPECT

The legal aspect of choosing to give birth at home is something you should know, especially so that you will not be intimidated by people who may be misinformed. *No state requires that childbirth take place in a hospital or forbids home birth.* There are laws about birth attendants, however, which vary from state to state. A doctor is legally free to attend a birth anywhere; the laws pertaining to certified nurse-midwives give the current, but frequently changing, regulations about lay midwifery. Standards vary widely among the states: in many states the responsibility for regulation is with state health or licensing agencies which determine the qualifications and training required.

***Your legal obligation to your child*** does not begin until he is born. If at that time he is in need of medical assistance and you do not make every effort to summon that assistance or get the baby to medical care, and the baby dies—that is considered manslaughter. It is *highly unlikely* that such charges would be brought against you, just as it is highly unlikely that parents would not go to a hospital or doctor if their baby were in trouble. When efforts have been made to summon appropriate medical care, no charge of manslaughter has ever been brought.

## THERE IS NO CRIMINAL LIABILITY FOR STILLBIRTH

***Nonprofessionals involved*** in home birth have no legal liability unless there is death or permanent disability. In that case the two possible consequences are a civil suit (money damages being sought) or a criminal suit (somebody wants to fine you or put you in jail). The "somebody" in these cases would presumably be the local authorities and, although it is highly unlikely that any action would be taken, nevertheless, legal grounds do exist. It is conceivable that there could be enough fear and resentment toward home birth (i.e., toward people who are challenging the status quo of the medical establishment) to generate at least talk of such proceedings. Therefore it's important that you know your legal rights beforehand.

***If the mother dies*** there is no legal liability as long as the mother knew what she was doing. It is her right to assume the risk of home birth. No one in the United States has to go to a hospital for anything, including childbirth.

# PSYCHOLOGICAL CONSIDERATIONS IN HOME BIRTH

In a home birth the responsibility for labor and delivery and the outcome of the baby rest entirely with the expectant couple. The positive aspect of this is that it gives you a sense of power and control over the situation, a feeling that you are running your own life. This responsibility also means that if anything goes wrong there is no one else to blame . . . you can't pin the fault on other people or factors that are out of your control. For many people it may be necessary to be able to do that and you should carefully consider and resolve this aspect of home birth ahead of time.

You will probably encounter a fair amount of social pressure directed against your decision to give birth at home. In most cases it is in your best interest not to get dragged into emotional and potentially destructive discussions—no purpose is served by them. If it is important to you that particular people *understand* your position then you should make the effort to explain it to them. But do not set out to persuade them you are "right" or to get their sanction: it will frustrate you and them and perhaps cause problems with your relationship. If you find that it is vitally important to you to get validation from other people, then you should talk again with your mate about your decision for home birth until you are sure it is what *you* want.

Giving birth outside of a hospital is not the norm in America. You have to prepare yourself not only for a lack of support for your decision but also negative feedback. There is a societal value judgment that will be directed against you for choosing home birth if anything goes wrong, even if it's something that could not have been prevented even in a hospital. Our society does not hold it against you if your child is damaged or her intelligence is stunted by too many drugs or other procedures in the hospital. However, if a baby is born at home with a birthmark or a clubfoot or cleft palate you will be held to blame. Even though you can *objectively* know that this is senseless reasoning, *subjectively* it can be upsetting. Recognizing these potential psychological problems ahead of time and discussing them with your mate is the best way to protect yourself.

## FEAR

Fear is the greatest problem a woman can have and it is the worst enemy you can have in home birth. It can prolong your labor and even impede it to the extent that you have to transfer to the hospital. The way to avoid this kind of fear is for a couple to be truly committed to birth at home. Even the man must feel at ease or he will transmit his doubts and fears to the woman. *Communicate* your fears and fantasies when you are discussing home birth. Talking about them may resolve some fears; other fears can be eliminated or lessened by making all the "just-in-case" arrangements listed in the preceding section.

*Our social conditioning* says that birth is dangerous and painful. We have all been taught that and people who choose to give birth at home cannot simply repress that conditioning—they have to *un*learn it. Taking excellent care of yourself during pregnancy, having regular prenatal examinations, choosing a qualified birth attendant, and making careful preparations for any eventuality, all help to inform and prepare you. It is vital to acknowledge that we are all deeply conditioned by social attitudes. There is a direct correlation between one's expectations and the realization of them: if you believe that birth is dangerous and painful, you will contribute to making it so. People who want to give birth at home have to make a conscious choice to experience it differently . . . which is to say, as a *positive* event.

*Pain in labor* may be related to fear. A woman who is frightened and tense is going to create the fear/tension/pain cycle that childbirth training attempts to avoid. If you are giving birth at home and the pain becomes unbearable and you cannot cope, it is advisable to go to the hospital. The pain may be the result of extreme fear that you were not conscious of before birth. At the hospital they can give you an artificial relaxant. You also may not have been as committed to home birth as you'd thought; just being in the hospital may relax you. Great pain may also mean there is some physical pathology, so going to the hospital is best for that reason also.

*A prolonged and difficult* labor may be the result of fear and tension on your part. Home-birth attendants find they can sometimes relax a woman be repeating over and over, "Let your baby come down, let your baby come out, let your baby get born." The need for physical contact is also a factor and being held or stroked by your mate and other attendants has also brought successful results where labor was impeded. There is always the possibility that labor is prolonged because of physical impediments to the baby's descent and these must always be taken into consideration—however, the issue here is the psychological aspect, particularly fear, in birth at home.

*See a home birth* or a film of one beforehand. This will give you and your mate a sense of what to expect even though every birth is different. The more information you have the greater sense of control you will have over your own birth experience.

## UNEXPECTED HOSPITALIZATION

Going to the hospital is a possibility that all home-birth couples must consider. Practical and emotional preparation will make it less traumatic.

*Psychologically the first step* is that you and your mate should be allowed and encouraged to *express your sorrow and disappointment* that you could not complete the birth at home. You should avoid feeling guilty.

*A woman feels let down by her own body* just as people do in cases of heart attacks, kidney failures, and other physical problems. Part of your self-esteem derives from the adequacy of your own body, and when it fails you, it can lead to feelings of anger, reduced self-worth, and disappointment in yourself. This can lead to depression if it is not seen for what it is; then eventually you can accept the fact that bodies do sometimes break down. Where home birth is concerned there is a great deal of emphasis on a woman's self-reliance and freedom from dependence on the medical establishment. The contention of the home-birth movement is that birth is a normal physiological process. However, it will help you if you concede that nature is unpredictable and that bodies do not function like well-oiled machines. If you don't make allowance for this going in, then you will feel like a failure if you have to be hospitalized.

*The primary concern* of loving parents is *the baby's well-being.* A woman may have to give up the satisfaction of the natural process of birth and go to the hospital. In doing this she is putting the baby's welfare before her own needs—which can make her feel good as a woman and a mother.

## REASONS FOR CHOOSING HOME BIRTH

*To be in a relaxed, familiar environment* for birth so that it can be a positive personal event with family and perhaps friends present.

- To choose who will be present at the birth.
- To choose supportive birth attendants who will remain with you throughout the labor and delivery.
- To be free to move around during labor and have food and drink as you desire.
- To wear what you want as well as to keep on jewelry, eyeglasses, or other personal effects often removed in the hospital.
- To be free to use your own bathroom as often as needed without waiting to be taken or having to use a bedpan, as in a hospital.
- To labor and deliver in the same room and same bed in whatever position you find comfortable.
- To have family members together during birth and afterward, which may lessen the jealousy of siblings, whose

bonding to the baby may be enhanced if they have participated in or witnessed the birth.

- To be free to reach down and touch the baby before he is fully born and assist in the rest of the birth if desired and/or to allow the father to be the first person to touch the baby.
- To be able to breast-feed immediately and on demand.
- To feel as if your baby belongs to you rather than feeling she belongs to a hospital staff, who bestow her upon you at certain times, or to have to ask permission for you or your mate to hold her.
- To be able to follow your own natural rhythms and those of your baby after birth so that you can rest, get up, nurse, and eat when you want and have visitors, including children, whenever you want; to not be awakened to have your temperature taken or to be given pills to sleep, for pain, or to dry up your milk as is routine in the hospital.
- To promote paternal bonding so that a man is there because he wants to be and is an integral part of the entire experience, on his own territory, without feeling he is imposing; so that he doesn't have to be condescended to or humored by hospital personnel who may not care how vital his presence is to the woman. And so that a man doesn't have to view his baby through a pane of glass or be considered the bearer of bad germs and have to scrub and change clothes or put on a gown before touching his baby.

*To avoid the overbearing environment of the hospital,* which, like the culture outside it, undermines women's confidence in their own bodies.

- At home a woman is encouraged to get in touch with her own body and she is listened to when she describes what is going on—good or bad—with her body and baby in labor. The hospital clouds most women's abilities to tune in with their bodies during birth or no one listens to them.
- To avoid excessive routine intervention in a natural event such as fetal monitors, I.V.s, shave, enema, synthetic oxytocin.

- To avoid routine episiotomies but instead to be attended by someone practiced in the methods which minimize the need for episiotomies and the possibility of tears.
- To avoid aggressive obstetric intervention, such as routine cesarean section of breech babies, routine induction after 24 hours of ruptured membranes, and routine induction of labor at 42 weeks gestation.
- To avoid the feeling of basic distrust of scientific practices in maternity care and to challenge many of the technical interventions which may be proven unsafe in time, as was oxygen, once used in large doses for premature babies until it was found to cause blindness.
- To avoid the feeling of being pressured to "perform" according to preconceived medical notions of what "normal" labor is, and to be made to feel inadequate or to have technical intervention if your individual labor does not fit the standard description.
- To avoid the temptation of drugs during labor, particularly during transition, when you may be tired and frustrated and your resolve may be lowered.

## SUPPLIES NEEDED FOR HOME BIRTH

*A very firm bed* is necessary; this can be achieved by putting a board under the mattress. Otherwise, your hips may make a depression so it is harder for the baby to get out. Also, a puddle of amniotic fluid may form under your hips which the baby will emerge into, with the danger that she will breathe in some of the fluid. Some elevation may be necessary anyway (pillows, for instance). If you are not able to stiffen the bed sufficiently, then you should lie on your side with your knees drawn up for delivery so that your genital area will be up and out of the soft mattress. A water bed is comfortable for first-stage labor but is not recommended for birth for this reason.

*A plastic sheet* should go over the mattress. You can use an old shower curtain or a plastic tablecloth—anything that will be large enough to protect the mattress.

*Old linens* can be tucked in over the plastic sheet and then can be discarded after birth or soaked in cold-water detergent.

WASH THE SHEETS and any towels you'll use in hot water using chlorine bleach. Tumble-dry in a clothes dryer at the hottest possible temperature. As soon as the dryer stops, fold the sheets and towels *while they are still hot* and put them in new, unused plastic bags. Seal them completely with tape and store in a closet until labor begins.

THE MOST CONVENIENT WAY TO ARRANGE THE BED is, once labor has begun, to make the bed as you normally would with fresh sheets. Then put on the plastic sheet. Get out the sealed old linens and put them on over the plastic. This way the old sheets and the plastic can be stripped off the bed after birth, leaving a freshly made bed for you and the baby.

*Newspapers* should be collected for several weeks before your due date. Newsprint is considered clean and even inhibits the growth of germs. The newspapers can be used for extra protection instead of or in addition to the plastic sheet on the mattress. They can also be used to make a pathway to the bathroom from the bed to catch any drippings. And if you don't object, they can even be used under you as bed pads.

*Disposable bed pads* (Chux or Johnson & Johnson) will be necessary for absorption under your buttocks. They resemble large disposable diapers and during labor will absorb amniotic fluid and then can be changed.

*A Fleet enema* should be used if there is any chance that you have hard feces in the lower intestine. Most women go into labor having had several bowel movements or diarrhea, which is nature's cleansing process, but sometimes women are constipated. In this case an enema makes labor easier because the baby has more room if there are no feces in the lower bowel.

## STRICT HYGIENE IS VITAL

*A small bottle of rubbing alcohol* is used to soak any instruments that the attendants need sterilized. The alcohol can also be used afterward on the stump of the umbilical cord.

*A saucepan or Dutch oven* is needed to boil instruments although you can check first with your birth attendant(s) who may bring presterilized equipment with them.

*A bottle of antiseptic solution,* either pHisoDerm, pHisoHex, Betadine, or Zephiran Chloride (which must be carefully diluted according to directions on it), is needed for washing up. A broad-spectrum antiseptic surgical soap can be used instead. Washing up should be done by the mother and birth attendant(s) at the beginning of labor and *again* during the pushing stage of labor when many hours will undoubtedly have passed.

BIRTH ATTENDANTS SHOULD SCRUB THEIR HANDS and arms up to the elbow with either an antiseptic solution or surgical soap and plenty of water. *Use repeated sudsings and rinsings for at least four minutes.* Make sure that fingernails are short.

THE MOTHER SHOULD WASH HER HANDS past her wrists in the same way, especially if she thinks she might want to reach down and touch the baby before he is fully born. In addition, at the beginning of labor you should wash your pubic region, including your pubic hair and the inside of your thighs, with the same careful sudsing and rinsing.

*Before the birth* do it again. Your thighs should be washed 12 inches down on either side. This time when you wash your pubic area you should finish with the antiseptic soap or solution on a fresh sterile cloth or gauze pad, making one clean motion from the top of your vagina downward. Repeat with a second *fresh* sterile cloth in the same way.

THE HYGIENE OF ATTENDANTS CANNOT BE STRESSED ENOUGH. Everyone at the birth should wear freshly laundered clothes. Anything coming into contact with your vagina needs to be kept scrupulously clean. No one with any infected sore on their hands or a sore throat should attend you.

ANTISEPTIC SOLUTION IS ALSO A GOOD LUBRICANT for perineal massage as it is antibacterial.

ANTISEPTIC SOLUTION IS NECESSARY IF THE ATTENDANT IS GOING TO DO VAGINAL EXAMS to determine how far dilated you are, but as a precaution against infection, *vaginal exams should not be done at home.* An alternative way to determine full dilation is to try a few pushes when you have the bearing-down urge. If it hurts it means your cervix is not quite fully dilated but will be soon, perhaps when your breathing has a "catch" in it during contractions.

*Two large boxes of sterile 4″ × 4″ gauze pads* have a variety of uses, including as compresses to support, relax, and soothe the perineum while the baby's head is crowning to prevent tearing or lacerations. Instead of sterile pads you can prepare 10 or more washcloths or old towels or flannel cut to washcloth size, washed and stored, especially if they're new, as described under Old Linens, page 429.

*A work area* can be a cleared tabletop or a dresser within easy reach of the bed for the attendant's supplies.

*A place for attendant(s) to lie down* is something to think ahead about, because labor can go on for many hours.

## EQUIPMENT FOR THE BABY

*Infant ear syringe* is sometimes used to suction excess mucus from the newborn's nose and mouth.

SOME HOME-BIRTH ATTENDANTS DO NOT SUCTION, contending that the mucus stimulates the baby to breathe. The argument is not a good one because even after suctioning a lot of mucus remains. *If you do not suction* then *at least* hold the baby's head lower than her feet so that gravity helps the mucus drain out.

THE EAR SYRINGE SHOULD NOT BE BOILED—rubber loses its retractability and sucking power when boiled. Wipe it off with alcohol before use.

*One pair of infant shoelaces* to tie the umbilical cord. They should be boiled for five minutes anytime before labor begins and then soaked in alcohol until needed.

*A large bowl* is needed to catch the placenta. If you line it with a plastic bag it will make cleanup easier.

*Receiving blankets* are needed to cover the baby and maintain her warmth. Even with skin-to-skin contact, a newborn's "thermostat" doesn't work efficiently yet. Towels can be used but flannel blankets are softer. Launder them several times before labor so that they are comfortable to the touch and then seal in plastic bags until they are needed to wrap up the baby.

*Clothes and diapers* for the baby after the birth, and a fresh change of clothes for you.

*Hospital-size sanitary napkins and belt* are difficult to locate but some drugstores carry them. They are slightly more expensive than regular napkins but they are more absorbent. If they are unavailable, the regular size is all right but will have to be changed more often. *Do not use Tampax* (although the way your vagina may feel after birth you probably would not consider it anyway!).

*It is mandatory* by law to protect your newborn baby's eyes with antibiotic ointment at birth. The issue of whether it is necessary or not to guard against the blindness which gonorrhea may cause is discussed in Chapter Nine. However, be advised that even late-pregnancy gonorrhea tests are not conclusive. The ointment can be applied after the baby's initial bonding with you and your mate has taken place.

*Scales* are necessary because you need to know the baby's weight for the birth certificate and registration. If there are no baby scales available, someone can step on a bathroom scale alone and then step on holding the baby; the difference in the two weights is the baby's weight.

*Relaxants* at home should never be drugs but it is a good idea to have some liquor around in case you get tense and need some aid relaxing. A mixed drink is best: your metabolism is working so rapidly in labor that there is little chance of your getting drunk or of depressing the baby's system. Ginger ale or cola are excellent mixers because they soothe your stomach and the sugar gives you energy. If you don't like hard liquor, have a glass of wine, a pleasant and effective tranquilizer.

## THE PLACENTA

The placenta is dealt with in various ways at home birth.

*Some people plant it under a tree* so that it symbolically nourishes the earth and so they can watch the tree grow as their child does.

*Some women eat a small portion of the placenta raw.* If there's any bleeding it stops as soon as the placenta comes in contact with the mucous membrane of the mouth.

*Most people dispose of the placenta* in a plastic garbage bag.

## CHOOSING A LAY MIDWIFE

Most people choosing home birth will be attended by a lay midwife because they are the birth attendants most willing and available. The area comprising the southeastern portion of the United States has the highest number of lay midwives

(Alabama, Florida, Georgia, Kentucky, Mississippi, North and South Carolina, and Tennessee), but the number is decreasing all the time. The legality of lay midwives is different in each state, where the legislatures rule on whether attending a birth is the "practice of medicine." The legislative trend has been to make it illegal even for a licensed certified nurse-midwife to attend home birth unless accompanied by a doctor.

The Maternity Center Associates in Bethesda, Maryland, is a unique home-birth service offering certified nurse-midwives with a doctor on call. In normal pregnancies and deliveries the primary care is given by the nurse-midwives; the doctor is notified when the woman goes into labor and is on call by telephone or in person. The definition of "normal" is the same as for any home birth or birthing room. If the pregnancy or labor is abnormal the nurse-midwives and doctor jointly manage the birth in a hospital. A woman choosing this service must agree to a hospital transfer in case of complications. Unfortunately there aren't any other organizations in the United States at present which offer trained medical attendants at home. But you can at least get information about what home-birth services are available in your community by contacting childbirth instructors, the La Leche League, birth-control and feminist health clinics, Jehovah's Witnesses, and the Christian Science Church, which often have connections to home-birth attendants because their religious doctrine shuns doctors and medication.

However, this has not stopped home birth or lay midwives, although many of them are cautious about how they work and with whom. The important thing to realize is that many lay midwives have had no *prior training*. In some areas where there are not enough attendants for home births, there are women who have been at one or two births who are calling themselves midwives. If you have a woman like this at your birth it is the same as having an *unattended* home birth—beware that this is what you are opting for if you don't find out a midwife's qualifications.

Try to meet with several midwives with the following questions in mind. Then ask around locally about each woman's reputation and even write to national home-birth organizations (listed in Appendix II, page 776) to see if she is known outside of your area. Then choose one midwife after careful deliberation with your mate and notify the other(s) you met with that you won't be needing their assistance.

## WHAT IS HER TRAINING AND HOW MANY BABIES HAS SHE "CAUGHT"?

*If a midwife has caught fewer than 50 babies* or is doing fewer than 2 or 3 births a month, she probably qualifies more as a helpful and knowledgeable assistant than as a professional midwife. Her presence can still be valuable but she may not have yet acquired some of the skills and techniques you might need. It is really a question of evaluating the risks and the degree of service you feel you need; 90 to 95 percent of births are normal, so if all goes normally, you might not desire more than a friendly helper. However, often problems do not arise until you are already in labor.

There is no formal training available for lay midwives, so one way to judge expertise is to find out whether a midwife has worked on an apprenticeship basis with a more experienced midwife and has been present at 50 to 100 births. Of course, it is possible to attend many births without gaining practical knowledge of how to cope with problems or prevent difficulties from becoming dangerous.

*Training for dealing with infants in distress* is also very important. There are textbooks in hospitals and the Red Cross offers courses in mouth-to-mouth and cardiopulmonary resuscitation; a midwife can get instruction from these sources. A midwife who knows the basic ways to resuscitate a baby in distress can make the difference between life and death or damage.

*A midwife who subscribes to professional newsletters* and journals in the childbirth and home-birth field and/or attends local or national conferences shows her interest in broadening her knowledge. A midwife becomes more competent by staying in touch with other midwives and childbirth organizations and reading new publications.

## WHAT COMPLICATIONS HAS SHE SEEN AND HANDLED?

It is a great advantage to have a midwife who has handled breech birth or other unusual presentations or complications. At the least she should have the experience and knowledge to recognize the danger signals and know when she is out of her depth. A midwife is fulfilling her role if she is honest about her limitations, can identify problems, and can get you to appropriate care in time.

A midwife should discuss the possibilities of complications and give you detailed information about what is happening in your pregnancy and labor. Beware of a midwife who does not explain to you what she sees or is looking for—or who seems afraid of facing the reality of complications and death. A midwife has to be strong and intelligent enough to share her knowledge and help you to comprehend the possible consequences of your choices. You and your mate have the final decision and responsibility and cannot choose wisely unless you have reliable information. There are no guarantees in birth. A midwife who tells you nothing can go wrong, or that she can handle whatever does occur, is doing you a disservice.

## DOES SHE HAVE MEDICAL BACKUP?

Ideally a midwife should have a working relationship with a physician so that if complications arise she can supply him with a written pregnancy and labor record. If you have to be admitted to a hospital she can also continue supporting you through the birth. This is rarely possible; most doctors are antagonistic to home birth and many lay midwives are antagonistic to doctors. A midwife should be familiar with local hospitals and public health facilities and be able to transport you there in case of an emergency and know the procedures required to admit you for care. You should also inform yourself and take responsibility for these precautions—if a midwife is well prepared it is a measure of her professionalism.

Pediatric backup is also very useful. It is probably preferable for you to find your own pediatrician who will agree to check the baby but it can be helpful if the midwife has access to phone or office consultation if it is needed. If not, she should know how to obtain care for a baby through public health facilities.

## DOES SHE DO PRENATAL CHECKUPS?

Good maternity care is based on thorough prenatal care, careful screening of high-risk mothers, and good nutrition. A midwife should either refer you to prenatal care facilities or be able to follow your pregnancy herself. She should check your urine for sugar and protein, your blood pressure, general health and appearance, and follow the growth of the uterus and the position of the baby and placenta. As with any prenatal care, you should be examined once a month until the 7th month, every 2 weeks until the 9th month, and then weekly until the baby is born. Beware of a midwife who does not invest or help you arrange for this time and effort in your prenatal care. It is also helpful if she is knowledgeable about nutrition and breast-feeding.

At some point in early or mid-pregnancy you should have a lab screening done to determine the following: what your blood type and factor are (A, B or O, and Rh negative or positive); whether there are abnormalities or infection in your urine; whether there is evidence of syphilis in your blood and whether you are anemic (hemoglobin less than 10.0, hematocrit less than 33 percent). If you show problems in any of these areas you should be retested during the last 2 months of your pregnancy so that if any severe problem is found you can get medical care for it. A midwife should require that you get this lab work done and should be able to interpret the lab findings and assist you in dealing with any problems.

## WHAT DOES SHE CARRY IN HER BIRTH BAG?

Her minimum equipment should include a thermometer, blood pressure unit, stethoscope, clamps and small scissors, sterile string or other means of tying off the cord, alcohol, antibacterial agent for cleaning and scrubbing up, and small bulb syringes to clean the mucus out of the baby's mouth and nose if necessary.

*Does she have any drugs to stop bleeding?* Although there is antidrug sentiment among home-birth couples and attendants, it only takes one experience with postpartum bleeding for a midwife to carry synthetic oxytocins which can usually stop bleeding by contracting the uterus, either ergotrate tablets or pitocin with disposable syringes. A midwife may not have access to these drugs because they are available by prescription only. She—or you—may be able to get some from a friendly physician. It is worth the trouble to have this drug on hand just in case.

*Does she use tetracycline or erythromycin ointment in the baby's eyes?* The purpose is to prevent damage or blindness to the baby's eyes from infection picked up from gonorrhea, which can be unsuspected and without symptoms in your vagina. Discuss this with a midwife ahead of time and be sure that you are in agreement about using a preventive substance. In some states, public health facilities are required to supply the ointment; in others it can be obtained by taking the baby within 3 or 4 hours of birth to a hospital emergency room, laboratory, doctor's office, or similar facility. A midwife can also get a supply from a friendly physician or over the counter.

## DO YOU FEEL COMFORTABLE WITH HER?

*Does she charge a fee?* If she does and it seems fair to you, pay it. If you think she charges too much, then you may disagree with her about other things as well. If she doesn't charge a fee but you don't feel right taking her help for free, devise a monetary or barter exchange that seems equitable. The area of payment is one in which you have to feel comfortable with a midwife or it can interfere with a good working relationship.

*Do you feel confident, open, and trusting* with her? Listen to your own instincts about this regardless of how well trained or how highly recommended a midwife is. She might be great for someone else, but you may not feel comfortable with her. Discuss your feelings with your mate and see if perhaps you can overcome them; if not, try to talk to the midwife about what is bothering you. There are some lay midwives, for example, who "manage" a home birth with the same dominance and authoritarianism that is often found in hospital management of birth. That may be reassuring to you at home or, more likely, it may put you off. If you don't determine what is making you uncomfortable, it is bound to cause a problem sooner or later.

*Is she dependable?* Does she make and keep appointments with you, for instance? Is her car in good running condition and does she live at a reasonable distance from you? It is important that you feel a midwife is organized and responsible so that you can depend on her.

## COMPLICATIONS AND WHAT TO DO ABOUT THEM

### EARLY RUPTURE OF MEMBRANES

This happens when the bag of water breaks and you don't go into labor. It can be an indication that the baby is in a bad position for delivery. The safest time for rupture is when the baby is well down in your pelvis, labor is advanced, and your cervix is fully dilated.

*Remain in bed after your membranes rupture.* If labor has not begun within 24 hours call a doctor; the infection rate rises dramatically after this 24-hour period, so the traditional decision is to deliver the baby before that time. However, less conservative doctors will let you wait 48 or even 72 hours at home as long as you stay in bed to avoid infection.

*The most dangerous possibility* with early rupture is that you can have a *prolapsed cord*—the umbilical cord comes down before the infant and can *mean death for the baby*. If your membranes rupture and a loop of umbilical cord washes out with the fluid and is protruding from your vagina, get into a knee-chest position (head down, behind in the air) and rush to the hospital or call the Rescue Squad. *The baby's oxygen supply is being cut off.* If the cord is still protruding in the knee-chest position it should be gently supported (not compressed) with warm wet gauze pads or any damp clean cloth. Stay in this position on the way to the hospital—it reduces pressure on the cord.

## BLEEDING PRIOR TO BIRTH

Any bright red bleeding of a tablespoon or more is a sign to rush to the hospital. It can indicate a placenta previa (the placenta is covering the baby's exit) and can mean death for you and the baby. Bleeding is clearly different from the "bloody show," or blood-tinged mucus plug that comes out before labor begins.

*Under no circumstances should you allow anyone outside the hospital (including a doctor) to do a vaginal or rectal exam on you if you have bleeding in the third trimester.* Bleeding can be an indication that you have a placenta previa and an internal exam can cause a major, life-threatening hemorrhage.

## BLEEDING AFTER BIRTH

This has two possible sources: from the *uterus* (darker blood that comes in gushes and starts a few minutes after the baby is born) or a *vaginal tear* (brighter red blood that starts right after the baby is born and is a continuous trickle). It is normal in birth for there to be blood-stained water (amniotic fluid) and perhaps some blood on the baby from vaginal tears. If there's going to be bleeding it usually occurs with third-stage labor: the birth of the placenta, which pulls off from the uterine wall where it has been anchored. It is normal for there to be a gush of about one cup of blood (sometimes as much as 2 cups) following delivery of the placenta. Then the uterus contracts and the blood vessels close off.

*If there is more than two cups of blood* this is considered excessive bleeding: the other symptoms are paleness, faintness, slowed pulse, and other symptoms of shock. Lie flat with your feet elevated, covered enough to avoid losing body heat but not enough to add extra heat as you are better off cool than too warm. Drink plenty of fluids, preferably mild saltwater—1 quart of water to 1 teaspoon salt—with ½ teaspoon baking soda added. Rush to the hospital. Encourage the baby to nurse on the way there; this will release oxytocin, which helps the uterus contract.

*Do not panic.* Hemorrhage after delivery rarely kills a mother quickly. A massive hemorrhage following delivery is usually very brief and shuts off before a dangerous quantity of blood is lost. Fatal hemorrhages are usually those that are slow, continuous bleeding.

*Control of excessive bleeding:* If the placenta has not been delivered and the uterus is soft, massage it with gentle downward pressure until it gets hard. Do not massage to the point of extreme pain: this can increase instead of decrease bleeding. Within the limits of comfort no damage can be done to a hard womb.

If the placenta has been born and there is excessive bleeding, *compression of the womb* will stop it. An attendant should push down with the edge of one hand, in a fist, beneath your uterus on the abdominal wall just above the bone which marks the lower limit of the abdominal wall. Her other hand should be placed above your womb: she is now holding your womb externally between her hands. After gentle massage has caused it to harden, she can hold your uterus pressed very firmly between two hands for at least 5 minutes. If bleeding starts again when the pressure is released, she should resume holding it firmly.

***Do not stuff gauze or cotton packing*** into the vagina: this should be done only by a doctor.

***Causes of postpartum hemorrhage*** are (1) trying to hurry the placenta by pushing on the uterus and/or pulling on the umbilical cord, (2) a long labor which leaves the uterus too tired to contract properly after birth, (3) a full bladder during second and third stages of labor, or (4) an unhealthy mother.

## PROLONGED LABOR

This is usually defined as (1) more than 20 hours of labor-breathing, (2) transition that lasts longer than a couple of hours without full dilation occurring, or (3) a second stage (pushing) that lasts longer than 2 hours with no sign of progress. Most long labors are not a result of physical obstruction to the baby's birth, but may have an emotional or nutritional cause. Prolonged labor is *not* damaging to the infant *as long as there is evidence of some progress, however slow*. A change in position, walking around, or stroking and other relaxing support from attendants may all speed things along. No progress may be a result of undiagnosed cephalopelvic disproportion (the baby's head is too large to fit through your pelvis), or the baby may be malpositioned. If either of these things is suspected you should transfer to the hospital.

## UNUSUAL AMNIOTIC FLUID

Any deviation from the normally clear fluid indicates that the baby is in distress. If it is foul smelling, yellow, green, or brown, you should get to the hospital. The abnormal color and/or smell comes from meconium in the baby's bowel, which is passed by the baby when the anal sphincter relaxes during stress. Although the baby is fine at birth in many cases of meconium staining, *there is no way of being sure of this at home.* You need to be near sophisticated infant resuscitation equipment in a hospital in case your baby needs help.

## FETAL HEART-RATE DROP

This indicates that the baby is not tolerating labor well. Normally the fetal heart rate (FHR) is 120 to 160 beats per minute. During a contraction it normally slows and then returns to normal after the contraction is completed. An increase or decrease of 20 beats per minute may indicate that the baby is not receiving enough oxygen. A rate of under 110 per minute or over 160 per minute is a cause for alarm. Also, a change in the rhythm (a long first sound and a short second sound instead of the reverse, or an intermittent or irregular FHR) is a sign of distress.

## BREECH PRESENTATION AT HOME

This is not something you should attempt if you know the baby is in this position. Some home-birth advocates believe it is not dangerous but their belief is based on ignorance.

Here is a simple explanation of why you should not purposely deliver a breech baby at home. In a normal vertex (head-down) position, a baby's head is an effective dilator of the cervix. The baby's head is the widest part of his body and is equal in width to the shoulders, which it precedes through the cervix and birth canal, making room for them. A breech baby comes down buttocks first: the buttocks are not as wide as the head and shoulders and therefore are not as effective in dilating the cervix or in molding the birth canal. A common problem is that the baby simply does not descend far enough down in a breech presentation for a vaginal delivery to be completed. The great danger is that in a fairly small baby *the buttocks can go through the cervix before it is fully dilated.* This means that even if the shoulders can also get through, the head cannot and the baby is trapped, with the partially dilated cervix like a collar around his neck.

*Just because you have heard that other people have successfully given birth to breech babies at home does not mean you should try it.* There are women who smoke two packs of cigarettes a day and eat poorly and manage to have large, healthy babies . . . that is no rationalization for you to try the same thing. The odds are against you. However, if you are unaware that your baby is in a breech position or if he flips into it during labor, the first indication will be the appearance of buttocks or feet instead of the head.

**Get into a hands-and-knees position.** This adds the baby's weight to the pull of gravity. *No one should try to support the emerging baby*—allow his body to hang down freely so his own weight is pulling him down. One attendant should stand by to steady you from falling and another attendant should take responsibility for the baby.

**When a breech is born to the point where the navel and cord can be seen** this means the umbilical cord blood supply is shut off and with it the baby's oxygen supply from the mother. *The baby must be delivered to the point where his nose and mouth can get air within the next 8 to 10 minutes or he suffocates.* Usually, the mother's bearing down accomplishes this.

**Never try to help a breech until after the navel appears** and the mother has had two more contractions with strong bearing-down.

**Never pull on the legs or buttocks before the navel is born.** If birth from the navel to the baby's armpit takes more than 2 contractions, then gentle pulling on the legs is all right. The pulling should be in a general downward direction so that the baby's back is kept toward the mother's belly or side. Do not allow the baby to turn toward the mother's back.

**The arms should be brought out before the head.** When the armpit appears, use one finger to push the baby's shoulder blade over toward his spine—this usually helps the arm to drop down. If this doesn't work then slide two fingers up along the baby's arm and sweep the arm down across the baby's chest and out. It is usually easier to do this with the arm nearer to the mother's back because there's more room in that part of the birth canal.

*When two arms are out, insert a finger in the baby's mouth* in order to flex his head so that his chin is bent down on his chest. The head cannot exit if the chin is raised and can get caught.

*When the head is flexed, strong pressure from above* on the mother's abdomen will often deliver the head. *Pulling from below may permanently injure the baby's spinal cord, the nerves of the arms, and his breathing apparatus.*

*If the baby can't be helped to deliver without using undue force,* then help him to breathe by creating and maintaining an air passage to his nose: use two fingers or your whole hand to press back the wall of the vagina from the baby's face. In this position he is able to breathe and can live for an indefinite amount of time until a doctor can complete the delivery.

## HAND-FIRST PRESENTATION (TRANSVERSE LIE)

This makes delivery mechanically impossible unless the baby is very tiny. In this position there is no sign of the baby's head because his body is wedged crosswise in the birth passage with one shoulder and hand pointing downward, his head shoved off to one side of the passage and his body to the other. You must get to the hospital if the baby is in this position.

## CORD AROUND THE BABY'S NECK

This is a common occurrence and happens in as much as 25 percent of births. The cord can usually be felt as soon as the head is delivered and can be slipped over the baby's head. If the cord is too tight to slip over the baby's head an attendant can cut it between two clamps but then the infant must be *delivered quickly.* The umbilical cord is the baby's lifeline—if you cut it, the baby must be ready to breathe with his lungs.

## SHOULDER DYSTOCIA

This happens in less than 1 percent of births and means that the baby's shoulders can't be born without help. In a normal birth there is a gap of 2 or 3 minutes after the birth of the head and the next contraction. With that next contraction the baby's anterior shoulder slips under the pubic bone, the posterior shoulder is born (the one toward the mother's back), and then the rest of the body slips out. If the baby begins to breathe after his head is born, an indefinite amount of time can pass before the shoulders are born—so you can summon medical assistance.

However, if the baby does *not* breathe after his head is born then the attendant should wait for only two contractions before helping the shoulders. Shoulder dystocia is a rare complication and is listed here only for thoroughness. *Do not be hasty.* After the birth of the head the mother must push through two contractions with verbal assistance. If the shoulders still have not been born, then for the next two contractions an attendant must put pressure on the uterus: push on the top (fundus) of the uterus during the next two contractions. Only if that doesn't work should the attendant insert a finger and hook it into the armpit that is toward the mother's back and then pull it gently out in a spiral fashion, rotating the hooked shoulder toward the baby's own face.

## THE BABY DOESN'T BREATHE PROPERLY

There may be fluid or mucus in his airways. You may have had too many drugs during labor (unlikely at home) or because the baby is brain-damaged (this is a major cause of improper breathing, although lack of breathing can also *cause* brain damage).

*If a baby is crying, this is good*—do not get sentimental and think it means the baby is upset. Let the baby cry until he's pink—this is the way the newborn's breathing and circulatory systems start working. If the baby is silent you want to stimulate him to cry to take in oxygen.

*First place the baby on his stomach* over your thigh, lowering his head and chest. Suction out his mouth again as thoroughly as possible with a syringe. Cover him with a warm blanket and massage his back and flick the soles of his feet. Gentleness is very important in trying to stimulate breathing in a newborn. An occasional shallow gasp means the baby is taking shallow breaths, although they may be imperceptible to an observer.

*If the baby still is not breathing,* tie and cut the cord if the blood has drained and it is blanched. Wrap the baby warmly and turn him on his right side. Holding him securely in both hands rock the baby *slowly and gently* by tipping first his head down and then his feet. Shifting the weight of the internal organs is often sufficient to compress and release the lungs, facilitating breathing.

*Artificial respiration (mouth to mouth or rib compression) is not a good idea.* The air capacity of a baby's lungs is only a mouthful of adult air so it is easy to blow out a baby's lungs accidentally. He can also contract pneumonia from contamination. With rib compression you can apply too much force and damage the ribs and internal organs.

*Artificial respiration you can use* is to hold two hands under the baby, one under his shoulders and head and the other under his hips. Keep his head level. Bring your hands together and gently raise them, turning them so that you gently bend the baby's body in the middle like a hinge to the point where the stomach is decidedly compressed. Then straighten your hands so that the baby's body straightens out again. This produces movement of air in and out of the lungs. The approximate rate should be 12 per minute, or once every 5 seconds.

*A pale, limp baby is in danger.* A baby with no facial expression, no limb movements, and no resistance to outside efforts to move his arms and legs has little hope of survival. If gentle efforts do not succeed, he cannot be helped.

*Even if baby is breathing,* check the breathing. Normally a baby will breathe about 60 to 70 times a minute for the first couple of hours after birth and then will slow down to 40 to 60 times per minute. Although a newborn's respirations are frequently irregular and easily altered by internal or external stimuli, the baby's breathing should be fairly regular and it shouldn't seem as if he has to work hard to breathe. If the baby has any of the symptoms on the following chart it may be suffering from respiratory distress syndrome (RDS) *and should be taken to a doctor or hospital immediately to be checked.*

---

**CHART 31. SIGNS OF RESPIRATORY DISTRESS SYNDROME**

- Respiratory rate of more than 70 breaths per minute in the 2nd or 3rd postpartum hour
- Chest retraction—the chest drops down (is sucked in) right under the rib cage or between the ribs while the baby is breathing
- Grunting on exhalation
- Gasping for breath
- Flaring of nostrils while breathing
- Cyanosis—a blue color, especially at the lips and ears (indicating the baby is not getting enough oxygen)

---

## EXAMINE THE UMBILICAL CORD STUMP

Be sure that no blood is oozing and be sure that there are *three blood vessels in the cord;* if there are only two you should have the baby checked by a pediatrician right away. Sometimes an abnormal number of cord vessels is associated with certain kinds of gastrointestinal tract, heart, and kidney abnormalities.

## RETAINED PLACENTA

This means that the placenta does not detach from the uterine wall or doesn't detach fully. Normally the third stage of labor lasts anywhere from 20 minutes to 2 hours long. If there is bleeding and cramping and the placenta is not delivered, you have to go to the hospital right away for manual removal.

When the placenta is born lay it flat and examine it. Any torn piece should fit together with another piece like a jigsaw puzzle. If there is any missing piece it may still be in the uterus. *Go to the hospital* because a retained placenta can lead to hemorrhage.

# 9

# Labor and delivery

The labor that your body goes through to result in the birth of your child is divided into well-defined stages. First there are indications of *prelabor,* then perhaps a stage of *false labor* (when your uterus is contracting but not effectively opening up your cervix), and then there is *early first-stage labor. Late* (or *active) first-stage labor* culminates in *transition,* the hardest part of labor, when your cervix completes the process of dilating (opening to the fullest). *Second-stage labor* is the time when you push your baby down the birth canal; this stage ends with the birth itself. *Third-stage labor* is the expulsion of the placenta, the organ that has nourished your baby in utero for nine months.

## THE SIGNS OF PRELABOR

*Lightening* (also called *engagement*) usually takes place 2 or 3 weeks before the onset of labor if this is your first baby. The baby's presenting part (in most cases her head) settles down into your bony pelvis: it is "engaged" in the pelvis. If engagement takes place more than 4 weeks before your due date it may mean that the baby will be early, although the head may also dislodge.

The degree to which the baby has descended is measured in "stations." Before the baby's presenting part is engaged it is at a negative ( – ) station. A baby may engage in your bony pelvis and then dislodge which some babies do even during labor, so that she is floating again. It might go back to a −1 or −2 station, meaning that the presenting part is that much above the ischial bones of the pelvis. Each station is approximately one centimeter. As the baby moves down through your bony pelvis she is at plus (+) stations.

    1. IN A WOMAN WHO HAS ALREADY HAD A BABY, lightening may not occur until early in labor. The abdominal muscles may not be as firm; thus the uterus tends to bulge *out* rather than being pushed down by those muscles.

    2. YOU WILL KNOW WHEN ENGAGEMENT HAS TAKEN PLACE: Breathing may be easier because the baby has settled lower down. You may feel pressure behind your pubic bone and you may need to urinate more frequently because of the increased pressure on your bladder. After engagement, walking becomes more difficult because of the increased pressure on your hip joints.

*Braxton-Hicks contractions* increase in strength and frequency. These are "practice" contractions which are more common in first pregnancies. The uterus is getting ready for labor, flexing its muscles to prepare for the work of labor. You can use them to practice your childbirth training: test your release of tension, your breathing techniques, and light massage of the hardened uterus, and get used to how a contraction feels at its peak and when it is falling off (although with Braxton-Hicks there is rarely any discomfort).

*Increased vaginal mucus* is another sign of prelabor. Vaginal discharge may increase the day before active labor begins. Then the tiny mucus plug blocking the cervix breaks loose: it is called "pink show" or "bloody show" because it may be blood-tinged from the blood capillaries that attach it to the cervix. Although "show" is usually a sign of early labor it can occur as much as 12 days before active labor begins.

*Weight loss* of 2 to 3 pounds often occurs three to four days before the onset of labor.

*A spurt of energy,* which can be considered a "nesting instinct," affects some women and motivates them to rush around doing chores and the like. *Resist* this urge: you have to conserve this energy and save it for the hard work of labor to come.

*Premenstrual feelings* may precede labor—the same sort of physical and emotional changes that often precede a period. You may also feel crampy with pressure in your rectum or the need to urinate frequently.

## FALSE LABOR

False labor is also know as "prodromal phase" labor—the symptoms of labor without any noticeable changes accomplished in the cervix. Prodromal contractions are different from true labor contractions: the uterine muscles contract differently and they can be quite painful—more so than true labor contractions. It can be discouraging to be hurting yet told that it's a "fake": it can make you worry if it's this bad and is "false labor" that you'll never make it through true labor! Don't despair. Although it can be embarrassing and discouraging to be examined and sent home, you are *better off there*—you can relax, drink, and move around. Especially with a second baby it really shouldn't be called "false labor" anyway: it is prelabor, during which the cervix is softened so that it is ready to thin and dilate.

Some people say that if you have to ask yourself whether you're in real labor then you probably are not—that you will know you are when the time comes. This is not always true: some women go through much of the first stage of labor without really knowing it. As your due date nears, you become understandably anxious and excited—when contractions begin you have every reason to suspect you are in labor. Early labor is, in fact, ill-defined and hard to distinguish between "warmup" contractions and true labor.

*In false labor, contractions won't occur in a regular 15- to 20-minute schedule.* However, this is not always true. For some women nonregularity of contractions is not a reliable measure; their contractions *never* become regular and last a specific amount of time with regular intervals in between.

***Contractions may subside*** if you walk around, whereas true labor usually worsens when you get up. To test if you are having true contractions, change your activity: they will stop or decrease if they are false contractions, whereas the opposite will be true if it's the real thing.

***One big difference in contractions*** is that in true labor they get stronger and longer as the interval between them shortens. In warmup labor, after maintaining a plateau of intensity, the intensity diminishes as time passes. However, contractions feel different to each woman and are different in each pregnancy: they can be like menstrual cramps, gas pains, a mild backache—some women think that early contractions are indigestion.

***Call your doctor, midwife, or childbirth educator*** because often they can tell from your voice during a contraction whether it's the real thing. True labor usually requires your full attention and you will stop your end of a conversation during a contraction.

***A good rule of thumb*** is that if you have to use your breathing techniques to stay comfortable during a contraction, you're probably in labor.

***One and a half ounces of liquor, liqueur, or a glass of wine*** will relax and stop prodromal contractions. It cannot do you any harm and will only help to relax you if you are in true labor, in which case the alcohol will not stop the contractions. A warm bath, if your membranes are still intact and have not yet ruptured, is also excellent. If you have a drink in the bathtub it can really relax you and separate prodromal from real labor! Your energy will be conserved and you can rest at home until labor commences in earnest.

*Get medical reassurance* if you want it. Go to the hospital and have them check you to see if your cervix is opening. If you are told it is not true labor, *do not be embarrassed*—this happens to many people. But *do* go home rather than staying in the hospital, where you may be confined to bed without fluids and may get tense and tired. Unless you live very far from the hospital, go home and rest there.

## WHEN TO CALL THE DOCTOR OR MIDWIFE

*If, during the space of an hour,* the contractions are one minute in duration and occur approximately 15 minutes apart and don't go away when you move around, call. The doctor will probably tell you to come to the hospital (or your midwife will come to your home) when the contractions are 5 minutes apart.

*Don't rush to the hospital.* The average first stage of labor lasts 8½ hours with a first baby. If you are unsure of the doctor's and/or hospital's attitude toward prepared childbirth wait as long as you can before going there. The other problem with going in early is that you won't be allowed any liquids and, for example, you won't be allowed to use a hands-and-knees position to do pelvic rock if you're having backache. Of course, if you live far away from the hospital or have a special fear about not getting there in time, then go as soon as you want to.

*A rule of thumb about when to leave for the hospital* with a first baby is when contractions are between 55 and 65 seconds long and when the first level of breathing is no longer adequate: this means your cervix is probably 4 to 6 centimeters dilated. This is a good time to go in because it's early enough to complete all procedures but doesn't leave you with too much time to kill in the hospital.

You should know how to get to the hospital and how much time is needed for the trip. It is wise to have thought of an alternate route in case of heavy traffic, construction, or other impediments. Choose smooth roads when possible for a more comfortable journey. Be sure you know which hospital entrance to use during the day and whether it is necessary to use a different one at night. Although in most cases your mate will probably drive you to the hospital, *you should know all this information* too, in case he is not available and you have to call a taxi or ask a friend to take you.

*The car trip to the hospital* will be more comfortable (if it's longer than 15 minutes) if you lie down on the backseat. If you want to sit in front, you may be more comfortable with a pillow behind your back; it allows your uterus more room to contract.

*What to bring to the hospital with you* in the bag you've packed ahead of time:

- **2 nightgowns** that open in front if you're breast-feeding and robe and slippers for walking around
- **2 nursing bras**
- **baby clothes:** diapers with pins and plastic pants if you're using cloth, nightgown or stretch suit, receiving blanket, something warmer if it's cold out
- **sanitary pads and belt** if you don't want to pay the hospital charges for each one they issue you
- **washcloths** for your face during labor and to suck on if there are no ice chips. Some hospitals don't supply washcloths
- **radio or cassette player** for music during labor, to relax you, to drown out other noises
- **camera, tape recorder** if you have gotten permission
- **heavy socks** as it can be cold in the delivery room
- **watch or clock**
- **books, baby announcements,** for your hospital stay

## FIRST STAGE OF LABOR

In the first stage of labor your cervix is effaced and dilated by the uterine contractions: "effacement" is the softening and thinning of the cervix, which is the lower, necklike part of the uterus. Effacement is measured in percentages; for example, your doctor or midwife may tell you that you are 30 percent effaced before you ever go into labor. By the time that you are about three centimeters dilated your cervix is usually 100 percent effaced. "Dilation" is the opening up of the cervix so that the baby can pass through it into the birth canal. Dilation is measured in centimeters and the cervix is completely open at 10 centimeters; some attendants speak in terms of how many "fingers" dilated you are—in this case, 1 finger equals roughly 1 centimeter. When your cervix is fully dilated, the first stage of labor is complete. The diagram on page 457 shows the stages of dilation. The circles are the actual sizes that your cervix opens up to.

## THE SIGNS OF FIRST STAGE

The signs of first-stage labor are sometimes the same as the signs of false labor. The important difference is in the contractions and whether they increase or decrease if you change your activity and walk around.

**YOUR MEMBRANES MAY RUPTURE.** Have a plastic sheet or a double mattress pad on your bed during the final weeks of pregnancy. You might want to wear a sanitary pad if you are out of your house a lot and are nervous about the possibility of your membranes rupturing. Most often the membranes of the amniotic sac do not rupture until late in first-stage labor when the cervix is opened up. It does not hurt when the membranes rupture: you will have a sensation of a warm flow of water. There may be a lot or a little fluid depending on the location and size of the break; usually once it ruptures there is continuous leaking with gushes during contractions until the baby's head is far down enough to act as a stopper. When you are standing up the baby usually pushes against the cervix like a cork and when you lie down fluid may escape. You can lose as much as 1 quart of liquid, although amniotic fluid continues to be manufactured at a rate of about ¾ of a cup per hour.

**CHART 32. DILATION OF THE CERVIX IN CENTIMETERS**

This is a life-size diagram of how much your cervix opens.

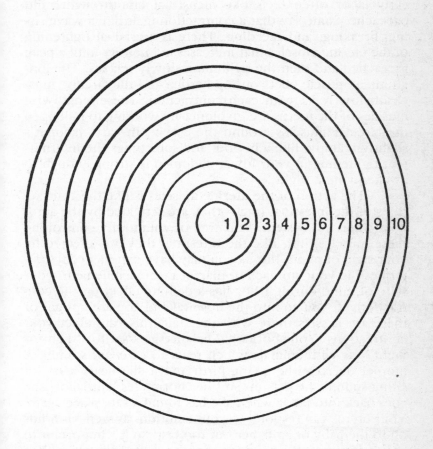

**PINK SHOW** (also called bloody show) may appear. This is the blood-tinged mucus plug that was blocking the cervix and that breaks loose before labor or at the onset of labor.

AN ACHY FEELING IN THE PELVIC FLOOR, similar to the feeling of sore muscles from exercising, is a sign that dilation is beginning.

CONTRACTIONS feel different to every woman, but early labor often feels like menstrual cramps with mild backache. Some say that a contraction feels like a wave rising, breaking, and receding. There is a gradual tightening of the uterine muscles that increases in intensity until a peak is reached and then the tightening slowly relaxes. The longitudinal muscle fibers on top harden and the circular muscles below relax with each contraction. These lengthwise muscles of the uterus are involuntarily working to pull open the circular muscles around the cervix. In early labor it's slightly crampy, like a period, and sometimes the intermittent tightening in your lower abdomen is strong enough to awaken you at night.

The action of the uterine muscles is like the contractions of the intestinal tract—they are activated by the autonomic nervous system. You are not voluntarily controlling these muscles, but, like the intestine, they are affected by your state of mind. Just as you may have experienced "butterflies" in your stomach or diarrhea from excitement, your state of mind during labor has a definite effect on the contractions. If you go into the hospital and you are uptight or there are hassles there with the staff, this can affect your contractions. Your hormonal balance gets set for "fight or flight," as with animals which react to *external* stimuli. A mother deer can be giving birth and if she hears a frightening sound, she gets up and her hormones halt labor; she goes back into labor when she has found a safe place again. Your uterus can respond to your emotions as well—it holds on to the baby or spits her out too fast. So it's important to create and protect a good atmosphere around yourself when you're in labor.

A common misconception about labor is that contractions start out weak and get stronger and stronger, ending in birth. But there is an ebb and flow to contractions, like waves on a beach. There will be a strong contraction and then a weak one, each contraction doing the work that is necessary at that time. Each contraction consolidates the work accomplished by the preceding one, slowly stretching and pulling open the cervix.

*The length of contractions* is timed from the *beginning* of one contraction to the *beginning* of the next one. In early labor contractions are 30 to 60 seconds long with 5 to 20 minutes between contractions. This is the stage of labor that lasts an average of 8½ hours for first babies. In the *active phase* of labor, which accomplishes dilation from 4 to 7 centimeters, the contractions are 45 to 75 seconds long and 2 to 4 minutes apart.

*The length of labor* varies but the average total length of labor is 12 to 14 hours for a first baby and an average of 7 hours in subsequent labors. The longest part of labor is the easiest part—in a first pregnancy it takes an average of 9 hours to get to 3 centimeters of dilation. Generally, the longer the labor, the lighter the contractions will be. Fast labors start with long, strong contractions and usually without much preliminary labor. The optimal length of time for labor is 11 to 15 hours: this is long enough for your tissues to stretch, long enough for the fetus not to be traumatized by a too-fast birth, but short enough so that maternal fatigue doesn't cause stress for the baby.

*Late first-stage (or active phase) labor* is when the cervix is opening from 4 to 7 centimeters. After about 5 centimeters dilation your prepared breathing techniques usually become necessary to maintain comfort. For many women this is when they will go to the hospital. Dilation from 4 to 10 centimeters is usually more rapid in women who have had childbirth education. They are able to relax so that their contractions can have maximum effect in dilating the cervix.

*Frequent position change* is important, especially in early labor. Try to walk around as much as possible. Moving around is discouraged in U.S. hospitals, but in other countries it is strongly recommended. Walking takes your mind off contractions and encourages more rapid engagement of the fetal head, meaning that it settles into your pelvis, which helps to dilate the cervix. Walking is restful because it aids circulation, which is better for you and the baby. Walking can also increase the intensity of contractions . . . *that is good*. You want good, strong contractions. Your goal in labor is to get your cervix open and get that baby out—so if the contractions get harder when you walk, think of that as *positive*.

## BACKACHE

Backache during labor is experienced by a majority of women but it is severe only for a minority. It is felt as abdominal tensing with an ache in the back. It occurs more frequently and with more persistence if the baby is in a posterior vertex position during labor (her head is pressing on your spine) or is a breech presentation. There are three techniques for relieving backache:

*Counterpressure* is the most effective: you "counter" the pressure the baby's head is putting on your spine. You can make fists, put them under your back where the pressure is worst, and press down on your fists during a contraction. Tennis balls are recommended by many Lamaze teachers to be used in the same way. You can also stuff a pillow or two behind your lower back and press back into them. Both these techniques should be done in a sitting or semi-sitting position. You can also have your coach apply counterpressure with his hands if you lie on your side.

*Position changes* can help. *The worst position for backache is flat on your back:* the baby's head presses hardest. You can lie on the side toward which the baby is rotating (usually the left) or you can try tailor-sitting, knee-to-chest, forward-leaning, or pelvic rock. Any position that gets the baby off your spine will relieve or reduce the pressure.

*Application of heat,* either during or between contractions, helps some women.

## EXAMINATIONS DURING LABOR

Examinations during labor are done periodically to check for cervical effacement and dilation. The attendant also checks for the position and station of the baby. The "station" is how far down the baby's presenting part is in relation to the ischial spines (the two bony projections of the pelvis). A "minus station" means the baby is that far above the ischial bones—a "plus station" means that the presenting part is below. Each station is approximately one centimeter. At a +4 or +5 station, the baby's presenting part is out in the world. These examinations are done vaginally or rectally by an attendant who puts on a sterile rubber glove and inserts two fingers.

*Ask how you are progressing after each exam* if you are not told. Each time that an attendant begins to examine you, ask what s/he is doing, so you are prepared. Some attendants use the term "fingers" to describe dilation, but it is a less accurate measure; if you are unclear ask for your progress in terms of centimeters.

*If contractions are getting longer and stronger* and you haven't been checked for quite a while *ask for an examination.* It can boost your morale if you find you have dilated substantially.

*Examinations can be quite painful,* so you will need your relaxation and breathing techniques while you are being examined. Some attendants are more gentle than others: if you are being hurt, say so. The back-lying position is the most common for exams, but if it's particularly uncomfortable for you, ask if the exam can be done with you in a side-lying position.

*In each contact with a new staff member* tell them that you have taken childbirth classes: they may not be accustomed to women with a positive attitude toward labor who want to be given information about their progress. *If a new staff member enters and begins to examine you without saying anything* have your mate interrupt the attendant by saying, "Excuse me . . . I'm Simon Harrison and I don't think we've been introduced." This is particularly effective with male interns. The point of this is that it is *your* labor and your labor room: anyone coming into it should introduce himself, explain any procedure he is going to perform, and then tell you the results. Members of a hospital staff are busy and they are often accustomed to just walking in, sticking their hand up a laboring woman, and leaving! If you want to be treated differently, you may have to work for it.

***Questions asked during a contraction*** should be ignored by you. Keep up your concentration and breathing. If your coach is there he can explain that your concentration is essential during contractions but that you will be glad to answer their questions between contractions—otherwise you can explain this when your contraction is over.

***Your coach may be asked to leave*** during examinations for no reason other than it is customary. Despite the fact that staff members who are strangers to you go in and out of your room and see your legs spread open there is a residual "modesty" in some hospitals about a woman's mate being present for examinations. In fact, you may need your coach more than ever because the exams can stimulate stronger contractions. The best way to deal with this is *not* for the coach to assert that he has every right to stay. It is better for the woman to say pleasantly, "I need my coach here during contractions. I know it's not routine, but we have Dr. Ray's permission so I'd really appreciate it if you could let us stay together."

***Forced accouchement*** is also referred to as a "vaginal hysterectomy" or a "vaginal hys" for short. It is what some doctors do during an internal exam in labor to speed things along: they force open your cervix with their fingers. One way to tell if a doctor is trying to do this (he certainly isn't going to tell you himself) is if a vaginal exam is especially painful. Some doctors' internal exams are painful anyway because they are somewhat rough. But if one exam feels more painful than the others he's given you, say, "Get your hand out of there—I can't tolerate it." He may be in the process of ripping open your cervix to hurry things up. The other sign that a doctor may have performed forced accouchement on you is if you go from 6 centimeters to complete dilation in a very short time (especially in a first labor). If the doctor then takes more than 15 minutes for the episiotomy repair and asks the nurse for a lot of sutures it may mean he is repairing your cervix as well as the incision.

## ADVICE TO THE COACH IN LABOR

In most cases a woman's mate will be with her during labor so the coach is referred to as "he" in this section. However, *anyone* can be a coach—friend or relative, male or female—as long as you feel comfortable and they are committed to going through childbirth training with you. Since this section is intended for the coach, the "you" will refer to the coach, not the pregnant woman (as in the rest of the book), who is referred to here as "her."

### EARLY LABOR

During prelabor you should encourage her to sleep or conserve her energy.

*There is often a burst of energy,* a sort of "nesting instinct," before labor really begins and often a woman needs someone to *tell* her to put her feet up. If there is some chore she insists is essential, *do it for her* even if it doesn't seem important to you.

*Suggest that she take a warm bath* to relax or a shower if her membranes are intact—once her membranes have ruptured, there is a chance of infection. Help her getting in and out of the bath as she can slip.

*Unless she is nauseous suggest that she drink.* Natural fruit juice, which has fructose (natural fruit sugar), is good.

Tea with honey or even toast with honey on it has natural energy. Jello-O has gelatin which is protein, although not readily assimilated by the body and sugar which gives energy but is not as healthful as honey, or fructose. You can make some "slush cubes" in an ice-tray—frozen orange-juice concentrate mixed with honey and a little water. Dairy products are a bad idea—they are hard to digest and remain in the digestive system for a long time. You want to give her fluids and quick energy but you don't want to burden her digestive system, because her body's attention is focused on the uterus. Be sure to eat something yourself—coaching is emotionally and physically strenuous.

*When contractions begin* you should time them. Note the interval between contractions and how long they last: they are timed from the beginning of one contraction to the beginning of the next. Also note when the peak of the contraction comes. Also note when/if she has any "bloody show" or her membranes rupture. This information will be useful for the doctor or midwife.

*When you leave for the hospital* bring your childbirth class certificate in case they require proof that you have completed the training. Bring this book with you if you feel more comfortable having the reminders with you. Bring a sandwich or other snack for yourself. Don't choose tunafish or anything with a strong odor because a woman in labor can be hypersensitive to smells.

*When you arrive at the hospital* don't get hung up filling out forms if she is having trouble with contractions and is finding it hard to cope. Just sign the essential documents and *go directly to the labor area.* You can fill out the forms later. The important thing is to get her comfortably settled so that the move to the hospital does not make her anxious or upset her control of labor.

*The father's waiting room* is where some hospitals send a coach while a woman is being "prepped" (hospital gown, shave, enema, I.V.). Although she may say to the nurse that she wants you to stay with her, some hospitals may be strict about excluding you. If you do go to the father's waiting room *do not wait there longer than 20 to 30 minutes.* They may forget to come get you and she may be waiting for you, increasing her anxiety. Identify yourself to a nurse and ask to join your mate—or if you know where her labor room is, just go there.

## REMINDERS TO THE COACH

Coaching her through contractions is your primary task, along with the basic comfort and support of your presence.

*Use positive words*—don't criticize her and don't point out negative things. Don't say: "You aren't relaxing properly." Use supportive phrasing, for instance: "You seem to be having trouble with _____. Would you like to try _____?" Some phrases which are particularly comforting and supportive are: "Good"; "Go with it"; "Easy, easy"; "Let your *shoulders* (for example) loose"; "Breathe, breathe"; "Steady, steady." These last two phrases can be used while you tap or count a rhythm to help her breathing.

*Make sure each breath is complete* with the emphasis on the *exhalation,* not the inhalation. A breath that is completely blown out makes way for the next complete breath and the complete exchange of gases in her lungs.

*Place your hand* on her abdomen so that you can feel when it begins to tighten and you can help her anticipate a contraction. A fetal monitor can tell you when a contraction is beginning if you ask a nurse to show you how to read the tracing coming out of the machine. When her uterus starts to harden and rise up, tell her to take a deep cleansing breath. By helping her anticipate contractions you can insure that she won't be caught off guard by them and will maintain better control.

***Encourage her to maintain each breathing level*** for as long as possible. She should only change from deep chest breathing *when it is no longer working* to keep her comfortable. Each successive breathing technique is more tiring and more demanding and should only be used when it becomes necessary. You want to get maximum effectiveness out of each breathing technique and not "use up" the effectiveness of a higher level of breathing before it is needed.

***Breathe with her when the going gets rough,*** "in stereo." In order to do this you have to establish *eye contact,* sometimes referred to as "catching eyes." As a culture we are not comfortable with prolonged eye contact so this is something you should practice before labor. It can give a transference of power and a feeling of "oneness" between two people whose gazes are locked and are breathing in rhythm. It can have this effect even if a stranger does it with a laboring woman, so it is that much more powerful if it comes from her mate.

If a woman is struggling with a difficult contraction and loses her perspective she may feel as if she is "disintegrating," or losing her center. Say to her—and you may need to make it a "command" if she has become agitated and distracted)—*"Open your eyes and look at me—*I'll breathe with you." Keep your face as close to hers as is comfortable and take deep, calm breaths along with her. If a woman will do this and trust you enough to maintain eye contact, you can get her through almost any kind of contraction just by the power of being there and experiencing it with her.

***Hyperventilation*** can occur if she is not making a complete exchange of gases in her lungs during breathing. The signs of hyperventilation are dizziness, tingling, and numbness of the nose and extremities. Cup your hands over her nose and mouth while she is breathing to correct the problem.

***Shaking*** during labor can be strange and overpowering to a woman. If a woman does not know this, the shakes can be more upsetting than the contractions. Do not let yourself be thrown by this shaking, which can be powerful in some cases. Soothe the woman, remind her that it is normal and that it will pass.

*Touching*—any skin-to-skin contact—can help a woman immeasurably. There is an emphasis on touching and stroking in home birth, and a saying that touching is worth at least 75 mg. of Demerol an hour to ease a woman's discomfort! Don't underestimate how soothing it is for a woman to be fondled during labor—wiping her face, massaging her back or abdomen, holding hands, etc.

*Watch for signs of tension* during *and* between contractions. Her forehead, neck, shoulders or feet will be the first places to show tension. You should constantly be on the lookout for tensing in those areas—you can remind her to relax an area of tension before it builds up and interferes with her relaxation and breathing.

*Remind her to keep her mouth loose between contractions.* There may be a correlation between tension around the mouth area and the pelvic area—keeping her mouth and jaw loose may influence the relaxation of her vagina and allow her cervix to dilate unhampered by tension.

*Remind her to empty her bladder every hour.* A full bladder can cause pain during contractions. Standing up and walking may increase her contractions, so stay near her when she goes to the bathroom. You can coach her, even through a closed bathroom door if necessary. Try to start her to the bathroom at the end of a contraction so she has the maximum amount of time.

*Follow her moods*: Talk if she wants to, play cards or any game you may have brought; or let her read or doze between contractions if she wishes but alert her to upcoming contractions so she isn't taken off guard.

*Medication* is an area in which you can be helpful, although you can't really presume to tell her that she shouldn't have any. If she asks for drugs, ask the nurse what a particular drug is for, how long before it will take effect, and how it may change her behavior. Be sure that she knows this information before she accepts the medication.

- TRY TO GET HER TO WAIT 15 MINUTES or, if possible, half an hour after the time she requests a drug. A great deal of dilation can take place in that time, particularly in the active phase of labor. You may be able to breathe with her through a rough time and help avoid unnecessary medication.
- MEDICATION IS DEFINITELY INDICATED when contractions continue, but effacement, dilation, and descent of the baby do not occur *or* if the doctor needs to use forceps and needs the vagina to be totally relaxed. *There is no reason to refuse medically indicated drugs*.

## TRANSITION

*Transition* is the hardest part of labor for a woman.

- TRY HARD to get her to relax.
- DON'T ASK QUESTIONS that require verbal answers.
- WIPE HER FACE if she seems warm.
- IF SHE TELLS YOU TO GET YOUR HANDS OFF, do so but *stay near the bed*. Her moods will swing and she may need you momentarily.
- IF SHE FEELS SICK or wants to vomit get a basin and encourage her to. She'll feel better afterward.
- EXPRESS AFFECTION AND PRAISE—continue coaching her through contractions with simple, firm commands. She may be confused and may also be irritated by talking. *Remind her to take it one contraction at a time.*
- IF HER LEGS ARE TREMBLING, put socks on her, cover her with blankets, and hold her legs firmly, stroking them.
- IF SHE GRUNTS OR MAKES PUSHING MOVEMENTS during a contraction, notify the nurse or doctor immediately. These are signs that the "bearing-down reflex" is starting and her cervix may be fully dilated. However, before she can

push she must be internally examined to be sure that none of her cervix is in the way. Use "don't push" techniques until an attendant has examined her and says it is okay to push.

- **A WOMAN MAY TURN TO A SUPPORTIVE FEMALE INSTEAD OF YOU.** Don't be offended or take it as a personal rejection or sign that you have "failed" her. A professional female who has years of experience may give her more confidence at some point during labor. Whatever gives her the most strength in labor is in your mutual best interest.

## THE DELIVERY

The delivery itself is imminent when the baby's head has crowned (is visible at the lips of her vagina). Your role changes going into delivery. The teamwork is now between the woman and her doctor or midwife. You are more of an observer, although you can still be involved.

- **CHANGE QUICKLY** when you know that delivery is near or, better yet, try to change before this time. Some hospitals give you a sterile gown to put on over your street clothes; others require you to remove them and put on hospital pants and top. It is important that you do this before the transfer to the delivery room takes place—it is very hard for her to make that move and keep her attention on contractions if you aren't with her.
- **REMIND HER TO RELAX HER PELVIC FLOOR DURING PUSHING.** She should take two or three deep breaths and push her hardest at the peak of the contraction—it is less tiring and makes fullest use of the force of the uterus. The pushes should be long, strong, and steady.
- **REMIND HER TO LOOK IN THE MIRROR AT THE BABY EMERGING**—in all the hard work and excitement she may forget. Don't forget to look yourself!
- **IF ASKED TO LEAVE THE DELIVERY ROOM, DO SO WITHOUT QUESTION.** In a medical emergency they have to move fast and you will be in the way. Go outside the delivery room but *stay nearby.* The problem may be handled quickly and you can go back in.

# LABOR POSITIONS

In most U.S. hospitals the lithotomy position is used, also called the supine, or lying-flat-on-your-back position. However there are a number of drawbacks to the supine position so it is advisable for you to practice and try different positions. The squatting and hands-and-knees positions are rarely allowed in most hospitals, but they may be more comfortable for you as well as beneficial to your labor. You can also try lying on your side. If you are laboring at home or in an alternative birth room in a hospital you should try a beanbag chair placed on the bed—it is very popular because it gives you support but also molds to your shape.

## SUPINE (ON YOUR BACK) POSITION

*The supine (lithotomy) position* has so many drawbacks that you might want to try a sitting, semi-sitting, or sidelying position for at least part of your labor. Some problems with the lithotomy position are:

* THE UTERUS IS COMPRESSING THE AORTA, a main artery supplying blood to the fetus, and the inferior vena cava. This causes a fall in maternal arterial blood pressure which can lead to fetal asphyxia: the baby doesn't get enough oxygen because its blood supply is reduced.
* THE NORMAL INTENSITY OF CONTRACTIONS is decreased.
* IT INHIBITS THE VOLUNTARY EFFORTS TO PUSH the baby out spontaneously because gravity is not working in your favor. This increases the need for forceps to assist delivery.
* IT INHIBITS THE SPONTANEOUS EXPULSION OF THE PLACENTA for the above reason, increasing the need for cord traction (pulling on the cord), manual removal of the placenta, and related procedures that increase the possibility of hemorrhage.
* IT INCREASES THE NEED FOR AN EPISIOTOMY because it increases tension on the pelvic floor and the stretching of the perineal tissue.

## OTHER POSITIONS

*The dorsal position* has many of the same drawbacks as the lithotomy. In this position you lie on your back with the soles of your feet flat on the delivery table. Contraction intensity and effective pushing are not hindered as much as in the lithotomy position and it is more comfortable because it gives you more freedom of movement. Also your feet are not spread as far apart, so there is less tension on the perineal floor. This position permits your spine to curve so you are working with gravity in pushing the baby out.

*The side-lying (left lateral) position* takes the weight of your uterus off the main blood supply to the baby and also reduces tension on the perineum. During the pushing stage of labor either you, your coach, or another attendant has to hold up your right leg during a contraction. If you are in the delivery room your right leg can be placed in the stirrup usually used for the left leg in the supine position—this is less tiring and more comfortable for some women. The problem with the side-lying position is that it is difficult to see the birth in the overhead mirror because your upper (right) leg blocks your view. You can solve this by having someone adjust the angle of the mirror.

*The semi-sitting position* is physiologically very good for birth. The contractions are not hampered, the perineum is not stretched, and the force of gravity aids the descent of the baby. Your upper torso is propped at a 45-degree angle with your knees flexed and your feet flat on the table. Some labor beds and delivery tables can be adjusted to support your back, otherwise you can use pillows.

*The hands-and-knees position* is good because it gets gravity to work for you, especially with babies in a breech or posterior position. It also takes the weight of the uterus off your back just as in the pelvic rock exercise, so it is good if you are having painful back labor. This position can be dangerous for delivery, however: the baby emerges face up, horizontal to the floor, and just as his head is fully born, the afterwaters flood over his body and into its mouth and up his nose. The afterwaters are the amniotic fluid that remain in the uterus. It would be like lying on the edge of the surf and letting a wave break over you. The afterwaters can surge in any delivery position, but if you are sitting or squatting, the baby's face is toward the floor and therefore doesn't get the full force.

*A birthing chair* may be available in some hospitals. It is a chair specially designed for labor and delivery. Some women like the idea of sitting up for delivery, while some doctors dislike the difficulty in doing episiotomy repair. If there is a birthing chair available where you intend to give birth, then by all means give it a try if you'd like to. However, if you find it doesn't suit you, get out of it and find another position in which you can get comfortable. It is important to keep in mind that devices like the birthing chair tend to be something of a fad. Labor is hard, slow work. No bed, no chair, no particular piece of equipment is going to change that substantially. Use whatever facilities are available to you wherever you give birth, but remember that in the end you are the one who makes it happen.

## TRANSITION

This is the time in labor before you are fully dilated: it is the transition from the end of first-stage labor to the beginning of second-stage labor when you will be pushing out your baby. Transition is the hardest part of labor, but it is also the shortest. It occurs when you are 7 to 8 centimeters dilated and may last only 10 to 30 contractions. The *average* length of transition with a first baby is 1½ hours but it usually lasts only 30 to 60 minutes and maybe less.

*The signs of transition* are important to look for because you will need extra encouragement during this stage, and in addition it signals that soon you will be ready to push. There are many signs of transition and a woman may have only a few or many of them: discouragement ("I can't go on"); shaking, shivering (which you should not resist or be frightened of); irritability ("Don't touch me"); nausea (to the point of vomiting, which you should not resist because you'll feel better afterward); restlessness, excitement, disorientation, anxiety for your safety and the baby's; dizziness, prickly skin (especially on the fingers) or sleepiness between contractions. Oxygen is being concentrated in the uterus rather than the brain, which means there is an increased need for breathing coaching during contractions and to alert that a contraction is coming.

*Transition is the emotional booby trap of labor,* the time when many women lose faith in their own abilities and take drugs. They get the feeling that the contractions are just going to get worse and worse until it is unbearable.

- A WOMAN NEEDS ABSOLUTE SUPPORT to get through transition. Do not leave her alone. Encourage her—she is more dependent now on outside feedback.
- EXPLAIN TO HER THAT HER LOSS OF FAITH IS NORMAL and that she is in transition—remind her that transition is short and a temporary discomfort indicating that first-stage labor is almost over. Tell her how well she has done until now and that it's only a little longer.
- IT IS ESSENTIAL TO MAINTAIN CONCENTRATION because when contractions come very close together and may have 3 or 4 peaks they are hard to manage. If she is worrying about the previous contraction she may lose control. If she isn't ready for a contraction she may panic and feel she cannot go on with her prepared techniques. Transition is the ultimate test of how well the woman and her coach work in unison.
- CONTRACTIONS ARE ERRATIC IN TRANSITION: they can last anywhere from 50 to 120 seconds, with 3 or 4 peaks, and can be anywhere from 30 seconds to 3 minutes apart.

*Eighty percent of women have continuous backache* during transition, which makes relaxation more difficult. The remedy for this is to lie on your side and have your coach apply counterpressure to your lower back. This is what the tennis balls and paint rollers recommended by

Lamaze instructors are intended for. You can get up in a nearly-sitting position with pillows behind the small of your back: bend your knees up with the next contraction and press the small of your back into the pillows. This releases some of the pressure of the baby off your spine. You can also try a hands-and-knees position during a contraction, arching your back to take pressure off your spine and breathing through the contraction in this position.

The psychological hazard of transition is that you may be afraid to move into another position on the theory that it's bad where you are but it might get worse if you move. You may be much more comfortable sitting upright or in these other positions during transition—so help yourself by ignoring the little voice in your head that says, "Stay where you are."

***The end of transition*** is often marked by a catch in your labor breathing. It may be a hiccuping sound, as if your vocal cords have gotten in the way of your breathing. This means that the bearing-down reflex is beginning to be established and you will have the urge to push soon. From this time on you should be propped up if you aren't already so that gravity helps you move the baby down and out. Your coach must listen to hear if you begin to grunt or to push involuntarily and *alert the staff that you are ready to push*. You may be able to tell him that you have the bearing-down urge or it may come as a surprise to you. When you have the urge to push, transition is over and second-stage labor is about to begin.

## SECOND-STAGE LABOR

The second stage of labor lasts from complete dilation of your cervix until the baby is born. This is the pushing stage of labor and it usually lasts 1 to 3 hours for a first baby and 30 minutes to an hour for women who have already had a child. It is routine procedure in most hospitals for forceps to be used if you have not been able to push the baby out after 2 hours of strong pushing.

## PUSHING

***The urge to push,*** also called the bearing-down reflex, is an instinctive urge caused by the pressure of the baby's presenting part on the perineal floor and the rectum. Many women feel an overwhelming urge to bear down while others are not overcome by the feeling. Notify your coach when you feel this urge *but do not push until you have had an internal exam* to determine that your cervix is fully dilated. Sometimes you can get the urge to push and a vaginal exam will reveal that you "still have a lip"—that there is a little lip (small portion) of the cervix that still has to recede. If you were to push before a complete 10 centimeters dilation you could rip your cervix. If the urge to push is very strong you may have to use a "pant" or "blow" breathing technique to avoid pushing until you're told it is safe.

***Coach should put on greens (sterile covering)*** around this time in labor. Usually the coach is sent to get changed when the baby is ready to be born and you are being moved to the delivery room. His absence at that point can be upsetting to you and may even mean that he will miss the actual birth depending on how long it takes him to get changed and how quickly the baby comes. By changing around this time he avoids a last-minute rush and he can be with you during the sometimes disorienting transfer from labor to delivery room.

***Pushing*** is the most strenuous work of labor but also the most satisfying. Once it's okay to push it can be a great relief, not only because the discomfort of the first-stage labor is over but also because you are no longer passive: finally you can *do* something. Pushing usually does not hurt if the baby is in a good position. The reason that pushing is such hard work and often takes quite a long time is that you have to move the baby down the birth canal. This means pushing the baby around the bend formed by your tailbone in back and your pubic bones in front which is a tight squeeze and explains why a newborn's head is often molded into an elongated shape in order to fit through. The pushing stage takes less time in a woman who has already had babies because her birth canal has been stretched before and is more pliable.

CONTRACTIONS in this part of labor are further apart than in transition, usually 4 to 5 minutes apart although they can be in the 2-to-8 minute range. Each contraction lasts about a minute (60 to 90 seconds) and it is *during* a contraction that you push. The uterus is the strongest muscle in the human body: during a contraction the uterus exerts about 50 pounds of pressure; so even if you didn't push, the uterus could expel the baby itself. This is why you want to take advantage of that great natural force and work *with* it. You should begin your pushing effort with the peak intensity of each contraction, not before.

IT MAY FEEL LIKE AN ENORMOUS BOWEL MOVEMENT but you do not push the same way as you would for a bowel movement. Moving your bowels involves muscles in the buttocks and pushing lower down. Pushing a baby out uses your lungs and diaphragm. When your lungs expand they push on the diaphragm, which in turn pushes the fundus (top) of the uterus.

SMOOTH PUSHING is very important. All your muscular effort should be down and out, toward the birth canal in a smooth and gradual curve. Think to yourself, "Baby down and out," to remind yourself of the bend around which the baby has to move. If your pushing is not smooth and the baby comes out too quickly, you can get a vaginal tear even if you've had an episiotomy to make more room.

RELAXATION OF THE PELVIC FLOOR AND ANAL AREA is very important during pushing. You may be unconsciously tensing your anus to keep fecal matter in—even if you've had an enema. The urge to push can feel as if you have to make an enormous bowel movement. Make a conscious effort to relax this part of your body when pushing or you won't get the maximum benefit of your efforts. If there *is* any fecal matter in your bowel don't worry about it—birth attendants have seen it all before!

**YOU MAY URINATE** during a push. Don't be embarrassed by it; this happens to many women especially if they've forgotten to empty their bladder in the late part of first-stage labor.

**TWO CLEANSING BREATHS** before and after a push are very helpful. You need more oxygen at this point and the cleansing breaths also help you to relax.

**DON'T RELAX TOO QUICKLY** at the end of each contraction. Don't let your coach lower you too quickly from a semi-sitting position after pushing. The baby will retain more of her forward progress if you relax slowly and gently.

**POSITIONS FOR PUSHING** are the same as those listed for first-stage labor. The hospital usually encourages back-lying or semi-sitting but if you have tried other positions at home ahead of time and would prefer kneeling, squatting, hands-and-knees, or side-lying, tell the attendant(s).

**PUSHING CONTRACTIONS ARE GOOD FOR THE BABY.** The contractions squeeze the water and mucus from her breathing passages. They also massage the baby's skin, which has been fairly free of stimulation in the amniotic fluid and will soon be rubbed and held by people. Contractions also increase the baby's circulation.

**AFTER TWO HOURS OF PUSHING** most doctors intervene. It usually takes 45 minutes to 2 hours of good pushing to get the baby's head to crown (to be visible at the lips of your vagina). At the end of 2 hours you may be too exhausted to continue, it is hard on the fetus to stay in the birth canal that long, and the baby may be hung up somewhere and need help getting out. In this case a forceps delivery is indicated.

## THE BIRTH ITSELF

The birth of the baby is imminent when she has crowned. If it is your first baby you will probably have done most of the pushing in the labor room, but if you have already had a baby you will most likely be moved to the delivery room before the baby crowns because a second (or third) baby will exit more quickly.

*Giving birth in the labor room* is an option you should discuss with your doctor and check out hospital policy ahead of time. This choice is mentioned on page 409 under questions to ask of the hospital. One benefit is that you are spared the rushed transfer to the delivery room which can be emotionally disruptive. Also you save money—the birth itself can cost half as much if you stay in the labor room. However, if there is any indication that your baby is having any distress or if you or your doctor feel anxious about giving birth in the labor room, it is preferable to make the move.

*The transfer onto the delivery table* can be awkward but there will be attendants to help you: your labor bed is pushed alongside the delivery table at the same height and you have to shift sideways. This move is clumsy and the delivery table is narrow. This may make you lose your pushing rhythm for a few contractions afterward or may even slow down your contractions. Try to relax. It is best not to make the move during a contraction.

*Face masks* will probably be worn by everyone in the delivery room except you and you will all probably be wearing caps to cover your hair. It may give you a slightly creepy feeling that things are now depersonalized and seem serious with everyone masked. Your mate may look strange because you can see only his eyes, but smile at him: his eyes can smile back!

*Arm straps* are used in some hospitals to keep your arms strapped down so that you don't touch the sterile area into which the baby is being born. This procedure comes from the days when women were so heavily drugged that they could not be counted on to control their own hands. You should discuss arm strapping with your doctor and the hospital *ahead of time,* but if you get into the delivery room and an attendant does try to strap your arms say that you understand the need for a sterile field and that you will keep your hands away. Then be very careful not to touch any of the sterile area, including the drapes over your legs and your perineal area which has been swabbed with antiseptic.

**Stirrups** are used in most delivery rooms but you can ask to have them adjusted lower so that your legs are more comfortable and there is less strain on your perineum, thus decreasing the chance of tears. Once your legs are put into the stirrups, which are actually molded supports for the entire leg, your vaginal area will be washed down with antiseptic solution and sterile drapes will be placed over your legs and abdomen.

**The mirror** above and in front of the delivery table makes it possible for you to watch the baby emerging. Make sure it is adjusted at an angle that gives you the best view. Even if you think you or your mate may not want to watch have the mirror tilted at a convenient angle—you may very well change your mind(s). Be sure to push with your eyes open . . . many women squeeze their eyes shut when they are pushing hard and they miss the sight of the emerging baby.

**If your doctor or nurse-midwife has not arrived** and the baby is ready to be born you may be told to "pant" or "blow" until they arrive. The urge to push, plus the baby's head crowning, can make it hard to pant for even 5 minutes. *Do not let anyone hold your legs together to delay the birth:* this can lead to brain damage. If your baby wants to be born and you cannot comfortably delay it, do not let anyone interfere. A nurse, intern, or resident can catch the baby—they have undoubtedly done this before when doctors were delayed or babies were more eager to be born than was expected.

*The birth itself* begins with the first sign that the baby is coming: your anus and perineum begin to bulge, distended from within by the baby's head. With each contraction more and more of the head shows, receding back into the birth canal between contractions. Don't get discouraged: you push the baby down two steps and she slides back one step but this is the normal pattern.

When the baby gets around the curve in the birth canal formed by your tailbone and pubic bone the baby's head stays in sight. When the whole top of her head is visible it is called crowning and the next contraction or two will bring the baby's head out into the world. The baby is born facing your backbone but as soon as her head is out it turns toward one thigh or the other, depending on the position of her body, which is still inside. This puts the baby's shoulders in a position to be born easily with the next contraction or two.

*A stinging, burning sensation* is normal as the baby stretches the outlet of the birth canal. This is your signal not to bear down with the contraction. When you feel the burning and stretching, stop pushing, lean back, and go completely limp. It is especially important to let go of the muscles of the perineal floor: tensing at this point can cause a perineal tear. This burning sensation is short-lived and is followed by a natural anesthetic effect caused by the baby's head. It is at this point that an episiotomy can be cut without injection for pain. Thus the birth itself is not painful but feels like a sliding sensation. Some women are actually surprised by the baby's first cry because they don't realize that she's actually been born.

*A feeling of being split apart* is something a woman may feel as the baby is stretching the birth canal. It may feel that way but it won't happen! If you get the feeling that you're being split open do not tense up—it will cause you discomfort and hinder the baby's exit.

## THE EPISIOTOMY

An episiotomy is an incision made in the perineum, between your vagina and your anus. If an episiotomy is cut when the baby's head is stretching your perineum there is a natural anesthetic and you won't feel it; if a doctor cuts an episiotomy before the baby gets that far out then he will inject a local anesthetic.

In the United States almost every woman giving birth in a hospital gets an episiotomy. There are some women who are rebelling against the routinization of episiotomies: they say that women are treated like links of sausage on an assembly line, as if no woman is capable of giving birth without a tear. There are four reasons given by the medical community for routine episiotomies. It is asserted that a clean, straight incision is easier to repair and it heals better than a laceration or tear, which can happen if the baby's head doesn't have enough room to get out. It is claimed that there are fewer third-degree lacerations following episiotomy. Second, it is stated that the episiotomy prevents fetal brain injury because it reduces the pressure of the fetal head on the pelvic floor. Third, it is said to shorten the second stage of labor, which in turn helps prevent damage to the pelvic floor. Finally, is is claimed that an episiotomy will keep a woman from becoming "stretched out," which would presumably lessen her sexual pleasure and that of her mate.

Studies that have been done give no clear indication, however, that episiotomy prevents third-degree laceration, which is an incision or tearing of the tissue that extends into the anus. In fact, the data even shows that sometimes episiotomies tear further and can extend into the rectum.

In hospitals in the United States, episiotomies are performed nearly 99 percent of the time, whereas in birthing centers where nurse-midwives have primary responsibility, the rate runs between 15 and 25 percent. In hospitals in other countries, the rate is around 10 percent. Detractors of the "American way" claim that it is the positioning of a woman for delivery (in a supine position, in stirrups, and in a rush) and especially the lack of perineal massage which *creates* the need for routine episiotomies. The technique of massaging the perineum with warm compresses and oil is used by many midwives worldwide to help gently stretch the perineum and decrease the laceration rate. Doctors in the United States are not taught perineal massage in medical school: they are trained to cut episiotomies. Therefore although there may be no scientific support for cutting an episiotomy on every woman in labor, it is done since that is all that American doctors know how to do.

The reasoning is faulty that a woman's sex life will be adversely affected if she doesn't have an episiotomy. Under the influence of pregnancy hormones, your whole vagina softens and stretches. If you do the Kegel exercise during pregnancy and exercise those same perineal muscles after birth they regain their tone quickly. For example, French women have a reputation as wonderful sexual partners . . . yet the French do not have routine episiotomies.

---

#### CHART 33. REASONS FOR AN EPISIOTOMY

- The perineal tissue hasn't had enough time to stretch gradually, even with the help of massage.
- The baby's head is too large for the opening.
- The woman's pushing isn't in perfect control and coordination with the person catching the baby so that she is able to stop pushing when necessary and be smooth and gradual when she does push.
- A speedy delivery is necessary, i.e., there are signs of fetal distress.
- A laceration seems imminent: a tear is more difficult to repair than a cut.

---

The basic point about episiotomies is that they should be done *if and when* necessary. It is not really possible to know *until delivery* just how elastic and yielding an individual's perineal tissue is. For this reason you should not

decide ahead of time that you absolutely refuse an episiotomy: once you state your desire to avoid one you have
to be flexible and trust that your caretakers have your best
interests in mind. However you should know that the perineal muscles have an 8-to-1 stretch ratio which means that
your perineum has been designed to stretch considerably.
Ideally, an episiotomy should be used on the small group
of women who have unusually tight perineums.

It's all very well to suggest that you trust your doctor's judgment about whether you need an episiotomy when
the time comes, but realistically you will probably get one
because American doctors are taught to believe that every
woman does need one. The following true anecdote describes the current medical thinking in the United States on
episiotomies. An obstetrician frantically called a childbirth
educator, very upset because Rachel Miller (his patient and
her student) was firmly refusing an episiotomy. Thinking
that the doctor was calling from the delivery room, the
teacher asked, "Is an episiotomy indicated?" "Absolutely,"
the doctor replied. "Then tell Rachel not to be foolish,"
the teacher answered. The teacher was then astounded because the following week Rachel Miller came to class as
pregnant as ever. The teacher realized that this doctor, like
so many others, did not wait for a baby's head to crown
before deciding whether an episiotomy was indicated.

There are two types of episiotomy incision: a "medial lateral" which goes off to the side at an angle from your
vagina downward and a "lateral" which goes straight down
from your vagina toward your anus. The lateral heals better, whereas a medial lateral can cause permanent muscle
scarring. If the repair on an episiotomy is not good a woman
can suffer spasm upon entrance in sex later on. The healing
period for episiotomies is very uncomfortable: the wound
can cause so much soreness that it is painful to sit down
and the stitches usually cause annoying itching.

## CUTTING THE CORD

***Clamping/cutting the umbilical cord*** is routinely done
at 45 seconds to 1 minute after the baby is born. The cord

is clamped in two places and is cut between the clamps. The cord pulsations cease after about 4 minutes. It is often a nice symbolic ritual for the baby's father to cut the cord: you should discuss this ahead of time with your doctor to see if he will agree to it, assuming all else is normal.

At birth there are two major changes which must take place in order for the baby to survive. First he must start to breathe, filling his lungs with air. Then his circulation must accordingly change from the fetal to the neonatal pattern. At birth, oxygen is reaching the baby via the umbilical cord while his lungs are taking over the breathing. The ductus arteriosus—the small vessel which links the venous and arterial blood flow while the baby is in utero—seals itself off and the lungs take over fully.

There is a controversy going on between the traditional practice of clamping and cutting the cord right away and the practice of late cord clamping which is advocated by Dr. Frederick Leboyer, of the Leboyer technique of delivery. Delayed cord clamping gives a large placental transfusion of blood to the baby. Twenty-five to 30 percent of the placental blood volume is transferred to the infant in the first 10 to 15 seconds after birth. The remaining 70 to 75 percent is transferred partly at 1 minute and almost completely at 3 minutes. Those who favor late cord clamping state that the baby receives an additional 25 percent of his blood supply if the cord is clamped late and that the red cell volume in these infants can increase by as much as 50 percent.

Regardless of claims about late cord clamping, it is vital to point out that this additional blood transfer only takes place *if the infant is held below the uterus,* in which case gravity allows more blood flow. But if the infant is held above the uterus it almost completely prevents this blood transfusion regardless of whether the cord is clamped or not. It must be noted that an essential component of the Leboyer delivery, for example, is to place the newborn immediately on his mother's stomach to be massaged. Obviously this means the baby is higher than the uterus and is not getting the additional blood anyway. Therefore the blood transfer is something of a moot point.

There are effects on late-clamped infants that have been noted in scientific studies. The additional blood volume distends the circulatory systems of normal newborns. The newborn has a great capability to adjust to this circulatory overload but late clamping does cause increased effort and duration in respiratory and circulatory adaptation. There are no ill effects but it does force the baby to compensate for the increased blood volume: a late-clamped baby will have a greater urinary output, for example. He will breathe faster during the first 2 to 6 hours and have some difficulty breathing. Both full-term and premature babies have a higher serum bilirubin count at 72 hours than babies whose cords are cut right away, and the incidence of jaundice is higher in late-clamped prematures. Late-clamped infants are red, more irritable, and cry more. There is a higher percentage of "quiet sleep states" and fewer "quiet awake states" after birth than with an early-clamped baby that has more "quiet awake" periods. This means that a late-clamped baby spends less time awake during the day and therefore may have less time to develop a close relationship with his mother after birth.

## THE NEW BABY

*The newborn at birth* is wiped off immediately to prevent cold stress. The baby is wet with amniotic fluid, perhaps some blood, and with vernix, the white cheesy substance that protected its skin in utero. Wetness increases cold—the same way that adults feel cold coming out of a shower until they dry off.

*Suctioning with a rubber bulb* is usually done when the baby's head is born, even before the body is fully out. The baby's mouth and nose are filled with mucus and amniotic fluid and when they are cleared out the baby can breathe more easily. The baby is then suctioned again when he is wiped off. If you have a Leboyer delivery the baby is covered and wiped off a little while lying on your stomach. After this skin-to-skin contact has been made, his nose and mouth are often suctioned out again.

Some home-birth attendants say that suctioning a baby is a bad practice. They say that mucus in the nose and mouth is desirable because it irritates and forces the baby to cough and spit, reminding him to breathe, which a baby can forget to do at first. The majority of doctors do suction a newborn and say there is still a good deal of mucus and fluid in the baby's breathing passages even after suctioning. Removing some of the fluid helps the baby, who has to cope with learning a new skill: breathing.

*Apgar rating* of the baby is done at 1 minute after birth and again at 5 minutes. This is a 2-point test that rates 5 aspects of the newborn: heart rate, respiratory effort (or "cry"), muscle tone, reflex irritability, and color. Dr. Virginia Apgar developed this test when she was an anesthesiologist to judge how well and how quickly a baby adapts to his new environment and as an indicator of how well he will continue to adapt. The chart on page 487 shows that 0, 1, or 2 points are given for each of five signs, depending on their presence or absence.

The 5-minute score gives a more accurate prediction of a baby's survival and normalcy. A low score at 5 minutes is much more serious than a low score at 1 minute. However, the problem with the Apgar rating is that it is subjective—and therefore unreliable. Each birth attendant might give a different score to the same baby, and often their evaluation is based upon their own egos. Some obstetricians view the Apgar rating as a reflection of their own competence and therefore they would be more apt to give a higher score. Many anesthesiologists or pediatricians have their egos wrapped up in "saving" babies and therefore they might unconsciously be prone to give a lower 1-minute score and a higher 5-minute score, reflecting their skill at resuscitation. A nurse or midwife might give the most accurate rating because she has nothing to gain personally, but it will nevertheless be her personal evaluation and everyone sees things differently. Thus the Apgar rating is only *one* indicator of a baby's well-being. Many birth attendants have a broader checklist by which they evaluate a newborn.

| CHART 34. APGAR RATING | | | |
|---|---|---|---|
| **Sign** | **0** | **1** | **2** |
| *Heart Rate* | Absent | Slow Under 100 | Good Over 100 |
| *Respiratory Effort* | Absent | Slow Irregular | Good, "Crying" |
| *Muscle Tone* | Flaccid | Some Flexion of Extremities | Active Motion |
| *Reflex Irritability* | No Response | Grimace | Cry |
| *Color* | Blue Pale | Body Pink Extremities Blue | Completely Pink |

*Antibiotic ointment* is always applied to the baby's eyes, a treatment required within 2 hours of birth in most states. Tetracycline ointment or erythromycin ointment is used, with delays of up to one hour after birth before applying them and the cautionary reminder not to flush the baby's eyes after any of these agents are used.

The purpose of these agents is to guard against eye infection that can lead to blindness. This infection can be caused by a mother who has gonorrhea, which often shows no symptoms in a woman who has it and often cannot be detected even by repeated tests before birth. It is therefore virtually impossible to be sure that a mother does not have gonorrhea, and thus much safer to medicate all babies as a precaution.

The ointments may not be irritating, although most babies shut their eyes after these agents are applied. Since this interferes with maternal-infant and paternal-infant bonding because it eliminates eye-to-eye contact, it is a good idea to delay applying the medicine until the baby has had a chance to look around and perhaps nurse. Then the baby will be less likely to cry and the drug won't interfere with bonding.

*Vitamin K* is routinely given by injection to newborns. The reason for this is that all babies are deficient in vitamin K because they have inadequate intestinal flora-bacteria. There are parents who object to this shot because they reason that if all babies are deficient in vitamin K then that is *normal* and should not be tampered with. Also, babies that breast-feed do have intestinal flora-bacteria. You should discuss this with your pediatrician before birth if you do not like the idea of the vitamin K shot.

*A band will be put on your baby* with your name and the doctor's name. Banding a baby at birth has replaced the old system of footprinting infants, so that the baby you give birth to is the same baby you take home!

*Stabilization nursery* or the central nursery is where most babies are sent very soon after birth. The issue of separating mothers and babies at birth is discussed on page 395 but it deserves more time here. The stated reason for not leaving a baby with her parents after birth is that she will get cold: her temperature has to stabilize at 98.6°. Hospitals may point out that the highest mortality rate for infants is in the first 24 hours of life—but that has nothing to do with a normal baby, who needs only to warm up.

Studies have shown that normal newborns who are dried, swaddled, and held by their mothers for up to an hour after delivery arrive in the nursery without significant cooling. The difference in temperature between these babies and those who were put in heated cribs was *less than half* a degree Fahrenheit.

There are strong reasons for keeping a mother and baby together after birth. If the hospital's routine procedure does not have a valid, provable reason, then it should be challenged, if you wish. Home-birth advocates who are opposed to babies being taken away and put in heated containers have been saying for years that, "a mother's arms are the best baby warmers." There is now scientific proof to support what they knew instinctively was right.

Discuss with your doctor the possibility of keeping your baby with you after birth if all is normal. If you cannot find any support for keeping the baby with you, there is an alternative you can try. *Just don't give the baby up.*

First you must make sure that everything is normal and the baby is okay. Ask the doctor or nurse, "Is the baby okay? Is there anything wrong?" It is natural for any new parent to ask this. If they say the baby is fine and they hand him to you after drying and swaddling him, don't let them take him away. Tell them that they can come and look at the baby anytime they *want* to—but that your baby belongs in your arms. If anyone tries to pull the baby away, say that you will sue them for assault and battery. You *would* have legal grounds for this, so it is not just an idle threat, but the practical intent is to intimidate anyone who tries to take your baby.

## MATERNAL-INFANT BONDING

Maternal-infant bonding is the process of a mother and newborn getting to know each other and to "bond." Doctors M. H. Klaus and J. H. Kennell of Case Western Reserve University's Department of Pediatrics studied maternal-infant bonding and determined that its importance is far-reaching. They contend that this bonding process with the mother is the wellspring for all of the infant's subsequent attachments and will affect the quality of future bonds to other individuals.

The newborn sees, hears, and moves in rhythm to your voice in the first few minutes and hours of life. He will turn his head to the spoken word; mothers seem instinctively to use a high-pitched voice to a new baby. A newborn alerts and attends best to a high pitch, perhaps because his ears are still filled with amniotic fluid so he may not be able to hear a lower pitch. In turn, the infant's appearance evokes responses from you. Seeing this little person you've been waiting to meet for nine months starts your feelings of loving and wanting to care for him. Eye-to-eye contact, in particular, establishes the baby as a reality, which is a rewarding feedback for you. When you look in your baby's eyes you begin to perceive him as a person. Skin-to-skin contact is yet another way of establishing these channels of communication which are essential to the attachment process.

*The "sensitive period"* is defined by Drs. Klaus and Kennell as the first hour of life: the infant is alert and quiet during this time and after that goes into a deep sleep for 3 to 4 hours. A baby in a "quiet alert" state is at his most responsive and thus this crucial time right after birth is ideal for attachment. The 30 to 45 minutes immediately after birth are the most rewarding for skin-to-skin and eye-to-eye contact.

*It is important to ask* that the application of antibiotic ointment to the baby's eyes be delayed until after this meeting has taken place.

*You may not want to face the baby instantly*—you may want a few minutes to compose yourself after the baby is born. No one should insist that you take the baby right away. Your mate can hold him until you are ready.

*Bonding should be a private session* with a minimum of interruptions. Affectional ties can be easily disturbed and may be permanently altered during the immediate postpartum period. Medical attendants may not be aware of this so you should protect yourself: any questions or procedures that are not essential can wait until after you and the baby have gotten to know each other.

*A heat panel* can be placed over you and the baby so that he doesn't get cold during this sensitive period. The radiant heater usually found over the newborn warming tray can be shifted next to the delivery table just as it can be placed above the bathtub in a Leboyer delivery.

*A Leboyer delivery* might interfere with the bonding process because the baby is taken away from you in order to have a bath. It is probably best to wait and see how you feel after the birth and decide then whether to give the baby the bath. If you and the baby are lying next to each other, touching and watching each other, then it may seem arbitrary to take the baby away and disrupt your communication just because a Leboyer bath seems like a nice idea. On the other hand, if you want the baby to have the bath or your mate wants very much to give the bath, it is equally arbitrary *not* to let that happen just because you know that the baby is in the "sensitive period" and his bonding with you can be so easily disturbed. *Do not get hung up on rigid ideas about what is "right," what you "should" do.* The most important thing is to know the facts and then be spontaneous—do what feels right to you *at the time.* If you try to go "by the book" with Leboyer, bonding, or any other technique, you'll be falling into the same trap as the hospital with its rigid routines.

*Anesthetics* and analgesics may depress the infant, depending on how soon before birth you were given the drug. This is not true of an epidural. A newborn with drugs in his system from labor and/or delivery is going to have depressed responsiveness which will influence the first mother-baby interchanges. If you did have drugs and your baby is somewhat groggy at birth, at least recognize that *this can affect you adversely.* If your baby doesn't respond to you—doesn't look at you or react alertly to your voice— you won't be getting the positive feedback that you would be from an unmedicated baby. Your affectional ties may be delayed to a baby who is groggy from drugs.

*The reciprocal action of baby and mother* is beneficial to both of them. The more contact you have with your newborn—and the sooner you touch, hold, and fondle him—the less bleeding you will have, and the better and stronger you will feel. It has not been scientifically proven but it appears that contact with the baby causes the release of maternal hormones which help your body return to normal. Studies have shown that a newborn's physiologic adaptation is easier when it is soothed, held, and given the opportunity to suck at will. Thus a baby who is allowed to bond with his mother at birth and then stays with her may have a smoother time adjusting to life outside the womb.

*Later development* is affected by maternal-infant bonding. Klaus and Kennell's studies show that mothers who were given extended contact in the postpartum period with their babies were involved later on with their children in a more constructive way. These women asked more questions of their children and used more informative speech with them than the control group of mothers whose babies were taken away at birth, as is routinely done in hospitals. At five years of age these "extended contact" children scored higher on intelligence tests than the control group.

The point here is not that maternal-infant bonding necessarily makes you a better mother or assures you of a smarter child. The outcome of this study implies that early and close contact with your baby makes you a *different* kind of mother—that you may interact with your child in a more stimulating way.

*Paternal-infant bonding* is as important as the mother's attachment to the baby, but in the rush to the delivery room and the procedures after birth, the father may be forgotten. However, eye-to-eye and skin-to-skin contact with the newborn has the same effect on the man and his baby as it does with the mother. But, unlike the mother, the father may not be biologically or culturally primed to be responsive to cues from the infant. A man may require longer exposure to the infant or more infant cues to elicit the same degree of responsiveness as the mother. For this reason, opportunities of extended early contact between a father and his baby is *particularly important.*

The way that a man relates to the mother of his baby during labor (touching, soothing, responding, etc.) is an indication of how he'll relate to the infant. Birth can help a man to learn to express emotions in a society where men are encouraged to repress their feelings. Thus a father should be involved in bonding for his personal growth as well as that of his relationship with the baby.

*The foundation for maternal-infant bonding* is laid during pregnancy. There are certain events that are important to the formation of your attachment to the baby.

*During pregnancy* these steps are (1) confirming the pregnancy, (2) accepting the pregnancy, (3) fetal movement (the baby first asserts his presence), and (4) accepting the fetus as an individual in utero: you begin to think of the baby as a separate person even before he is born. *After birth* the events that affect bonding are (1) the birth itself, (2) seeing the baby, (3) touching the baby, and (4) giving care to the baby. If you skip any of these steps it can alter the bonding process.

Anxiety about your baby's health or survival in the first few days—even when the problems are resolved—may affect your relationship afterward. Sometimes women who are heavily drugged and do not see their babies at birth wake up and believe something is wrong with the baby or he has died and no one is telling them. Even after they see the baby this feeling may linger—and it can affect the delicate bonding process. If your baby has trouble breathing at birth or another problem which is cleared up, your anxiety and negative fantasies may influence your initial interaction with the baby.

## THE THIRD STAGE OF LABOR

The third stage of labor is the expulsion of the placenta, which normally takes a few minutes to an hour or more; 30 minutes is about average. In hospitals, doctors often give pitocin, a synthetic hormone, to increase your contractions in order to expel the placenta more quickly. This can be painful and cause cramping later on. Some doctors even pull on the umbilical cord to hurry the expulsion—this is a common cause of hemorrhage and can cause excessive bleeding in the hours after birth. It can also mean that a woman has to return to the hospital for a D&C (dilation and curettage) for suspected retention of a fragment of the placenta which may have remained in her uterus when the doctor pulled the placenta out.

The average length of third-stage labor at home, where there is no interference in the natural process, is 21 minutes . . . at the hospital the average time for third stage is 4.6 minutes, because doctors so frequently intervene.

What happens in third-stage labor is that at the site where the placenta was attached it detaches and pencil-thick blood vessels are torn across. Women usually do not bleed, however, because the uterus is constructed with muscle fibers running crisscross, with blood vessels in the spaces in between, like lacing the fingers of one hand between the fingers of the other. The blood vessels of the placental site are shut off when the walls of the vessels are squeezed together by the tightly contracted muscle bundles surrounding them on all sides. This is why it is essential that the uterus remain firmly contracted after the third stage of labor. This is usually done by kneading the uterus periodically for an hour after the placenta is expelled.

*A hormone shot as the baby is being born* is given in many hospitals to stimulate the uterus to contract and to decrease the possibility of hemorrhage. Sometimes the uterus contracts so violently that the placenta is retained. In this case the doctor has to remove the placenta by hand, reaching up into the uterus, detaching the placenta and scraping or scooping it out.

*Doctors are often impatient*—they are accustomed to "improving" on nature and getting the placenta expelled in a few minutes even though it is normal for a placenta to take 20 to 30 minutes to be born. If a doctor says that he has to perform a manual removal of the placenta after only 10 minutes without a medical reason (i.e., that you are bleeding), then ask him to wait. Manual removal can cause hemorrhage.

*If the placenta doesn't detach spontaneously,* the doctor and nurse will push on your abdomen. This can be uncomfortable and you may need to use the breathing techniques you used during first-stage labor. There are cases of a *retained placenta* which have nothing to do with the hormone shot which can sometimes create this problem. In a case like this a doctor should explain to you that your placenta is not detaching and that he has to go in and get it. This is different than a doctor who rushes in to perform manual removal because he is impatient.

***The placenta is examined*** to make sure it is complete and none of it was left behind. If any piece of placenta is left in your uterus it can cause hemorrhage later on. Ask to see the placenta when the doctor has examined it so that you and your mate can see the amazing organ that nourished your baby inside for nine months.

***Shaking after birth*** can sometimes be quite strong. It is caused by a combination of the adrenaline that your system has released, from the sudden change in your circulation (the 25 percent of your blood volume which was directed to the placenta is suddenly routed back into your circulatory system) and from the adjustments your body is making and the big stress it has just gone through. Don't be frightened by this shaking; ask for a blanket and try to relax.

***Nursing on the delivery table*** reinforces the baby's instinctive rooting and sucking reflexes; it releases hormones into your system which cause the uterus to contract and it is an important aspect of bonding. If you think you might want to nurse on the delivery table discuss it with your obstetrician ahead of time. It also helps to have written orders from your pediatrician. When you are uprooting deeply ingrained routines and traditions it helps to have the approval of the most powerful voice in a hospital: a doctor.

Some pediatricians object to nursing on the delivery table. They say that the newborn has too much mucus in her nose and mouth to nurse properly, which may also make the mother insecure about her ability to breast-feed. The objection is also made that a baby won't be warm enough—but remember, a swaddled baby in her mother's arms is in the "best baby warmer on the market." Some doctors also feel that the hospital should give a test feeding of glucose and water to a baby before she ingests anything else to make sure that her digestive system works properly. You should discuss all this with your pediatrician ahead of time and make sure you are in agreement.

*The recovery room* is where you are sent for 1 to 3 hours after delivery. The nurse there will check your pulse and blood pressure frequently and knead your uterus to make sure it remains firm. If you have arranged ahead of time to keep your baby with you in recovery if all is normal, this can be a peaceful time together. If you cannot have the baby with you, you should try to arrange ahead of time for your mate to stay with you. Otherwise the recovery room can be lonely and frustrating if you are elated about your baby's birth, feeling fine, but cut off from your baby and mate.

*Hunger* may overtake you after the baby is born. You probably will not have had anything to eat for many hours and—particularly if you're unmedicated—you'll most likely be ravenous. Try to get the hospital to bring you some food, although this is fairly difficult—they only serve food at designated mealtimes. Maybe you'll be able to persuade your mate to go out and bring you back a wonderful "birthday treat."

## THE PSYCHOLOGICAL ASPECTS OF LABOR

The way you *feel* and *think* before you go into labor and while you are in it have a considerable influence on how labor progresses physically. If you understand how your mind may be functioning—or how it may play tricks on you—there is a better chance that you will have a positive experience.

*However you get through, labor is an accomplishment.* This has to be said before anything else. Repeat it out loud before, during, and after the birth.

*Human birth may be more protracted, difficult, painful, and dangerous if the mother is fearful.* The most anxious time precedes labor itself. You fear the unknown and you fear that you will lose control. Sometimes these fears are the reason that a woman chooses to have labor induced—it gives her a feeling that she has control over at least *when* labor will happen. But induced labor is dangerous; even if it weren't, it cannot really reduce fear.

The more meticulously you know and understand every step in advance, the less possibility there is that you will be surprised—and the less subsequent anxiety you will feel. In turn, the less anxiety you have during birth and the immediate bonding period after birth, the better your initial relationship to the baby will be. This alone is reason enough to take childbirth education classes so that you fully understand and anticipate the various changes your body will go through in labor.

Your attitude toward pain is a major factor once you are in labor. Do you have a high or low tolerance for pain? Does the idea of pain make you frightened? Don't get trapped in an ideology that is inappropriate to your experience and your personality. If you have unrealistic expectations of how you're "supposed" to handle labor or if you let your mate or childbirth teacher intimidate you ahead of time about accepting medication, you're setting yourself up to fail. Try to learn as much as you can, practice your childbirth exercises, and keep an open mind—say to yourself and your mate that you're going to "wait and see" how you feel once you're in labor. This way you won't feel locked into any promises or high standards you feel you have to live up to.

Your anxiety level is high during the end of pregnancy and especially high right before and during labor. No matter how calm you feel, how prepared you are, how positively you feel about the birth, your anxiety level is high. You may forget breathing techniques, you may forget how to push; you may forget a lot of the information you learned during classes. This is normal. Ask for help. Do not expect perfection from yourself.

Studies have shown that stress, fear, or anxiety are known to increase levels of substances in the blood called *catecholamines,* which can counteract the work of natural hormones like oxytocin that help labor progress. The possibility exists that interference with oxytocin production from stress reactions may affect not only your labor but the "attachment emotions" and maternal behavior after birth.

Maternal anxiety has been shown to result in increased catecholamine levels in the mother's circulation, which can adversely affect the progress of labor and also can decrease circulation to the placenta, thereby affecting the baby.

Another proven physical consequence of stress and/or anxiety during labor is the uterine muscle tension which can result, thereby converting simple contractions into painful cramps. Research indicates that women with higher levels of anxiety may be more likely to have complications in pregnancy, including dysfunctional uterine contractions—painful contractions which do not accomplish their function, which is to open the cervix.

The reason to point this out is not to alarm you, but to make you and those attending your labor aware of how important it is to conquer your fear and anxiety so that it does not physically manifest itself and impede your child's birth.

*Depend on those around you for support.* Turn to your mate and any attendants you feel comfortable with for advice, encouragement, and just plain friendship during this difficult, exciting time in your life. If a woman feels neglected, persecuted, or ill-used during labor or delivery it can mar her experience. *Never be left alone when you're in labor.* Births at home tend to have shorter labors in part because of the constant support, encouragement, and reassurance from the people who are in attendance.

There is a good reason not to separate a woman from her mate, not to surround her with strangers, not to annoy her with noise and bustle, and not to stress her with unnecessary procedures. The reason is that it interferes with a positive emotional and physical experience of birth.

*A feeling of autonomy* is an important aspect of birth for a woman. Just as you need people to depend on, you also need to feel you have some control over a rather frightening life crisis. Your feeling of strength and self-reliance come in part from feeling that you *have a choice* about what happens to you and your baby during birth. This feeling of autonomy, a feeling that you are able to handle your own life, may be a critical force in your personal development. If you are denied that perception of yourself during labor it can make you fear that you are losing your identity or that you are inadequate.

It is easy to feel overpowered by the authority of the physical building, its equipment and procedures and its efficient, uniformed staff. The criblike bed, the parental figures, and the imposition of routine procedures can make you feel childlike and powerless. The nurses support the hospital and its policies and can often be intimidating without realizing it.

When you're in labor it's common to be hypersensitive to care-givers' reactions to you. If a nurse simply says, "Is this your first baby?" it can make you feel judged and incompetent although it wasn't meant that way. This can be your reaction to the unrealistic standards you have set for yourself—therefore you imagine that everyone else is judging your "performance." If you find yourself saying things during labor like: "I'm sorry," or, "I'm doing terribly, aren't I?" you will know that you are in danger of wrapping yourself into an emotional pretzel. There is no "right" way to cope with labor; no one is keeping score. If you see that you're doing this to yourself, rip up your scorecard and relax.

Some women feel so overwhelmed by the authoritarian atmosphere in a hospital that they are afraid to "disobey." If a nurse gives you an enema, takes you to the toilet and says to stay there until she comes back, you're a fool if you wait any longer than *you* feel is needed to empty your bowel. Nurses get very busy and you could wind up spending a lot longer than necessary in a cramped stuffy bathroom. It's your body and your baby—even if your anxiety level *is* high you still have the power to reason. So do what seems reasonable and right and don't fall into the trap of feeling you're back in grade school and have to do exactly what you're told.

*A feeling of inadequacy* affects many women after birth, although some may not want to talk about it. This feeling occurs more often in hospital birth, perhaps because women feel less "at home" and therefore feel as if they should be on their "best behavior." Childlike perceptions of yourself can occur during birth. The feeling of inadequacy can be strong for women whose labors start at home and have to be transferred to the hospital: they have the problem of feeling they've failed because they wound up in the hospital, which they were determined to avoid. The way to protect yourself against feeling inadequate is not to set up rigid expectations that will mean you have "failed" if you don't meet them. A small example would be if you were laboring in the hospital and you gripped the bedrail during a contraction. That may be what works best for you, but it contradicts what you learned in childbirth education, where you were taught that total relaxation is the "right" way to deal with a contraction. Once you're locked into an inflexible belief system like that, you are a failure if you deviate at all. This can also be true of accepting medication or of making grunts, groans, or screams, which may startle other people but can be relieving for you—there is no relationship between the amount of noise and the amount of discomfort or pain you feel—but you will have "failed" if you start out believing that it is admirable and desirable to "control" yourself. Once again, however you get through labor is an accomplishment.

***Romantic notions about togetherness with your mate*** are sure to trip you up. Don't either of you get your expectations high about staying in loving unison, eyes locked throughout labor. You may withdraw from everyone—the force of the physical changes may consume all your energy. Or when the baby starts to descend, you may tune out everything but getting that baby out—and after that you may care only about holding him.

Beforehand you or your mate may have fantasies about intensely sharing every magical moment, about how this powerful experience will bring you closer than ever. It's fine to fantasize but don't let it become an *expectation*. Do not feel guilty that you ignored your mate or forgot about him during intense moments. Childbirth can be enhanced by being a shared experience but that doesn't mean you have to be totally tuned in to each other every minute—just being there together is sharing it. Don't try to second-guess how it will be. There's enough pressure on you to perform without adding the additional burden on yourself of a spiritual experience of closeness. You may very well have it anyway.

*Labor is not just a physiological preparation for birth,* it is also a readying for the postnatal functioning of the infant as a social being. At birth babies have many communications to make, principally to the mother, secondarily to the father, and then to siblings and others. These interactions begin immediately at birth—the way you touch the baby, put it to your breast and look at it, all influence the way the infant responds. It becomes a chain of reactions because you are in turn influenced by the baby's behavior.

Labor is a dramatically binding event—and in a hospital there is the danger of regarding the labor process and the result of it (a baby) as a sickness or disease. Drugs during labor reduce or suppress the infant's ability to communicate with you. This retards the physical as well as psychological recovery that you and the baby have to make. You will benefit most fully if you are aware of the psychological importance of labor to your relationship with your mate, to the beginnings of perceiving yourselves as parents, and to your relationship to the new baby.

## DRUGS DURING LABOR AND DELIVERY

The American Academy of Pediatrics recommends the least possible medication during childbirth. It is best for your baby if you do not take any drugs during birth; sometimes it is best for you to have drugs. But do not believe or trust anyone who tells you that drugs during labor cannot harm your baby—*all drugs except epidural anesthesia reach your baby* and even an epidural affects your labor, and therefore can affect your baby.

*Learning disabilities are increasing among American children.* At this point there is only circumstantial evidence that this is a result of medication used during labor. Eight-five percent of women in the United States are medicated during childbirth and our country has more infant deaths due to birth injuries and respiratory diseases than other developed countries. Learning disabilities or some form of minimal brain dysfunction affects 1 out of every 8 American children. One out of every 4 U.S. high school graduates is functionally illiterate: can't read beyond the 5th-grade level. One out of every 35 U.S. children will eventually be diagnosed as retarded and in 75 percent of the cases there is no genetic or sociological predisposing factor.

The National Association for Retarded Children predicts an annual increase of 100,000 retarded children as well as a rise in children with perceptional and behavioral problems. Obstetric medicine is thought to play a part in the high incidence of neurologic disability. For the temporary relief you may get during labor, you may suffer—via your child's disability—for a long time.

There are many women who come into the hospital in labor and ask for epidural anesthesia right away . . . they have been told it cannot harm their baby. Often the hospital staff offers a laboring woman a small dose of analgesia to "take the edge off the contractions"—more often than not that drug is Demerol. Demerol can drop maternal blood pressure, which reduces the blood supply, and with it, the oxygen, to the infant. It is not known the degree of oxygen deprivation an unborn or newborn baby can tolerate before permanent brain damage sets in—if more women knew this they might be slower to accept drugs. Studies using fetal monitors have shown asphyxiation patterns in the fetuses of medicated mothers. In mothers given oxytocin, synthetic hormones to speed up contractions, 25 percent of fetuses showed these patterns; when the mothers had epidurals 20 percent of fetuses showed these patterns, some moderate, some severe; when oxytocin and anesthesia were used together, which is often the case, a full 50 percent of the fetuses showed asphyxiation patterns.

According to the United Cerebral Palsy Foundation

there are 15,000 new cases of C.P. a year. Our country has the greatest percentage of cerebral palsy in proportion to the population of any other nation: 500 per 100,000 births. *The major cause is a lack of oxygen before and after birth,* which can be caused by the injudicious use of obstetric anesthesia and analgesia.

## ARE DRUGS SAFE DURING LABOR

***Consider the "price tag" of drugs*** before you take any. There can be a domino effect in which one drug necessitates using another—often an epidural "knocks out" contractions and oxytocin has to be used. When your bearing-down reflex is lost through anesthesia, forceps are often necessary to get the baby out. If you are a prepared mother, even a minimal dose of some drugs can cause you to lose control of your techniques and therefore need more drugs to cope with the contractions.

**YOU HAVE A LEGAL RIGHT TO REFUSE ALL MEDICATION.** Some doctors have standing orders for routine medication of their patients in labor. Some nurses may make it sound as if you have to take the drugs—make sure your doctor is aware of your wishes about drugs and ask him to write that information on your chart.

**WAIT BEFORE ACCEPTING DRUGS.** A few encouraging words and some physical contact with your mate can get you past a tough time. Have an attendant examine your cervical dilation—knowledge that you are making progress can be as good as drugs to sustain your strength. *Find out how far dilated you are* before taking any drug in labor: if taken early in labor it may stop the contractions. If you are almost fully dilated you have gotten through the worst of it and only have a little longer to go. If you take drugs without careful thought you may regret it later, so be cautious. Try to wait 15 minutes to half an hour after you think you want drugs before taking them. You may make considerable progress during that time, particularly in late first-stage labor, and may find you can manage without them.

ALERTNESS IS IMPAIRED by any drug. Even a minimal amount of Demerol, for example, offered to "take the edge off contractions" can affect your childbirth techniques. All medications alter your ability to work with contractions. A common problem is that a drug may make you fall asleep between contractions and you may be panicked if you wake up in the middle of one. Perhaps you will temporarily forget how to breathe and will therefore experience more pain. The domino effect here is that you would then request more medication, further impairing your ability to cope with labor.

THE BABY'S BODY TAKES LONGER TO BREAK DOWN DRUGS than yours does. If you take a drug your kidneys and liver rid your body of it in several hours. But the drug reaches the baby, whose organs are too immature to eliminate the drug from his system. This is true even of a healthy, full-term baby—it is harder for a premature baby or one that has any kind of complications. The drugs will affect the baby at birth, often making her groggy and unmotivated to suck; it can take several days for the effects to wear off completely.

*There are times when drugs can be helpful during labor.* Despite all the drawbacks to medication in childbirth you should try to keep an open mind about it. Be aware of the dangers but leave an open mind for the possibility that you may want or need drugs.

The foremost reason for accepting drugs is if you become very tense and cannot relax with the techniques you were taught. If tension mounts it not only increases your perception of pain but it can even slow down labor, which can cause fetal distress. In a case like this drugs to reduce tension may be beneficial.

There is a growing belief among physicians that prolonged pain in the mother has ramifications for the fetus as well. Long periods of pain can lead to chemical problems and hormonal imbalances that can compromise blood flow to the uterus. For example, pain can release two related hormones, epinephrine and norepinephrine, which can reduce the blood flow that reaches the fetus.

***Advances in technology permit*** a more subtle use of drugs during labor. Much more is known about how drugs interact with the fetus. For example, doctors are using one-fourth the dosage that was used 15 years ago of Demerol, the narcotic most commonly used for women in labor. Many physicians feel that the dosages of drugs used today do not cause problems in the normal, healthy fetus and that the dosage can be adjusted for a fetus showing distress.

Even more significant is the ability to deliver the epidural block on a continuous basis, either through a pump or by injection. In the past, the epidural was given in a single shot. With the newer continuous administration, the anesthetist can lighten the dosage and stop giving the drug as the mother is ready to push—and then give it again as the baby emerges.

***Your doctor may want you medicated.*** You may find yourself having to withstand pressure from your doctor who wants to give you drugs. There are some doctors who feel drugs are "more humane" and make it easier on a woman. They assume that all women want medication since so many women have in the past. These doctors want to relieve "unnecessary suffering": their intentions are good . . . but misguided. No man can fully understand the experience a woman goes through in labor—but obstetricians stand by and watch hundreds of women give birth and they *imagine* what it feels like. Based on these projections—and the fact that they've seen many unprepared women crying and screaming in labor from the vicious cycle of fear/tension/pain—doctors want to protect women from that. You can insure your chances of not needing drugs by taking classes—and you can protect yourself from an overprotective doctor by explaining your desire to avoid drugs.

Try not to be too rigid about drugs, however, or you may be irrationally upset afterward if you *do* find you want them or your doctor advises them for medical reasons. There are some women who just cannot tolerate the pain of labor. It is better for those women to have an epidural, for example, than to start a relationship with a baby following a painful and traumatic labor and birth. This can be very bad for maternal-infant bonding because a woman can feel as if the baby has violated her, has assaulted her body, and this will affect her attachment to it. A bad birth experience for you can also terrify a man and be detrimental to *his* bonding with the baby.

## THREE KINDS OF LABOR DRUGS

There are three basic types of drugs used for labor. *Analgesia* is used to relieve pain. These drugs inhibit the reception of pain stimuli and therefore raise your threshold for pain. There are several kinds of analgesics—tranquilizers, barbiturates, narcotics, amnestics and inhalation analgesia—all of which are listed on pages 507 and 508. *Anesthesia* is used in late first-stage labor and during expulsion of the baby to block sensation in an area of the body or to block consciousness. *Oxytocics* are the third type of drug used during labor, synthetic hormones given to stimulate contractions. The various forms of anesthesia are listed on pages 510–513. And oxytocics are explained on pages 508–509.

CHART 35. DIRECTORY OF ANALGESIA DURING LABOR

TRANQUILIZERS (examples: Miltown, Vistaril, Phenergan, Largon, Sparine): Reduce anxiety. Good for long labors if tension mounts. May have little effect on fetus. DRAWBACK: Too much hampers alertness, e.g., loss of control over contractions, e.g., narcotics necessary for pain.

NOTE: Valium should not be given in labor because of the length of time it remains in the newborn's body.

BARBITURATES (examples: Seconal, Nembutal): Sedate and produce sleep. DRAWBACK: Cross placenta in 1 minute if given I.V., 5 minutes if given intramuscularly. Are stored in midbrain of infant; effects last at least one week postpartum.

NARCOTICS (examples: Demerol, Phentinyl, Dolophine): Relieve pain to some degree. Sedate, relieve anxiety. DRAWBACK: Severe depressant on neonatal respiration. Reach fetus in 1 minute I.V., 5 minutes intramuscularly. Phentinyl, which is short-acting, is the narcotic most frequently used in labor. Morphine, sometimes used, has a less long-term effect on baby. Demerol (meperidine) is rarely used any more for labor, although smallest possible dose is effective relaxant. Demerol can drop maternal blood pressure, reducing blood (oxygen) supply to fetus. Some women find it ineffective in relief of powerful contractions. Can interfere with ability to relax or concentrate, giving feeling of being drunk or can cause sleep (e.g., loss of control). Is better I.V. because it goes through your system and wears off in an hour. Intramuscular okay in early labor for first baby or to bring blood pressure down. If Demerol ineffective in lowering pressure, woman diagnosed as preeclamptic.

AMNESTICS (example: scopolamine): Used in combination with pain-relieving drugs. Hallucinogenic. DRAWBACKS OUT-WEIGH ANY ADVANTAGES: Causes violence, odd behavior—"scoped" women become so irrational nurses cannot recognize legitimate requests behind wild, often savage behavior. Woman has no memory of her acts later on but embarrassment at vague recollection of her undignified carryings-on.

---

**CHART 35. DIRECTORY OF ANALGESIA DURING LABOR**
*(continued)*

---

INHALATION ANALGESIA (examples: nitrous oxide, Penthrane, Trilene): Inhaled during peak of contraction. Self-administered—if you get lightheaded you'll drop the mask, regain full consciousness in a few seconds. No clinically significant respiratory depression or other side effects on mother or fetus. Does not interfere with contractions. DRAWBACK: Trilene can cause "twilight sleep" like scopolamine. Necessary to learn to time self-administration so maximum effect coincides with peak of contraction.

---

**OXYTOCICS** are used to induce labor and to speed up a slow labor or one that has been slowed down by other drugs. There is the possible danger of violent labor because the amount of labor hormones secreted naturally by you is not known. If the pitocin does stimulate very strong contractions there are two ill effects. The contractions may be so hard, intense, and unpredictable, both in frequency and length, that you lose control and are not able to handle the labor with the techniques you have been taught—and therefore will require drugs for pain.

The even more dangerous possibility is that these more intense contractions with shorter intervals between them can asphyxiate the baby. This is logical when you recognize that with every contraction the baby's blood supply and therefore his oxygen is cut off—he is strangled, in a manner of speaking, during each contraction. As a contraction tapers off the blood flow returns to the uterus and the baby is nourished again until the next contraction. But with the unnatural pitocin-induced contractions the baby often does not have time to replenish his oxygen supply.

There is also the rare but possible danger that if oxytocin is administered and you are not carefully watched, the contractions can become violent enough to burst your uterus. Most hospitals have a rule that there must be constant surveillance of a woman who "has been pitted" (the medical slang for it)—but the reality often is that there is not enough staff for uninterrupted surveillance.

PITOCIN (posterior pituitary extract) is the most commonly used oxytocic. It is often given intravenously through the I.V. fluid you may already be receiving. The drug is diluted in the glucose and water solution and drips into your vein along with it—the doctor cannot predict to what degree your uterus will respond to the drug and he cannot easily control the dosage when administered this way. The alternate method is to give pitocin in your vein via infusion pump. With this method the doctor can increase or decrease the dosage instantly depending on how your body reacts.

ERGOTRATE is an oxytocic given in pill form post-delivery to contract your uterus. If you are breast-feeding, the hormones which will contract the uterus are naturally excreted—if you are given ergotrate in addition it can create painful "after pains" because uterine contractions are overstimulated.

## CHART 36. DIRECTORY OF ANESTHESIA DURING LABOR

GENERAL ANESTHESIA: Inhaled to produce unconsciousness. Administered only very close to delivery. SELDOM USED IN NORMAL BIRTH—crosses placenta causing neonatal depression. Increases chance of postpartum hemorrhage. Forceps necessary. Side effects: grogginess and amnesia. Most people excrete from their bodies within 24 hours; others are groggy for days. Overweight women are affected more because anesthesia is fat-soluble and readily absorbed by the fat tissue.

ALL OTHER ANESTHESIA IS REGIONAL

CAUDAL: Administered after 6 centimeters dilation in lower back at tail of spine. You are turned on your side while a small catheter—a thin tube—is inserted and taped in place; takes 10 to 20 minutes to insert and give dosage, which can be continuous or one-shot. In *proper dose* has little effect on length and strength of contractions. Does not mix with spinal fluid so no spinal headache. DRAWBACKS: Transfers quickly to fetus. Can produce drop in maternal blood pressure which can effect amount of oxygen fetus receives. Blocks sensation but you can usually move after administration; removes bearing-down urge but trained woman can still push. Forceps often required. Risk of puncturing rectum or head of fetus.

EPIDURAL: Administered after 6 centimeters dilation in epidural space surrounding spinal cord in similar procedure to caudal but higher in back. If administered before 5 centimeters dilation can stop contractions. ADVANTAGE OVER CAUDAL: Less drug required; takes effect more quickly; less risk of infection; does not cross placenta (is protein-bound so it does not enter maternal bloodstream); no risk of puncturing rectum or head of fetus. DISADVANTAGES COMPARED TO CAUDAL: Requires greater skill: only an experienced anesthetist should administer; risk of puncturing membrane surrounding spinal cord greater. Might cause spinal headache—5 percent to 10 percent do get a headache postpartum.

**CHART 36. DIRECTORY OF ANESTHESIA
DURING LABOR** *(continued)*

EPIDURAL *(cont.)*
<u>DISADVANTAGE COMPARED TO SPINAL:</u> Takes 10 to 20 minutes
to take effect; spinal takes only 3 to 4 minutes.

Epidural called "Cadillac of anesthetics" and thought to
be safest drug with minimal side effects. However, it may
not reach fetus directly but *can* affect labor. <u>DRAWBACKS:</u>
Can cause drop in maternal blood pressure reducing amount
of oxygen fetus receives—25 percent of fetuses show dramatic slowdown in heart rate when given in early labor. Has
made forceps delivery almost routine and episiotomy required for forceps; 75 percent of epidural deliveries use forceps; you can feel pressure but no pain yet lose urge to push.
A few women have sore backs postpartum. Epidural causes
chain of intervention—it mandates the following procedures:

* I.V. HYDRATING SOLUTION
* BLOOD PRESSURE GAUGING every 15 to 30 minutes
* FETAL MONITORING especially necessary if epidural is
  administered continuously—to monitor baby's reaction
  and tolerance to it.

SPINAL: Injected into spinal fluid at 8 centimeters or often
after full dilation, i.e., no relief of first-stage labor, the only
part of labor usually associated with pain. Administered in
sitting position or lying on your side with your knees pulled
up to your chin; necessary to lie flat on your back for 4 to
8 hours after delivery to avoid spinal headache. Used when
mother too tired to push any longer: often given with only
a few pushes left. Removes urge to bear down but trained
women can still push. No placental transfer of anesthesia.
Relaxes tense perineal floor for forceps delivery. <u>DRAW-
BACKS:</u> Does not just numb but paralyzes to waist. Slows labor; contractions lose full force as uterus relaxes. Blood
pressure drops, reducing oxygen to fetus. Forceps often necessary. Also can lead to incomplete rotation of fetal head in
delivery increasing the likelihood of forceps.

---

**CHART 36. DIRECTORY OF ANESTHESIA
DURING LABOR** *(continued)*

---

SADDLE BLOCK: Spinals often referred to as saddle block, although a true one is injected into spinal fluid lower than a spinal. Given close to delivery. Less drug required than for spinal. Drug does not cross placenta. Deadens area you would touch on a saddle; somewhat anesthetizes legs also. DRAWBACKS: Can lower maternal blood pressure. Necessary to lie flat on back afterward to avoid spinal headache (20 percent of patients get them anyway). Spinals and spinal blocks less popular than caudals and epidurals.

PARACERVICAL BLOCK: Administered on side of cervix—cannot be given before active labor well under way but must be enough cervix remaining to inject into. Stops pain from uterus and cervix. Good for a cervix not dilating well. Easy to give: doctor rather than anesthetist can administer. Effects last approximately 1 hour: return of sensation can be overwhelming if not anticipated. DRAWBACKS: Anesthesia crosses placenta in 2 to 4 minutes: fetal heart rate can slow. Can be accidentally injected into fetus. Can cause temporary decrease in intensity and frequency of contractions but rarely slows labor.

PUDENDAL BLOCK: Injected into pudendal nerve in vagina or into buttocks, aimed toward pelvic region. Numbs vagina and perineum; good for forceps delivery. Easy for doctor to administer. Urge to push usually lost but you can feel baby moving down birth canal and can push when told. DRAWBACK: Anesthetic transfer to baby in 15 minutes.

**CHART 36. DIRECTORY OF ANESTHESIA
DURING LABOR** *(continued)*

LOCAL INFILTRATION FOR EPISIOTOMY: Xylocaine or procaine injected into perineum. Is "local" only as far as administration—reaches entire system instantly. DRAWBACK: Will affect baby slightly because her head is near point of injection. There is natural anesthetic action produced by baby's presenting part so preferable to wait until after baby is born when local can be given for episiotomy repair rather than for incision.

# 10
# Complications in pregnancy and birth

## TESTS FOR COMPLICATIONS IN PREGNANCY

### ULTRASOUND

Ultrasound (or sonography) can be used to detect many complications of pregnancy. It is a quartz crystal placed on a woman's abdomen; high-frequency sound waves, 2 million cycles per second, are beamed toward the fetus and the ultrasound machine produces a picture of the fetus in utero. Unlike X rays, ultrasound can depict soft tissue in detail and offers none of the hazards of X rays.

This device is used to investigate development of the fetus: its exact placement, the location of the placenta, and the size of its head. Ultrasound is used before amniocentesis is done so that the doctor knows precisely where the baby and placenta are and won't touch them with the needle. It can identify disorders like hydrocephalus (fluid on the brain), uterine tumors, and ectopic pregnancy (pregnancy in the fallopian tube rather than in the uterus). It can detect fetal life or death and measure the growth of the baby.

Ultrasound can be used to measure the biparietal diameter (BPD) of the fetal skull, a measurement that gives a general correlation with gestational age. There is minimal risk to the patient with this test, but the errors of results in predicting lung maturation are too large to be acceptable in managing high-risk pregnancy. A BPD of 9.0 + centimeters indicates gestational maturity, but is unreliable as the *sole* indicator of fetal lung maturity, the most important consideration is whether a fetus is ready for extrauterine existence. The BPD can show a full-term baby when the lung maturity test (L/S ratio, see below) indicates otherwise.

## AMNIOCENTESIS

Amniocentesis is a test in which a painless needle is inserted in your abdomen and extracts some of the amniotic fluid for microscopic examination. This test has potential complications of pain, bleeding, infection, and premature labor, *but* it is the most reliable test for determining postmaturity syndrome—whether a fetus is postterm and should be delivered. Late in pregnancy this test may not be possible or can be hazardous for some women because the quantity of amniotic fluid decreases after 42 weeks.

***Determination of whether there is meconium*** in the amniotic fluid is best done with amniocentesis, although it is also possible to determine it with the use of an endoscope, a device inserted into the vagina and placed against the cervix to view the amniotic fluid.

***Fetal lung maturity*** is the most accurate indicator of gestational age and is determined by the lecithin/sphingomyelin (L/S) ratio in the fluid. Lung maturity is reached when the L/S ratio reaches 2.0 or greater. Research has shown that the fetal lungs must contain enough "surfactant" to allow oxygen to pass in and carbon dioxide to pass out. The transfer of these gases will be inhibited—and the baby may develop RDS—if the lungs don't have enough surfactant. The L/S ratio measures this. There is a "shake," or "foam," test which measures surfactant activity and may be a more precise indicator.

***Determination of estriol levels*** is yet another indicator of whether a baby is postmature. Certain substances excreted by your body are converted by the baby and then the placenta into a hormone called estriol. The amount of estriol in your urine can be measured, giving an indication of the condition of the baby and the placenta. If the estriol level is low or not increasing as it normally does, it indicates the need for delivery.

## FETAL MONITOR TESTING

Three kinds of fetal monitor testing are used antenatally: the nonstress test, the oxytocin challenge test, and breast stimulation.

In all three cases the woman is made comfortable with a monitor belt around her waist. This belt measures the fetal heart rate (FHR) as well as uterine activity, and the results are printed out on a video screen and simultaneously on paper.

In a *nonstress test,* the mother makes a mark on the monitor printout when she feels the baby move. This will normally be accompanied by an acceleration of the baby's heart rate.

In the *oxytocin challenge test,* an I.V. has to be started and the mother is given a synthetic hormone similar to the one her own brain makes to cause uterine contractions. Abnormalities can be detected if there is a deceleration, or slowing, of the FHR following each contraction.

*Breast (or nipple) stimulation* is a combination of the previous two tests. The mother is asked to stimulate her nipples until they become erect and create uterine contractions. She is asked to mark the monitor when she feels the baby's movements. The monitor will detect acceleration of the FHR with movement, which is normal, as well as detecting deceleration of the FHR after a contraction, which is abnormal.

### OXYTOCIN CHALLENGE TEST

Oxytocin challenge test (OCT): In the management of pregnancies at risk, stress testing of the fetus may be performed in an attempt to evaluate fetal well-being and placental function. Some indications for doing the test are hypertension, diabetes, toxemia, falling estriol levels, millitus, suspected postmaturity, and suspected intrauterine growth retardation. Currently the most widely used method is probably the OCT, which simulates the stress of labor by means of induced uterine contractions in order to measure the response of the fetal heart. If there is no significant change in the FHR before, during, and after the contractions, the blood supply to the baby is considered sufficient.

An OCT is done before labor begins, at 31 to 44 weeks gestation. A weak oxytocin (usually pitocin) infusion is used to start contractions and a fetal heart monitor is hooked up to observe the FHR response to this simulated labor. The dosage of pitocin is increased every 10 to 20 minutes until contractions are elicited at 3 per 10-minute period. "Late deceleration" patterns in the fetal heart response are watched for on the monitor. If these patterns are recorded it indicates placental insufficiency and the likelihood that the fetus will not tolerate "real" labor well. A positive stress test is designated at 3 successive late decelerations (decelerations in the FHR) in a 10-minute period.

A positive OCT is an indication for immediate delivery, usually by cesarean. A negative stress test is one that shows no ominous FHR changes in response to contractions; negative OCTs are often repeated to assure accuracy. However, it is possible for there to be a false-positive OCT—in which the fetus subsequently tolerated labor well despite the OCT prediction that it would not. Also, some experts postulate that the increased strength and length and shorter relaxation periods between induced contractions create stress, and that the OCT then records it, often resulting in an unnecessary C-section.

## FETAL NONSTRESS TEST

Fetal nonstress testing has recently been devised. It is an alternative to the OCT, which has several disadvantages. The OCT requires the constant presence of trained hospital staff and may have to be repeated on several occasions, resulting in increased cost and inconvenience. The OCT is also contraindicated in some high-risk pregnancies.

In nonstress and stress testing the terms "positive" and "negative" indicate a reaction or lack of reaction by the fetus, but their significance is different in each case. "Positive" in a nonstress test means a normal *acceleration* of the fetal heart in association with movement or some external stimulus; a lack of acceleration is "negative." In stress testing, "positive" means an abnormal *deceleration* of the fetal heart in response to uterine contractions; the test is "negative" if no deceleration pattern is observed.

## PROBLEMS WITH THE MOTHER

### MISCARRIAGE (SPONTANEOUS ABORTION)

Miscarriage is a fairly common occurrence: some studies show that it occurs in 1 in 10 pregnancies, others show that it happens in 1 in 6. Your own chance of miscarrying depends on certain factors: the chance is 1 in 400 if you are under 25 years of age, conception took place within 3 months of trying, and you have no previous history of abortion; the chance is 40 in 100 if you are over 35 years old, conception took 6 months or more, and/or you've had previous abortions.

#### SYMPTOMS OF MISCARRIAGE

An early miscarriage can feel no worse physically than a heavy period. With a late-first-trimester miscarriage there can be bleeding and cramping on and off for days until the contents of your uterus are completely expelled. If you miscarry in the second trimester it is a mini-labor, with strong, regular uterine contractions that dilate your cervix.

*Go to bed and phone the doctor* if you have cramplike pains in your lower abdomen and bleeding (not necessarily heavy) from your vagina, although not necessarily both symptoms. The pain and bleeding *can* disappear and the pregnancy continue, but if the fetus is definitely aborting, the cramps and bleeding will worsen, with large blood clots in the flow. There is not much the doctor can do but he may ask you to save some of the clots for examination to determine the cause of the abortion.

***Collect the fetus and afterbirth in a clean container.*** This is a difficult task but it will yield information about why you miscarried. It may show a "blighted pregnancy," which is a random natural event. If it shows genetic abnormalities or suggests you have illness or infection, the doctor may be able to help correct the problem. There are also treatments available if you had insufficient hormone levels or an incompetent cervix (see Causes of Miscarriage below).

***The miscarriage is complete*** when a large clot is expelled and the bleeding stops. You'll be physically fine in a few days. If bleeding persists it means placental tissue remains in the uterus and a D&C (dilation and curettage) is necessary: the doctor must dilate your cervix and go into your uterus and scrape out the tissue remaining.

### CAUSES OF MISCARRIAGE

***Blighted ovum*** is the most common reason for first-trimester miscarriage, and most miscarriages take place in the first 3 months of pregnancy—75 to 90 percent of them. The fertilized egg never develops into a normal fetus: 80 percent of miscarriages reveal a deformity or biological malfunction. This is a random mistake of nature and the chance of a repeat is highly unlikely.

***DES daughters***—that is, women who were exposed to DES in utero—will often have malformations of the cervix and uterus that make them at higher risk for premature labor and habitual miscarriage. If your mother took DES while she was pregnant with you, your doctor will want to check you more frequently than is usual during the first half of your pregnancy. Being a DES daughter is an important factor to mention to the person giving you prenatal care. For more information about DES daughters, please see page 30.

*Hormonal deficiency:* If the estrogen or progesterone levels diminish in your uterine lining, then the attachment of the embryo is jeopardized. The hormonal status of a woman threatening to miscarry can be the cause *or* the result of it and the risks to the fetus of drugs, including hormone treatments, must be considered.

*Ordinary tap water* may contribute to miscarriages. According to the results of studies released in California in 1988, women who drank bottled water had fewer pregnancy complications than those who drank tap water, even in neighborhoods where the tap water was not polluted. In the groups studied, the miscarriage rate for women drinking bottled water was about half of that for women who drank at least some tap water. Refer to page 142 for more information. You may want to consider drinking only bottled, distilled water during your childbearing years.

*New research has linked HLA* (human leukocyte antigens) to spontaneous abortions. Doctors have found that if the mother and father have similar types of HLAs the pregnancy has a higher than normal chance of aborting, usually around the 12th week of pregnancy. Both the mother and father should be tested to pinpoint the cause of repeated miscarriages, and the aborted fetus should be tested as well. Medical front-runners advocate obtaining a full-body X ray of the fetus, as well as karyotypes (chromosomal tests) and tests on skin or lung tissues. Studies in which these tests were done have shown that half the aborted fetuses were physically abnormal, and of those, half were also chromosomally abnormal. This helps provide a diagnosis so the family can be advised about the next pregnancy.

*Anatomical problems of the uterus* such as a bicornuate uterus (divided inside with a central wall) or fibroid tumors in your uterus can cause miscarriage.

*Anatomical problems of the cervix* are relatively rare. The cause may be a congenital defect, most commonly in women who were exposed to DES in utero. Or an "incompetent cervix" may have been caused by a previous pregnancy, too many dilations of the cervix for tests, previous miscarriages, or elective abortions. The result is that the cervix does not stay tightly closed and weakens with the increased weight of the fetus. A doctor can do a cervical circlage: he threads a ring of stitches around the cervix to keep it closed until labor, when he takes the stitches out.

*Incompatible blood type:* An Rh-negative sensitized woman or a woman who has an antagonistic blood type with the baby's father may develop antibodies to the hostile blood type. This can cause fetal death and miscarriage.

*T-mycoplasma virus* is a microscopic organism that infects a man or woman without giving any symptoms. This virus may be a factor in habitual miscarriage (more than three), but antibiotics can easily eliminate it.

*A late habitual aborter* is a woman who has had three or more miscarriages. The problem may be due to maternal systemic factors like thyroid or another endocrine imbalance or a major disease like syphilis or renal-hypertensive disease. Some doctors find that dietary instructions plus thyroid treatment help some women; some doctors use hormones, others prescribe psychotherapy plus liberal amounts of vitamins B and C. There seems to be a strong psychic component in repetitive abortion and if a woman is reassured by a doctor's authoritative attitude it may eliminate this psychological element of habitual abortion.

*Second-trimester miscarriage:* an autopsy should be done to determine the cause and indicate any necessary treatment to prevent the problem from recurring.

### THE IMPACT OF MISCARRIAGE

*The sight of blood,* especially a heavy flow of blood with clots, can be unnerving and frightening. There is also the intensity of the cramps—if it is a second-trimester abortion the woman is actually in labor and it can take several hours of strong uterine contractions to dilate the cervix sufficiently to expel the fetus.

*Fear of the unknown* can affect you. Was there something wrong with you or your mate? Did you do something wrong? There is also a common fear that a hysterectomy will be necessary after miscarriage—this is never done unless it is impossible to stop the hemorrhaging any other way, which is highly unlikely.

*Miscarriage is considered an obstetrical admission* if you have to go to the hospital. *This is very hard on you.* You are taken to the labor area to miscarry and the maternity ward to recover. Hospital staff and others don't know your situation and are bound to ask about your baby. Every effort should be made to isolate you from these insults to your feelings—if possible, you should have a room on another floor. Most important, your mate should have unlimited 24-hour visiting privileges—speak to your doctor about arranging this or just do it. Unlimited access to each other and privacy from all but the essential care-givers will facilitate the grieving process.

### MOURNING A MISCARRIAGE

*Mental health experts* used to underestimate the depth of grief that a woman can feel for her lost infant. Friends and relatives of the bereaved may try to downplay the importance of the event, thinking this will lessen the intensity of the parents' grief. Now health professionals recognize that these couples had been left to suffer in silence, perhaps thinking there was something wrong with them for mourning so deeply. Parents who lose a baby before, during, or soon after birth can have equally profound grief.

Health-care providers are realizing that grief is not related to the length of a baby's life, and that unresolved grief over a miscarriage can leave lasting emotional scars. Many women say they are still grieving over miscarriages that happened many years ago, which they have not been able to come to terms with. Both parents can get very attached to their unborn baby; other people never got to know the baby and therefore may not be able to appreciate the depth of your affection and subsequent grief.

*Please refer to the section* on "Death of a Baby" (pages 595–599) for more information and advice about how losing your baby can affect you and how to understand and deal with those emotions. On page 778, Appendix III: Help for Grieving Parents, there is a state-by-state listing of support groups to help you deal with the experience of losing your baby. At least five groups have hundreds of chapters all over the country which offer counseling to parents who have lost infants.

*Naming a baby can be important.* Women who lost fetuses or babies many years ago have found that even giving the lost child a name now can help them put the grief behind them. It can also help to do something tangible, such as plant a tree. Do anything you want that helps you to deal with your sadness.

*Having a funeral or memorial service* is suggested by some self-help groups, which encourage parents to view miscarriage as the loss of a family member. The ritual involved in a small funeral can be an important part of a healthy grieving process, as well as encouraging the compassion and support of loved ones. A funeral for a lost fetus may seem bizarre to others, but it can be important as a way for some people to express their love for that child. There is more about funerals on page 597 in the section on Death of a Baby.

*A man will react differently* than his wife to the loss of a baby. Men in our society are taught not to cry or otherwise show grief, yet a woman who is grief-stricken may mistakenly perceive her husband's lack of tears or signs of grief as an indication that he does not share her sadness. He may throw himself into his work or a sport after losing a child, which can be his way of handling grief. A man's ability to bounce back right away and return to his normal life pattern can be upsetting to his wife if she perceives him as uncaring or unsympathetic. Exerting control over his life can be one way a man copes with feeling powerless and helpless: he may behave in a controlling or authoritarian manner to mask what he's feeling underneath.

*A **woman's reaction to a miscarriage*** can include all the obvious signs of grief, from crying to not eating to difficulties in sleeping. There are also psychosomatic ways in which your body may symbolically grieve for the lost baby. A mother's arms may hurt at some point after the miscarriage, which can be a natural part of grieving—it may be your body's way of wanting to hold and cradle the baby you lost. You might think of it as the searching and yearning phase of your grieving process.

*Hopes and dreams are lost* when you lose a baby. Your fantasies and plans for the baby and her future life are lost with the planned-for child. Many parents become very attached to their unborn babies from early in the pregnancy, even giving the child a name from the beginning. The father may talk to his baby through the mother's abdomen, and the mother may sing or talk to the unborn infant and stroke the child through her belly.

*Anticipate the components of the grief process* so that you recognize the normalcy of your reactions during the period of acute grief. Some of these are: loneliness, depression, guilt, anger, irritability, insomnia, psychosomatic complaints, difficulties with friends and relatives, feeling a sense of unreality or that life has no meaning, inability to get through your normal tasks in a day, preoccupation with thoughts about the infant you lost.

You may have "roller coaster" shifts in your emotions, from high to very low. And even when life seems to have gone back to normal, there may still be some painful reminders—for example anniversaries of the due date or the date of the loss.

***The reactions of friends and relatives*** is important after a miscarriage—it can help you recover or add unnecessarily to your grief. Some psychologists believe that people who are mourning need to have their grief acknowledged by others, yet there is a natural impulse to deny that death occurs or to be uneasy talking about it. You may have to be the one to raise the subject and explain to those close to you that they can help you by listening. You may find comfort and release in talking to a few very close friends about the details of the pregnancy and miscarriage.

Friends may be sympathetic to your pain and want to help, but they may not know how. Some will say the wrong thing and hurt you without meaning to; you may think others don't care about your pain because they say nothing at all—when they're remaining silent because they just don't know what to say.

The easiest and most helpful thing for a friend to tell you is that she is sorry you miscarried. You may be hurt by the thoughtless clichés people utter, which are listed below. However, if you're prepared for these comments, they may have less negative impact and you won't resent the well-meaning friends who leave you feeling even lonelier in your grief.

## *HURTFUL CLICHÉS ABOUT MISCARRIAGE*

- *"It's normal, people miscarry all the time."* This doesn't make you feel any better: miscarriage is hardly a "normal" event for you.
- *"You'll get pregnant again in no time."* Whether you can or will conceive again has no bearing on the traumatic experience you've been through, which this comment invalidates.
- *"There was probably something wrong with it anyway."* It is not comforting to be told that a fetus was probably defective and you've been having a handicapped child. A doctor can tell you that half of all miscarried fetuses have genetic defects—hearing it from friends is no consolation.
- *"It was God's will."* This is a variation on the previous comment, and is equally unsympathetic. It's like telling

you not to be sad over the death of a beloved grandparent "because he was old, anyway."

- *"You have other child(ren), be grateful."* This comment is infuriating because children you may be blessed with have nothing to do with the baby you have lost. Children are not interchangeable—it can be maddening to be told "to go home and love the son you already have" when your heart is breaking for the one you'll never know.

### WHEN TO CONCEIVE AGAIN

You can resume sexual relations again as soon as your cervix has closed, which prevents infection, usually 4 to 6 weeks after a miscarriage. Check with your doctor about attempting another pregnancy, but usually it is considered best to wait for 1 or 2 normal menstrual cycles after a miscarriage.

*Some doctors* say that if a defective germ plasm (blighted ovum) was proven responsible for the miscarriage, attempts for another pregnancy should be made immediately after the first period—which usually comes 4 weeks to the day after the abortion. The reasoning here is that the miscarriage was just a natural random event and implied nothing wrong with you—and that psychologically it may be better to try again right away.

*Some doctors* believe it is best to wait about 3 months before trying to conceive again. You should correct any known medical problems, go on an excellent diet, get plenty of rest and exercise—in general, build yourself up.

*Doctors are more conservative* in cases where there was no known cause for the miscarriage, i.e., the fetus and placenta were normal. They say that a 6-month wait is best, hoping that whatever the cause was will correct itself in that period of time.

### ECTOPIC PREGNANCY

Ectopic pregnancy occurs when the egg is fertilized in the fallopian tube and, rather than passing into the uterus, remains in the tube. This is dangerous because if the pregnancy is allowed to continue, the tube will burst. A pregnancy test and a physical examination can determine whether you have an ectopic pregnancy.

***If you suspect you are pregnant and have any of the following symptoms, call your doctor immediately:***

- Vaginal bleeding
- Pain in the lower abdomen (often on one side)
- Weakness and/or fainting

### TREATMENT

Surgery must be performed. Sometimes the fallopian tube can be rebuilt, other times it has to be removed on the side where the pregnancy occurred. A woman treated for one ectopic pregnancy tends to be infertile. There is a 50 to 60 percent chance of not conceiving again. You *can* have a normal pregnancy the next time but you have an increased risk—a 15 percent chance—of having another ectopic pregnancy. This means that if you are able to become pregnant again the risk of another ectopic is 40 times greater than in a previously healthy woman.

### BURSTING OF THE TUBE

***The tube usually bursts between the 8th and 12th weeks*** of the ectopic pregnancy. If it does, you get the symptoms already mentioned.

***It is difficult to discover an unruptured early tubal pregnancy*** unless you have gotten a pregnancy test that measures HCG (see Pregnancy Tests, page 17.) Even so, an ectopic has a lower level of HCG than a normal pregnancy, so it still might not register.

***Try to be aware*** that the first sharp abdominal pain might mean a rupture. Go quickly to the doctor.

*You are bleeding internally* when the tube bursts. It may be a sudden, acute bleeding or, more frequently, a slow trickling of blood into the abdominal cavity. You might feel an aching pain in your diaphragm or a sharp shoulder pain caused by blood flooding up to your diaphragm.

*If the bleeding is greater,* you might be in shock. The symptoms are: hot and cold flashes, nausea, dizziness, fainting.

*Bleeding can be misleading.* Before or after a ruptured tube you might have a late period with mild menstrual-type bleeding or fragments. You—and the doctor—might misinterpret this as an early natural abortion (miscarriage). If uterine lining is passed with the blood it should be examined microscopically. If there is no evidence of early fetal (trophoblastic) tissue, then an ectopic pregnancy should be suspected.

## DIABETES IN PREGNANCY

There are an estimated 10 million diabetics in the United States, one-half of whom are unaware of their condition. Women are 50 percent more likely to become diabetics than are men. There is a great risk of complications in a diabetic woman's pregnancy: she is more prone to toxemia, infection, and congenital malformations in the baby. Even though all diabetic pregnancies are dealt with as "high risk," there are still many problems that even advanced obstetric science cannot resolve. The best results during pregnancy and delivery occur if you are under the joint care of an expert in diabetes and an obstetrician who specializes in high-risk pregnancy.

The *earlier* the onset of diabetes and the *longer* you've had the disease, the worse the prognosis for pregnancy. The risks are greater for insulin-dependent diabetics. Maintenance of a normal glucose concentration in the blood brings the best fetal and maternal results—but this may be extremely difficult and require frequent hospitalization.

Even under constant care there is no certainty that your baby will be born alive and healthy.

RISKS TO THE BABY

***The characteristics of the offspring of diabetic women*** are: hypoglycemia, low serum calcium levels, elevated bilirubin level, large fetal organs (the heart and adrenals), and relatively small brain and thymus.

***The risk of respiratory distress syndrome*** (RDS) is 5.6 times greater in a diabetic pregnancy. There are maturity studies which can be done; RDS usually affects a baby whose lungs are not yet mature enough, which can be determined by the L/S ratio in the amniotic fluid. Even an L/S ratio of 2.0—which is normally considered a measure of fetal lung maturity—doesn't necessarily guarantee that a diabetic's baby will *not* have RDS. In a normal pregnancy a 2.0 L/S ratio is usually reached at 35 to 36 weeks gestation. In a diabetic pregnancy it is safest—in order to minimize the risk of neonatal RDS—to wait, if possible, for a gestational age of at least 36 weeks and an L/S ratio of 2.5 or higher.

***The fetus of a diabetic woman has a tendency to die.*** The risk of death before labor is greatest in the last 2 or 3 weeks of the pregnancy. The optimal delivery time is 36 to 37 weeks: most doctors terminate a diabetic pregnancy by cesarean or induction 3, 4, and sometimes 6 weeks before the calculated due date. Insulin-dependent diabetics cannot go to term and are nearly always delivered prematurely.

***Toxemia*** is an indication for prompt delivery. Early delivery is required in the occurrence of preeclampsia, repeated ketoacidosis, marked hydramnios, advancing retinopathy, and preexisting renal disease with hypertension or albuminuria.

***Early delivery is indicated*** in all the above cases *regardless* of the results of fetal maturity tests. The hazard of intrauterine death is a greater risk with the above complications than the risk of neonatal death from prematurity.

## TOXEMIA OF PREGNANCY

Toxemia is a complication of pregnancy which usually happens from the 20th to 24th weeks. It used to be blamed on gaining too much weight during pregnancy but that is now known not to be true. *Poor nutrition* is thought to play an important—perhaps the most important—part in causing toxemia, but the full causes are not known. Toxemia is also called preeclampsia, and if it reaches the severe stage is known as eclampsia. In the latter case, a doctor may decide to deliver the baby by cesarean to eliminate the additional stress of labor.

*The signs of preeclampsia* are: swelling, vision disturbance (from cerebral edema, usually a sign of second-stage toxemia), high blood pressure, and protein in the urine. The signs of second-stage are abdominal pains, vision disturbance, severe headaches, and mental dullness. The last three result from cerebral edema, "water on the brain."

*Water pills (diuretics)* are sometimes prescribed to treat toxemia, but they deal only with the symptoms, not the cause. They should not be used to "cover up" the swelling of toxemia, which is one of its danger signals. Along with the fluid they force out of your tissues, diuretics also cause the loss of essential nutrients and can deplete the amniotic fluid.

*Malnutrition*—insufficient protein in particular—has been linked to toxemia in various studies. The best way to prevent toxemia is to eat a well-balanced diet with a focus on high-quality protein.

*The signs of the eclamptic (severe) stage* of toxemia are convulsions and coma, but this stage is rarely reached if you are under medical care.

*A psychosomatic basis* for toxemia is being studied. The effect of the mind on the body is being examined more fully in all aspects of health care and there is an apparent link between high blood pressure and stress and anxiety. Toxemia may fall into this category but more investigation needs to be done.

*Toxemia affects the baby* because the placenta does not function as well, which may cause a small-for-date baby or fetal death. Since labor must be induced early in some cases of toxemia, prematurity is another danger to the baby. There is also a higher incidence of placenta abruptio along with toxemia.

## HYPERTENSION (HIGH BLOOD PRESSURE)

Hypertension is one of the signs of toxemia, but it can also exist in a pregnant woman as a separate complication. There is usually some sign of high blood pressure in the last trimester of pregnancy, but some women having a first baby develop it during labor with no prior indication. This is one of the reasons that blood pressure is monitored in the hospital during labor—because if it does develop, it gives no warning until the woman goes into convulsions. It can cause temporary or permanent blindness if the blood pressure is not lowered.

Blood pressure is usually not monitored in most out-of-hospital birth settings, but it would be of little use anyway because there is no medication at home to correct the problem. In the hospital a ''magnesium drip'' is started (magnesium is added to an I.V. hydrating solution), which has an excellent ability to lower the blood pressure.

A blood pressure of 140/90 is universally recognized as hypertensive, especially in a first pregnancy. Some doctors will hospitalize you before labor for observation and bed rest with this pressure reading. But it is possible to be hypertensive with a lower reading than this. A doctor knows what your blood pressure has been during pregnancy and uses that as a base line—you will be diagnosed as hypertensive if there is a 20-point rise during labor in either the systolic (top) number or the diastolic (bottom) number. For instance, if you are 130/80 during pregnancy, you can have a slightly higher pressure in the late stage of active labor without any concern. But if your baseline blood pressure was 100/60, you may be having a problem in labor at the 130/80 or 140/90 reading.

A diastolic rise is more significant because this is the "resting" pressure of your heart. Your system is under maximum pressure when your heart is working hardest, which is the systolic, or "pumping" measurement. Thus, when the diastolic number is high it may be a sign of problems because theoretically this is when your heart is supposed to be resting. For example a 110/60 rise might be normal in labor, whereas a 110/65 rise to 120/90 might indicate problems.

### HERPES SIMPLEX VIRUS II

Active vaginal or cervical lesions at the time of birth can pass the virus to the newborn—50 percent of infants that pass through an infected birth canal will get herpes. This means they will die or have severe nerve and/or eye damage. A woman who has had herpes II *at any time* must be examined for recurrent infection in the cervix and birth canal as delivery time nears. Infection of the fetus before birth can occur if the membranes are ruptured for a prolonged time. It is believed that the virus passes through the placenta; this hasn't been proven, but other, related viruses do pass through. If a woman has herpetic lesions in the genital area at the time of delivery, it is essential for the baby's well-being to be delivered by cesarean section before the membranes rupture or within 4 hours after they do. With this precaution, only 1 in 16 newborns becomes infected.

### SYPHILIS

A pregnant woman with infectious syphilis can miscarry at any time after the 4th month or have a stillborn. Early diagnosis and treatment of the mother will cure infection in the unborn baby. If the mother is treated with drugs before the 18th week the disease will not cross the placenta and affect the baby. Most states require a syphilis test for pregnant women even though they may have had a premarital test which was negative.

One-quarter of syphilis-infected babies die before birth and nearly one-third more die after birth. Babies can be born with congenital syphilis. They can also have such abnormalities as saddle nose (lacking a bridge), blindness due to an opaque cornea, deafness due to syphilis of the auditory nerve, abnormal pegged teeth, and internal problems. These babies can also have three symptoms known as Hutchinson's triad: baldness, rashes, and lesions.

## COMPLICATIONS DURING LABOR

Around 5 to 10 percent of women can be diagnosed as high-risk before labor and delivery so they and their doctors are prepared for possible complications. However, 50 to 60 percent of all complications during labor, birth, and the immediate postpartum period occur in women with no indications during pregnancy. Some studies have shown that during labor itself one-third of all women who were designated "low-risk" become "high-risk."

The problems that arise vary in seriousness, but the medical community points to this one-third proportion as an argument for birth in the hospital; advocates of the fetal monitor cite these figures as a rationale for routine fetal monitoring of all women, since it isn't possible to know ahead of time who will develop complications. There is another side of the issue, as pointed out by those who favor out-of-hospital birth. They question what proportion of complications are a *direct result of aggressive obstetric procedures.* Some examples are inducing labor by starting it or speeding it up with synthetic hormones for the woman's or doctor's convenience; keeping the woman comfortable at the expense of jeopardizing the integrity of the fetal brain; artificially rupturing membranes to speed labor or to insert an internal fetal monitor; and other procedures that may provide a learning experience for medical students, interns, and residents.

## LABOR IS BEST LEFT TO NATURE UNLESS NATURE FALTERS

There *are* times when nature falters and only medical intervention can correct the problem. However, there are several ways in which you can insure that labor will not falter and several things you can do if problems arise.

*A peaceful emotional state* is essential for a successful labor. The peak time for delivery is from 3:00 to 4:00 A.M., and the onset of labor signs occurs more frequently during the nighttime hours. This is when you are most likely to be in a calm state of mind. If you realize the importance of your emotional condition, you and your mate can do everything possible to protect it.

ENVIRONMENTAL DISTURBANCES may affect the timing, strength, and efficiency of your contractions. Contractions often decrease or disappear temporarily in the move from your home to the hospital and from the labor room to the delivery room. Medical care-givers usually ignore the psychological component of labor complications, so you have to be aware of them and try to improve your emotional state so that it doesn't interfere with labor.

ANXIETY, either overt or covert, may be related to the length of your labor. Also, uterine dysfunction may be associated with concealed anxiety. If you are feeling frightened or worried during labor, *talk about it.* Share your feelings with your mate; ask the doctor or nurse for information that may reassure you. If you simply try to "forget" the anxiety it may assert itself by slowing down your labor or undetermining the efficiency of your contractions.

REACHING A PLATEAU, in which dilation slows or stops, is a common occurrence but can be discouraging if you are having strong, regular contractions but dilation is not progressing. Do not let this upset you. Take cheer—and don't take artificial relaxants or stimulants right away. When the plateau has passed your dilation often progresses rapidly. Try to keep a positive outlook, stay calm, and try some of the suggestions below.

### HELPFUL SUGGESTIONS FOR LABOR COMPLICATIONS

*Change positions often*—moving your position or walking around may cause the baby to move into a more favorable position. Moving may engage her head more firmly in your pelvis, which is a better wedge to dilate the cervix.

*Check your release of tension.* You may be getting tense although you're unaware of it and this can slow your dilation. Use all your relaxation techniques. Have your mate give you a light massage. Concentrate on a feeling of floating in water.

*Massage or pull on your nipples*—this will increase contractions that have stopped or slowed. By stimulating your nipples you trigger the release of oxytocin into your system. This is the natural form of the hormone pitocin, with which labor is often medically stimulated, but can have side effects which mandate other medical procedures as a result.

### NONCOMFORMING LABOR— THE PROBLEMS THAT CAN ARISE

*Hypotonic contractions* are weak, infrequent, and do not produce normal labor progress. They can occur any time in labor but are more frequent in advanced stages. Oxytocic stimulation usually works.

*Hypertonic contractions* are severe but with little or no progress. They may occur in early labor, in which case you can be sedated to rest before resuming a more normal labor or you can be given an oxytocic to regulate the contractions.

*Incoordinate uterine activity* resembles hypertonic labor in that the contractions are difficult to predict or control and bring little progress. A change of position is the most helpful treatment, along with a mild sedative and analgesia if the pain is severe.

*Prolonged latent phase* (0 to 4 centimeters dilation) is considered anything longer than 20 hours for a first baby or 13½ hours for subsequent pregnancies. This complication may be the result of excessive analgesia, a breech presentation, a large baby and small pelvis, or if your membranes rupture when the cervix is still unripe and has not yet effaced (thinned out). A mild sedative can help you rest or oxytocin can be used to stimulate the efficiency of the contractions.

*Prolonged active phase* (above 4 centimeters dilation) is usually caused by a malposition of the baby—either his head doesn't descend into the pelvis, he is a breech, or there is cephalopelvic disproportion. Patience and close supervision are often the best means to deal with the problem.

*Secondary arrest* is when the progress of labor stops altogether in the active stages. This may be from cephalopelvic disproportion or from too much medication. Oxytocin can be used to stimulate contractions or a C-section can be performed if the problem is an inadequate pelvis that isn't large enough for the baby to pass through.

*Precipitate labor* starts out with very strong, frequent contractions with rapid dilation—more than 5 centimeters per hour for a first baby or complete dilation within an hour in later pregnancies. Labor can last a few contractions to a few hours but things are happening so fast that it will be hard for you to stay in control. Do not let anyone hold your legs together: it can cause brain damage in the baby. Do not push with contractions: the uterus does not need any help—keeping the baby from coming out *too fast* is desirable. If it happens when you're in the hospital the doctor may try to slow labor down because a gentle birth is easier on you and the baby who needs the hours of contractions to stimulate its skin and lungs; she can also suffer oxygen deprivation from the hard, frequent contractions. The reasons for precipitate labor are now known, but there is a tendency for it to recur—so be prepared for the next time you get pregnant!

*Soft tissue dystocia* is a rare occurrence that may follow previous treatment or an operation on your cervix, or there may be no discoverable cause. The cervix dilates at an abnormally slow rate despite strong contractions, a normal pelvis, and an average-size baby in a satisfactory position. It may prolong labor many hours and the very last stages of dilation may have to be completed by some operative means. Sometimes a doctor or nurse can massage your cervix during contractions to help it open up. The treatment is patience—on your part and that of the doctor.

Resistant vaginal tissues may prolong second-stage labor (pushing). It is especially common for women over 35 who are having their first baby. Strenuous athletics, especially riding, can thicken vaginal muscles, which can produce soft-tissue dystocia. An episiotomy can overcome this problem.

---

### CHART 37. SOME SIGNS OF ABNORMAL LABOR

---

- *Continuous and severe lower abdominal pain,* often accompanied by uterine tenderness
- *Discontinuance of good strong contractions* during first-stage labor
- *Excessive vaginal bleeding*—some reasons could be a cervical laceration, placenta abruptio, or delivery before full cervical dilation
- *Abnormality in fetal heart rate,* in which case you should be moved onto your left side to take pressure off the major blood vessels on the right
- *Abnormally slow dilation* of the cervix, which is a subjective judgment made by attendants based somewhat on your pain tolerance and the strength of the contractions
- *Abnormal presentation or prolapse* of the cord, placenta, or an extremity of the baby
- *Adverse change* in the condition of the mother (fever, high blood pressure) or the baby (fetal heart rate, meconium staining)

---

## CESAREAN BIRTH

One out of every 10 women reading this book is going to have her baby by cesarean section—depending on the particular area of the country and the hospital involved it may be as many as two out of every ten pregnant women. It may mean you. Many women don't know they are going to have a cesarean until partway through labor. Cesareans are not something that "happen to other people"—*every* pregnant woman should know about cesareans. *Please* read this section and inform yourself ahead of time.

Understanding what procedures will take place and why (the preparation, the catheter, the operation itself) will make it less frightening and less emotionally wrenching if you have to be sectioned; a cesarean section is often referred to as a "C-section" or a "section," and the verb "to be sectioned" has grown out of that. Many childbirth classes and books don't discuss cesareans, but preparation for the possibility makes it much smoother. You and your mate should know enough about the whys and wherefores of cesareans to be able to participate with your doctor in the decision to have a cesarean. You should talk to your doctor *ahead of time* about what options are available if you have to be sectioned. Don't accept a doctor's reply of "Why worry about that now? Everything's going to be fine." Most of the time a doctor doesn't know any better than you do whether you'll need a cesarean until you're in labor. There are several options available to you and you should negotiate them beforehand with the doctor. It may be possible to have your mate in the operating room with you; you should also have the choice to be awake and have regional anesthesia or to be unconscious under a general anesthetic. Sometimes medical factors determine this, but often it's decided by a doctor's or hospital's habits.

## THE INCREASE IN THE CESAREAN RATE

The high cesarean rate sounds ominous until you look at the reasons for it. Cesareans now account for 15 to 20 percent of all births in the United States—the number has doubled over the last decade. Some people "blame" the increased cesarean rate on fetal monitors, but this increase predates widespread monitoring. There are a number of reasons for the increase:

*The operation is safer.* Although a cesarean is major surgery, and therefore carries with it the risks of any surgery, the operation has evolved to the point where it is a relatively safe procedure. This means that a doctor can decide in favor of a cesarean when its risks are low compared to the alternative—which may be a high-forceps delivery, a baby in a breech position, or signs of fetal distress. A cesarean has become so safe that it can be considered more risk-free than many complications of vaginal labor and delivery.

*Women are waiting until their late 30s and early 40s* to have their first baby. They are approaching the age where the risks of a deformed child increase and when there can be complications in labor. These women often want only one or two children and they are demanding that nothing be wrong with the baby—they have waited a long time and don't have the leeway of many childbearing years ahead of them. Thus if things are not going smoothly a cesarean will be performed rather than riding it out and taking chances.

*Ultrasound and electronic fetal monitors predict* which babies might be compromised by the rigors of labor, indicating a cesarean rather than attempting a vaginal delivery. Monitoring also detects which babies do not tolerate labor well once it has begun. The stillbirth rate has been cut in half at many hospitals since fetal monitors were introduced there. It is also true that cesareans are performed before they are really necessary by doctors who are newly introduced to monitoring and do not read the monitor properly. *A fetal monitor is only as good as the person reading the tracing:* reading the monitor properly is a skill that has to be developed. Often the cesarean rate will rise at a hospital when fetal monitors are first introduced and the rate will drop back down once the personnel have become more practiced in deciphering the information correctly.

*Defensive medicine causes many cesareans.* Doctors are afraid of malpractice suits. They are afraid of the dangerous effect on the baby of prolonged labor, in which there can be oxygen deprivation. They are afraid of being sued for failing to do everything possible to deliver a perfect baby. It is the attitude and actions of prospective parents that have backed doctors into a corner so that the only way they can deliver what people demand is to do a cesarean and eliminate the risks of the unknown. Nature is whimsical and wasteful—yet many Americans are not willing to accept that. They expect a doctor to present them with a "perfect" baby and they often feel justified in blaming him if he does not. Doing a C-section gives him more control over the outcome and therefore a greater chance of meeting parents' expectations.

One study showed a higher cesarean rate for women

who had taken childbirth classes. Doctors have a greater fear of malpractice litigation from educated, affluent, sophisticated, middle-class parents than from clinic patients. The resulting irony is that those women who care the most about having a normal, natural birth may be more likely to have their baby by cesarean.

## INDICATIONS FOR A CESAREAN

There are two categories of reasons for performing a cesarean. The *absolute indications* are those in which there is no question or doubt as to whether a C-section is required—and the absolute indications listed here can sometimes even be emergency cesareans, in which immediate delivery is necessary to save the baby's and/or the mother's life. They involve the subjective opinion of your doctor, perhaps in consultation with another physician or with you and your mate. The decision depends on your body, the baby's condition, your desires, and your doctor's beliefs, based on his experience. *Relative indications* can be divided into two categories; determining factors which are known about before labor begins, and those which are evaluated once you are already in labor. All of the indications listed in Chart 38 are discussed in detail in this chapter.

Because some experts believe that a little labor is good even when a cesarean has been decided upon, your doctor may wait until you go into labor and then allow you to labor for a while before doing the cesarean. Cesarean babies sometimes have respiratory problems, and labor contractions help stimulate the fetus's lungs, compressing them to remove some of the fluid and to prepare them for breathing. Therefore, if you have a relative indication, you might want to discuss this possibility with your obstetrician ahead of time.

## CHART 38. DIRECTORY OF REASONS FOR CESAREANS

### *Absolute Indications*

- *Placenta previa* means that the placenta is preceding the baby; vaginal delivery is either physically impossible or you can hemorrhage. In the United States, 6 out of every 10 women with placenta previa are given a cesarean. A *total placenta previa* means that the placenta is completely covering your cervix, blocking the baby's exit. A *partial placenta previa* is sometimes not an absolute indication for a C-section, depending on how much of the placenta is covering the cervix. If the doctor can feel only a sliver of placenta, he may allow you to deliver vaginally, usually in the operating room so that a cesarean can be performed instantly if it becomes necessary.
- *Placenta abruptio* means partial or complete detachment of the placenta from the uterine wall before the baby is born. It normally detaches after the baby is delivered. There is grave risk to the mother from hemorrhaging, and to the baby, whose oxygen supply is cut off.
- *Prolapsed cord* means that the umbilical cord slips down in front of the baby's presenting part. Vaginal delivery would compress the cord in the birth canal, endangering the baby's life because her oxygen supply would be cut off.

### *Relative Indications*

### INDICATIONS BEFORE LABOR

- *Rh incompatability:* depending on whether your antibody titer is high or rises before your due date. With a vaginal delivery there would be a greater chance of your blood's mixing with the baby's.
- *Malpresentation of the baby:* If the baby is in a breech position (buttocks first) or transverse lie (sideways in the uterus), the risks may outweigh the benefits of vaginal delivery.
- *Previous cesarean:* depending on what the reason was for the previous C-section and what kind of incision was made (see detailed discussion later in this section).

CHART 38. DIRECTORY OF REASONS FOR CESAREANS *(continued)*

*Relative Indications*

**INDICATIONS BEFORE LABOR** *(cont.)*

- *Postmaturity:* If determined by tests that the baby is at least two weeks past the due date, and placental function is diminishing, then a cesarean may be better than the risk of waiting for spontaneous labor or the potential hazards of induction, which can place added stress on an under-nourished, postmature baby.
- *Maternal disease:* In some cases of *diabetes, renal disease,* and *toxemia* the mother's health may be further endangered by the stresses of labor. In the case of *herpes simplex virus II,* if the mother has active vaginal lesions at the time of delivery, this viral infection can be fatal to a baby going through the infected birth canal.

**INDICATIONS DURING LABOR**

- *Cephalopelvic disproportion:* if prelabor tests suggesting CPD are proven correct when baby does not descend.
- *Primipara over 40:* A woman having her first baby past the age of 40 may lack the elasticity in her pelvis to give birth vaginally.
- *Fetal distress:* which continues after changes in position and other corrective measures designed to improve oxygen supply to the fetus.
- *Ruptured membranes:* without the commencement of labor, or prolonged labor after the membranes break. The infection rate rises if a woman has not given birth within 24 hours of the time her membranes rupture.

## THE OPERATION ITSELF

### DECIDING WHEN TO HAVE THE CESAREAN

If you are going to have an elective cesarean (one you have decided upon beforehand), there is the decision as to when it should be done. The main concern is not to take the baby out before it is mature enough because premature babies are at risk for many complications after birth. There are a number of tests to determine fetal maturity, all of which are described earlier in this chapter. At about 20 weeks gestation, ultrasound scans are done to determine the baby's general size and the fetal biparietal diameter, which correlates, although imprecisely, to gestational age. Amniocentesis can be done to determine the L/S ratio—the amount of lecithin/sphingomyelin increases as the baby's lungs become more mature. Unfortunately, the more reliable amniocentesis is not done as frequently as ultrasound, because the latter does not have any risks. Thus there is almost always the chance that a cesarean may be premature.

Some medical evidence shows that even a little labor is good for the baby. Under some circumstances it may be best for labor to begin and then have the cesarean. You should discuss this possibility with your doctor.

## KINDS OF CESAREANS

There are two kinds of cesareans. A *classical* incision is vertical, a longitudinal cut made on top of the uterus. It is the quickest way to cut a cesarean and therefore may be done if speed is essential, or if you have a placenta previa located so it might be cut, or if the baby is especially large or in a transverse-lie position. The uterus is quite thin at the top and a classical incision is more difficult to repair and more likely to rupture in future pregnancies (a 2 percent chance). A *transverse* incision is also called a bikini cut because it is done right below your pubic hairline, allowing you to wear a bikini afterward without the scar showing. It is done if the doctor has more time. The horizontal incision is made at the bottom of the uterus and is easy to repair and unlikely to rupture in the future, only a 0.5 percent chance. A third incision, a low-flap vertical, incorporates the other two cuts. It is made in the lower portion of the uterus, but the incision is made up and down, so that it can be enlarged if necessary.

Although a cesarean is a relatively safe operation, it

still carries the risks of any major abdominal surgery. You are left with a scar on your uterus which can rupture before or during labor or delivery in a subsequent pregnancy. Uterine rupture carries a very high mortality rate for you and the baby, although this is highly unlikely. The uterus has an almost infinite capacity to stretch and is able to hold up to 15 to 18 pounds—the fetus and the other "products of conception."

**PREPARATION**

Most C-sections are scheduled for early morning so that the doctor can then go to his office and see patients. By knowing ahead of time exactly what will be done to you it makes a cesarean easier—just as childbirth education makes vaginal delivery less frightening. Be sure to *ask* about any procedures that are done to you—the more you know the less scary it will seem.

*You will check into the hospital* about 2 hours prior to the operation or the preceding night. If you feel jittery, nervous, and afraid, that's normal! Samples of your blood and urine will be taken and your abdomen will be "prepped"—a nurse will shave your stomach from about your belly button down through the upper portion of your pubic hair. You can request not to have your entire labia shaved because there is no need to shave *all* your pubic hair. Also, the routine enema is unnecessary unless you are constipated, so you can ask to forgo an enema. You may be given a sleeping pill to calm you so you'll get a good night's rest if you check in at night. If you *are* feeling uptight there is no reason not to accept this medication to make it easier for yourself. It doesn't usually compromise the baby because the drug is out of your system by morning.

*A sedative before the operation* may be given by injection. It is your right to refuse this medicine. This is something you can discuss with the anesthesiologist, who will probably discuss what he will be doing during the operation. This drug will reach the baby and may make him groggy, as drugs used in vaginal labor and delivery often do. It can have the same effect on you, too.

***The anesthesiologist is an important part*** of a cesarean—you should discuss with your obstetrician whether you have a choice of anesthesiologist or whether you simply have to use whoever is on duty at the time. The latter is usually the case. The man or woman administering the anesthesia is the only person during the operation who will be relating directly to you unless you're fortunate enough to be able to have your mate with you. Your doctor and the other staff will be too busy with their tasks. If an anesthesiologist is friendly and supportive of your feelings of fear and excitement, it can have a calming and cheering effect on you. The anesthetist is the person who has the final decision on what kind of anesthesia you get—general or conduction—and will probably use whatever he feels most comfortable administering.

***A catheter*** will be inserted into your bladder. This is usually done in the operating room. It is a rubber tube placed up your urethra and into your bladder so that urine is drained out of your body during the operation. The catheter is left in afterward, depending on how you are feeling after the cesarean and how soon you're ready to get up and walk. It doesn't usually hurt but feels strange when they take it out.

### HOW THE OPERATION IS DONE

***A cesarean takes 45 minutes to 1 hour*** to perform. Right before it begins, you will be given oxygen by mask to insure that the baby has plenty. The mask may smell medicinal, but they are giving you pure oxygen, not gas. If you had a previous C-section the first step is to cut around the skin scar and excise the old scar so that the normal skin edges can be brought together at the end. After the initial incision the abdominal muscle fibers are separated and then the peritoneum (the lining of the abdominal cavity) is opened, exposing the uterus. If you are having a "classical" section a small incision is made in the lower midportion and is enlarged upward and downward to about 6 inches in length. In the low type of incision first your bladder has to be detached from the front of the uterus and then is pushed down in the pelvis beneath the pubic bone. A 6-inch longitudinal incision is made in the lowermost portion of the uterus, which was previously overlain by the bladder.

At this point the membranes usually rupture. The doctor then gets the infant's head out of the incision, extracts the body, and clamps the umbilical cord. From the beginning of the skin incision to delivery is the shortest part of the operation: 5 to 6 minutes. The repair of the uterine and abdominal walls takes the most time. The placenta is manually removed and an oxytocic drug (usually pitocin) is given intramuscularly or intravenously to encourage your uterus to contract. These contractions may be painful so if you know breathing techniques you may want to use them. Your uterus is not massaged, as it would be in a vaginal delivery, because it might bleed.

If stitches are used they will probably be of nonabsorbable silk and have to be removed between the 5th and 7th postoperative days. Some doctors use metal clips to close the skin, which can be removed in a week or less. There are 12 to 14 external clips or stitches.

***An epidural is the anesthesia most often used*** for a cesarean (see pages 510–511). After the baby's birth the mother is often given a drug called Duramorf, which is administered via the epidural catheter. This is a morphine drug which stays in a woman's body about 24 hours, during which time it will eliminate or greatly reduce any postoperative pain. Many women do not need any other pain medication in recovering from the cesarean. Duramorf has a few mild side effects, like itching and dizziness. The drug also has an uncommon but dangerous complication of respiratory depression: a woman has to be monitored carefully to be sure she's breathing normally during the 24-hour period after the drug is administered.

*General anesthetic after the birth* is still used by some anesthesiologists, who may put a new mother lightly to sleep after the baby is born. You might want to discuss ahead of time the possibility of *not* being knocked out since this can make you groggy or even sick at a time when you might want to be with your mate or baby if you can arrange it.

When the anesthetic begins wearing off in the recovery room, you will become aware of the pain from the incision. The return of sensation is more abrupt after general anesthesia. You will probably be given an injection of pain medication, and this—especially after general anesthesia—may make you nauseated to the point of vomiting. Retching is most uncomfortable after abdominal surgery, so if you are prone to nausea, you should ask your doctor before delivery about receiving an antiemetic drug. This is sometimes given routinely along with pain medication to prevent nausea.

## THE EMOTIONAL ASPECTS OF A CESAREAN

A simple thing like the choices of words used about cesareans can be negative. Some women feel it is dehumanizing to be spoken of as "a section" or having been "sectioned"—they say that grapefruits are sectioned but women give birth. Another example is when it's said that someone had a cesarean rather than a normal birth—this implies that a woman who had a C-section is abnormal, which can translate as "bad." The words you use can have a subtle influence on the way you feel about a cesarean; it helps to be aware of this.

To avoid potentially negative feelings about a cesarean, it is important to keep your perspective. The most important thing is that a baby is being born—a new family unit is forming. If this attitude can be kept foremost, without losing sight of the fact that a C-section is also major surgery with its risks, it allows you to focus on the joy of birth rather than the anxiety about the operation or the disappointment at not being able to have a vaginal delivery.

*Anxiety* often dominates a woman's feeling about a C-section. If the cesarean is planned, you may be apprehensive for the entire time beforehand. If it is unexpected, often following a long and arduous labor or a frightening alarm for the baby's well-being during labor, it can be emotionally shattering. In the second case your choices and participation are often eliminated so it can also make you feel helpless.

*Braxton-Hicks contractions* before your due date and other normal uterine twinges during a pregnancy can be frightening if you know you are going to have a cesarean— you can fear that your uterus will rupture. Talk to your doctor to get reassurance if you do have these fears.

*Another worry can be the expense* and separation from your other children during the traditional 5-day stay for a cesarean. Find out whether your insurance covers a cesarean: many that don't cover vaginal delivery do pay for a C-section. Try to have your other child(ren) visit you in the hospital once you are up and moving around.

*Get a second opinion* about whether you need a cesarean, if your doctor tells you it's necessary ahead of time. That way you and your mate can satisfy yourselves that the decision is justified; it eliminates the possible doubts later that the cesarean could have been avoided.

*Maintaining control* is a factor in making a woman feel positive about her birth experience. If you are self-sufficient and feel like an autonomous, active participant rather than a passive object of care, it can enhance your feelings about yourself and the birth. It is a great disadvantage to cesarean women—especially those given a general anesthetic—not to have the opportunity to participate in the experience in that way. Make an attempt to involve yourself as much as you can in the decision about the operation and the post-operative procedures to overcome this feeling of helplessness. Your mate may also feel this way, so encourage him to be as involved as possible.

*Negative feelings afterward* are fairly common. A woman's self-esteem often suffers. You may feel like a failure at mothering if you have trouble moving around and doing chores right from the start. You may also feel that your body didn't work "right," and in addition you have a scar as a constant reminder. Some women feel mutilated and no longer whole. If you feel this way you can take heart that the scar will be less and less evident as time goes on and may eventually disappear altogether.

*Your mate may feel inadequate* and like a failure after an unexpected C-section. He may interpret his banishment to the waiting room as a punishment for not having helped enough—although the feeling is usually not a conscious one. If a man feels he was inadequate during labor ("If only I had been more supportive, labor could have gone on normally"), these feelings may be carried over into the early fathering role. A man who subconsciously feels he failed his partner and his baby, may continue these feelings as a new parent.

*Discuss the reasons for the cesarean* with the doctor beforehand and also afterward if you still have any questions. Get any information you want and talk about your feelings as well as plans for future pregnancies. Often these issues are left up in the air. Repressed feelings and a lack of understanding can cause fears, frustration, uncertainties, and anxiety.

*Allow yourself to feel and express* negative feelings after a cesarean. You may feel jealous or resentful toward other women who talk enthusiastically about their nonmedicated birth and the ease of mothering. You may feel angry at the baby for having caused the cesarean; then you may feel guilty and blame yourself for "letting the baby down" because a cesarean was necessary. These feelings may be irrational but you have to confront them—there may be a "C-sec" group you can call in your area and talk to a member or join a discussion group. If you don't get these feelings out of the way they may haunt you or interfere with your relationship with the baby.

### SOME OPTIONS TO THE TRADITIONAL CESAREAN EXPERIENCE

There are some options you and your mate might want to consider in order to avoid some of the possible negative aspects of a cesarean and to enhance the experience for yourselves and your baby.

*Allowing the baby's father into the operating room* has gained popularity across the country. Birth is a time for togetherness, and this is especially true of a cesarean. You need each other at a time of stress for mutual support. Your mate may feel helpless, unneeded, and worried. You may feel lonely and scared. At the same time you may want to share the excitement and joy of seeing your baby's first minutes of life. For more information about how to make this option possible, see pages 381–383. "Prevailing practice" is what is considered in a hospital's decision to permit a couple to stay together. This means that if other hospitals have already allowed husbands to stay with wives, the path will be opened for the more cautious hospitals to try it. If they will not allow your mate in the delivery room they may allow him to join you in the recovery area—ask about this. If it is a general recovery room—with various postoperative patients and not just women recovering from childbirth— it is less likely they'll allow your mate and/or baby to keep you company.

*Lowering the screen* when the baby is born is done by some doctors to let you see the baby being born from your body. This eliminates the problem that some women have in making a connection between the baby they have been carrying inside and the one that is placed in their arms, usually many hours later. The baby can also be examined near your head rather than the routine of examining her over in the warming tray or in the nursery. This gives you a chance to see the baby and assure yourself she is all right.

*Holding the baby,* if only for a few minutes, can make a big difference. If the baby is not having respiratory distress (cesarean babies sometimes have trouble breathing right away), then ask if you can hold her for a little while. This is not routine in cesareans, but can make you feel closer to the baby, particularly if the hospital policy is to take it away for many hours. Unless the child needs immediate medical attention at birth there is no reason why the father cannot cuddle her, too. It is an important opportunity for paternal-infant bonding.

*Breast-feeding on the delivery table* or in the recovery room is possible if the baby is fine and you've discussed it with your obstetrician and pediatrician, preferably beforehand. Breast-feeding often has a special meaning for cesarean mothers who may feel "At least my body can do *something* right!" The sooner a baby sucks, the better the chances of successful breast-feeding, because its sucking reflex is reinforced at birth. A cesarean mother who experiences difficulty breast-feeding, perhaps because of an immediate and prolonged separation after birth, may have feelings of *two* failures.

    Don't forget that any drugs you take for pain relief after a cesarean pass into your breast milk. To whatever extent you can, try to avoid drugs, because they can affect the baby. To lessen your reliance on medication you should rest as much as possible. Overexerting yourself makes your incision hurt more. Use hot-water bottles on the incision, change positions, and get more comfortable with pillows—turn to whomever you can for support.

*Postdelivery observation of the baby* usually means separating you and the baby: you may want to do everything you can to minimize it. Bonding immediately at birth is particularly crucial for cesarean mothers and babies. Usually, the prerequisite for releasing you from the recovery area is that the anesthetic has worn off—this means you will be feeling pain, which will inhibit your first encounter with the baby if you cannot bond in the delivery room.

    Some hospitals require that a cesarean baby go routinely to the intensive-care nursery (ICN) or the central nursery for a minimum number of hours or days, regardless of her condition. There is no medical justification for this; a healthy baby is healthy no matter how she was born. Many experts now believe that some alternative to this separation is necessary. One-third of all battered children in this country were cesarean births—they were denied close and immediate bonding with their mothers, which is especially important in this type of birth.

Although the routine is to send the baby to the ICN or CN for a long observation there is no reason the baby and mother cannot be watched together postpartum. If it isn't possible to keep a healthy baby with you, *make every possible attempt to have the baby released from the ICN to the central nursery or to your room* as soon as possible. Just having your baby in the ICN can make you feel she is ill or there is something wrong, which in most cases is *not* so.

If that doesn't work, you and your mate should visit the baby and *insist upon touching her.* As soon as you feel able to, you should arrange for the baby to room-in with you. The possible trauma and separation of a cesarean birth are something you have to work to overcome.

## VAGINAL BIRTH AFTER CESAREAN (VBAC)

In 1980 the National Institutes of Health released a report recommending vaginal birth after cesarean (VBAC) when appropriate. In an effort to reduce the rising number of cesarean births, the American College of Obstetricians and Gynecologists (ACOG) adopted new guidelines in 1988 to encourage attempts at normal, vaginal births by women who had previously had cesareans. Repeat cesareans represent 23 percent of the recent increase in cesarean births. Data shows that 50 to 80 percent of women have successful vaginal births after a low-flap transverse incision (bikini cut).

Not so long ago it was believed "Once a C-section, always a C-section," but research has shown that a woman who's had a cesarean before doesn't necessarily have any higher risk in vaginal delivery. The ACOG changed its long-standing policy and declared that VBAC is perfectly safe for mother and fetus, even if the mother has had two or three cesareans, unless there is a medical indication for a repeat cesarean.

The basic rule of thumb now is that the only repeat cesareans should be for a repeat of the *reason that the first cesarean was performed.* In other words, you won't need another cesarean if the first C-section was for reasons of the baby—he was breech or transverse, it was a multiple birth, or distress showed on the fetal monitor, unless of course the same conditions apply with the next birth. Nor will you need another cesarean if your first C-section was for placenta previa or abruptio, toxemia, or infection, and you have no history of surgery on your uterus other than the first cesarean.

### *The new ACOG guidelines for VBAC are:*

* There should be only one fetus, with an estimated weight of less than 4,000 grams.
* The previous cesarean should have been transverse: VBAC is not safe with a previous classical incision, but vertical incisions are rare and occur in only 1 to 2 percent of cesareans.
* If your previous baby's head was too large for your pelvis, you can attempt labor this time if ultrasound shows that your pelvis is adequate for the head of the new baby. Studies show that subsequent trials of labor are successful for up to 70 percent of women who were originally given a C-section because of "failure to progress in labor." Remember that absolute cephalopelvic disproportion (the baby's head not fitting through your pelvis) is rare.
* There should be continuous electronic monitoring of fetal heart rate and uterine activity throughout labor.
* Staff and facilities should be able to respond to acute obstetric emergencies—in other words, should be able to perform an immediate cesarean if it becomes necessary.
* Blood of your type should be in the hospital blood bank and 24-hour blood-banking capabilities should be avail-

able. When you arrive for the delivery, your blood should be typed and screened for irregular antibodies.

## ARE YOU A CANDIDATE FOR VBAC?

***The kind of incision on your previous C-section*** is one determinant of whether you are a candidate for VBAC. If it was a low-flap transverse incision (bikini cut), then it's possible to try a vaginal delivery. A high "classical" incision, rarely used anymore except for emergency cesareans, would allow your uterus to rupture too easily. Since the incision on your skin may not parallel the internal incision on your uterus, your doctor has to find out how the previous surgery was done: if he wasn't the one to do it, he can contact the doctor who did or consult your medical records.

***Whether you're a candidate for VBAC*** depends on whether you meet certain criteria. While every doctor and hospital will have individual guidelines for making that decision, the chart below outlines most criteria used to determine who can be considered for a vaginal delivery.

---

### CHART 39. WHO IS A CANDIDATE FOR VBAC?

- Previous low transverse incision (bikini cut)
- Normal pregnancy
- Delivery within 12 to 24 hours after rupture of the membranes
- Willingness to avoid pain medications or use minimal amounts so that you have full feeling in case of pain due to rupture
- Avoidance of pitocin to induce or augment labor; pitocin (or other forms of oxytocin) to be used only in conjunction with an internal fetal monitor
- Understanding that general anesthetic may be used if a serious problem develops requiring an immediate cesarean

---

***Previous abnormal labor (dystocia)*** should not disqualify you for VBAC. Dystocia is a common diagnosis of labor that frequently results in cesareans—but it doesn't mean a woman shouldn't try a vaginal delivery the next time around. Dystocia includes cephalopelvic disproportion (CPD), prolonged labor, "failure to progress," arrested labor, uterine inertia, and prolonged second stage. Studies show that cesarean birth is being performed for abnormal labor far more often than in the past: it is estimated that the diagnosis of dystocia accounts for about one-third of the increase in the cesarean birth rate. Doctors today tend not to wait as long as in the past, nor to try more conservative measures to enhance labor, before resorting to a C-section. This is because cesarean birth used to be viewed as a risk to be avoided, whereas today the thinking is that a cesarean is safer for the fetus than a complicated forceps delivery. Also, the medical-legal climate has doctors practicing "defensive medicine" for fear of being sued if the baby is compromised.

Although some doctors screen out women who had abnormal labor before, recent research indicates that dystocia which previously led to a cesarean need not disqualify you to try a vaginal birth the next time. The conditions causing dystocia do not necessarily repeat themselves. In fact, some physicians feel that there is less chance of uterine rupture when the previous C-section was performed because of abnormal labor. This is because the uterus had a good chance to stretch during the previous labor, permitting the incision to be placed lower where it is least likely to rupture.

### RISKS AND BENEFITS TO VBAC

***There are multiple benefits*** to VBAC. You eliminate operative and postoperative complications and postpartum pain, and have a shorter hospital stay, which, depending on your insurance situation, can reduce your financial costs. Infection rates in mothers after cesarean birth range from 10 to 65 percent and are much lower after vaginal delivery. Also, labor can be beneficial to the baby, readying her lungs for life outside the womb. After cesarean birth, the infant is usually taken to the nursery for observation, severely limiting the time parents can have with their newborn at that special moment.

Finally, it can be psychologically important for you to have a vaginal birth. You may have had an emotional investment in having natural childbirth before, and you may have suffered from the "failure syndrome" after your cesarean. Also, your sense of control and participation in the birth are enhanced by attempting a vaginal delivery.

***The risk of VBAC is uterine rupture,*** but this is a term which can strike fear in your heart and rarely happens, literally. What uterine rupture actually refers to is any separation in the wall of the uterus. The most common ruptures are incomplete, which cause a window-like effect, or small separations of the previous scar in the uterus. However, rupture is highly unlikely: the statistical risk of rupture is less than 1 percent for a woman who had a lower segment incision (bikini cut) and is undergoing a trial of labor.

Massive uterine rupture, which is life-threatening, is extremely rare. The possibility of excessive strain on the uterus is feared only for those women who have weakened uteruses from many pregnancies and deliveries or who receive too much oxytocin during labor. Because of the potential risk of uterine rupture with the administration of oxytocin, some physicians choose not to use it to induce or augment labor in VBAC. However, several studies have shown that using oxytocin for women undergoing a trial of labor after a prior low transverse cesarean delivery carries no greater risk than using it to augment labor for women who haven't had previous cesareans.

***Finding a supportive doctor*** can be the most important element of VBAC. The best way to find one is by word of mouth: ask friends, ask childbirth educators, ask the OB/GYN department of your local hospital, contact local childbirth organizations or find out if there are going to be childbirth workshops or conferences in your area.

*Accepting the realities of VBAC* is important to the experience you will have. You're setting yourself up for disappointment if you expect a vaginal birth to make up for what may have been an unsatisfactory birth experience the first time. You might want to make a list of the things you liked and didn't like about your previous cesarean delivery and to become aware of how you want things to be different this time. If you and your mate can discuss these feelings and requests with your doctor, it gives you a chance to clarify what your priorities really are. If the physician has concerns about any of the items, listen and take this into account. You may have to be more realistic in the kind of birth experience you can expect with VBAC, and/or you and your doctor may be able to compromise so you're both comfortable.

*Making the decision is difficult*, and whatever you decide, you'll probably have moments of ambivalent feelings, wondering whether you've made the right choice. The important thing is to consider the option of VBAC. You may decide after talking to even the most open-minded and supportive doctor that you want to choose a repeat cesarean anyway. You may want the convenience of a scheduled birth to arrange child care and time off from work or other responsibilities. You may feel that a vaginal birth is too frightening a prospect for you, or that you have specific medical problems that make it an unacceptable risk for you. What it comes right down to is to trust your instincts. The most valid factor in making a decision is to think it through with your partner and respect your own feelings about what is best for you and your baby.

*What if you have another cesarean?* If your vaginal birth doesn't work out, will you be devastated and hurt? Or will you be disappointed but glad you made an attempt at labor? Most couples are able to accept a disappointing outcome of VBAC if they are well-informed and prepared before labor and have established a good line of communication with their physician. Be sure that your doctor understands that you and your mate want to be active participants in the management of the VBAC and that you want to be kept informed about the options available as your birth situation unfolds.

If a couple can participate in the decision-making process throughout VBAC, it can be a positive experience even if it results in another cesarean. A woman's feelings of failure—that she could or should have done more—can come from the feeling that the labor was out of her control and she had no say in what was being done to her and her baby. Even if the outcome is disappointing, by being involved you'll know you did the best thing for your baby and yourself under the circumstances.

## WHAT TO EXPECT IN THE FIRST POSTPARTUM DAYS AFTER CESAREAN

***The I.V. is kept in after surgery*** depending on your condition but it is usually 24 to 48 hours. The intravenous solution keeps down postoperative fever, which is especially important if you're nursing.

***The catheter*** that emptied your bladder during the surgery will be removed within 24 hours, but you may find it hard to urinate afterward. It is important to drink plenty of fluids. This keeps you from becoming dehydrated, encourages urination, and may shorten the length of time you have to stay on I.V. fluids. The catheter may increase your chances of getting a urinary tract infection and/or urethral irritation. If you develop any of the symptoms of such problems, notify your doctor.

***Bowel movements*** may be difficult following your operation. The operation itself, plus your postoperative limited diet and activity, may contribute to sluggish bowels or constipation. Straining in an effort to have a bowel movement is nearly impossible after you've had an abdominal incision. It is important to do everything possible to get your bowels moving and keep your stool soft. The first few postoperative days you'll be put on a liquid or very soft diet. Drink plenty of fluids, eat roughage and whole-grain cereals and bread as soon as you're able to, and get on your feet and moving around. Your doctor may prescribe a stool softener, which is a capsule that you swallow, to ease your first bowel movement. If you're having trouble moving your bowels, ask about taking a stool softener if it isn't offered to you.

*Gas and gas pains* are a sign that your intestines are beginning to function again, which will probably be about the third day after the operation. Although you may be upset by these sharp pains, your doctor will view them as a good sign that your body is recovering from the surgery. The fact that gas is being moved down the intestinal tract means there's no infection causing intestinal difficulties.

Getting up and moving around is the best prevention and cure for gas. Rolling from side to side in your bed and changing positions will also help your body get rid of the gas. Sleeping on your stomach may help, although getting into that position may be uncomfortable.

Try placing the baby on your upper abdomen when you give her a bottle, or put her on a pillow on your stomach if you are breast-feeding. In both cases the baby's weight will tend to push the gas down and bring you relief.

There are certain foods and drinks you should avoid until at least 10 days after the cesarean. Carbonated drinks and bubbly water can make gas pains worse. Some women find that apple juice, which is frequently given to postoperative patients in the hospital, can cause gas. The worst offenders for causing intestinal gas are leafy green vegetables and beans of any kind. Avoid these until your body is functioning normally or you may feel like you're going to explode!

*Pain in your shoulder(s)* may occur due to blood and air that collects under your diaphragm and irritates, pressing on the nerves that go to your shoulders. This shouldn't last very long.

*Medication* can be tailored to breast-feeding—some drugs will not harm the baby as much and are suited for nursing (see Chapter Eleven). The small amount of colostrum in your breasts the first few days won't have any appreciable amount of medication to pass on to the baby. However, when the painkillers wear off the pain may seem worse to you; try to take as few drugs as possible for as short a time as possible. Some doctors routinely prescribe tranquilizers in addition to pain medication. It is better not to have your perceptions and emotions blunted after birth. Be sure to ask what drugs you are being given and why.

*Walk around* as soon as you can. This will get your body systems like digestion and elimination working and start you on the road to feeling well. Walking may be quite painful at first and you'll have to take short walks with tiny steps. Your lower abdomen will probably feel bruised and tender—as if you've been beaten up. Try to stand upright, although your instinct will probably be to hunch over like an old lady because the incision will feel like it's pulling. Don't worry: the stitches will not come out.

*Belly binder* is a large bandage used by some hospitals to support your stomach after the operation. It may be uncomfortable, in which case you should ask to have it removed.

*Abdominal discomfort* will lessen within 7 to 10 days. On the 3rd day after surgery the intestinal tract begins to function normally again, and sharp gas pains may occur when you sneeze, cough, laugh, or hiccup. The involuntary movement of your abdominal muscles may hurt. Hold your hands pressed against the incision or press a pillow against it when you laugh or cough.

*Lochia* is the same as a vaginal delivery—it is a menstrual-like flow of the uterine lining that lasts for a week or two after delivery. If you are given a sanitary napkin with a belt, the metal clasp may irritate your incision. You should try beltless napkins that attach to your underpants or pin the napkin to your underpants with safety pins.

*Look at your incision* before leaving the hospital in case you have any concerns. Have your mate look at it too. The scar can be itchy, numb, it may pull or may ooze a little—all this is common and not a cause for alarm. If the stitches are nonabsorbable, they will be removed about a week after surgery. The procedure is uncomfortable, but there is no reason to fear that it will be very painful.

The incision bandage is usually removed a day or two postpartum. The incision can hurt a bit more afterwards because it has no support. Your clothes can rub your stitches or clamps, if you don't have the absorbable kind of stitches.

*The breathing exercise* to clear your lungs should start as soon as possible after the operation. Place a pillow over the incision: breathe deeply in, exhale, breathe deeply in and hold for 5 to 10 counts, then exhale and breathe in and out normally.

*Modified rooming-in* might be the best solution if you are feeling less than terrific and need to rest. A woman who has had a cesarean may have a hard time focusing on the newborn's needs instead of her own real and pressing needs. You should ask for lessons in infant care from the nurses and get accustomed to the baby as soon as you can.

*Nursing* may be uncomfortable at first—putting a pillow over your abdomen may be a solution. Remind the staff that you are breast-feeding and don't want the baby to be given bottles of glucose water or formula. Your baby may be sleepy from the effects of general anesthesia if that's how you were medicated for the delivery, or the baby may be placed in the intensive care nursery for observation, since cesarean babies have more respiratory problems—both these factors may interfere with initiating successful breast-feeding. You may have to be more patient than a woman who had a vaginal delivery. Also, don't forget that all medications enter your breast milk; see the chart on page 683. If you're taking pain medication, realize that it reaches the baby and may affect nursing.

*Emotions* in the first days can be depressed—you may feel tearful, cheated, or like a failure. Feelings are not right or wrong—they just *are*. Try writing your feelings down. Your mate may feel he was thrust out of the picture by the cesarean and may feel cheated himself. You two must *talk to each other* in order to overcome the feelings and recognize that you aren't alone—you're going through it all together.

## ADJUSTMENT AT HOME IS ESSENTIAL

*Help at home is essential.* Unless your mate has been a practicing house-husband for some time he cannot handle the household alone. A well-meaning man may try to stay home and handle everything, but he will exhaust himself and you'll probably feel obliged to get up and help him. That is the last thing you should do. You'll recover more quickly and fully if you take it extremely easy. Yet taking care of you postoperatively and taking care of a new baby and a house is a *big job*. If you have parents or in-laws who are willing and able to help out, that's great—if not, hiring someone for the first week or two would make a great gift from the new grandparents if you can't afford it.

Do not be a stoic—it will needlessly prolong your convalescence. Hired help might be less taxing emotionally than friends or relatives because if you are paying someone, you won't feel it's an imposition or that you have to help them.

*Avoid stair-climbing for the first week or two* if at all possible. Your abdominal muscles are healing and climbing stairs puts a strain on them that may cause you pain afterward, tire you out, and otherwise hamper your quick recovery.

*Avoid lifting* until about fifteen days after surgery, when the incision heals and becomes strong. This even means lifting the baby in the first postpartum days. Have someone hand the baby to you.

*Medication* for the first week at home will probably be the same kind you used during the end of your hospital stay, if you were taking painkillers then. Beware of codeine-based drugs, which are constipating.

**Wear a lightweight girdle,** a stretchy and inexpensive Lycra spandex type, if you get the unpleasant sensation that your belly is about to fall out. The girdle will give you support until your stomach muscles tighten up again.

**Try never to be left alone, at least for the first week.** It is really important to have someone there at all times, if only to lift the baby and hand him to you. Lifting anything is forbidden after abdominal surgery. Although guests are going to tire you out a lot the first week you can ask *certain* friends and relatives to come be with you in shifts—then you won't feel helpless or that you have to get up and do things you aren't ready for.

**Siblings** may be suffering from a feeling of jealousy and abandonment since you've been away a week or so. One good way to overcome those feelings without tiring yourself is to let the older child come into bed with you and read, draw, and cuddle.

**Sex** is something you probably won't be in the mood for right away. The sheer physical exhaustion and hormonal changes after birth may cause the lack of interest. Some women say it took 6 to 9 months for their previous level of sexual interest to return.

THE OBSTETRICIAN USUALLY GIVES THE OKAY for you to resume sex after your 6-week checkup postsurgery. However, your mate may still be fearful of hurting you; you should have him talk to the doctor to get reassurance.

YOUR VAGINA PROBABLY WON'T LUBRICATE as quickly as in prebirth days no matter how much foreplay you have. K-Y lubricating jelly can solve this problem until your hormones are back to their previous levels.

THE MAN-ON-TOP POSITION MAY BE UNCOMFORTABLE. Experiment with other positions for lovemaking that don't put a strain on the incision, which can still be tender.

YOU MAY BE FEELING UNATTRACTIVE, which would make you shy away from sex or feel negatively about yourself. Your new scar and bulging stomach may make you feel unsexy. Start exercises to get back in shape as soon as you can.

THE FEELING OF FAILURE can be overwhelming for some time after you get home. Some women feel incomplete as a result of having had a cesarean and some become obsessed with the feeling of failure. You can have periods of nonstop crying and depression. If this happens, seek professional help—these feelings are detrimental to your newly forming relationship with the baby.

## PROBLEMS WITH THE BABY

### PREMATURE LABOR AND DELIVERY

Premature labor is calculated on the baby's birth weight rather than the duration of pregnancy because the latter is so difficult to determine with exactitude. When a newborn weighs less than 5½ pounds (2,500 grams), it is considered to be a premature infant. Ordinarily a 5½-pound baby is about 4 weeks from its expected delivery date and at that weight has a greater risk of survival and an increased risk of cerebral palsy and mental retardation. There is a critical difference in the final 2 or 3 weeks of gestation for fetal development, particularly of the lungs.

Some causes of prematurity are multiple birth, toxemia, placenta previa, premature separation of the placenta, or maternal illness with severe infection such as pneumonia or untreated syphilis. But in 60 percent of cases there is no obvious reason: in an apparently normal pregnancy labor begins or the membranes rupture between 20 and 36 weeks.

When labor starts there is nothing that will stop it

for sure, but doctors can attempt to halt it. The drugs commonly used to prevent premature labor are beta-sympathomimetics, which stimulate the action of the sympathetic nervous system. The beta-sympathomimetic drug Nylidrin seems to have been the most effective in some tests. There are side effects to these drugs: hypotension, tachycardia, dizziness, and nausea.

Intravenous alcohol solution given by a continuous-drip technique over several hours is thought to inhibit labor by blocking the release of oxytocin. Evidently the alcohol acts on the pituitary gland; the high blood level of alcohol prevents the discharge of pituitrin, the chemical hormone that stimulates uterine contractions. In some instances when the alcohol is stopped it has shut off the trigger mechanism that initiated labor. The side effects of I.V. alcohol can be a headache and nausea. Alcohol can also have an effect when drunk—a glass of wine or a mixed drink can stop the contractions of prodromal labor (see page 453).

Several other drugs to stop premature labor—isoxyprine and ridadrine, for example—have had varying degrees of success. Terbutaline, a drug which is not yet FDA-approved for use in labor, is probably used even more frequently. Under the brand name Brethine it is currently prescribed as a drug for asthma. However, it has been found that bed rest may accomplish as much as any drug. If the membranes ruptured prematurely but contractions do not begin, a woman may be put flat in bed in the hospital, perhaps on antibiotics to guard against the infection that can develop with ruptured membranes in the hopes that labor will not begin for the crucial final weeks of pregnancy.

***Get to the nearest large medical center*** if you do go into labor prematurely. If your labor begins 6 weeks early, a community hospital is going to be inadequate to meet your baby's needs when it is born. Have your mate or the police rush you to the nearest perinatal center where they have specialists and facilities intended for the care of premature infants. Some of the equipment they may have is:

CPAP (continuous positive airway pressure): A tube is inserted into the baby's windpipe or a pressurized hood is fitted around his head so that a continuous supply of low-pressure air is directed to the sacs of the immature lungs, preventing their collapse.

BILIRUBIN lights detoxify the jaundice that often affects "premies."

SKIN SENSORS monitor oxygen and other blood gases.

BLOOD ANALYSIS is done with several drops pricked from the newborn's heel or from a plastic tube inserted into the umbilicus and left there (which eliminates the need to keep pricking the baby). Blood sugar, blood acidity, and blood gases are measured and analyzed for any changes.

ELECTRONIC THERMOMETER is taped to the baby's skin to insure that his temperature remains constant.

INFUSION PUMP is a tiny tube inserted into the umbilical cord to deliver intravenous fluids at a preset rate to the baby's bloodstream.

NASOGASTRIC FEEDING TUBE is a tube inserted into the baby's nose and breast milk or formula is fed through it if the baby is not strong enough to suck.

ALARMS SOUND if breathing or other rates become too fast or slow. Neonatal intensive care specialists are in constant attendance to correct any such problems.

**The survival rate of premies** depends on how early they are born. A premie is technically any baby born more than 3 weeks early. The most troubled babies are those born at the current limit of viability, about 24 weeks old. At this point, a baby's lungs have developed to the point where he can breathe with the help of a machine called a ventilator. Before 23 or 24 weeks the lungs are so rudimentary that the infants have virtually no chance of survival. Infants have been known to survive at a weight of about 500 grams or 1 pound; infants weighing less than about 2 pounds currently have about a 70 percent chance of survival. Larger babies do better: 90 percent of infants weighing from 2 to

3 pounds live, while in the 1960s more than half of them died.

Sex and race are important factors, too. Statistically, black girls seem to do best, while white boys are the least likely to make it. A premie's first hours are crucial, and if they are born in a hospital with a neonatal intensive care unit, they generally do better.

*Lung failure used to be* a major reason that premature babies died. In normal gestation, a substance known as surfactant provides surface tension in the air sacs of the lungs. Natural surfactant does not develop until 35 weeks into the pregnancy, so it has not developed in many premies: without it, the tiny air sacs collapse and stick together with every breath, the cause of respiratory distress.

The newborn's tiny lungs have to be expanded and contracted mechanically by a ventilator. With the increased use of this ventilator, more babies are surviving. However, there are side effects. Some infants' fragile lungs are damaged by the ventilator and they develop chronic lung disease. Others become ventilator-dependent. Researchers are working on methods of injecting natural or artificial surfactant into the babies' lungs at birth to aid pulmonary functioning.

A circulatory condition characteristic of premies is known as *patent ductus arteriosus,* which allows too much blood to flow into the lungs and poses the risk of collapse and hyaline membrane disease, a condition in which immature lungs are vulnerable to collapse. Although the infants may be capable of breathing on their own, they are placed on respirators as a precaution.

---

**CHART 40. DIRECTORY OF GROWTH PATTERNS OF PREMIES**

---

*24 WEEKS*
*Height:* 13 inches
*Weight:* 1¼ pounds
Lungs have just developed enough for mechanical ventilation. All babies have a dark red appearance because skin pigmentation has not begun. Skin is unable to help regulate body temperature or ward off infection. Eyes are often fused shut, earlobes are just skin flaps. Baby has a 5 to 20 percent chance of survival outside the womb.

*29 WEEKS*
*Height:* 14½ inches
*Weight:* 2½ pounds
Lungs have developed enough to increase chance of survival outside womb to 90 to 95 percent. Baby takes a more rounded, plump appearance because fat layer is developing. Pigmentation is present. Eyes partly open. Baby can follow objects with his eyes and has longer periods of alertness. Some babies begin to suck.

*35 WEEKS*
*Height:* 18½ inches
*Weight:* 5½ pounds
Baby sees almost as well as a full-term baby and shows a preference for a human face. Testicles in the male have descended. Baby can coordinate sucking, breathing, and swallowing, to allow nipple feeding. Skin is smooth because there is a substantial fat layer. Muscle tone is developed.

*40 WEEKS*
*Height:* 20 inches
*Weight:* 7 pounds
Baby is plump and fully developed. Baby has received from her mother: iron, calcium, vitamins and immunities against infection.

---

***Other problems premies face*** are usually suffered by the very smallest babies. Brain hemorrhages continue to be a major problem. Serious bleeding and lack of blood supply to the brain can lead to severe brain damage; in other cases, infants have cerebral palsy or are spastic. Premies can also become jaundiced because their underdeveloped livers cannot filter out dead red blood cells, although they receive a form of phototherapy (light treatment) that accomplishes that task.

Blindness in premature infants is on the rise again. New studies have shown that bright lights in hospital nurseries may damage premies' eyes, contributing to blindness and other vision problems. Research has shown that the smallest premature babies suffer considerably less eye damage when they are shielded from round-the-clock hospital lights, which have grown brighter over the past 20 years to make it easier to monitor premature infants.

### THE PSYCHOLOGICAL ASPECTS OF PREMATURE DELIVERY

A premature delivery robs you and your mate of the final weeks of physical and psychological preparation for the new baby. Then, aside from the physical risks to a premie, there is also a tremendous psychological impact on the parents. In order to understand and cope more constructively with those feelings it is necessary to know what they are.

#### BASIC PSYCHOLOGICAL STEPS

*The mother prepares herself for the possible loss* of an infant whose life is in jeopardy.

*She must face and acknowledge her failure* to deliver a normal, full-term baby.

*She must then reorient her perspective* from preparing herself for a potential loss to viewing the situation with hope and anticipation.

*She must learn the premie's special needs* and growth patterns, which will eventually become normal.

### ANXIETY

This is the primary emotion you will probably feel. Most premature babies do survive, however pessimistic remarks in the first hours of its life can cause you anticipatory grief. Medical caretakers can make negative remarks about your baby's condition that can set off initial feelings of grief in you; you prepare yourself for losing the baby. This stifles your attachment process to the baby—as an unconscious defense mechanism you repress the natural bonding to the baby because you fear she will die. This can cause *years* of anxiety; you may remain unconvinced for a long time that all is well with your child.

***Bring the baby's father into the situation*** as much as possible. Insure that he is included in nursery discussions of the baby's condition—this will lessen his anxiety and give you support. Often a woman can fear that developments are being kept from her by the doctor, who is telling "the truth" to the baby's father.

***Assure yourselves that the doctor*** is not being deceptively optimistic. But if he says, "Your baby may not live," the physician is not being sensitive to the irreversible psychological damage he is doing to you. Doctors are accustomed to dealing with life-and-death situations and to discussing them in a sometimes casual way. A doctor may not recognize that new parents are unable to hear certain comments without jumping to unwarranted conclusions. For example, some doctors might mention the general possibility of brain damage or eye problems with premies. However, it is not possible to tell what the outcome for *your* baby will be at such an early age and such negative predictions or speculations are often proven false. As parents, you would be upset by such discussions and they may be totally unnecessary. A doctor should certainly not withhold information or lie to parents, but he should only tell them negative information where it can be accurately predicted, such as with Down's syndrome. If your doctor is having these theoretical conversations with you, at least ask him the odds of such an outcome for your baby. You may find that they are quite small and the doctor has unnecessarily increased your anxiety.

***It is important for you to rebel against rigid visiting hours.*** In many hospitals if a woman is separated from her baby, which of course you would be with a premie, the visiting hours for fathers are shortened. But this is the time when *you need your mate the most.* Do whatever you have to in order to have as much time together as possible—whether it means getting special permission from the hospital administration or just ignoring the rigid visiting hours.

***Get yourself moved to a different division*** of the hospital or at least get a private room, so that you are not subjected to the routine care of full-term babies. It is hard enough to deal with the complex emotions of a premature delivery without having other mothers and babies right under your nose. You will probably have an empty feeling: your uterus is emptied but you have no baby to hold. It can only hurt more to be around normal babies and mothers.

### GUILT

Guilt can be a strong feeling: a premature delivery can make you feel like a failure and can be a blow to your self-esteem. You perceive it as a comment on your "inferiority" and feel guilty that it is your "fault." These feelings are irrational, clearly, but they are common feelings nevertheless. Unless you face these feelings they can affect your relationship with the child. This underlying feeling of your own "badness" translates to your being an "unfit mother" with the net result of distancing you from the child. The longer this withdrawal persists—and it can be subtle—the more the possibility arises of "deprivation syndromes" developing in the baby. Some such syndromes are "failure to thrive," in which a baby deteriorates physically because of insufficient affection, or a "battered" child.

It is very important to *verbalize* these feelings. Talk with your mate. Talk with sympathetic doctors, midwives, or nurses. Parent "rap sessions" can be most helpful. You have to face the difficulties of the small baby and wrestle with the guilt you are feeling because of the prematurity. Passivity and withdrawal mean that you will have an increasingly hard time adjusting.

### THE SHOCK OF SEEING A PREMIE

You should have a chair nearby the first time you see your baby in the neonatal intensive care nursery in case you feel faint. It is beneficial to see pictures of premies ahead of time and get a verbal description of the equipment that will invariably be attached to your baby. This will lessen the discrepancy—and therefore the shock—between what you expect, a chubby "Gerber" baby, and what you will see.

A premie bears little resemblance to a full-term newborn. Their earlobes are often just skin flaps at the sides of their heads and their eyes may be fused shut. Their skin is a dusky red color no matter what race the baby is: normal pigmentation comes about a month later. The infants have no ability to control their body temperature; their skin is like gelatin, not a good barrier to infection or water loss. Very premature babies are so delicate that their brittle bones can break easily: the amount of calcium a full-term baby naturally gets from her mother cannot be reproduced in the Intensive Care Nursery. The Directory of Growth Patterns of Premies on page 569 can give you some idea of what you might expect your premature infant to look like.

You may feel frightened and repulsed by the sight of your baby and those feelings toward your own child may make you feel guilty unless you know they are normal reactions. The baby will most likely be scrawny and naked with tubes coming out of her nose and/or umbilical cord, wires attached to her chest, labored breathing, ominous-looking equipment like a plastic hood around her head, flashing and beeping machines, and perhaps bandages over her eyes. She will hardly resemble the cuddly pink infant you had fantasized snuggling in your arms. The sight of all this equipment may not only stun and revolt you, but will probably also increase the anxiety you've already been feeling. There is usually one-to-one nursing in an intensive care unit, so ask the nurse assigned to your baby to explain all the contraptions. It will not only help you feel less put off by them, but you may be able to appreciate the good they are doing for the baby.

### PROBLEMS FEELING CLOSE TO THE BABY

*Your relationship to the baby will be influenced by your "coping attitude."* It is better to be worried, to ask questions, to *grapple* with your feelings than to repress these urges. Your coping attitude can be measured to some degree by the presence of four elements: high anxiety, seeking information, maternal feelings, even before seeing or holding the baby, and support from your mate. If you are going through the adjustment with these characteristics it is a good sign of effective coping.

*Feeling that the baby belongs to the hospital,* that the staff and machines control the baby, is common. Premie mothers and fathers often don't think of the baby as "mine" until they get her home—*but that is too long to delay your bonding.* There is a tendency, especially in the medically overwhelming setting of the intensive-care nursery, to feel inferior to the nurses. You may feel "bad" or "inadequate"; nurses should encourage your participation in diapering and other tasks. However, it is not uncommon for there to be jealousy between a nurse and a mother, and it's important for you to establish who's in charge—or at least who is the mother.

*Involvement will overcome these feelings.* Get confidence and lessons from the nurses in holding, feeding, and diapering your baby. Try to minimize your separation from the baby to whatever extent you can. Participate where possible and make a special effort to establish eye-to-eye contact with the baby—this gives you reinforcing feedback and is fundamental to maternal-infant bonding.

***Breast-feeding is excellent*** because it gives you a chance to make a tangible contribution. If the baby is not yet strong enough to suck, you can express breast milk with the help of a nurse if you want, and it can be fed to the baby through the nasogastric tube. When the baby gets stronger you can actually breast-feed. The breast milk can reduce infections and other complications, which is particularly important for a premie. Please see page 656 of the breast-feeding section for important information about the special qualities of breast milk for premature babies.

***The longer a woman delays in becoming attached*** to a premie, the harder it will be. It is *very serious* if a woman does not visit the nursery or ask about her baby. Delay in naming the baby and referring to him as "it" is also a critical problem. *The establishment of the mothering process is endangered.*

***Maternal-infant bonding is vital for premies*** and their mothers. Studies have shown that simply by touching and stroking a premie, a mother can improve the infant's breathing, physical development, weight gain, and relaxation. Hospitals that recognize this benefit allow a mother to hold her baby while she is being fed through a nasogastric tube—but *only* if a nurse or doctor has tried it first and there is no possibility of failure. If you hold the baby during feeding, she relaxes and digests more easily. You should bottle-feed the baby only if a doctor or nurse has successfully bottle-fed the child several times already—it can be devastating to your self-esteem about mothering if it does not go smoothly.

The child's development is positively influenced by close contact. She does better if the mother feeds and cares for her through the incubator. If a baby is touched, rocked, and fondled daily, she develops better and more quickly—and since there is a personnel shortage in any hospital, you should *fight* to get into the nursery if necessary.

A premie only has short periods of wakefulness, so it can be discouraging for you. If the baby is usually asleep you cannot establish eye-to-eye contact and other feedback;

you will need encouragement from the staff and your mate. But some alternative to separation of premies and their mothers is necessary. Twenty-five to 40 percent of all battered children in this country were premature infants. Child abuse and neglect are a severe social problem and are correlated with immediate and prolonged separation at birth.

## POSTTERM (POSTMATURE) PREGNANCY

Traditionally, a pregnancy prolonged past the 42nd week is considered postterm. At most, 4 percent of pregnancies are truly carried 2 weeks or more beyond the average time but in many cases the due date has been miscalculated.

There are two reasons for errors in calculating postmaturity. One is that ovulation took place several weeks later than the usual 14th day of the cycle—impregnation therefore did not take place until 40 or 50 days after the onset of the last period. The other reason is that there has been an error in menstrual dates. In some cases, however, a pregnancy actually does go beyond the usual 40 weeks. After 280 days in utero a baby gains little weight. In fact, he may lose weight: a typical postmature baby is thin, scrawny and old looking, with loose, baggy skin, long nails, an abundance of scalp hair and a very alert look. They gain back the weight after birth.

There are several tests which can be done (amniocentesis, ultrasound, OCT, etc.) to determine whether a baby is postmature. If these tests are not normal—if an OCT is positive or meconium is present in the amniotic fluid—delivery should be immediate. However, normal test results do not necessarily mean that there is no postmaturity syndrome. There is no clear-cut solution if, for instance, the OCT is negative and amniotic fluid is not available for testing.

The reason to determine whether a baby is postterm, and if so, to deliver him immediately, is because there is a risk of fetal distress in postterm babies in labor. Some studies show that the risk of waiting for spontaneous labor in a postterm baby is higher than the potential hazard of induction or a C-section. Other studies do not confirm that the postterm fetus has a special intolerance to labor. One solution might be to allow such a fetus to go into labor but then use fetal monitoring with particular care to watch for distress.

*Cervical ripening* by self-stimulation of nipples can be done at term. Some doctors recommend it for low-risk patients, as it may shorten labor and prevent the complications of postmaturity. The woman is instructed to stimulate her nipples until they are erect for one hour, 3 times a day for 2 days. WARNING: THIS SHOULD ONLY BE ATTEMPTED UNDER A DOCTOR'S INSTRUCTIONS.

*Prostaglandin gels* are used to stimulate prostaglandin production, which helps to thin the cervix in preparation for induction of labor.

## BREECH PRESENTATION

In over 96 percent of births the baby is in a cephalic (fetal head leading) presentation; in 3 percent of cases the baby is in breech position (buttocks lead). In less than 1 percent of pregnancies, a baby is in some other unusual position. There are several types of breech presentations: *complete* (the baby is cross-legged in the bottom of the uterus); *frank* (his legs are straight up with his feet near his face); *footling* (a rare position in which one foot or both come down first); and *knee* (an even more rare occurrence with the knee presenting).

Another presentation which can cause complications is *posterior vertex* in which the baby faces your abdomen on his way down the birth canal: normally he would face your tailbone. This can cause painful back labor. If the baby does not turn before he is born, the doctor may have to rotate his head with forceps. There are also two very rare versions of the cephalic position: *face* or *brow* presentation. The fetus's head, instead of being flexed down chin on chest, is extended so that he delivers with his face presenting rather than the top of his head. His features may appear swollen with contusions as if he's been in a fight, but this will disappear within 48 hours. The final unusual position is *transverse lie:* the baby is lying sideways in your uterus, and unless it can be manipulated into a cephalic position, he will have to be delivered by cesarean.

## CAUSES FOR A BREECH PRESENTATION

- A small or premature baby
- A large baby who may not have enough room to settle head-down into your pelvis
- Excess amniotic fluid, which allows the baby to float around instead of engaging in your pelvis
- Multiple pregnancy
- Placenta previa
- Contracted pelvis
- Uterine tumors
- A hydrocephalic baby with water on the brain, making the head oversize

## THE DANGERS OF A BREECH PRESENTATION

The danger is equal whether this is your first baby or a subsequent one. Because there are so many risks in a breech presentation the current medical practice is to deliver all breeches by cesarean section. There are *some* situations in which *some* doctors will attempt a vaginal delivery (see pages 580–582) but generally the dangers outweigh the benefits of a normal delivery.

In 1980 the National Institutes of Health (NIH) studied breech births and found that in 1970 only 11.6 percent of breech births were delivered by cesarean while in 1978 it had risen to 60 percent. There was concern about this trend toward routinely performing a C-section for full-term breech babies, since the outcome of the deliveries in terms of mortality was not improved.

The NIH task force did find that three categories of breech presentations did better if delivered by cesarean: the large fetus over 8 pounds, the fetus presenting as a complete or footling breech, and the fetus with marked hyperextension of the head. For babies under 2,500 grams the study found no consistent difference between those delivered vaginally or by C-section and hence made no recommendation for small breech babies.

The task force did recommend that vaginal delivery of the term breech should remain an acceptable obstetrical choice for delivery, when the following conditions are present: (1) anticipated fetal weight of less than 8 pounds, (2) normal pelvic dimensions and architecture, (3) frank breech presentation without a hyperextended head, and (4) delivery to be conducted by a physician experienced in vaginal breech delivery. See section on vaginal delivery on the following page.

*Labor can be longer or simply not progress* because the buttocks are not as good a wedge to dilate the cervix as the head would be. The birth canal cannot be as effectively molded open; when the head exits last it has no time to be molded in the birth canal and may not be able to descend all the way out.

*The after-coming head is usually larger* than any other part of the baby that has come down first. Therefore especially with premies or small babies, the cervix does not need to dilate fully because the body is small enough to get through—but the cervix may not have opened enough to allow the head to pass through *or* the cervix may close around the baby's neck after the shoulders have slipped through.

*Prolapse of the cord* occurs in 4 to 5 percent of breech births, which is 10 times the normal frequency of this dangerous complication in which the umbilical cord comes down before anything else. With prolapse there is a chance of the cord being compressed and cutting off the baby's blood supply. It necessitates an immediate cesarean section.

*The cord can be compressed* in its passage through the pelvis, cutting off the baby's oxygen supply.

*Fractures, dislocations, and nerve damage* are all more common in vaginal breech deliveries because of the already mentioned complications in getting out.

### VAGINAL DELIVERY WITH A BREECH PRESENTATION

This is an alternative to a C-section that some doctors will attempt if it is very important to you. If you are aware of the potential complications in a breech delivered "from below," yet a vaginal delivery matters to you, seek out a doctor who will try it. This does not mean seeking out a doctor who will deliver a breech vaginally because he does not know or respect the potential dangers or who has not had experience but needs your business, for instance. It is essential that you find a doctor who will do every possible examination ahead of time and then will know what to do in the possible event that labor does not progress normally.

You should also be aware that you may be disappointed if your motivation in attempting vaginal delivery is because you want a "natural, normal birth." A vaginal delivery calls for high-risk management. If you meet the requirements for a vaginal delivery you will have to be closely watched on a fetal monitor: the prevailing attitude will be "poised for emergency." You might even be required to go through labor and delivery in the cesarean section room with an anesthesiologist in attendance so that a cesarean can be done immediately if it becomes necessary. There are very real potential dangers and the atmosphere may be tense.

In a breech delivered vaginally the buttocks and genitals are often swollen and discolored. They can be black-and-blue because they came down first and were battered against your cervix and the walls of the birth canal. This clears up quickly and causes no permanent damage.

*Before you can attempt a vaginal delivery,* the doctor will want to know whether your pelvic structure will allow the baby's head through. What they want to learn beforehand is whether there is cephalopelvic disproportion—whether, given the baby's size and position, and given the shape and size of your pelvis, there may not be room for the baby's head to fit through. The problem with breeches is that this disproportion may not be discovered until the baby's body is born. Ultrasound can be used to get a measurement of the baby's head size, her "biparietal diameter." If you have what is known medically as an "inadequate pelvis" (a rather insulting term for it!) or if the baby's head is not well flexed, with the chin up rather than resting down on her chest), these would be contraindications for a vaginal delivery.

***The baby's weight should not be less than 5 pounds or more than 8 pounds.*** A baby over 8 pounds is likely to have a large head that may not be able to descend; a small baby's body can slip through a partially dilated cervix, which may then close around her neck. One reason that routine C-sectioning is done on breeches is that it isn't possible to accurately predict a baby's weight ahead of time.

***Once you are in labor*** if there is any fetal distress or labor does not progress well, the doctor will undoubtedly perform a cesarean. It is thought that a labor lasting longer than 16 to 18 hours may be risky for you or for the baby. There may be a halt in the progress of labor for any of the reasons already mentioned—the baby is "hung up" and cannot descend. Fetal distress can be caused by this lack of progress or problems with the umbilical cord. Meconium, a dark, tarry substance from the fetus's large intestine, may be expelled after your membranes rupture. More will be expelled with each contraction, so if you are not yet in the hospital when this happens, wear a sanitary pad or a clean cloth and report it to the doctor *immediately*. When a baby is not receiving enough oxygen (is "in distress"), his anal sphincter relaxes and passes meconium, which he can swallow.

***Gravity is the greatest helper*** in labor in breech and posterior presentations. You should be sitting as much upright as possible. If you can do it, sit bolt upright with your knees spread wide and the soles of your feet together to aid in the baby's descent. In home deliveries where vaginal delivery of a breech is attempted (which is not a wise idea) they often use a hands-and-knees position so that gravity helps pull the baby out.

*Piper forceps* are a special kind of gentle forceps used only for delivering breech babies. They are not used to pull the baby out but only to keep his head flexed down.

*Ways to try to turn the baby out of a breech position before labor.* You have nothing to lose; and if it is successful, you will be able to have a normal delivery rather than a C-section or a high-risk vaginal delivery.

1. THE DOCTOR CAN TRY TO ROTATE the baby from the outside. During late pregnancy or early labor a doctor can try to convert a breech to a head presentation. He grasps the fetus externally through your abdominal wall and turns her 180 degrees by gradually pushing the buttocks to one side with one hand and the head and shoulders to the opposite side with his other hand. Although this external manipulation can turn the baby, she will often revert right back to the breech position as soon as the doctor releases her.

2. THE TILT POSTURE has been successful for some women. It is an exercise you should start around the 30th week of pregnancy and continue for at least 4 to 6 weeks. Obviously this can only be used by women who know in advance that their babies are breech. You lie on your back on the floor with your pelvis raised to a level 9 to 12 inches off the floor by three large pillows under your buttocks. Your knees should be bent and your feet flat on the floor—the position is awkward: if it's not very comfortable you're doing it right! You should do this twice a day on an empty stomach and stay in the position for 10 minutes each time. Many babies have been encouraged to shift to a head presentation by this method.

## TWINS

Multiple births, of which twins are the most common, are included as a "complication of pregnancy" because they pose increased risks.

*Greater likelihood of premature labor* exists with twins and all premature babies are at greater risk for a variety of complications. If you are carrying twins you should avoid physical strain and if possible give up work at 24 weeks instead of the usual 34 weeks. You should also give up traveling at around 24 weeks, to be on the safe side. Some doctors recommend giving up sexual intercourse during the last 3 months of pregnancy because of the possibility of a prematurely dilated cervix or the early onset of labor.

*There is increased liability to toxemia* in a multiple pregnancy. Be sure you eat extremely well with a lot of high-quality protein, take long afternoon rest periods, and increase the number of prenatal visits to the doctor or midwife.

*Mortality risk* to twins is 4 times greater than in single births. The factor responsible is the large proportion of twins weighing less than 4½ pounds—any baby with low birth weight has a higher mortality rate and possibility of complications. Twin babies are sharing nutrition, oxygen, and pelvic quarters and thus are often premature or low birth weight.

*Greater proportion of sluggish labors* occurs with twins than in single births. There is an increased incidence of uterine inertia and poor, inadequate contractions. These problems are all probably because the uterus has been overdistended during pregnancy. The labor and delivery for twins is usually shorter than for single births because the cervix is often partially dilated before labor begins and the fetuses are usually smaller.

Spontaneous labor is preferable with twins. Analgesic

or anesthetic medications are especially dangerous to multiple births, as they are a risk to any fetus: it is desirable to have no (or minimal) medication. This decreases the chance of blood loss and the babies, which are usually smaller than average, are safer without drugs to interfere with their breathing. It is important that you know how to push effectively because the uterine walls have been stretched thinner so the contractions may not be as effective. Pushing properly will make the births easier on you and the babies.

It is also not uncommon for there to be a cord prolapse with multiple births—the cord descends before anything else, potentially cutting off the babies' blood supply. This necessitates performing a cesarean.

*Unusual presentations* of the fetuses are common. There are many combinations of fetal positions, with one baby vertex (head first) and the second baby breech as the most common presentation. The next most frequent is for both babies to be in a cephalic (head first) position. Five to 10 minutes are allowed to elapse before delivery of the second twin. The membranes usually have to be ruptured around the second baby, which is usually smaller. The doctor determines what the presenting part is and, if necessary, manipulates him to a better position by reaching up into your uterus and turning the baby.

*The discomforts of pregnancy are doubled.* Breathlessness, varicose veins, hemorrhoids, insomnia, and edema can all be twice as bad as in a single pregnancy. The twins take up more room and demand more from your circulatory system which can increase minor discomforts.

*The likelihood of producing twins* is a hereditary tendency. If multiple births are passed on in a family, it affects both men and women and such families have several instances of twins on almost every branch of their family trees, not just an occasional pair. This tendency to twinning does not skip generations—if it is true of your family, then it will be expressed in succeeding generations.

Twins happen 1 in 86 births. Women who are 35 to

40 years old are 3 times more likely to have twins than a woman under 20. Black women are more likely to produce them than Caucasians, and Caucasians are more likely to have twins than Orientals. A woman who has already had a pair of twins is 3 to 10 times more likely to have twins again than a woman who has had a single birth. It should also be noted that even with all the sophisticated tests available it is not uncommon for twins to remain undiagnosed and come as a surprise to everyone.

More twins will be born in the U.S. than ever before: more women are having babies at a later age, when the odds of giving birth to twins rises, and the increased use of fertility drugs and in vitro fertilization increases the chances of multiple births. Also, women who become pregnant soon after going off birth-control pills also have a higher chance of bearing twins.

***Twins can present health problems*** that result in developmental delays. Multiple births are a health risk to the babies, since half of all twins arrive prematurely, on the average 4 weeks early. The greatest risk for these children is underdeveloped lungs, although they may also have less mature nervous systems and be more likely to have ruptured blood vessels in the brain. The risk to the mother carrying twins is increased incidence of anemia, high blood pressure, and hemorrhage after delivery. Birth itself can be more complicated, and as a result, about half of all twins are delivered by cesarean section, as compared to 20 percent of all births.

Twins may not reach all the developmental stages "on time" because they are premature, but this is ordinarily only a temporary delay. By the time they are 3 years old, premature babies have generally caught up with other children in physical and mental development.

***Twins can cause stress in a relationship*** because of the added pressure they put on a marriage. There is the financial burden of having to provide two of everything at once: from high chairs to college educations. This stress on the family puts twins at greater risk of being abused children; there is also a higher rate of postpartum depression in the mothers of twins because of the exhaustion. However, if a couple is aware of these potential problems it can go a long way towards lessening the stress on the marriage.

*Identical twins (monozygotic)* are the result of one egg being fertilized by one sperm. The germ plasm of the 2 offspring is identical: they are of the same sex and exactly alike in skin, hair, and eye color. Identical twins are much less common.

*Fraternal twins (dizygotic)* are the result of 2 different eggs fertilized by 2 different spermatozoa. The eggs may be from the same ovary or opposite ovaries. If twins are a boy and girl, if their blood groups differ even slightly, and/or if they are nonidentical they must be from two different eggs. Fraternal twins each have a separate placenta or there are 3 or 4 membranes in the partition wall of a single placenta rather than the usual 2 membranes. Even if twins are the same sex they are most likely fraternal—and bear no greater resemblance to each other than regular siblings.

## POLYHYDRAMNIOS

This is a complication of pregnancy in which you have too much amniotic fluid. Normally there is approximately 1 liter (slightly over 1 quart) of fluid—if there is more than about 2 quarts it is considered polyhydramnios. The condition is often associated with diabetes, toxemia, or multiple births, but the cause is not known for sure. In 20 percent of pregnancies with polyhydramnios there is a congenital malformation of the baby, especially of the nervous system and gastrointestinal tract. A normal baby swallows amniotic fluid—which may be one way that the amount of fluid is controlled—but a baby with an intestinal obstruction, for instance, cannot swallow.

During pregnancy polyhydramnios can cause greater than normal edema (swelling) of the legs and vulva, difficulty breathing and sleeping, indigestion, heartburn, and constipation, all because of the extra pressure the additional fluid places on your system. The condition also has its effects on labor. The cord is more likely to prolapse. Premature labor can occur because your uterus is over-stretched. Unusual presentations are more common because the baby can float around more. Labor may also be slower because the uterine muscles are stretched out and the baby's presenting part may float around in the excess fluid rather than engage in your pelvis, which would help to dilate the cervix. The overstretched uterus may also result in post-partum hemorrhage.

There is a relatively high prenatal mortality rate associated with polyhydramnios; the rate increases as the amount of fluid increases. If you have a severe form of this condition, you should see an obstetrician who specializes in high-risk pregnancies.

## PLACENTA PREVIA

In this complication of pregnancy the placenta is situated low down in the uterus instead of at the top of it and blocks the cervix so the baby cannot exit. It is rare in a first pregnancy and occurs 1 in 200 births—the risks increase with subsequent births. The symptom is vaginal bleeding during the last trimester.

Blood transfusions can protect the mother but are risky for the baby, especially when she must be delivered prematurely. The mother is hospitalized, transfused as necessary, and observed until tests show that the baby is judged to be 5½ pounds. Then the mother is taken to the operating room. If the doctor can feel a lot of placenta blocking the cervix he will perform a cesarean. If he cannot feel any placenta or only a small sliver of it then he will rupture the membranes and induce labor. Six in 10 women with placenta previa are given a cesarean and 4 in 10 are delivered vaginally.

## PLACENTA ABRUPTIO

Placenta abruptio is the premature separation of part or all of the placenta from the uterine wall—normally it would separate from the uterus after the birth of the baby. It is a rare occurrence, most likely in women who have had 5 or 6 babies (grand multiparas). It is 3 times as common for them as women having a first baby. This complication has a tendency to recur: it repeats in 10 percent of subsequent pregnancies.

The symptoms are the same as for placenta previa: vaginal bleeding accompanied by abdominal pain in the last weeks of pregnancy before labor begins. As with placenta previa it can cause premature delivery. Although the mother is likely to survive the possible hemorrhage with blood transfusions, the danger to the baby is grave in placenta abruptio because his oxygen supply is cut off. A cesarean delivery may be indicated.

## CEPHALOPELVIC DISPROPORTION (CPD)

Cephalopelvic disproportion (CPD) means that the fetus's head is larger than your pelvic opening and therefore the baby cannot fit through and be born vaginally. Twenty-five to 40 percent of first-time cesareans are done because of CPD, or "failure to progress." However, there is a misunderstanding about CPD—some doctors may tell a woman before she has gone into labor that she has a "definite" cephalopelvic disproportion and must have a cesarean. The truth is that CPD is *not* a condition that can be determined absolutely before labor begins, because, in theory, *any fetal head can fit through any pelvis.* During pregnancy your body produces hormones, progestins, which allow your pelvic structure to expand, which is why walking may be difficult or you may be ungainly as your pregnancy advances. It is said that theoretically the female body is built to be able to deliver up to a 15-pound baby. Of course, in reality there aren't many babies that big, and some women's pelvises will not expand enough to allow passage of a baby of even half that size.

The point is that it is incorrect to tell you that you have *definite* cephalopelvic disproportion *before* you go into labor. Although it is possible to get a good estimate of the proportion of your pelvis compared to the size of the baby's head beforehand with ultrasound, there is no way of knowing for certain until you are in labor whether there is room for the baby's head to exit. It is your muscles and joints that have to expand in order for the baby to fit through: the size of your pelvic opening is not fixed, it will increase. It is a question of whether it will increase enough to allow the baby to exit vaginally.

The decision to perform a cesarean should be based on your progress in labor as well as the baby's position and size. Do not trust any doctor who tells you ahead of time that you *must* have a cesarean because of cephalopelvic disproportion. Once you are in labor, the effect of the hormone *relaxin* on your connective tissue may allow your joints to expand enough to permit the baby to pass through. If a doctor tells you before your due date that a C-section is necessary, seek a second opinion and *keep on practicing your prepared childbirth techniques.* Inform yourself about cesareans, see the section on Cesarean Birth (538–565), but don't give up hope of a vaginal delivery until it is clear during labor that a C-section is necessary.

## FORCEPS DELIVERY

Forceps are large, curved metal tongs. The two sides of the tongs are put into your vagina separately and slipped up inside on either side of the baby's head. The tongs are then locked together outside, something like a one-piece salad server, and the doctor pulls the baby out by her head. Some doctors use forceps routinely on women having their first baby—be sure to ask ahead of time whether your doctor practices this way. There *is* a use for forceps . . . but *not* as a routine procedure. Forceps can save a baby's life in a complicated birth but no other country uses them for as many normal births as in the United States. Judgment, caution, and skill are required.

## THE THREE KINDS OF FORCEPS DELIVERY

*High-forceps* is done very rarely nowadays. The cesarean section has replaced high-forceps as a way to deliver a baby that will not descend.

*Mid- or Low-forceps* is used only when absolutely necessary because it involves inserting the forceps quite high and exerting a lot of pull on the baby. Low-forceps delivery is defined as intervening when the baby's head has descended below your ischial spines. A low-forceps delivery may be necessary if anesthesia has made it impossible for you to push the baby out.

*Outlet or perineal forceps* is quite common and is used when the baby's head is visible at the perineum, or the scalp can be clearly seen if the lips of your vagina are spread open. The forceps are used to lift the baby out of the vagina.

### The usual reasons for a forceps delivery:

- To speed up second-stage labor if there is severe fetal distress.
- If the cord is wrapped tightly around the baby's neck, which occurs in approximately 25 percent of deliveries, or the cord prolapses.
- In case of unusual presentations.
- To shorten a very long second stage of labor.
- If regional anesthesia doesn't allow you to push the baby out.

### COMPLICATIONS

Complications of forceps delivery are rare—the common problem is that the forceps can bruise the baby's head but the bruises disappear in a few days. The rare occurrence is that the pressure of the forceps can cause intracranial hemorrhage and damage to the infant's facial nerves.

There are also some formerly unrecognized long-term effects that may not manifest themselves until early adulthood. Grand mal seizures in young adults are on the increase in this country. The theoretical hypothesis is that intracranial hemorrhage causes the process of gliosis to occur: as the glia cells (scar tissue) continue to accumulate over the years, eventually these cells thicken to the point where they may interfere with the normal functioning of the brain.

## CONGENITAL MALFORMATIONS

There is something wrong with a baby in 2 out of every 100 births. Depending on how severe the defect is, many of the usual reactions to birth will be suppressed. You can be reluctant to name the child and send birth announcements. People may be at a loss about the appropriate way to respond and may not send flowers or telephone you. It can be lonely.

There are 5 stages of reactions which parents usually go through and which you can expect to experience if your baby is born with a congenital malformation:

*Shock:* You will feel helpless, cry, and perhaps have an urge to run away.

*Disbelief (denial):* You cannot believe that it has happened to you.

*Sadness, anger, and anxiety:* These feelings will be directed toward yourself, the doctor or midwife, the hospital, and fate or God. Do not intellectualize the grief—do not put up a defensive wall and think, Aha, this is the third stage and it is predictable that I will feel angry and sad. If your baby has a defect, you and your mate will be mourning the loss of the "perfect" dreamed-of infant. You should allow yourselves to feel the strength and depth of that grieving.

*Equilibrium:* Within a few weeks or months you will reach a more even keel. However, this adaptation can be incomplete and you may find yourself in tears years after the baby's birth.

*Reorganization:* You accept the situation and go on with your lives.

These stages are something that you and your mate both have to go through—the danger is that this process can create a problem in your relationship. If you both don't go through the states of adaptation at the same speed it can isolate you from each other. And if you do not keep the lines of communication open it can split you apart. A trauma like this can magnify the weaknesses in a partnership, whereas the easy birth of a normal child more often highlights the strengths in a relationship. It is vital that you both recognize the potential problems a malformed baby can cause to your union. Either one of you may start drinking heavily to escape the situation or you may have an affair for the same reason. The sequel to this book, *Childbirth & Marriage,* covers this topic in depth.

*Take things day by day.* Try not to worry excessively. Tranquilizers are often prescribed, but you should try to refuse them. Drugs will only blunt your natural responses and slow your adaptation to the problem. If you cannot sleep at night you may want to accept a tranquilizer, but if at all possible, avoid using them during the day. A doctor may prescribe drugs because it is easier on him than having to cope with the full force of your feelings—he may also feel he's doing you a favor by lessening the blow. In the long run you are better off venting your feelings so that you can resolve them in due time.

*Have rooming-in* even if your instinctive reaction is to never want to see the child or to hope she dies. The sooner you adjust to the reality the better off you'll be. The sooner your maternal feelings develop, the easier it will become, and spending time with the baby will facilitate this process.

*Talk to the pediatrician* and elicit his support and advice. If you had already selected a doctor you liked and trusted before the baby was born, avoid the temptation to "doctor-shop." Sometimes parents will go in search of other diagnoses as to the reason for the child's defect. This may come from a sense of guilt on their part; this kind of quest will only delay your ability to face the situation and cope with it.

*"Chronic sorrow"* is experienced by some parents of malformed children. They are not able—or it takes them a long time—to overcome their grief about the baby's condition. Chronic sorrow may to some degree affect all parents of congenitally deformed children; it may be unreasonable to expect the painful impact on a family simply to disappear.

Parents of children with birth defects can now receive helpful information through a nationwide support group called Association of Birth Defect Children, Inc. (3201 E. Crystal Lake Avenue, Orlando, Florida 32806). ABDC provides support and information through a free quarterly newsletter for families of children with congenital malformations thought to be caused by the mother's exposure to drugs, chemicals, and environmental agents, as well as children with genetically linked defects.

*If you have a Down's syndrome baby,* it is important to have the baby tested. There are two kinds of Down's syndrome, also known as mongolism, and which one your child has will indicate what your odds are of giving birth to another baby with this abnormality.

The *sporadic variety* recurs in 1 percent of subsequent births. The *translocation variety* recurs in 8 percent of subsequent births. If a couple has a child with translocation-type Down's syndrome, both parents should have chromosomal tests. If the mother is a carrier, there is a 12 to 15 percent chance of recurrence in future pregnancies. If the father is a carrier, the chance of recurrence is only 2 to 4 percent. If both parents are normal, then the possibility of Down's recurring is the same as for people who had sporadic variety offspring: only 1 percent.

## FETAL SURGERY

This is a new science with thrilling possibilities for the future, although at present its applications are controversial and limited. It has been found that, while still inside the uterus, the fetus can tolerate corrective surgery, done either by opening the womb or not. However, the method is so new that the risks—and benefits—are still being weighed. There are only a few medical centers around the country equipped to perform prenatal intervention, and so far only a few fetuses have been treated.

With the aid of sophisticated prenatal diagnosis, obstetricians are able to detect serious conditions in the fetus early enough to treat some of them before irreparable damage is done. At the moment there are only four conditions that are considered correctable by experts. One is hydrocephalus, an accumulation of fluid under pressure in the brain that causes brain damage. A second is a urinary-tract obstruction called hydronephrosis, a blockage in the urethra. The third condition is diaphragmatic hernia, a hole in the diaphragm that allows the intestines to be pressed up against the lungs. Surgeons are able to drain excess fluid from fetal cavities and leave behind tiny draining tubes, called catheters, that stay in place until birth. Experts can also use fetal surgery to correct some of the heart defects that impair thousands of newborns every year.

However, there are many cautionary voices in the field. For one thing, it is known that an affected fetus often has a cluster of defects that may have damaged several organ systems. Doctors agree that it may not be wise to correct a heart defect, for instance, only to find out at birth that the fetus's brain is also severely damaged. And in the case of hydrocephalus, many times it is due to problems that may not be corrected simply by unplugging an obstruction—yet one cannot tell in advance. Also, no one yet knows whether relieving the fluid pressure actually prevents brain damage. In addition, even in the correctable form, hydrocephalus is often accompanied by other brain-development problems that may be beyond repair.

It is important for parents to realize how many unanswered questions there are in this field. If a couple is told that their baby is affected, they may be overly eager to accept these still-experimental procedures—without recognizing that their baby may still be very sick when he is born. Another issue rarely raised is the cost of fetal surgery. Even when fetal surgeons do not charge for their services, the corollary costs before, during, and after the surgery can easily run into tens of thousands of dollars, much of which an insurance company may not be willing pay since these procedures are experimental.

Doctors are still wrestling with the complicated questions of exactly which fetuses to treat and when. They do not yet know whether they are salvaging fetuses that will become profoundly retarded or otherwise handicapped children. They don't know whether they are operating on fetuses who would have survived intact without their help, or whether they are achieving their hoped-for goal of producing healthy, normal children who might otherwise have died.

## DEATH OF A BABY

Although the tragedy of a baby dying at birth or soon thereafter is an unlikely occurrence, it is still a possibility. Stillbirths are a reality of life even though they are rare in the socioeconomic group that takes childbirth education classes, for instance. There is the same lack of faith in a couple's ability to cope with death as there has been about their ability to cope with birth. This attitude—on the part of the medical community—is changing. The most responsive care-givers are aware that if a couple's baby does die, there are certain stages they will necessarily go through and certain steps they can take to cope most effectively.

Death is difficult for hospital personnel. It is important for them to help you confront and resolve your grief, but they rarely can do it. Even though you might think that care-givers have seen enough death to be able to deal with it, the truth is that it frightens, overwhelms, and saddens them—and they often withdraw from you because they don't know what to do.

Doctors also have trouble acknowledging death. Most doctors are not helpful unless they have had special training in helping people with the grieving process—which is unlikely, considering they don't even have training in the psychological aspects of *birth*. A doctor often prescribes sedatives for a woman whose baby has died even though this can actively interfere with the healthy resolution of grief. Some doctors do this routinely because they don't know what else to do. Regardless of the cause of the baby's death it can make a doctor feel guilty and inadequate—and your emotions afterward can just increase that feeling for him. Early discharge from the hospital is just one of the ways that care-givers protect themselves from sadness about death. If you and your mate are aware that you cannot realistically expect support and advice, then you will depend more on each other to get through this difficult time.

***The stages of your psychological reaction*** to your baby's death are fairly predictable. One thing you may feel is *somatic distress:* a feeling of tightness in your throat and a shortness of breath. These are ways that your body expresses the anxiety and sadness you feel. You may have a *preoccupation* with the image of the dead baby—it may "haunt" you when you are awake or asleep. You will probably also feel *guilt* and *hostility*. You will probably experience a *loss of the usual patterns of conduct*—you may feel disoriented, confused, and out of control of your life. These are the normal processes that people go through after a death.

***Grieving is a natural and normal process.*** You have to go through it one way or another. It will be better if you accept that grieving is something you must *do* rather than something that has happened to you. You and your mate have to talk, share tears, and not deny your own *or* other people's feelings.

A man's feelings might be ignored because American men are not trained to show their emotions. They often don't know how and others don't expect them to. A man may take on extra work in his business or increase other tasks so that he is constantly busy. A woman should try to draw out her mate—for her good as well as his. Feelings that are denied can surface in unexpected ways. A couple can find new strength together if they can face and fully experience the tragedy that has befallen them.

**Explain to siblings** why you are crying or are moody. It is good for both of you to express your feelings as openly as you want but it is very important to explain this to young children who see the world as revolving around them. Children may think you are upset and angry at them. They also may worry that they are responsible for the baby's death. It is not uncommon for siblings to have bad thoughts about an impending baby and they may be afraid they caused her death unless you explain what happened and why you are feeling as you do.

**When a dead baby is seen by both parents it facilitates the grieving process.** You can move forward from the same frame of reference to an eventual resolution of your feelings. If you wish, you should visit even a seriously ill infant in the intensive care nursery. Seeing him can help you deal with the reality. If you wish to see or touch the baby when he has died, do so. If you have that inclination, be sure to act on it—it can help make the death a reality. Even seeing a photograph of the baby after death can be beneficial to you and your mate. Holding the baby can help you accept the reality of death and thus allows you to begin the growing process of resolving your grief.

**Have a simple funeral.** The traditional rituals promote grieving and make the death real. Although you may fear that it will only make you feel worse, it can release and relieve many emotions. However, it should be a simple ceremony with *only family present.* The point of the ritual is to help you and the presence of even the closest friends may add to your already heavy emotional burden.

**People's comments** when they learn that your baby has died can be disturbing. People don't intend to upset you but everyone feels helpless and ill at ease when there is a death and they say whatever they can. One comment you can depend on hearing is "You can have another." Although that probably is true, it is quite beside the point when you are trying to cope with your feelings about the baby you have been awaiting for so long who has just left you. "The baby is better off dead," is often said if there was something wrong with the baby. As far as you're concerned, the baby—and you—would be much better off if the baby were well and alive. "You must pull out of this and get involved in life again," may be some people's way of giving "constructive" advice. Unfortunately they don't know that death and the grief it produces are something you must experience in order to go on with your life. The worst thing you can do for yourselves in the beginning is to throw yourselves into work or play as a way of "forgetting" about the tragedy. There's no way to forget it; only the possibility of denying it for a while.

People's comments may make you angry; they may also make you feel lonely because there is no one to turn to who really understands. You have each other—take advantage of that. Realize that people mean well and thank them for their concern however inappropriately they may express it. Try to protect yourself from outsiders in the early period after the baby dies.

*It is recommended not to conceive again* until the mourning period is complete. This can take 6 to 12 months, even though there may be times when you feel you are "over it" sooner. Grief takes quite a long time to work itself out and you'll be cheating yourselves and another baby if you don't allow at least that long. The processes of attachment and detachment cannot easily occur simultaneously. While you are grieving it isn't possible to care fully for a new baby. Give yourselves at least 6 months to emotionally give up the baby who has died. Only then should you attempt to replace her.

*Fetal death in utero* is defined as a fetus over 500 grams or more than 20 weeks gestation. If this happens to you,

you'll probably be aware that the baby hasn't moved during a 24-hour period. You should be examined: an absence of fetal heartbeat and an ultrasound test which confirms that growth has stopped both determine whether the baby has died inside you.

Perhaps the hardest part of a fetal death in utero is that it is best to await spontaneous labor. This means that you have to walk around with the dead baby inside you, which can be a grotesque thought for some women. If labor is induced it may cause contractions but no cervical dilation—this means your cervix can tear, causing problems in subsequent pregnancies.

The wait for labor to begin can be several weeks. It is thought that labor may start naturally by a hormonal process triggered by the lack of fetal growth. Blood tests are necessary twice weekly until labor begins. After a 6-week wait it is best to induce labor because the products of conception, the fetus, placenta, and amniotic fluid, are reabsorbed into your body and can cause blood clots. It may be best not to have natural childbirth, but to be sedated. Some people feel that if this is your first pregnancy that it's better not to associate this experience with labor. However, some women may want their mates with them for this difficult labor and delivery and they may want to be awake. As mentioned, seeing and perhaps touching the baby can facilitate your grieving process.

Guilt is something women often feel about a baby that dies inside them. It is similar to the emotional experience of a miscarriage, particularly a second-trimester one. This guilt comes in part because we all believe to some degree in our own potency—that we are in control of what happens in our lives. If we are in control it is something we did—or did not do—that caused this baby to die. Thus we feel guilty. In order to get rid of that feeling we have to accept that there are things we have no power over . . . for many people, giving up the belief that they are in control means that they have to accept the terror of "the unknown." The death of a baby can force people to see that.

## SUDDEN INFANT DEATH SYNDROME (SIDS)

SIDS is defined as the sudden death of any child, unexpected by history, where a postmortem examination fails to show adequate cause for death. There are 8,000 to 10,000 such infant deaths a year in the United States; SIDS occurs in 2 to 3 per every 1,000 live births. It is the largest single cause of post-neonatal infant mortality and accounts for one-third of all infant deaths from 1 week to 1 year of age. The peak incidence for SIDS is between the 2nd and 4th months of life and it accounts for one-half of all deaths in the 3rd and 4th months.

SIDS is a specific disease entity and a common cause of infant death but its *cause* is not yet known. It is not a new disease—accounts of it go back to Old Testament days. At present there is no way to prevent or predict crib death. Studies show that it is probably significantly related to sleep, since most cases occur during normal sleeping periods. Death is rapid and silent—it is not associated with an outcry and apparently the baby does not suffer.

The most recent research emphasis on SIDS, which has also been called crib death, is shifting to the brain. Even with 20 years of research into babies who have died of SIDS, studies of their organ systems, including the heart and lungs, have failed to explain why seemingly healthy infants die in their sleep. Lacking strong clues that would identify infants who might be at risk for SIDS, researchers are turning to fundamental theories of brain development.

Scientists are still far from knowing the underlying cause of sudden infant death, but most experts now believe that SIDS babies have a subtle brain abnormality. Some researchers believe the abnormality could lie in the brain stem, which controls breathing and heart rates. Others believe that the problem may lie in brain areas controlling sleep patterns or learning processes. Still others are looking at centers that control specific functions, such as tongue muscles or regulation of body heat.

It was originally thought that suffocation was the cause of SIDS, although research has shown this not to be true. Although thousands of babies have been fitted with monitoring devices that sound an alarm when their breathing becomes irregular during sleep, experts say that the incidence of sudden infant death has not fallen.

There is a lot of misinformation and speculation about what causes crib death. These myths and rumors can unnecessarily alarm the parents of newborns, and cause additional stress for parents who have suffered the loss of a baby from SIDS. The directory that follows is intended to dispel myths and lay out what few facts *are* known about the terrible problem.

The parents have no fault in SIDS, but sometimes they are treated as if they were criminals. In many communities crib death is viewed as suffocation, neglect, or deliberate infanticide. Autopsies are very important—although they must be interpreted appropriately. Many pathologists are reluctant to call a baby's death SIDS for fear of "missing" a case of infanticide. It is bad enough to have to suffer the horrible shock of your baby dying in his sleep—it then becomes gruesome to have to deal with accusations.

Fact sheets and other printed material are very helpful to parents of SIDS victims. If your baby dies and is diagnosed or suspected of having had SIDS, you should contact the National SIDS Foundation (310 So. Michigan, Chicago, Illinois 60604, 312–663–0650) and/or The International Council for Infant Survival, Inc. (1515 Reisterstown Road, Suite 300, Baltimore, Maryland 21208, 301–484–0111).

---

**CHART 41. DIRECTORY OF WHAT IS KNOWN ABOUT SIDS**

---

- Ninety-five percent of the infants who die are between 2 and 4 months old
- Most babies die between midnight and 9 A.M.
- The position in which the baby sleeps—back, side, abdomen—is not related
- Seventy-five percent of all SIDS babies are from well-to-do families with good prenatal care
- Low-birth-weight babies are more at risk (but all risks are higher for them)
- A majority of the babies have had a cold or the sniffles in the days or weeks before death
- It is slightly more common in boys (but male babies generally have a higher mortality rate)
- Some experts say that extremely passive infants, who do not fuss and squirm, may be more vulnerable
- Breast-feeding neither prevents nor reduces the risk of its occurring
- Parental age is not related
- Antenatal infection is not related

---

***There is a national SIDS hotline*** that you can call for information and support about crib death, as SIDS is also called. The American Sudden Infant Death Syndrome Institute has a toll-free number: 1–800–232–SIDS. This number is available for physicians, other health-care providers, or parents who wish to learn more about this tragic condition.

***Appendix III,*** Help for Grieving Parents, on page 778 has a state-by-state listing of groups to help you deal with the experience of losing your baby.

## SPECIAL SECTION: EMERGENCY CHILDBIRTH

*This is not intended as a do-it-yourself birth guide—this is an outline of what to do if the baby wants to be born before you reach the hospital or the doctor or midwife reaches you.*

**If the urge to push comes** and you are driving to the hospital, use your breathing techniques to avoid pushing. Remain calm. Assess the situation with your mate. If the urge to push is too strong for you to control, have him pull the car over and stop. If you are at home, call the paramedics, who may at least be able to get there to take you to the hospital to be examined after the baby is born. If you are in the car, stop, or at least slow down if there is nowhere to pull over. If possible, cover the backseat and car floor with a thick layer of newspapers. You can slump down and deliver the baby over the edge of the backseat into your mate's hands or you can lie across the seat.

**If a loop of umbilical cord** washes out when the membranes rupture—if you can see a piece of gray-blue, shiny cord bulging out of the vagina—this means you have a *prolapsed cord. This is potentially fatal to the baby*. Get into a knee-chest position: on your knees with your head down and your buttocks in the air. Call the paramedics immediately. When the cord prolapses (comes down before anything else), it is compressed and *the baby's oxygen supply is being cut off*. If the cord is sill protruding in a knee-chest position, then cover it with warm, wet sterile gauze pads or a very clean towel. Do not put any pressure on the cord, however. It is still the baby's lifeline. Stay in the knee-chest position even on the way to the hospital because it reduces pressure on the cord. A prolapsed cord necessitates a cesarean delivery.

**Under no circumstances hold your legs together** to delay the birth. Do not let anyone else hold your legs together. This can cause brain damage in the baby.

**Ease the baby out with contractions.** A baby coming out this fast does not need much pushing help. There is a greater chance that your vagina and perineum will tear if you push along with the force of the uterus. So pant lightly with each contraction.

*Deliver the head slowly.* It is best if you push it out *between* contractions. If possible, your mate should support the perineum with warm, wet compresses or a very clean towel to avoid tearing. If there is time for this, he should put the heel of his hand over the area between your vagina and anus.

*Never pull on the baby's head* to get it out. This may permanently injure the spinal cord, the nerves of the arms, and the baby's breathing apparatus. Although it's unlikely that your membranes would not have ruptured by now, if the head is still covered by membranes, then they must be torn off. Your mate can use his fingernails, a pin, or any sharp instrument, being very careful of the baby's head. If there is time, dip the pin in alcohol before using it. The membranes have to be removed in order for the baby to breathe.

*Put clean towels or newspapers* under you. Your mate should support the baby's head as she is born.

*When the head is out* your mate should check with his fingers to feel if the cord is around the baby's neck. Loosen it gently by pulling it over the baby's head or loosen it so the body can deliver through it.

*The head turns naturally* to one side so that the shoulders can rotate. When she first comes out, the head will probably be facing down and can be wiped off with a clean cloth. After her head has turned to the left or right you should push with the next contraction to deliver the shoulders.

*Do not pull on the baby.* Support her whole body as she is born.

*Dry the baby thoroughly* and wrap him in a clean receiving blanket. Be sure his head is covered to guard against heat loss. Keeping the baby warm is of utmost importance.

***Hold the baby with his head lower than his body.*** This position should not be exaggerated but his face should be down or to the side so that the mucus in his nose and lungs can drain out. *Do not wipe out the inside of his mouth.*

***Put the baby to your breast*** if the umbilical cord is long enough to reach without pulling on the baby's navel. Even if the baby does not want to suck, it will warm and comfort her. Be sure to keep her carefully covered, especially the head. The baby's sucking will stimulate oxytocin in your system which will help expel the placenta and contract your uterus.

***If the placenta is born*** before you reach the hospital or an attendant arrives wrap it up with the baby—this provides much-needed extra warmth for the baby.

***Do not pull on the cord. Do not cut the cord.***

***After the placenta*** is born your mate should massage your uterus *firmly* with a deep circular motion within the limits of your comfort. He should push down 2 to 3 inches below your navel and rub. This is important to make sure your uterus contracts and stays hard after the birth so that there is no hemorrhage.

***Less than 2 cups of blood*** when the placenta delivers and for a few minutes afterward is *normal*. Get the baby to nurse immediately if possible to help contract the uterus. *Gentle massaging of your nipples* can be a substitute way of releasing oxytocin into your system.

***The normal color of a baby at birth is blue.*** He "pinks up" in the first minute as oxygen enters his body. The hands and feet take longer.

# 11

# Taking care of yourself and your mate postpartum

There is a wide range of possible physical and emotional feelings you will have in the postpartum (after birth) period. You may feel a few or many of these bodily discomforts and mental upheavals—but if you know ahead of time what to expect it can make it easier. Forewarned is forearmed when you have to face the enormous adjustment of your body and mind postpregnancy as well as a new baby.

*Childbirth & Marriage is a sequel to this book* that focuses on what to expect after the birth of your child. I wrote the second book because I heard from so many couples who were struggling with the "transition to parenthood." That book goes into much more depth about how a baby impacts on your life. If you are interested in the issues that can affect your marriage after the birth of your child, have a look at that book.

## IN THE HOSPITAL

*Nurses can be bossy*—some of them have a naturally authoritarian attitude, other times they are simply busy because hospitals are often understaffed. Do not let negative attitudes of hospital personnel get to you, particularly where breast-feeding is concerned (see page 377–378, How to Cope with the Hospital). Some nurses may insist, for example, that you wash your breasts with soap and water before every feeding—not only isn't this necessary, but it may dry out and crack your nipples.

*The food may be bland* and unappetizing, as most institutional food is. Have "care packages" brought in or ask a friend to visit you around mealtime and bring food of your choice to you. For instance, if you ordinarily eat health foods you are going to be unhappy with the processed, refined-sugar, white-flour, and high-carbohydrate meals served at most hospitals.

*Visitors will tire you out* more than you imagine. You should try to limit each visitor to a half-hour stay. The other problem may be that the hospital restricts you to only one visitor during each visiting period. This means that you have to make the choice between your mate, your mother, or perhaps a sister or close friend. These kinds of hospital rules are a terrible way to separate families right from the start, but it is a policy you may have to contend with.

## CHANGES IN YOUR BODY AFTER BIRTH

Physical changes are the first thing you'll have to cope with after childbirth. Your body has to go through an enormous adjustment because of hormonal changes, tender and engorged breasts, and the processes of repair taking place in your uterus and vagina.

### VAGINAL DISCHARGE (LOCHIA)

*You will have a vaginal discharge* of blood, mucus, and tissue following the birth of your baby. This occurs because the site in your uterus where the placenta was attached has to heal. This process takes anywhere from 1 to 6 weeks after birth. Breast-feeding reduces the bleeding more rapidly. First the lochia is a menstrual-like red flow, which gradually turns pale pink or brown and then yellow-white or colorless.

*Use only sanitary napkins* for the first two weeks. The hospital will charge you a steep fee for each and every napkin they dispense to you while you're there, so you might want to bring a box with you to the hospital. The larger hospital-size napkins available at many drugstores can be helpful in the beginning. Many women find sanitary napkins awkward and irritating. Self-adhesive sanitary napkins that adhere to your underpants may be less uncomfortable: they are most suitable when the flow of lochia has decreased somewhat.

*After the second week* postpartum you can use tampons, as long as your doctor approves. Tampons may help you feel that your vagina is returning to normal. However, many physicians feel that tampons increase the likelihood of infection if used during the first weeks after birth, so this should be discussed. Putting a small amount of some kind of lubricating jelly, such as K-Y, on the tip of the tampon may make insertion easier.

*If the flow becomes bright red* any time after the first week, especially if it has turned brown and is suddenly red again, *notify your doctor.* It probably means you aren't giving the placental site enough chance to mend. If so, your doctor will most likely tell you to slow down, go to bed for a day, and get more rest.

*A continuing vaginal discharge* or an unpleasant vaginal odor may indicate incomplete healing of the cervix, or vaginal infection. You should let your doctor know about this so he can recommend treatment. *Do not use* feminine hygiene deodorant products, nylon underpants, or panty hose, all of which tend to aggravate the problem. Cotton underpants, which stay drier and allow oxygen to pass through, can help discourage persistent itching and infection.

*If you soak 2 pads in half an hour* call your doctor or midwife at once. Passing clots in the lochia is normal, but if you are bleeding enough to soak two pads in 30 minutes at any point during the healing process, you should be examined.

## CHANGES IN THE VAGINA AND CERVIX

*There may be changes in the size of your vagina* which may be disquieting. It is normal for the vagina to feel slack during the first couple of weeks after giving birth. One of the amazing things about a woman's birth canal is that it can expand dramatically to let the baby pass through, and then resume its usual size and shape. However, this doesn't happen overnight; for some women their vaginas never return to precisely their pre-pregnant size. By doing the Kegel exercise described on pages 190–191, you will be able to tighten your vagina considerably.

*Your cervix* is contracting too. After expanding enough to allow your baby to pass into the birth canal, the cervix returns to its normal size in several weeks. However, once you have given birth you will need a larger size diaphragm. See Birth Control on page 616.

## RECOVERING FROM THE EPISIOTOMY

*The episiotomy that was cut* in your perineum to make more room for the baby's head at birth can be sore and itchy afterwards. How big the incision is, and the skill with which your doctor made it, affect how much discomfort you feel. The soreness you feel is a result of the tissues swelling and pulling against the stitches. The swelling is usually worse the first 3 days after delivery and then lessens.

Some women find that recovering from the episiotomy is the most painful part of childbirth. For some women the soreness lasts for 2 to 3 weeks; for others it's gone within a week. There are several things you can try to ease the discomfort; however, *be sure not to use any ice or heat treatment if your genitals are numb from an anesthetic spray or cream.* If you are anesthetized, you won't be able to feel the burning sensation that would warn you if the temperature becomes too extreme.

- *Put an ice pack* on the area around your vagina as soon as possible after the birth. Ice is the most soothing treatment to reduce swelling and discomfort. Ask a nurse for a sterile glove and fill it with crushed ice, then apply this ice pack on your episiotomy wound. You may also find this helpful after you return home.
- *Do the Kegel exercise* immediately after the baby is born and continue to do it often during the postpartum period. It will pull the stitches together and begin the process of mending and strengthening the affected muscles.
- *Local anesthetic creams and sprays* can be helpful, so ask your doctor if he recommends them, perhaps along with some aspirin. These products will cost much more if the hospital issues them, so you might want someone to buy them for you in an outside drugstore.
- *Keep your genital area dry and clean* by bathing and changing sanitary napkins frequently. Notify the doctor immediately if you think the area is infected so that scar tissue is not allowed to develop.
- *Perineal pads* (a brand such as Tucks) can be put between your sanitary pad and the stitches to relieve itching and soreness.
- *Put a bottle of witch hazel* in the refrigerator or in an ice bucket. Dip a sterile gauze pad in the witch hazel, then apply it to the wound.
- *Some doctors recommend the use of alcohol swabs* after urination and bowel movements, to prevent infection and speed healing.
- *Wipe from the front to the back* when you have a bowel movement and then drop the paper in the toilet. Fecal matter can cause an infection if it enters the vagina or urethra.
- *Warm baths or showers* can soothe the healing perineum, although it may be best to wait until the swelling around the wound has subsided before you expose the area to

heat. Use plain water only: bath additives can be irritating to a wound.
- *Sitting can be painful,* and putting a soft pillow underneath you, especially on hard chairs, can ease the pain. You might also try a "donut cushion," intended for people with hemorrhoids.

## URINATION AND URINARY TRACT INFECTIONS

***Birth is a trauma*** to your entire pelvic floor, which includes the muscles and tissues surrounding your urethra, vagina, and rectum. Your body may feel different and uncomfortable when you have to perform such simple functions as urinating. In the process of being born, the baby was pressing on your bladder as he descended through your vagina. It will take some time before this area recovers from the trauma of childbirth.

***Difficulty in passing urine*** is not uncommon after childbirth. It may be the result of swelling in your perineum, which may close the urethra. Or if you had a spinal anesthetic, it may have made your bladder less sensitive to how full it is, and made it temporarily unable to empty completely. Women who are unable to urinate within 6 to 8 hours after delivery are usually catheterized to allow the urine to pass out of their bladder.

***An increased need to urinate*** is not uncommon during the first week after delivery. The extra fluid you retained during pregnancy is being eliminated.

***Postpartum urinary tract infections*** are fairly common. Notify your physician promptly if you think you have an infection so you can take care of it before it becomes more serious. There are several signs that you might be developing such an infection, although you probably will not experience all of them:

---

### CHART 42. SYMPTOMS OF URINARY TRACT INFECTION

---

- Fever
- Chills
- Discomfort when urinating
- Inability to empty the bladder completely
- Urinating frequently in small amounts
- Abdominal or back pain

---

## BOWEL MOVEMENTS AND HEMORRHOIDS

*Giving birth affects your intestines* and rectum because of the pressure exerted on that area during delivery. Your bowels may be sluggish after childbirth and you may not feel able to have a bowel movement. You may also develop swollen, tender lumps in your anus; these dilated veins are hemorrhoids, which can make bowel movements uncomfortable.

*If the pain and swelling* of hemorrhoids are bothering you, try sitting in a shallow tub of warm water. Your doctor can also recommend local anesthetic creams or compresses. Tucking hemorrhoids back in after a bowel movement can be helpful, although be careful that your fingernails aren't long or sharp.

*You may be worried* about being constipated after giving birth, especially if the hospital staff keeps asking whether you've had a bowel movement. Don't strain to move your bowels, just relax and allow your body to find its way back to normal.

*How to deal with constipation* during pregnancy is discussed on pages 159–160, but there are several things it's important to do postpartum. The first is to get up and walk as soon as possible after the birth, which gets your system going. Drink plenty of fluids and eat a lot of fresh fruit, vegetables, and whole-grain cereals and bread to help keep your stool soft.

*Prunes or prune juice* in the morning, followed by coffee or any other hot liquid, works for some people.

*A mild laxative* may be necessary if everything else you try doesn't work, although you should check with your doctor, who may recommend an enema, suppositories, or a stool softener, instead. *For Nursing Mothers:* If you are breast-feeding, a stool softener (which does exactly what its name says), *not a laxative,* may help without affecting your milk.

## MISCELLANEOUS POSTPARTUM PHYSICAL CHANGES

*Your hair may thin out* after the baby is born. During the postpartum period you may lose 50 to 100 percent more hair daily than before your pregnancy. You can see the evidence of this not only in your hairbrush but also on your pillow and clothing. Your placenta and the rich proteins in it were responsible for your hair being thick and shiny during your pregnancy. Without the placenta, you no longer have adequate protein in your system to sustain the previously rapid hair growth and you may find your hair falling out. Other reasons for thinning hair can be postpartum stress or a hormonal imbalance. But take heart: there is a remedy! Hair is composed almost entirely of protein, so concentrate on getting a lot of protein in your diet.

Your hair may be dry and brittle after your pregnancy. If so, check your shampoo: detergent-based shampoos can strip your hair of vital oils and cause the scalp glands to have to work harder to replace these valuable natural oils. Switch to a cream-based shampoo made of natural proteins and such vegetable oils as wheat germ oil. Use a good conditioner, too.

If your hair is dry postpartum, don't wash it every day. Give it a rest and wash it only 3 to 4 times a week. Don't use rubber bands or sleep in curlers, both of which can break hair. Avoid dying your hair, getting permanents, or using a hair dryer frequently.

*Dry skin is a common problem* postpartum, although a few women may find that their skin becomes more oily. After birth, the fluid balance in your body is disturbed by hormone production. Breast-feeding women are even more susceptible to dry skin: your body is using all available fluids to produce milk.

There are remedies for dry-skin problems. Try to drink a lot of fluids, at least 2 quarts a day, preferably in the form of water and juice. Drinking liquids will help replenish the moisture lost to hormone imbalance and milk production. However, drinking will probably not be enough; you'll also need to treat the surface of your skin with moisturizers. Although it's good to take steamy hot baths, do not use bubble baths, which often contain detergents and perfumes that can further dry your skin. Any product you use in your bath should be oil-based.

*Your teeth and gums* may have problems postpartum. Since pregnancy depletes your body's natural supply of calcium, you may find that your gums are inflamed, or that there is grayness at the gum line of your lower teeth. Bone-meal, other calcium supplements, or foods high in calcium are just as important for your health after delivery as they were for the baby's growth during pregnancy. Vitamin C is also helpful for gum problems. When you brush twice a day use a soft-bristle toothbrush to massage your gums in a circular motion.

*Your uterus should feel firm,* like a grapefruit in the middle of your stomach. Immediately after birth the nurse or midwife will knead your uterus every 15 minutes for the first hour to help the involution process, so the uterine muscles stay firm. They may show you how to knead the uterus yourself. Especially if you are leaving the hospital on early discharge, or if you've given birth at home, it is important for you to know if your uterus is remaining hard.

Postpartum hemorrhage can be very dangerous, but if the uterus remains firm, everything is okay.

Just after the birth your uterus is about 3 finger-widths below your belly button. After 24 hours it will have risen to the level of your umbilicus and then it continues to shrink, until by the end of the first week you probably won't be able to feel it when you press on your belly. By 6 weeks postpartum the uterus should be back to its prepregnancy size.

*Your breasts may feel congested.* If you are breast-feeding you can hand-express milk and wear a supportive bra day and night to help relieve congestion. Applying very hot washcloths may also help. If you are not breast-feeding and lactation has been suppressed with medication, do *not* hand-express milk and do limit your fluid intake. A feeling of feverishness can also accompany breast congestion.

*There are controversial drugs* available to stop maternal milk production. Hormones such as estrogen and certain forms of testosterone continue to be used by some doctors, even though a Food and Drug Administration advisory panel called for an end to this practice long ago. Consumer advocate groups have been petitioning the FDA to ban the use of hormones and drugs to stop milk production and breast engorgement. It is estimated that each year 700,000 women are given these drugs, which are only marginally effective and can cause serious side effects. Health advocacy groups say that the drug bromocriptine can cause sharp drops in blood pressure, as well as nausea and dizziness. However, the manufacturer of the drug, which is marketed under the name Parlodel, claims that the drug has been used by up to 5 million women since 1980, with few major side effects reported.

*Chills and hot flashes* can occur simultaneously and can be frightening if you aren't aware that this is a common occurrence. As with many of the physical reactions after birth, it is one of the body's ways of readjusting to the powerful hormonal changes going on.

*Profuse sweating* is the body's way of ridding itself of the excess fluids accumulated in your body during pregnancy. It can be especially bothersome at night so put a towel on your pillow.

*Thirst* can be quite marked postpartum because your body is losing fluid. Drink plenty of liquids. This thirstiness will pass as soon as your body has recovered its normal balance.

*Weight loss* postpartum is something most women welcome. It is normal to lose between 10 and 20 pounds immediately at birth, depending on how much weight you gained and how much of it was water weight. Although you will undoubtedly have more weight to lose, *do not go on a severe diet right away,* regardless of whether you are breast-feeding. Your body is recovering from the stress of birth in the first month or so and it requires a nutritious, well-balanced diet to do this.

*Menstruation recurs* anywhere from 2 months to 4 months postpartum. There is some variation but it is usually 8 weeks after the birth if you are not breast-feeding. For several months the interval between periods and the amount of bleeding may be unusual. Painful periods (dysmenorrhea) are almost always improved by pregnancy—for many women who had even incapacitating pain before, it never returns after birth. Most women do not ovulate when they are nursing *but some do.*

*Birth control* is necessary as soon as you're ready to have sexual intercourse. *Do not rely on breast-feeding or the lack of menstruation* to protect you against conceiving. You can get pregnant the first time you ovulate, which will be before you have a period. Your old diaphragm will not fit—you will have to be refitted with a larger size by the doctor or midwife about four weeks postpartum. *This is true even if you had a cesarean.* Many doctors will want you to return four weeks after that to check the fit again. *Do not use the birth-control pill while breast-feeding.* Your mate can use condoms with lots of spermicidal foam or jelly.

# FATIGUE

*Total exhaustion* is common after childbirth, but many women are surprised by just how fatigued they feel in the first weeks. The drastic reduction in your blood volume (it decreases by 30 percent) can be felt as exhaustion, although some women experience it as exhilarating. In either case it is *important to continue taking your iron pills for 6 weeks postpartum.* If you feel unusually weak or tired during the first 2 weeks after birth, it may be from anemia.

*Fatigue is the most common complaint* of new mothers. The newborn baby has no conception of day and night. The average newborn eats every 2 hours if breast-fed and every 4 hours if bottle-fed. Although the period of sleeplessness for the new mother is usually greatest in the first 6 weeks to 2 months after birth, *you should expect to be up at least once a night for the first year of the baby's life.* Some women find it is many months, even a full year, before they sleep well again after the arrival of their child.

*There is a fatigue cycle* that can be self-perpetuating. Once you are tired, you get more irritated by chores and the things you do not have time to accomplish. You may feel inadequate and overcompensate by trying to do more, which only tires you out further. Here are some suggestions on ways to avoid creating a fatigue cycle:

• Good nutrition helps fatigue, so be sure to eat properly
• If you are unable to sleep at night because you are over-tired, try to make sure that the hour before bedtime is peaceful
• Half an hour before "bedtime," get into bed with warm milk and read, watch TV, or listen to music
• Don't eat heavily or drink caffeine or other stimulating drinks before bed

*Do not ignore the signs of fatigue.* Tune into the signs that your body gives you about being tired or having little energy. Take a nap when the baby naps—don't do chores in that time. For the first week try to limit stair-climbing to once a day and avoid heavy lifting. Visitors can be very tiring—if you want company do not try to be super-hostess. People can take care of themselves—they can go get a drink for themselves from the kitchen and there's no reason for them not to get one for *you* while they're up! If you do not want visitors and want to be alone just tell people that your doctor or midwife has forbidden you to have guests for the first week.

*Sleep is essential* in the immediate postpartum period. Studies show that in the last weeks of pregnancy women have a loss of REM (rapid eye movement) sleep. Rapid eye movements are associated with dreaming, which occurs in the deepest sleep. REM sleep is necessary for both physical and psychological replenishment. The loss of REM sleep and the associated disturbance in dream patterns may be related to the impending crisis of childbirth.

*This loss of sleep can and must be made up.* If you continue to lose sleep after the baby is born, it can lead to physical and emotional disturbances. You *may* feel fine even though your usual sleep pattern is interrupted. However, you may be someone who sleeps the most soundly in the 6th or 7th hour of sleep—if you feel sleepy during the day then you probably are. In this case you should have someone else give the baby a bottle during the early morning feeding so that you can get the sleep you need. Another alternative is to have someone give the baby a bottle while you take an afternoon nap—either way, the intention is to give you more than a 3- to 4-hour stretch of sleep between feedings so that you can get that deep sleep necessary to your well-being.

---

**CHART 43. SIGNS OF POSTPARTUM PROBLEMS
(NOTIFY DOCTOR AT ONCE)**

---

- Unusually heavy bleeding on any day, more than a menstrual period, or if you soak more than 2 sanitary napkins in half an hour
- Vaginal discharge with a strongly unpleasant odor
- A temperature of 101° or higher. If you develop a rise of temperature to 100.4°F. [38°C.] or higher on any 2 of the first 10 postpartum days, exclusive of the first 24 hours, the assumption is that you have puerperal fever, unless there is an obvious other source like an inflamed breast or bronchitis. Bacterial cultures are taken of the interior of the uterus, your blood, and urine, and wide-spectrum antibiotics are begun immediately.
- Breasts are red, feel hot or painful

---

*If you are not feeling well, call the doctor.* Do not wait for the 6-week postpartum visit. Although it is common to feel tired you should not feel poorly after birth. If you have *pain* anywhere call the doctor right away—it may be a sign of infection, which can occur easily postpartum. If you have a loss of appetite for an extended period, call the doctor. If there is a sudden increase in vaginal bleeding—if you are passing large clots in the lochia or it turns a sudden bright red color—these may be signs of problems.

*Your mate may not understand* the changes your body has to go through. He has nothing in his physiological life which can correspond to pregnancy and postpartum. He may not understand that you look healthy and beautiful and can receive visitors but just don't have the energy to cook or do things around the house. If you are a first-time mother, unsure of yourself, you may feel silly not pitching right in with chores and a skeptical mate can make this worse.

The fact is that it takes a full 6 weeks for your body to return to its prepregnancy condition. No matter how good you feel, you should still be kind to your body and take it easy. Your mate has to protect you, rather than question why you have less energy. A man should help around the house, encourage you to forget about chores for now, or do both.

## GETTING HOUSEHOLD HELP POSTPARTUM

It is important that you have a good chance to rest after the baby is born: it will affect your early relationship with the child and will also mean that you will recover *fully* from the birth as soon as possible. The kind of help you get will depend on what you can afford and who is available. The essential thing is for you to recognize that although it is humanly possible for you to handle everything alone it will be a great deal more pleasant to have an extra pair of hands around.

You don't actually need help for the baby—the first postpartum week is a special time for you and the baby to spend time together, particularly if you are breast-feeding. Household help is most useful to cook, clean, answer the phone, fend off visitors, and run errands. It isn't going to be a big help if you have someone to tend to the baby, whose needs are basically to be fed and changed, leaving *you* to run the house.

*Paid help* is preferable if there is room for it in your budget because when you are paying someone it's a lot easier to ask them to do things. With a friend or relative it can feel awkward to ask them to go to the post office or prepare dinner while you lie in bed with the baby. Two weeks help would be ideal, but if you can only afford 4 or 5 days, that's certainly better than none at all. It will give you a chance to get your bearings.

*Interview* possible candidates *before* the baby is born. It will be too hectic—and too unpredictable—afterward. If you are going to get professional help it is a good idea to contact an employment agency that specializes in domestic help or in baby care. You might also ask women who have had babies in the past few years whether they used anyone they would recommend.

*A trained baby nurse* is good if you feel ill-at-ease taking care of a newborn and don't think you'll gain enough confidence through the infant-care classes offered by the hospital or the American Red Cross in your community. A trained nurse can show you how everything should be done—but beware of a domineering, bossy woman who seems as if she'll want to take complete charge of the baby and have rigid, set ideas about the "right" way to do things. And also remember that unless you have other help in the house, a trained nurse will do no housework or cooking—she may even expect to have meals prepared for *her*. Professional nannies are scarce and in demand so they can pretty much "write their own ticket"!

*A practical nurse or professional baby-sitter* can also be located through an employment agency. These women will usually be willing to do light housework, some cooking, and can also look after the baby and show you the ropes. In the case of these women or trained baby nurses you should check out their references and find out about them from mothers who have used them recently.

*A student* can be quite a bit less expensive—although perhaps also less efficient. You should call the local high school and college and see if they have any young women available for light housework or baby care. Some of these students may have cared for younger brothers or sisters at home and may have as much practical experience as professionals. It may also make for a more informal arrangement, which might suit you best if you are not comfortable with the idea of having an older woman around who may have an authoritarian air.

*Grandmothers* can be wonderfully helpful with a new baby. They can also be a pain in the neck. It depends partly on your relationship with your mother or mother-in-law, as well as her attitude about a newborn. She may have been unhappy or dissatisfied with her own birth experience and may try to work out her feelings by participating in yours. Or she can be rigid in her ideas about baby care, which will put pressure on you to give in to avoid a confrontation or to contradict her and start arguments.

If you have a less-than-terrific relationship with your mother—or if you fear she might be more dominating than you'd like—make other plans for postpartum care ahead of time. You can keep her at a distance if you have specific plans already set up and tell her tactfully. If you happen to have a close, easy relationship with your mother-in-law and would like her to be with you after the baby is born, you have to weigh that choice against the insult your own mother may feel. You may be able to finesse it—with reasons of geographic distances or economics—but it can cause hurt feelings. In either case, if you don't want to have your mother or mother-in-law in residence, it may be easier on you if you can delay her arrival until the baby is 2 or 3 months old. By then you will have settled in, gained confidence, and won't be as vulnerable to being dominated, something many women worry about.

*Neighbors and friends* can do you the greatest service by bringing over a cooked meal. If anyone asks what they can do for you, say that a casserole you can freeze would be a wonderful gift. This way you can count on having a few meals taken care of, which takes some pressure off you. If any of these women are familiar with babies they also might be willing or even eager to stay with the baby for a few hours if you want to do things out of the house and don't want to take the newborn along.

*Stock up on disposable plates* and napkins, even if you don't ordinarily use them for aesthetic or conservationist reasons. You can also use frozen foods, takeout food, and any other possible shortcut in the postpartum period. You should not feel guilty about this legitimate use of convenience products. You deserve all the help you can get.

# THE EMOTIONAL ADJUSTMENT AFTER BIRTH

The birth of a child is one of the more stressful events in a person's life. One study showed that a death in the family was the most stressful life event and that childbirth was the second most. Regardless of how much you may have wanted the baby, how ready you are for it, and how positive your birth experience may have been—it is still an enormous upheaval of your life.

In the immediate postpartum period you may feel exhilarated by the baby's birth and then perhaps experience some "blues" (see Postpartum Depression, page 633–637). The second stage of postpartum adjustment is the reality of actually coping. There is the incredible fatigue from the lack of uninterrupted sleep, the stress of incorporating the new little person into your life, your changing role with your mate, and the baby's constant needs.

New motherhood can create a conflict nowadays. Our society makes it difficult for women to pursue their own goals while providing good care for their children at the same time. A woman may want to get out and work or do something more with her life than housewifing—but there are still the dishes to do, the baby to feed, and no easy solutions for how to incorporate both. You may feel caught between the heavy responsibility of your child and your personal interests and drives. These are all problems you have to begin to face and solve in the postpartum period.

***Do not try to be supermom.*** If you try to live up to whatever idea you have of a "perfect mother," you are bound to feel inadequate. There are aspects of caring for a baby that may bore or annoy you. *Accept yourself* and what you do and do not like about baby-tending. If you can do that, then others—the baby included—will accept it, too. It is not "bad" to dislike constantly changing a baby's diapers. Don't trap yourself with some image of Supermom: who enjoys the endless tasks of baby care, can give a splendid dinner party, and is also a well-organized interior decorator. For instance, you may enjoy breast-feeding but be annoyed that you have to get up twice in the night to do it, which is a legitimate reaction.

***Differentiate between your "fantasy" mother and reality.*** A fantasy mother is what you're "supposed" to be like. You form your ideas about a fantasy mother from the fairytales you heard as a child, from television and movies, and from books and magazines. Everybody's fantasy mother is some form of Supermom, but what they all have in common is that they are unrealistic—no woman can live up to those expectations. If you have a demanding fantasy mother, always "telling" you how you should be doing things, you won't ever do things "right." It doesn't give you a chance to be kind to yourself—to give yourself strokes for the things you *have* done "right"—to let yourself off the hook from unnecessary and unrealistic demands.

Try to recognize the fantasy mother within yourself and *listen only to the good messages.* For instance, if your fantasy mother says you should always look lovely, no matter what, then *do* set time aside for a hot bath, a nap in the sun, or a pedicure. It is important for your sense of well-being to pamper yourself at times. But if your fantasy mother says that your *house* should always look lovely, so that if anyone were to drop in everything would be tidy, tell her to buzz off! Decide for yourself which messages are good and then disregard the ones that don't make sense or have any real value.

***Tune out everybody else's theories*** about caring for a newborn and parenting. If you get into discussions with people—about breast-feeding, about when to introduce solid foods, about whether a baby should wear shoes or not—everyone knows what is "right." It is not unlike childbirth itself, when everyone knew the Right Way and tried to convince you of it. If you disagree with any of these well-meaning advice-givers they may make you feel like a "bad mother." Get all the facts you need and then trust your own instincts and judgment.

*Criticism* of any kind may be very hard to take in the postpartum period. You may be hypersensitive to any critical comments. This is part of the adjustment period, and although it helps to know that it is not uncommon, understanding it intellectually may not lessen your feelings of anger and defensiveness.

*A feeling of motherhood* is something you may not experience right away. It has to grow on some women and that takes time. However, there is a social image that says a woman is automatically infused with a joyous desire to love and nurture a new baby. You *might* feel that way, but you also may be slow to warm up to this new role. Do not feel guilty or as if something is wrong with you. It takes time for you and the baby to get to know each other. Motherhood is not unlike an old-fashioned prearranged marriage: you've never met each other but all of a sudden you're "stuck" with each other for the rest of your lives! It's understandable that you might want to ease into it slowly; feelings of loving warmth, protectiveness, and involvement in the baby's development will grow eventually.

*A fear of incompetence* is perfectly normal. In America, most girls and women are isolated from birth and babies— they don't have a chance to learn baby care by watching. Just because you are a woman does not mean that you instinctively know how to care for a baby. Experience is essential—seeing someone else do it, or doing it ourselves is how we learn.

You do not have to perform perfectly. Tell yourself this when you start to get anxious or feel inept. Everyone feels uneasy at first. A newborn is tiny and fragile and mysterious—but if you are reasonably intelligent there's very little you can do to harm him. By trial and error you'll figure things out. The important thing is to ease up if you're making unrealistic demands on yourself. It is really okay not to know how to handle a new baby. Call someone and ask for help. Read a baby-care book. One thing's for sure— before long it will be second nature to you.

*Allow yourself to have negative feelings about the baby.* There will be ways in which you feel put-upon by the burdens of baby care. It's all right not only to have those feelings but to voice them. A baby turns your life upside down and you're more than entitled to resent that. It is okay to feel jealous that your mate may come home and go directly to the baby instead of to you. Just as it is normal and healthy to have ambivalent feelings about getting pregnant, it is equally healthy to have misgivings about motherhood. It's not all fun or exciting—there's a lot of drudgery. It is fine to feel negative at times and it's good for you to admit that. If you try to swallow these feelings they will undoubtedly surface in your relationship with the baby. It would be much better to get it off your chest by talking about it—or by rearranging your schedules or priorities—than to be a martyr with bottled-up resentment.

## TAKE CARE OF YOURSELF

*Nurture yourself*—it is too easy to fall into the trap of feeling that everything is more important than your own "selfish" needs. "Selfish" is *not* a bad word. In fact, it's important for your own well-being and that of your family that you are selfish at times. If you are not rested and satisfied with your life everyone will be cheated. You will have less patience, feel resentful, and it will come out in the way you deal with the baby and other children, your mate, and your career if you're working. Everyone loses out if you aren't good to yourself.

*Be a baby yourself* when you feel like it. Especially in the beginning you may feel overwhelmed by the responsibilities and constant demands of a newborn. It may all seem like too much for one person to handle and still keep her sanity and sense of humor. Listen to those feelings. Turn to your mother or your mate or a close friend and let them baby you a little. It's important to get your perspective on this new role of motherhood and realize that it does not mean that you have to be on top of things all the time— caring for the baby, running the house and perhaps also a job. There are people to take care of you, too, if you let them.

**Set aside time for yourself and no one else.** Use it however you want to—and don't feel it has to be practical or constructive. Use your private time to write letters or in a journal, to do exercises, to read a great novel or a trashy magazine, to make yourself a dress, or to take a walk. Or just to nap. You may be amazed at how all-consuming a new baby can seem—unless you make a point of protecting a certain piece of each day for yourself. Ask yourself, "What can I do for fun every day?" Listen to music, read while you nurse the baby, dance in front of the mirror—whatever gives you pleasure.

**Set up priorities for yourself.** Unless you have help, it is not going to be possible to run an organized household with everything tidy, washing and ironing done, great meals, a well-loved baby, and time for yourself. Something has to give. Decide what you will give up: it might be ironing. It might be that you used to cook elaborate meals and now will simplify cooking. You might give up the idea that it's necessary to have a kitchen floor that is always spotless. Something has to go: you have to make a purposeful decision what it will be and then really let it go. Do not be a slave to your house or baby—skip certain chores. Leave things until "tomorrow." You'll drive yourself nuts otherwise.

Now decide what you will *not* give up. There may be activities in your life that are not essential, but in determining your priorities there will be things to protect. It might be playing the piano; it might be planting a flower or vegetable garden; it might be going to an exercise class; it might be cooking a fancy dish. Whatever nurtures you is what you should be determined not to lose in the midst of the new responsibilities a baby brings.

## ISOLATION

***You may feel horribly isolated*** after the baby is born. A new mother needs support and guidance in learning baby care and also holding on to her identity. You may find yourself home alone for eight hours or more. You will be deprived of adult recognition and the strokes and interchange that take place during an intelligent adult conversation, for example. It can be depressing if you are stuck at home all day without any support and only a tiny baby for company.

***Loving helpers,*** guidance from experienced women, and the exchange of affection are all at least as important as good food and rest in the postpartum period. A woman can experience sensory deprivation if she is cut off from other adults; it can lead to apathy. Many women feel sad in the immediate postpartum period, but if they have close contact and support, the stroking they receive can end the sadness that could progress to depression. The hormonal imbalance and physical adjustments after birth can affect your emotions—you have to work to overcome that.

***Before the baby is born,*** you should seek out friends who have had experience with babies. If you don't know any, then you should try to find an organization of parents. Some childbirth instructors hold postpartum classes and the La Leche League and others have parent "rap sessions." You can also arrange to visit women from your childbirth class after birth. You are all going through the same stage of adjustment together and just knowing you aren't alone is a big help.

***For those women who have or want their mother around,*** she can be a wonderful source of love and encouragement.

***It is important to get away*** from the confines of your house, either with or without the baby, for a short or long outing every day. It helps you maintain a sense of identity— that you still interact with the outside world even though the main focus of your life right now is at home with the baby. Get used to using baby-sitters early on—it's good for you to have the independence and it's good for the baby to get accustomed to not having you around constantly.

## THE MAN'S REACTIONS

*The father's adjustment postpartum* has many of the same elements as your adjustment although in most cases a man will be away at work all day whereas you'll be home with the child at least in the first weeks. Perhaps the most common feeling a man has is that the baby comes first and gets all the attention—in some relationships the man may have had that position and now feels displaced. The truth is that the baby *is* getting most of your time and attention, especially at first—and then you may be so tired by the time your mate gets home that you just want to lie down. There are several ways to insure that your mate doesn't feel slighted and to make time for yourselves apart from the baby. It's as important for you as it is for the man.

*If you find you're exhausted* by the end of the day, which is when your mate probably comes home from a fairly demanding day himself, why not take a nap together? It can give you a lovely sense of closeness and intimacy while replenishing your energy.

*Set aside certain special time* together—it may seem a little contrived, but it also may be the only way you're sure to protect your need to have time alone. A new baby can turn your lives so topsy-turvy that it *seems* as if it just isn't possible anymore for you two to go off together. It is possible—it just takes some planning.

Nothing can be as easy and spontaneous as it was before the baby was born. Everything you do now has to take the baby into account. Either you have to take the baby along or you have to arrange for someone else to look after her. Do not make the mistake of feeling that it's more effort than it's worth—it is extremely important for you and your mate to have times to yourselves. A baby puts a big strain on a relationship and you can't just sit back and expect that everything will fall into place on its own. You have to do it. Making time for yourselves doesn't necessarily mean elaborate planning—once you are committed to the idea it can be quite simple.

Decide what you most enjoyed doing together pre-baby or what you would like to start doing now. It might just mean setting aside the forty-five minutes when your mate comes home as a time to put your feet up, have a drink, and talk about the day or play cards. Maybe you like to go out to the movies once a week. Perhaps it means going for a drive on Saturday afternoon and having an ice-cream soda. If you play tennis together, make a permanent "date" to have two hours to do it on Sundays. It really isn't important what you do—all that matters is that you recognize that the health of your relationship depends on sustaining some of the intimacy and closeness that a new baby can disrupt *if you let him*.

*Two is company, three's a crowd.* Think of that cliché as it applies to you and your mate and the baby. It's fine to take the baby along on certain outings and it's nice if you want to include him. But there is a difference between just the two of you window-shopping and what it's like with a baby and all the paraphernalia along. Having a baby in your lives changes the way you feel about yourselves individually and how you relate to each other—welcome the change, but also hold on to the way you were beforehand. Many marriages suffer soon after a baby is born because the partners are not aware that the need for *twoness* continues.

*There are five factors* which influence a father's adjustment in the postpartum period.

1. PREPARATION FOR PARENTING can make a man more relaxed and confident about the new baby and able to enjoy her more. If at all possible you and your mate should see infant-care demonstrations either at a hospital, through the American Red Cross, or wherever they are offered in your community. Most men feel shut out of their baby's early

months because they don't know how to do anything and are afraid to make mistakes. Men can feel inadequate because they don't know how to feed, bathe, or diaper a baby—they're afraid the baby will cry because they aren't doing something right and then they won't know how to stop it.

A terrible mistake made by many new mothers, who are anxious themselves, is to give all sorts of instructions to their mate when he's got the baby and then to criticize the way he's doing it. If you watch a new mother and father you're apt to hear her saying, "No, you're squeezing her leg, hold her head up," or: "Hold her higher up to burp her." It's no wonder that fathers feel so inept and fearful—how would you feel if every time you went to pick up your baby or feed him there was someone giving you orders ahead of time about how to do it and then giving you negative feedback?

Keep in mind that it is the man's baby too. The implied message of the way many women treat their mates is, "Okay, you can have my baby for a little while but you better not mess up . . . Oh no, you messed up, I was afraid of that." Keep your mouth shut. Your mate isn't going to harm the baby—he's as protective of her as you are and is reasonably intelligent. He is not going to choke the baby or drop her on her head. So what if he doesn't keep the bottle of juice at the exact angle *you* think is best? He'll work it out by trial and error if you leave him alone and let him pick up the cues from the baby.

If you find you simply cannot button your lip—that you just *have* to butt in with some important tidbit of advice—then leave the room while he's with the baby. It's quite common for women to cluck and complain that the baby's father doesn't share care, yet those women will not recognize that they have driven the men away. But the most important reason to let a man get used to his baby is *not* so that he can change a diaper or play patty-cake when you want to take a bath. The more essential reason is that a man deserves the opportunity to be intimate with his child. *If you badger him you are depriving him of his rights.*

It is lovely for the baby to receive care from her

father and that nurturing can be wonderful for the man too. He will be able to experience himself in a new way—expand the ways in which he gives and receives love, setting the foundation for the kind of parenting that men have often been excluded from. Given a choice, most fathers would want to have greater involvement with their child than bouncing her on their knee for 10 minutes at the end of the day. When a man learns that he can "mother" too—that this enriching experience is not the private territory of women—it can give him much pleasure and satisfaction. It is within your power to give your mate that chance—the same chance you have.

2. AGREEMENT ABOUT ROLES is another aspect of a man's adjustment. Couples who discuss and agree on the ways to share and divide basic family tasks have an easier time. Couples who don't make an agreement usually fall into the pattern of woman-does-everything-in-the-house-and-for-the-baby, man-does-his-thing-outside-the-home. More often than not this unplanned arrangement makes the woman feel resentful—which she lets the man know in both subtle and overt ways—and makes him defensive or guilt-ridden in return. It also can make the man feel excluded from the baby's care yet burdened with the responsibilities of his work, which may pressure him more with the added expense of the child.

Men tend to adopt either the Breadwinner role or the Equal Parent role. In the latter, infant-care is shared, although usually not 50–50, since he's not home during the day. Both are effective patterns to cope with the stresses and strains *as long as both partners feel comfortable*. That is at the heart of the matter—and you won't straighten it out unless you both discuss how you feel, what you'd ideally like, and what can realistically be done.

3. SUPPORT FROM HIS WORKPLACE is important to a man's adjustment. For instance, the option of flexible-hour scheduling, so that a man can come home early to give the new mother a break, can mean the difference between success and failure at creating a situation that works well for all three of you. A man should talk to his employers before

the baby is born and try to get some flexibility from them, at least in the early postpartum period.

4. **SUPPORT FROM FAMILIES** is important to good beginnings for a new family. If the baby's grandparents have respect for the new parents' wishes to be alone—yet also visit, bring gifts, and give steady encouragement—it can be an important support structure. Nowadays people live so cut off from each other and the nuclear family is so isolating that to have the support of one's family and extended family can be a great comfort. It can give you the feeling that you aren't out there all alone, struggling to make order out of the instant chaos that a baby creates.

5. **THE HEALTH OF THE BABY** and his disposition can be an important factor in the ease with which parents adjust. A baby that isn't healthy can cause feelings of rage, guilt, desperation, exhaustion, and helplessness. A fussy baby that cries often can create these feelings on a smaller scale. There really isn't much you can do to improve these situations. Hopefully a sickly baby will gain his health and a less-than-sweet-tempered one will grow more mellow.

## POSTPARTUM DEPRESSION

"Baby blues," or postpartum depression, affects anywhere from 15 to 80 percent of women. It usually lasts 1 to 7 days and is marked by tearfulness, anxiety, depression, restlessness, and irritability.

*Hormones* are a major reason for this emotional unpleasantness. It is caused by the precipitous drop in the amount of estrogen and progesterone in your system after delivery or by an imbalance in the two hormones. Women who have difficulty adjusting to changing hormone levels in the premenstrual period tend to have greater difficulty adjusting to hormone levels postpartum—meaning that they are more sensitive to hormonal fluctuations.

*Lowered thyroid function* may be related to postpartum depression. The psychosomatic nature of pregnancy (the way in which your body affects your emotions) should not be ignored. If you're feeling low for quite a while after the baby's birth you should have your thyroid levels checked. There may be a relation between low thyroid and emotional/social stress—which childbirth certainly is. In one study it was found that third-time mothers had lower thyroid levels in their blood than first-time mothers—indicating that pregnancy may inhibit thyroid activity, which in turn is linked to how you feel.

*A woman's psychological makeup* influences postpartum blues. The way that you deal with new situations in general and the way that you feel about yourself will be reflected in how you handle a new baby. The incapacity to master and control a new event in your life can bring on a depression. If you are a very dependent person, or are preoccupied with meeting your own dependency needs, or if your sense of identity is not clear, you may have difficulty adjusting to maternal responsibilities. If you are a chronically anxious person you are more likely to have anxiety-stress reaction in the postpartum period. If you have ambivalent feelings about femininity or mothering you may get depressed. And a woman who has had long-standing life-adjustment problems will deal differently with postpartum than a woman for whom this is the first major stress in her life.

*It is difficult to predict* postpartum adjustment by the way that you adjusted psychologically during pregnancy. Sometimes a serene pregnancy can lead to a rough postpartum. This can be true of a woman who hasn't fully faced what is happening—if she has trouble relating to her sex role she may admit she is pregnant but deep down refuses to believe that she'll actually have a child. Perhaps she hasn't prepared herself for motherhood but has sailed through pregnancy as if she didn't have a worry. A postpartum disturbance may reflect her inability to accept her womanhood.

Many women have negative or ambivalent feelings during pregnancy but don't seek help, hoping that childbirth will solve everything. It is safe to say that for women like this the arrival of the baby just makes things more complicated. If these women finally face their problems once the baby is born they may feel it's "too late" to do anything about it—which can lead to depression unless they get help working out their feelings.

*A lack of support for new mothers* can lead to depression. In "the old days" a woman was surrounded by helpful kinfolk and neighbors when she had a new baby. In our society today a new mother not only has no actual support but is additionally cut off from the mainstream of life when she is alone at home with the baby.

Postpartum blues may also come from the loss of the supportive relationship with her doctor or midwife. During pregnancy a woman may have turned to them for support—in fact, a woman might have been using complaints of physical symptoms to mask emotional problems—and now that support system is gone.

## "MISSING PIECES"

"Missing Pieces" is a psychological syndrome which affects some women after birth. They repress or forget aspects of their labor and delivery and experience frustration, anger, and tears when they try to remember and are unable to. **Some signs of this "missing pieces" syndrome are:**

- *You are obsessive:* talking and asking about your birth experience over and over. Other people may make fun of you or become annoyed.
- *You may have dreams* with a recurrent theme and hope that the missing components will come to you this way.
- *You may feel you haven't slept well,* feel fatigued when you wake up, and feel lethargic during the day.
- *You may be unable to focus* on the present situation and be preoccupied with finding the missing links in your birth experience. You may have little or no interest in the baby.

## The reasons for "missing pieces" are:

- *A long labor,* which may result in confusion and a loss of a sense of how events took place.
- *A rapid labor,* which makes it hard to put sequences in a logical order or understand what is happening at the time: a sensory overload. Because labor was going so fast you may have gotten less information from your attendants about your progress at the time.
- *Any high-risk condition* during labor causes stress and anxiety so that you do not hear what's said to you or may forget it later. Especially when there is an unexpected cesarean, a woman is vulnerable to forgetting important areas of the experience.
- *Unfulfilled expectations* which don't integrate with the actual outcome of the birth may mean that your energies were directed to coping with your grief over your unmet expectations rather than focusing on the events of the birth.
- *Medications which are administered* can affect your alertness and sense of the passage of time. Also the conditions requiring the use of drugs—complications or a lengthy labor—may cause you anxiety. You also may have been upset because you felt strongly about avoiding drugs but you accepted them because you couldn't cope with the contractions.

There are several ways to deal with the "missing pieces" syndrome. Get information from your mate and the medical personnel. Do not accept the attitude that your requests are silly, stupid, or unimportant. Fill in the gaps you can't remember by talking to those who shared the event with you. The important thing is to integrate the birth experience for yourself so that you are satisfied.

***Get professional help with any postpartum disturbance that lasts longer than 1 to 2 weeks.*** "Baby blues" are caused by all the reasons listed (pages 633–635) but do not normally last longer than a week or two. If you find yourself depressed or unable to cope well with your changed life after the baby is born, seek outside help. If you don't do this, problems can become magnified and a depression can get deeper and have dangerous repercussions to your physical health as well as the health of your relationship with the baby and your mate.

## BREAST-FEEDING

It was difficult to decide whether breast-feeding belonged here or in the final chapter, Taking Care of Baby—but it is included here because breast-feeding involves your body and life as much as it does the baby's.

Breast-feeding is an important issue and this section gives you all the available information. You can decide for yourself whether or not you will breast-feed, and if so, which of the options you will choose in how long to nurse or how to breast-feed partially to fit into a busy life-style. Each set of parents has to weigh the physical, psychological, and emotional factors, and come up with a decision about breast-feeding that is right for them.

This section will cover the supportive atmosphere necessary for breast-feeding, general information about how the breasts work and what breast-milk does for an infant, a discussion of both the advantages and drawbacks to breast-feeding, and advice about breast-feeding while working outside your home. There is also a section on diabetes and breast-feeding and a chart indicating which drugs are harmful if used when nursing.

### WHY IS BREAST-FEEDING LESS POPULAR THAN THE BOTTLE?

Since 1950 only 30 percent of babies have been breast-fed, with slight fluctuations from year to year. There is a higher level of breast-feeding among college-educated women but generally it has declined in popularity ever since the introduction of the bottle about seventy-five years ago.

*Status symbol:* Originally only upper-income women bottle-fed their babies. There is a residue of this which is part of the influence to bottle-feed, even though people may not be consciously aware of it.

***More women are working:*** Although it is possible to breast-feed and have a career, it requires an energetic commitment and maneuvering. All the same, many working women do not return to their jobs when the baby is less than six months, so this is not as strong a reason as it might seem.

***Vigorous promotion of infant formula:*** Advertisements and free samples to doctors and women leaving the hospital greatly influence the decision not to breast-feed. In fact, this pressure is so potent that the International Pediatric Association recently made recommendations about the commercial promotion of formula: ''The dissemination of propaganda about artificial feeding and distribution of samples of artificial baby foods should be banned from all maternity units.'' This international group found that the promotion of formula undermined breast-feeding, which they recommend. Also, many mothers who introduced solids into the baby's diet early—which the association disfavors—first used the baby food samples from the hospital.

***The breast as sex symbol:*** Some men and women can think of breasts only as they relate to sex and have difficulty acknowledging their lacteal function. They have been so conditioned in their attitudes toward bosoms that they are repulsed by the thought of breast-feeding.

***Lack of profit from breast-feeding:*** Commercial interests cannot gain by promoting breast-feeding—which is another reason for its decline. Since no money can be made from breast-feeding, there has been no organized effort to educate or encourage women. Since there are comparatively few women breast-feeding, encouragement from one's peers is rare.

The La Leche League was started in 1956 to fill this gap. Some women complain that the LLL is too fanatic: they are so enthusiastic that when you go to them for support and information you feel bulldozed. It is important to understand that this small, volunteer organization with local groups nationwide is working against a cultural mainstream. They are David fighting Goliath: women who believe that breast-feeding is best for mothers and babies versus huge corporations that make millions of dollars from promoting formula. It is a hard task requiring almost fervent dedication.

La Leche League is the only group that exists for advice and encouragement about breast-feeding, so it is recommended several times in this section. It is necessary right up front to caution that the ideology of many LLL members is not the "right" point of view and may, in fact, turn off some women. Their philosophy is that a mother should have sole responsibility for feeding her child, which means that breast-feeding has to pretty much dominate her life. The League's book, *The Womanly Art of Breastfeeding,* has this point of view and does not acknowledge the mother as an independent person with demands which may exclude her baby. This concept of Total Mothering, also referred to as "natural mothering," may seem suffocating to you—the righteous attitude that often goes with it can also be off-putting. However, if you keep in mind what the La Leche League represents and their uphill battle, perhaps you won't be as critical.

## SUPPORT IS ESSENTIAL TO SUCCESSFUL BREAST-FEEDING

Especially because we live in a society where the majority of women do not breast-feed, those who want to have to be aware that other people's attitudes have a direct effect on breast-feeding. Particularly a first-time mother is acutely sensitive to other people's reactions. Verbal, nonverbal, and even unconscious judgments by those around her can influence a mother who is trying to breast-feed. The attitudes of her mate, obstetrician, pediatrician, nurses, her mother, immediate or extended family, and friends are all important. Even subtle criticism—a grandmother's comments or a doctor who mentions that a baby is at the bottom of the weight-gain graph for his height—can inhibit a woman's milk supply for a feeding or two.

Therefore if you do want to breast-feed you should

be aware of how powerful other people's attitudes can be. Let others know ahead of time that you're going to breast-feed only when you're prepared to hear negative reactions without getting discouraged. You can also protect yourself from problems in advance of the baby's birth by talking only to those people you cannot avoid having contact with in the early weeks postpartum. Explain to them that their support is going to be essential to the ease and success of breast-feeding. If they have questions or are against it then ask them to read this section or other material so that they are fully informed about the subject.

*Your own negative presumptions* and partial-information can mitigate against breast-feeding. You may be interested in trying it, but you've let yourself be negatively influenced by bits and pieces you've heard. Learn everything you can ahead of time—if you decide to breast-feed, give it your full commitment, or you'll be your own worst enemy. You may say, "I'm too tense a person to breast-feed," or "I doubt I'll have enough milk," both of which are erroneous statements. You may have heard that a friend had trouble breast-feeding and you don't want to have to go through it. That's ridiculous—would you not have had a baby for that reason, too? Someone else's experience has nothing to do with yours.

*The initial 1 to 2 weeks* of breast-feeding are the most frustrating. You are learning a new skill, you may feel insecure, and there is often a lack of knowledgeable people to help you. Your baby may also not be fully cooperative—she may be groggy from drugs you had during delivery or she may not have had a chance to reinforce the sucking instinct at birth. The important thing is to anticipate that the first couple of weeks are going to be difficult—if they're fairly easy, you have a nice surprise. At least you won't give up because you didn't *expect* to be frustrated.

## THE HOSPITAL AND NURSING

*Choose your hospital well* because breast-feeding can be sabotaged by an unsupportive staff and a rigid feeding schedule. Try to get a hospital that permits the baby to stay with you immediately from birth or at least has the shortest possible observation period after birth. Some hospitals will release your baby from the stabilization nursery within 4 hours but many still have a strict 24-hour observation period, despite all the evidence about the importance of immediate maternal-infant bonding and nonseparation.

Ask the hospital what percentage of mothers breast-feed—if it's at least 40 percent, they will probably be flexible to your needs. If it is under 25 percent the hospital is not oriented to breast-feeding and may make it harder for you. Talk to your doctor about the hospital's policy on breast-feeding and try to arrange for support if it isn't already there (read Choosing a Hospital, pages 374–411). It is routine at many hospitals to give a baby glucose and water during the observation period, yet if a baby were not separated at birth she would be getting colostrum from your breasts. Your efforts at breast-feeding are undermined right from the start with a baby that has sucked from a rubber nipple—it is so much easier that the baby may refuse your breast. Have your pediatrician write on your chart, *No bottles by request* or *No artificial nipples*.

A great problem with giving birth in a hospital is that you are so cut off after the baby is born. You are separated from your mate and your family—important sources of emotional support—and unless you have rooming-in, you are also separated from your baby. This isolation can contribute to postpartum depression, as well as to problems with breast-feeding. You should know the specific areas in which a hospital is going to make breast-feeding more difficult—and the ways you can try to overcome the obstacles.

**SCHEDULES, ROUTINES, AND ALLEGIANCE TO THE CLOCK:** Breast-milk digests in 2 to 3 hours, yet hospitals have a 4-hour feeding schedule. This means that your baby is going to get hungry and cry in the nursery: he will probably be given a bottle of glucose and water to quiet him. The rubber nipple undermines breast-feeding, the baby's hunger will be satisfied, he will fall back to sleep and he won't be interested in your breast when he's brought to you. If your chart says *No artificial nipples,* the baby will cry from when he gets hungry until he exhausts himself, falls to sleep, and is too tired to nurse properly when you get him.

Many hospitals have a policy of not allowing a baby to have anything to eat for the first 12 hours of life. However, the advantages of early sucking are known: a baby whose sucking reflex is reinforced at birth and frequently thereafter is going to learn to nurse well. Also, frequent sucking insures you will have a good milk supply which will come in sooner and helps prevent engorgement of your breasts. The hospital schedule makes frequent sucking difficult, thereby increasing the chance that breast-feeding will be compromised. If you cannot get rooming-in, at least try to get your baby every 3 hours. That hour can make a big difference in the success of your breast-feeding.

NURSES ARE RESISTANT TO CHANGE: The hospital staff is accustomed to having things a certain way—the way they have always been. Special requests upset the smooth routine. For example, if you want your baby an hour sooner than all the other babies are brought to their mothers, it means that a nurse has to remember this out-of-the-ordinary request and stop whatever she's doing to bring your baby to you. That may throw off the way she has organized her tasks for the day, especially if the hospital is understaffed, as most are. Another example is extended visiting hours—if all fathers are allowed unlimited visiting, it disrupts the staff. This may mean nurses have to alter when they bathe and change babies and it means extra work for them if the hospital requires that fathers wear sterile gowns and "scrub up" when they're in the rooms: the nurses are the ones who make sure this is done.

NURSES ARE NOT TRAINED TO TEACH BREAST-FEEDING: Often a nurse will bring your baby, retreat to the nursery, and reclaim the baby 20 minutes later. If the baby was too sleepy to suck or nursed poorly, you didn't benefit from any advice. When the baby wakes up hungry in the nursery an hour or so later she'll probably get a bottle of glucose and water. The solution would be to assign nurses who are interested to work with groups of breast-feeding mothers. Another alternative would be for the maternity floor to have a nurse who is a breast-feeding advocate to help when problems arise and to work closely with new mothers who are nursing.

Unfortunately, many nurses believe they can't help if they themselves have never breast-fed. It may be that some of these women are uncomfortable with their own sexuality or have uptight feelings about the sexual implication of breasts. Needless to say, if nurses review the anatomical aspects of breast-feeding and learn the psychological aspects for a new mother, they could give great support. But this doesn't exist in most hospitals, so *you have to fend for yourself.* Read as much as you can, and the moment doubts or problems arise, seek help from wherever you can get it: friends who have breast-fed, your pediatrician (whose support is essential), or the La Leche League, which volunteers help over the phone or in person.

## LACTATION CONSULTANTS

*A lactation consultant,* also known as a lactation educator or specialist, is a new kind of health-care provider. If you are having difficulties breast-feeding, you can get direct care through a clinic designed expressly to provide this service, or more likely through a private consultation with a specialist.

Lactation consultants can be found through the hospital by contacting the head nurse of the *newborn unit—* usually not through the maternity nursing staff. Many pediatricians also provide the names of lactation consultants to breast-feeding mothers with problems.

A consultation usually runs about an hour and a half, beginning with an extensive questionnaire to fill out. Then the specially trained consultant will check your breasts, evaluate your ejection reflex and milk supply, and examine the baby's position and way of sucking. Then she will suggest techniques to correct your breast-feeding problems or at least reduce them.

A lactation consultant usually rents or sells breast pumps, loans or sells books, and has a doll on which to demonstrate correct and incorrect techniques of nursing. She may also operate a telephone hotline for information and support.

Appendix V, page 786, is a listing of lactation consultant organizations, which may in turn be able to direct you to local help in your area.

## PREPARATION FOR BREAST-FEEDING

In the last weeks of your pregnancy you should prepare your breasts with a *daily routine* to "toughen them up" and open the milk ducts.

**Rub your nipples** gently with a towel. This friction accustoms your nipples to the stimulation they will get from the baby. Rub them until they are uncomfortable but never to the point of pain.

**Pull out your nipples** firmly, using some kind of oil or cream as lubricant.

**Flat or inverted nipples** are those which don't stick out by themselves—they fold back into the breast and need additional preparation. If you aren't sure whether you have inverted nipples, pinch the areola (the darker circle) just behind the base of the nipple. If it comes out, even a little, it is not a true inverted nipple. If your nipples react to pressure by retreating, they are inverted, which is rare. One treatment for bringing out truly inverted nipples is to use breast shields. The La Leche League International sells them—the address is on page 777. However, nipples are only guides for the baby—they don't really need to protrude for successful nursing. Try to breast-feed on demand from birth to make it easier on yourself.

*"Nipple-rolling"* is a good preparation for both inverted and normal nipples. Pull out the nipple with your fingers and roll it between your thumb and forefinger for a few minutes to make it stand out. Do this automatically when you get dressed and undressed during the final weeks of your pregnancy.

*Go without a bra* for part of each day—or wear a nursing bra and open the front of it—so that your nipples get friction against your clothing.

*Expose your nipples* to the air and sun.

*To open your milk ducts* you can hand-express a few drops of colostrum during the last 6 weeks of the pregnancy. This may reduce engorgement, which sometimes happens when your milk first comes in and can be very uncomfortable.

1. CUP THE BREAST IN ONE HAND. Use your other hand to place your thumb above and the forefinger below the nipple on the edge of the areola, the brown or darker area—the milk ducts are under here. Press inward toward the chest wall, squeeze the thumb and forefinger together gently, release and repeat.

2. DO NOT SLIDE THE THUMB AND FOREFINGER out toward the nipple or you will cause soreness. Shift your fingers to new positions to reach all of the milk ducts, which radiate out from the nipple in a circle. If you think of the areola as a clock, the ducts are at all points of the clock. Alternate where you squeeze every few minutes so that all the ducts get a workout.

3. DO THIS VERY GENTLY and only once or twice a day. It may take some time to get colostrum and some women never do, but it is still good preparation for breast-feeding.

*Redheads and women with fair complexions* are the most prone to difficulties with soreness and tenderness because their skin is so tender. They should follow these preparatory steps carefully to minimize problems during breast-feeding.

*Nursing bras* are a good idea during breast-feeding because they support your breasts and also protect your clothes if you leak. You will need a minimum of 3 bras—one on, one in the laundry, and one in the drawer.

*Smaller-breasted women* find that stretch bras give enough support, are comfortable and convenient. They can just lift the entire bra up over their breast while they're nursing.

*Disposable nursing pads* absorb any leakage and also protect your breast from any detergent residues which can irritate it. An economical alternative to ready-made pads is to cut a disposable diaper into 9 sections, with the plastic backing removed. *Avoid plastic-coated pads:* they can cause a rash, especially in hot weather.

*Breast shields* can be used to catch leaking milk. *Do not save the milk* that leaks into the shields—it can turn bad very quickly. Also, wash the shields frequently in hot soapy water and dry thoroughly.

*Breast-feeding does not make your breasts sag.* Sagging breasts are more often caused by not wearing a bra in pregnancy when your breasts are heavy and need support. Although more women who have nursed have sagging breasts than those who didn't, not all or even most breast-feeders do sag. *You can prevent or minimize sagging:* wear a proper nursing bra, don't nurse for too long a period (more than 6 months) and limit the number of children nursed.

*The size of your breasts* has nothing to do with your ability to produce milk. The amount of milk you make is determined by how much your baby stimulates your breasts—the more sucking, the more milk is produced.

## NUTRITION

*Nutrition* is very important during breast-feeding. Your diet during pregnancy can affect lactation. If you cut down on salt, calories, and protein during pregnancy it is unlikely that you will have enough stored fluid, fat, and protein to sustain a good milk flow.

     Lactation is a greater nutritional stress on your body than pregnancy was. Progesterone, which is secreted throughout pregnancy, acts as an appetite stimulant. This seems to be the main factor in the additional weight most women gain over and above the "products of conception." If you are breast-feeding *you need this energy reserve.*

*You should have no caloric restrictions.* You should use the same daily food guide as when you were pregnant with the addition of one daily serving from the milk/milk products group. When nursing you need an extra 500 calories and extra 20 grams of protein a day.

*Continue taking an iron supplement* during breast-feeding—30 to 60 mg of elemental iron daily.

*No oral contraceptives during breast-feeding.* Consult the chart on pages 683–687 to see which other drugs are unsafe during lactation.

*You need to drink plenty of fluids* in order to produce milk. You have to drink 2 to 3 quarts of liquid a day—and more if the weather is hot and you're perspiring. One way to meet this need for fluids is to get in the habit of having a large glass of any liquid beside you while you nurse—you can sip on it while the baby drinks. You may be aware that you get thirsty soon after nursing starts—have a glass of milk, juice, water, or beer beside you.

*Fluoride: Experts disagree* about when to begin supplementation and how much is necessary to prevent cavities. Some say that 0.25 mg of fluoride should be given beginning at 6 months, regardless of the local water supply, since fluoride is not readily transferred into breast milk from water you drink. Others say to give 0.5 mg of fluoride from birth if the fluoride content of your water supply is less than or equal to 1.1 ppm. Ask your pediatrician what he recommends. But in any case, your local water supply may be irrelevant—after you read the section on industrial pollutants in the water and how they contaminate breast milk, you may switch to drinking bottled water.

## How the Breasts Work and the Content of Breast Milk

*Colostrum* is a watery or creamy yellow liquid that precedes your milk supply. The colostrum has twice the protein of mature breast milk, which comes in within 5 to 7 days, and colostrum is high in vitamins A and E. A baby is not born hungry; by the time he needs more nourishment than colostrum, your milk will have come in.

Colostrum has an enzymatic effect to break down the mucus in the baby's digestive tract so that when the milk comes in, no mucus remains and the passageways are prepared for milk. The laxative effect of colostrum clears meconium, the dark, tarry substance in the baby's lower intestine at birth, from the bowels. Meconium contains bilirubin, which can be reabsorbed by the baby if the meconium remains in the intestines. Too much bilirubin causes jaundice. The early appearance of milk is also important because it hydrates the baby and helps prevent high-level jaundice.

Perhaps the greatest benefit of colostrum and breast milk is the antibodies it provides the baby. During the first 6 weeks of life a baby is most vulnerable to infection, but she doesn't manufacture many antibodies. Colostrum (and milk to a lesser extent) contains IgA, a rich source of antibodies that protect against allergy and pathogens and enter through the gastrointestinal tract. Colostrum and mature milk contain maternal antibodies against various bacteria and viruses: protection against anything you have had or have been immunized against is transferred to the baby (e.g., *E. coli,* polio, mumps, influenza, etc.).

**Breast milk** is the most easily digested and best balanced food you can feed a baby. The protein content of the milk is highest in the first few weeks following delivery when the baby's need for immunoglobulins is highest.

There are certain antibody protections which human milk provides. The immunity given by the milk during the first 6 weeks may last beyond that time so even a short nursing period is advantageous. *Human milk contains: enzymes* (lactoperoxidase, lysozyme), which promote chemical reactions that kill bacteria; *leukocytes,* which are cells that limit or prevent the spread of infection; *lactoferrin,* milk protein that binds the iron that bacteria need for growth, and *antistaphylococcal* agents that guard against staph infections.

Milk, often thought of as a living tissue, contains living white cells which not only make antibodies but also can actually engulf and destroy disease-causing bacteria and viruses in the infant. A breast-fed baby's intestines are inhabited primarily by *lactobacilli,* "harmless" bacteria, while the intestines of a bottle-fed baby contain high levels of *E. coli,* potentially disease-causing bacteria. There is a lactobacillus-promoting factor in human milk which aids the growth of this kind of bacteria. The bacteria cause an acid environment to develop which in turn discourages the growth of *E. coli.*

*The fat content of your milk* changes, leading to speculation that it adjusts to the child's needs. The fat content decreases after 5 to 6 months of lactation, which may be what a child requires in the second half of his first year. The evening feeding has an increased fat content, perhaps promoting longer sleep at night. The low milk-fat content in the morning may allow for a more alert baby.

**The *"let-down reflex"*** allows your milk to be released when the baby sucks. You have no conscious control over the let-down reflex but it can happen when you hear your baby cry or even when you're away and *think* of the baby— your milk starts flowing. Tension, distraction, and embarrassment all inhibit this reflex, so you should try to make things peaceful during the first few weeks of nursing.

**You may get very strong uterine contractions** when you breast-feed during the first few weeks. This is because the baby's sucking releases the hormone oxytocin into your system, which makes your uterus contract. These contractions can be stronger after a first baby; you may need your childbirth breathing techniques to stay comfortable.

**If you are accidentally given medication to dry up your milk** you can still breast-feed. In some hospitals hormone shots are given routinely on the delivery table to inhibit milk production. However, the effects wear off and although it will *delay* your milk supply coming in, the baby's sucking will bring it back anyway. (See page 615 for more on these drugs.)

   CAUTION: In some cases the drug used to suppress lactation is the hormone DES (diethylstilbesterol). *This drug is a known human carcinogen and could increase your chances of cancer in later years.* There is also evidence that the risk of thromboembolism is increased tenfold if DES is used to dry up your milk supply. *Even if you don't plan to nurse,* you'd be better off nursing for the first week and then gradually drying up your milk supply to avoid using this potentially dangerous drug.

**The length of a feeding is around one hour.** It takes the baby about 10 minutes to "empty" your breast. He gets the most milk in the first 5 minutes, but then the stored milk is depleted and richer, creamier milk is produced on the spot. Therefore the last part of the feeding is more nutritious.

**Demand feeding** is the most successful. This means that you let the baby nurse whenever she is hungry. Some doctors prescribe a schedule on which you're supposed to feed the baby but this may make the baby fretful and diminish your milk supply. The more a baby sucks, the more milk you produce—demand feeding stimulates milk production that is appropriate to the baby's needs. It focuses you on the baby instead of on the clock.

However, demand and scheduled feedings are not really opposites. A baby fed on demand will settle down to a schedule soon—her own schedule, though, not one predetermined by a doctor.

*You can skip a feeding regularly* and still breast-feed successfully. Many people say that arranging for child care is easier with bottle-feeding, but you might consider an alternative—after a month or two of breast-feeding, alternate with regularly scheduled bottle-feedings. Try not to miss more than one breast-feeding daily in the first two months. *Regularity* (missing the same feeding[s] daily) is the key to successful part-time breast-feeding. This is one way to maintain independence—which may include working—and still nurse.

*There is a nasal spray with oxytocin that can help* if you're having problems with breast-feeding. This spray has no side effects and will help speed up the let-down reflex. If you are still in the hospital, any nurse can phone your doctor's office and get permission to give you the spray; it has been a great help to women having trouble with early nursing. One quick spray into each nostril a few minutes before nursing can make the milk flow easily and alleviate much of the pain from the baby's sucking. You probably won't need the spray after you are fully lactating (your milk has come in), but it can be a great aid during those first few days.

## How to Breast-Feed

It will be easiest to have someone show you how to breast-feed and be there with you when you first attempt it; this is a general description of what to do.

• Hold the baby in the crook of your arm. If you're right-handed begin on the left side so that your right hand is free to direct your breast.

• Depress the breast with your index and middle fingers, the nipple protruding between them, so that you give the baby a good place to latch on.

• Touch the baby's lips with the nipple. He will open his mouth. The baby's natural "rooting" instinct makes him turn when touched on the lips or cheek. You will confuse the baby if you push his opposite cheek toward your nipple or pull both cheeks at once. Then place the breast as far into his mouth as it will go and the baby will begin sucking. Be sure the areola is in his mouth and not just the nipple or the milk ducts will not be stimulated and your nipples will get sore.

• If you have soft, small nipples a young baby may open her mouth and shake her head back and forth at your breast, trying to locate the nipple. So that the baby doesn't have this trouble finding the nipple you can put a cold, wet cloth on your nipple for a moment—this will cause the areola to shrivel and the nipple to protrude and become firm.

• For the first feeding stay on the left breast about 10 minutes and then switch to the right breast and let the baby stay there as long as she likes.

• Milk flows in both breasts at every nursing and it is better to use both at each feeding. Start with the heavier of the two breasts: let the baby suck 10 minutes on that side and then switch to the other.

• If your breasts are large you may need to use your index finger to maintain an air hole to the baby's nose until she gets experience and knows how to do it alone.

• To break the suction of a nursing baby put your finger gently into the corner of her mouth until she releases.

Never *pull* a nursing baby off your breast—it will hurt you!

## HOW TO HAND-EXPRESS MILK

Hand-expressing milk is necessary if you have to stop breast-feeding temporarily because you are ill, you have to take medication, or if you want to go away or if you want to breast-feed while working and want to keep a store of your milk at home. You can have a weekend away alone with your mate, for example, and pick up breast-feeding where you left off when you come home—if you express a little milk by hand each day to remind breasts of their function. If you anticipate your departure you can express a couple of ounces in a bottle before each feeding, freeze it, and thus leave food for the baby while you're away.

*In the back of the nipple* under the areola are the ducts through which the milk flows. To get it flowing, support your breast with one hand and place the thumb and forefinger farther apart, at the same time pushing them gently into your breast. Then squeeze them gently together, pulling the areola out toward the front.

*Milk should spray out* if you're pressing the right area. If it doesn't, don't worry. Keep trying until you massage the milk ducts correctly toward the nipple.

*While expressing, shift your fingers* to slightly different locations every couple of squirts. Do not slide your fingers on the skin because that can cause soreness. By changing the area of impact you give all the milk ducts a workout.

## BREAST-FEEDING OUTSIDE YOUR HOME

This may seem awkward at first. Our culture is hostile to breast-feeding in public. Breasts are connected to sex in most people's minds and seeing them—especially used for a different purpose—can make people uncomfortable. You should take people's discomfort into consideration when you breast-feed in public, but it should not be a deterrent. *Discretion* is all that is necessary—once you get the hang of it people won't even realize you're nursing. Wear knits or tops that can be unbuttoned from the bottom and lifted up. Wearing a jacket or sweater that partially covers the baby works well also.

## THE ADVANTAGES OF BREAST-FEEDING

A report from the Rockefeller Foundation suggested four ways in which the food habits of Americans need to be altered: their diets should contain less salt, less sugar, a lower fat content, and there should be a *return to universal breast-feeding of infants*. This impressive recommendation is but one more piece of evidence that breast-feeding is better both physically and emotionally than bottle-feeding. The only *disadvantage* to breast-feeding is the environmental pollutants that can reach your baby through breast milk. This consideration is covered in the following section.

The choice that you make about how to nourish your baby is the first decision you make about parenting (outside of circumcision) that has a long-lasting effect on your child's life. Don't just throw that decision away—you may come to regret it. It is every woman's right to decide how to feed her child, just as it is her right to determine where and how she will give birth. Just as with that decision, it is her duty to herself and the baby to make an informed, thoughtful choice. Please do not decide against breast-feeding or conversely feel you're "morally obligated" to breast-feed until you have all the facts.

## THE ADVANTAGES TO THE BABY

**Breast-fed babies have been shown healthier** in certain studies. One study concluded that there was a 3 times greater incidence of illness in bottle-fed infants. These infants were compared to an equivalent group of breast-fed babies and the bottle-fed babies had twice as many episodes of otitis media (an ear infection) in the first year; 16 times more acute lower respiratory illness; 2½ times more significant vomiting or diarrhea; 8½ times more hospital admissions. This study also showed that while the average child gets 6 to 8 respiratory infections per year, that bottle-fed babies get more seriously ill, because human milk and colostrum supply antibodies to viruses. It was also concluded that the length of time a baby is breast-fed is correlated positively with health. Infants that were breast-fed longer than 4½ months became ill *one-half as often* as those that were breast-fed less than 4½ months and those that were bottle-fed.

There are certain diseases that are considered problems chiefly for bottle-fed babies. *Many of these diseases can apparently be avoided if the newborn is breast-fed for at least the first 2 weeks of life.*

- **NEONATAL TETANY** is a newborn disease caused by a deficiency of calcium in the blood. It causes convulsions and a loss of consciousness.
- **HYPOCALCAEMIA** is a diminished amount of calcium in the blood which can lead to convulsions. Infants at the greatest risk are low-birth-weight, those born to diabetic mothers, and those subjected to a long and difficult delivery. There is also a high incidence in premature infants, particularly those with respiratory distress. The onset of the disease usually occurs within the first 5 to 10 days of life.
- **HYPERNATRAEMIA** is an abnormally high sodium level in the blood causing dehydration. It is frequently responsible for brain damage and later intellectual retardation.

*Human milk is more digestible.* A baby's stomach learns gradually to digest. In the first days after birth the colostrum precedes the true milk, which gives the stomach and digestive juices time to learn how to function. The chemical composition of the colostrum is the same as what the baby was fed before birth because both are derived from the mother's blood. A breast-fed baby usually spits up less and the vomit doesn't have the harsh smell of "spoiled milk" as with bottle-fed babies.

***Breast-fed babies are rarely constipated*** because the curd of breast milk is smaller and more easily digestible than the curd of cow's milk. Breast milk contains proteolytic enzymes which aid digestion. A breast-fed baby's bowel movements have a less offensive odor and the baby is less likely to have diaper rash.

***Human milk has 20 mg of cholesterol per 100 mg.*** Most formulas have 1.5 to 3.3 mg per 100. The amount of cholesterol needed by infants has not been established but animal studies show that low-cholesterol in infancy meant *higher* serum cholesterol levels when they got older, as compared to animals fed diets with moderate amounts of cholesterol in infancy. The higher cholesterol content of breast milk appears to promote lower serum cholesterol levels in adulthood. The implication is that low-cholesterol formulas may contribute to atherosclerosis in later life, which is a big national health problem in the United States.

***The small content of iron*** in breast milk is bound to the protein lactoferrin, which enables virtually all of the iron to be absorbed by the baby. Lactoferrin also acts as an antibacterial agent.

***Taurine is a nonprotein nitrogen compound*** that is two times more abundant in breast milk than in cow's milk, which is the base for most artificial formulas. The importance of taurine or the harm of a deficiency in bottle-fed infants has not been proven but it is known that a newborn has only 25 percent of his mature brain weight at birth. After birth a baby is still in a phase of rapid growth and there is a great demand—which may be critical—for specific essential nutrients.

***The breast milk of mothers of premature babies*** has only recently been discovered to differ from that of women with full-term deliveries. The milk of mothers of premies has been found to contain substantially higher concentrations of protein, sodium, and chloride. Studies show that premature babies fed this preterm milk tolerated their diet much better.

These new findings contradict a widely held belief that premature infants fed formula grow more quickly than those fed mother's milk. Premies who breast-feed and get preterm milk grow as well, but most important, they are more apt to avoid the intestinal infections that are associated with some premature babies who take formula.

These findings also call into question the controversial issue of feeding preterm infants. Because they are not developed enough to breast-feed, premature infants who do receive mother's milk normally are fed from a milk bank—human milk pumped from several mothers, all of whom had pregnancies that went a full nine months. It was this milk that was found to be deficient for premature infants. This new research suggests that when premies receive mother's milk, it should be pumped from the natural mother only.

## The Problems with Cow's Milk

*Cow's milk has three times the percentage of salts* as breast milk. In the first weeks of life the baby's kidneys are not sufficiently developed to handle this high phosphate content. Convulsions sometimes occur between 6 to 8 days after birth in children who have been fed cow's milk.

*Cow's milk proteins are foreign* and quite allergenic to babies. During the first 6 weeks of life, the intestine is rather permeable and may allow absorption of foreign proteins. These absorbed proteins may sensitize the infant and lay the foundation for food allergies. After about 6 weeks the local immune response of the baby helps prevent the absorption.

*If the baby's immediate family* has a history of allergies, breast milk will reduce the baby's exposure to foreign milk proteins and possible allergy. Allergies seem to be a familial condition. If a parent or sibling has an allergy of any type the baby is more likely to develop allergies as well. Moreover, once an individual is allergic to one substance other allergies become more common.

It has been estimated that between 0.3 and 7 percent

of American babies develop an allergy to cow's milk. Symptoms of this allergy are: vomiting; colic; skin irritations like dermatitis, hives, or eczema; gastrointestinal infections; respiratory illness; stomach bleeding; growth retardation; and central nervous system damage. Allergic reaction to milk can be life-threatening for an infant. Severe vomiting and diarrhea are symptomatic of this allergy: if it is not treated promptly it can lead to rapid dehydration and death.

When there is a family history of allergy the baby should not be given cow's milk formula from birth. A baby's allergic reaction may be minimized if cow's milk is withheld during the first months of life. Most pediatricians recommend soymilk formula instead, but one study showed that 30 to 50 percent of children who were allergic to cow's milk developed an allergy to soymilk as well. In such cases you can substitute either a meat-base formula or a predigested milk formula (Nutramigen) if you don't breast-feed.

***There is less likelihood of overfeeding*** when you breast-feed. You don't know the amount the baby is getting—he just nurses until satisfied. There is a theory that breast milk is so perfectly suited to a baby's needs that it first satisfies thirst and then gives more substantial nourishment. The milk at the beginning of nursing is more watery; higher calorie milk comes naturally at the end of the feeding. Cow's milk formulas do not satisfy thirst. A baby's thirst may be misinterpreted as hunger so he might get more calories than he needs or should have.

A mother's encouragement to a baby to drink the entire contents of a bottle is probably responsible for the higher caloric intake of bottle-fed babies. Research suggests that consuming a large amount of calories early in life can lead to the development of an excessive number of fat cells. Later on these fat cells can be reduced in size—but not in number—by dieting. Bottle-feeding mothers have to be cautioned against pressuring infants into finishing each feeding and to avoid a similar attitude toward their eating throughout childhood.

**Strong sucking develops correct palate** formation. A breast-feeding baby has to suck harder to get milk. A bottle does not require a baby to use the same strength when he sucks. Nursing from the breast also develops muscles that are used later for speaking.

**Breast-feeding is a continuation of the intimate physiological relationship** that began when your baby was in utero. During nursing, bottle-fed babies do not seem to receive the same intimate physical contact—skin-to-skin contact, close holding, eye-to-eye contact—that breast-feeding babies get.

If you watch a woman bottle-feed her baby you'll notice that she often doesn't hold her close to her body with firm contact. Sometimes bottle-feeding mothers even feed a baby while she's in a plastic chair or they prop her up, encouraging the baby to hold her own bottle. Some parents have the misguided notion that this is "progress"— that the sooner a baby is separated from close physical contact, the more quickly she is developing. Regardless of what you feed your baby and what container it comes in, a baby deserves the warm, close, secure feeling of being held in your arms when she eats. All too soon a baby *does* grow up and become increasingly independent. The physical and emotional pleasure of being held next to your body helps a baby develop into a secure, self-reliant person.

There are tangible results of the close contact which breast-feeding babies enjoy. A breast-feeding mother doesn't have to think about how to hold the baby—she has no choice but to snuggle the child against her. Studies have shown that breast-fed babies that were *not separated* from their mothers after birth averaged a half-pound over their birth weight at 6 to 7 days of age. Bottle-fed babies are expected to fall below their birth weight and take 7 to 10 days to regain the weight they had when born.

**It has been said that breast-feeding** is "the first way to tell the truth to a baby and keep a promise." At the breast a child commences to learn how to relate to another person as a warm, loving, caring human being.

## THE ADVANTAGES TO THE MOTHER

*Breast-feeding immediately* after birth promotes uterine contractions and reduces the risk of postpartum hemorrhage. Further suckling helps the uterus return quickly to its prepregnancy size.

*Some experts say that there is a decreased incidence of breast cancer* in women who breast-feed.

*There is a value in being forced to sit or lie still* while breast-feeding. The early weeks postpartum are when the baby makes the heaviest demands to nurse. This corresponds to the time when you should be resting and allowing your body to rebuild. The sitting-still time that breast-feeding demands protects you from the tendency to overexert yourself in the first weeks after birth.

*Prolactin is the milk-making hormone.* It is believed to be important in promoting maternal attachment. Some studies have shown that prolactin increases motherliness.

*Breast-feeding is important for the reciprocal development* of you and your baby. Each time a baby is born a mother is born too—and your further human development is enhanced by close, intimate contact with the baby.

*Breast-feeding is less expensive* than formulas, which are very costly. The extra 500 calories and extra 20 grams of protein that a breast-feeding mother needs a day can be provided by a peanut-butter sandwich on wheat bread and a glass of milk.

*Breast-feeding is more convenient.* There are no bottles to clean or formula to worry about. Traveling is much easier; when the baby is hungry you just put her to your breast. There is none of the hassle of trying to sterilize bottles and have enough formula while traveling.

**Breast-feeding requires only one arm,** so it leaves you freer to do other things simultaneously. You can hold a book, write a letter, or talk on the telephone while nursing.

## COMPLICATIONS OF THE BREASTS AND NIPPLES FROM BREAST-FEEDING

**If a baby is not allowed to breast-feed immediately** at birth, it can cause complications. Babies not allowed to suck at the breast when they first have the need, tend to forget the sucking instinct in the hours of frustration that follow. There can be a deep psychological trauma to you when the baby is finally brought to you and won't take your breast.

However, if you were heavily medicated during labor and delivery you may not be able to hold the baby. Also, the medication is secreted into the colostrum and it may be better not to add it to the system of a baby already struggling with the labor drugs.

If your baby has been given a bottle before he breast-feeds, he will not know how to nurse at your breast, which requires stronger sucking. First of all, make sure the baby gets no more bottles. And don't feel rejected. You'll just have to show the baby how to do it. If your breasts are still soft enough to put way into the back of his mouth, prop the baby on a pillow in your lap under your left breast, if you're right-handed. Express some milk into the baby's mouth. Compress your breast between your fingers, put it as far back into the baby's mouth as it will go and express more milk. Eventually the baby will coordinate the right movements to latch onto your breast.

If the baby gets upset, comfort him over your shoulder, and when he's quiet, try again. You can alternately put some breast milk on your knuckle and when the baby sucks well on that, transfer him to your breast. Or you can use a breast pump and have the baby drink directly from it like a cup. It is messy but preferable to an artificial nipple, which miseducates the baby's sucking technique.

**Engorgement** of your breasts can happen on the 3rd or 4th day postpartum with the onset of lactation. Your breasts will feel hard and tender. One cause of this can be that the baby did not start nursing from birth. If you don't get the colostrum flowing before your milk supply comes in this can result in hard, painful breasts. Make sure that your bra is supportive but isn't too tight; 15 minutes before you put the baby to your breast take an aspirin or a glass of wine or beer to lessen the pain. Ice packs or heat can help lessen the discomfort; alternate the two, depending on which feels best. A warm shower is good, or applying a washcloth that is as hot as you can stand. Once your milk starts flowing the engorgement will pass.

One remedy is to get in the shower and turn a gentle stream of water warmer and warmer until it's as hot as you can stand. Once the blood is circulating well, massage your breasts gently one at a time. Have one palm underneath supporting the breast and working upward toward the nipples. The other palm should start at your collarbone and work down toward the nipple. Then your upper hand should massage the side of the breast, working from your armpit in toward the nipple, then from your breastbone toward the nipple. The lower hand should massage on the opposite side of the breast. The object of this massaging is to get the milk flowing and to continue working the lumps caused by backed-up milk down toward the nipple.

There are several preventive steps you can take to avoid painful breast engorgement. The first is that the baby should be nursed soon after birth to facilitate lactation. The wait of 6 to 12 hours in some hospitals is too long a fasting period for successful breast-feeding. Second, no bottle should be given to the baby, of either water or formula. It will interfere with the natural establishment of lactation. It is easier for the baby to nurse from a bottle: some may simply wait for the post-breast-feeding bottle, which sabotages nursing. The mother's milk will collect in her breast, so there will be diminished milk production, which depends greatly on emptying the breast.

To help prevent engorgement, become aware of how the breast works and fit your nursing schedule around that. In the first 2 hours after nursing, the breast produces most of the milk for the next feeding. Breast engorgement will be more likely to occur if the breast is kept from the baby for longer than 2 hours. One hour after a woman's breast is emptied, it has already produced 40 percent of the supply for the next feeding. Two hours afterward she may have as much as 75 percent. Although it might seem sensible to wait until a higher percent of her milk capacity has been re-gained, that kind of schedule can lead to breast soreness.

Because breast milk is quickly digested (maybe in 2 hours, but certainly sooner than the 4-hour interval for breast-feeding that is often recommended), the baby be-comes overly hungry. A very hungry baby is going to suck more vigorously. Also, if the mother has waited the extra hour for her breasts to fill to capacity, congestion of the areola becomes a problem. The baby cannot put the nipple and areola into the back of his mouth and his abnormally vigorous, hungry sucking will cause pain.

A good way to facilitate nursing if your breasts are engorged or even if they aren't is to express a little milk at the beginning of each feeding. This will soften the areola, allowing the baby to get the nipple to the back of his mouth easily. With two fingers placed around the areola, you can gently press against your chest, emptying the sinuses and making the areola soft. This will be a great help for the first couple of weeks of breast-feeding.

*Mastitis* is an infection of the breast caused by a clogged milk duct or a staphylococcal infection. It is not to be con-fused with engorgement, which occurs on the 3rd or 4th day postpartum. True mastitis rarely occurs before the end of the first postpartum week and usually not until the end of the 3rd or 4th week. It is believed that the infant harbors the bacteria (staphylococcus auereus) in her nose and throat and the organism enters the breast at the time of feeding through the nipple, via a fissure or abrasion which may be quite small. The baby may have gotten the bacteria in the hospital from the partially washed hands of one of the staff but there are many other ways it could have been picked up.

The symptoms of mastitis are sudden: you will feel poorly, have a fever, headache, and engorged breasts that feel warm. The tender area will be hard and red. If you contact the doctor promptly, the condition won't become serious. A drop of your milk is sent for bacterial culture and penicillin G or another antibiotic is given in the meantime. If your temperature and inflammation don't subside within 48 hours, an abscess usually forms, but this is quite uncommon. In this case the baby must be completely weaned and the doctor has to drain the abscess.

It is not necessary to stop breast-feeding if you get mastitis. If your doctor says to stop, call the La Leche League, which will give you information about nursing and mastitis. They usually recommend that you continue nursing from the affected breast, that it will heal more quickly. The baby will not get sick, as was once thought. Stay off your feet as much as possible and apply heat to the breast with wet washcloths. Offer the sore breast first at each feeding—that way it will probably be emptied and the clogged duct will unclog.

The other alternative is to breast-feed only from your healthy breast and express enough milk from the infected side to relieve pressure. You can then supplement your breast milk with a bottle, being careful to use only "premie" nipples, which have small holes. This way your baby cannot get milk too easily from the bottle and learn to prefer it over your breast.

## SORE NIPPLES

Sore nipples can occur even if you prepared your breasts before nursing. Be sure to let your nipples air-dry and never keep on a wet bra or a wet pad. *No nursing bra should ever have waterproof backing:* tear it out or get rid of the bra. This is a cause of sore nipples. Also, make sure the baby has the whole areola in her mouth.

*Do not use soap,* alcohol, tincture of benzoin, or petroleum jelly on your nipples. If you choose to use an ointment, do so sparingly: these substances can keep out the light and sunlight, which are important to healing. There are several substances which are commonly recommended to minimize nipple discomfort: vitamins A and D cream or concentrate, oils, aloe vera, and expressed breastmilk or colostrum. Massé breast cream is also commonly used—although based on new information about the danger of lanolin (see below), you should check the ingredients to see if a product contains lanolin.

***New research indicates that pure lanolin may be contaminated*** with pesticide residuals. Although lanolin has been recommended for years as a natural remedy for nipple pain, analysis of several lots of anhydrous lanolin United States Pharmacopeia (USP) showed contamination. The tests were done by the Division of Colors and Cosmetics of the Food and Drug Administration (FDA) and the Environmental Protection Agency (EPA) National Toxicological Program. Although the reports stated that "the levels of pesticides did not present an immediate toxic hazard," breast-feeding mothers who apply lanolin to their breasts may be unnecessarily exposing their babies to toxic chemicals. We do not know the potential effects on a newborn who ingests lanolin products—but why run the risk?

***Warm, dry heat*** is the best cure for sore nipples. Leave your breasts exposed to the air as much as possible. To make an ultraviolet lamp just buy an ultraviolet bulb and put it in any light socket. Sit 3 feet from the lamp: expose your nipples a half-minute the first day, 1 minute the 2nd and 3rd days, and 2 minutes the 4th and 5th days. If your skin does not redden you can increase to 3 minutes on the 6th day and maintain that level until the soreness is gone. If there *is* redness at the 2-minute level, cut back to 1 minute for several days and increase by a half-minute if possible. Be sure to use a towel or other cover for your eyes. The bulb gets *very* hot after use. Time yourself carefully with a kitchen timer.

***Do not curtail nursing***—this will just prolong the problem. In fact, continuing to nurse frequently is the best solution. Leisurely nursing every 2 or 3 hours is easier on tender nipples. This way your breasts don't get overfull and the baby doesn't get ravenous. Give the least-sore breast first because the baby sucks hardest when she is hungry. You may limit nursing to 8 to 10 minutes on the sore side, but no less than that. Change nursing positions at each feeding. If your nipples are very sore and you limit sucking time to 10 minutes on each side the baby's sucking needs may not be satisfied and you may have to offer a pacifier.

A mother who has a *great* deal of pain from a sore nipple may have to limit nursing to only 5 minutes on that side. Actually, the first 5 minutes empties most of the milk from the breast and 10 minutes will empty it completely. You have to decide for yourself how bad the pain is and whether it's better to have the baby suck for more than 5 minutes even if the nipple is very sore, because you get the benefit of emptying the breast completely.

If the baby seems satisfied, she can certainly manage for 5 or 6 days while the nipple is sore with only 5 minutes' nursing time. Remember to put the baby first on the breast that is not sore, or less sore. The baby is more likely to take the sore one gently in her mouth because she's less hungry by then. A good rule of thumb is to nurse a sore nipple second, but to nurse a sore breast first, to empty it.

*Apprehension* may be related to sore nipples. Slightly tender nipples may cause enough tension to hold back the let-down reflex. This delay in the milk may make the baby angry so he pulls and tugs on the nipple. This makes it even sorer and causes you greater concern. Try to make a conscious effort to relax before nursing.

To ease the discomfort while nursing take an aspirin or glass of wine or beer 15 minutes beforehand. This will help relax you and encourage the let-down reflex. If you're having a problem with the let-down reflex, you can hand-express some milk before the baby starts nursing. If you're having real difficulty with your let-down reflex when your nipples are sore, talk to your doctor about prescribing some oxytocin.

*Ice water or ice* eases the pain of sore nipples immediately. Crush the ice, wrap it in a washcloth, and apply it to the nipple area.

*Fungus infection* can cause sore nipples. The baby may have thrush, which is common and bothersome, but not serious. If the nipple soreness persists and there are white spots inside the baby's mouth, or if the baby has persistent diaper rash or you have vaginitis, or if you have been fine and suddenly develop sore nipples again—call the doctor for treatment.

*Cracked nipples* can be caused by anything that keeps the baby from getting his jaws on the areola. Most hair around the nipple doesn't bother a baby, but sometimes he will react by pulling back and chewing on the nipple. Trim the hairs if this happens. Treatment is the same as for sore nipples, but more so. Sit in the sunshine by an open window, letting the sun bake your breasts—but not burn them, obviously. In the winter the sun coming through the glass is helpful. For some women, a sunlamp is too strong: in this case the heat of an ordinary naked lightbulb is good.

*A blood blister* on the tip of your nipple is caused by vigorous sucking. It is not significant and you should just leave it alone when it is in the blister and scab stages. It will go away by itself.

*Hemorrhage (bruising)* in and around the nipple during breast-feeding is often found as a result of abnormal sucking with painfully engorged breasts. This bruising is often caused by the mother waiting too long between feedings, allowing the breasts to get engorged and the baby to become so hungry that he sucks abnormally vigorously.

Hemorrhage into the nipple is caused by palate sucking. There is rarely a problem on the sides of the nipples because the sides of the baby's mouth are more gentle on the nipple than the upper or lower portions of the mouth. The top part of the baby's mouth sucks with the greatest force. Sometimes the bruising appears right on the edge of the nipple, a clear indication that the baby is not getting the nipple to the back of his mouth. Be sure that the whole areola goes into the baby's mouth when nursing.

## PROBLEMS WITH THE BABY AND NURSING

AFTERNOON FUSSINESS AND HUNGER are a common complaint in the first month of breast-feeding. The baby nurses well in the morning and sleeps 3 or 4 hours between feedings; in the afternoon she cries and wants to be fed nearly every hour. The reason this happens is that as the mother goes through the day she tires, and milk production suffers as she runs around. One way to overcome this problem is to do most of your chores and errands in the morning and by early afternoon relax, preferably with the baby near you.

STRENUOUS EXERCISE can create difficulties in nursing. If a breast-feeding mother does intense exercise it can result in higher lactic acid levels in her milk, which may influence its taste and quality. If your baby is having difficulties related to nursing, you can experiment for a few days and see if less exertion on your part results in the baby feeding more easily.

INSUFFICIENT MILK SUPPLY is a common complaint during the first postpartum days. A major cause for this is a delay in starting breast-feeding postdelivery or infrequent feedings afterward. The breast has to be stimulated by the baby nursing often, more than the every-4-hour schedule at some hospitals. The baby has to nurse several times from each breast in every 24-hour period; if the breasts are not emptied frequently, milk production will suffer. Supplementary formula feedings will reduce the milk supply because they reduce breast stimulation.

Another reason for a low milk yield is the emotional factor of a new mother being told her milk supply is poor or that her baby is hungry. This can make a woman feel guilty and anxious, which will lead to reduced milk production and a poor let-down reflex. If you are aware of these potential problems, you can avoid them. You might want to try the oxytocin nasal spray described on page 651 to help your let-down reflex.

***If you're worried about your milk supply,*** there are a couple of things you should know about breast-feeding babies. Generally speaking, a baby who is breast-feeding will eat every 2 to 3 hours. She should gain ½ to 1 ounce a day in the first six months of her life. Babies tend to lose a little weight after birth, but by the time she is two weeks old she should be at least back to her birth weight.

      If you feel your baby is constantly wanting to eat— she's still hungry after feeding and a pacifier doesn't satisfy her—you may suspect your milk supply is low. Have a breast-feeding consultation with your pediatrician or better yet, a lactation specialist.

***The baby may refuse to nurse.*** A baby may be sensitive to your diet and can be fussy about particular foods which impart a flavor to your breast milk. Some foods to avoid or eat sparingly if your baby is fussy are: onions, garlic, cabbage, brussels sprouts, and chocolate. When you're menstruating your milk may be offensive to the baby. If so, you can cut down the nursing time until your period is over.

***A teething baby*** can refuse to nurse. Rub whiskey or gin on her gums or dissolve a baby aspirin in water and rub it on. If your let-down reflex requires vigorous sucking, which may be hard for a teething baby, you can use a nasal-spray oxytocin before difficult feedings or hand-express some milk first so the baby doesn't have to suck so hard.

***The baby may bite*** when nursing. This usually doesn't happen until around 3 months and ordinarily occurs at the end of a feeding. Say "NO!" loudly and suddenly; terminate the feeding right then. At the next feeding don't continue nursing after the baby begins to play around, and she will learn soon enough.

***You cannot see how much the baby is eating.*** This may bother some women who feel the need to know the quantity that the baby consumes. Don't worry about it. The beauty of breast-feeding is that it is a supply and demand system—you produce milk in response to how much the baby sucks. A breast-fed baby eats until satisfied. As long as the baby has frequent wet diapers, is alert, and looks healthy, she's getting enough. You can always check intake by output: except in very hot weather a baby will wet a lot of diapers. This is one way to verify that the baby is getting enough.

**The baby will be hungry sooner** than if you feed her formula. Breast milk digests more quickly—cow's milk is hard for a baby to digest and the large curds stay in her stomach longer. If your baby won't sleep through the night once you've got a good milk supply, after the early postpartum period, you might consider giving some formula before bed.

**Breast-feeding takes longer than bottle-feeding,** which some women consider a disadvantage to nursing. You can give a baby a bottle in about 10 minutes, but breast-feeding realistically takes about an hour. However, with a bottle you and the baby may miss out on that contact with each other which is so important for both of you. Breast-feeding forces you to sit still and enjoy. If you are accustomed to having a superefficient, rushed, very organized rhythm you may have to change it temporarily. It may be good for you to have a change of pace—and you shouldn't undervalue the time you spend in an intimate embrace with your baby. All too soon your baby will be changing and growing—try to make whatever adjustments you can in your life so you can enjoy every stage of the baby's life without thinking of it as "wasted" time.

## PSYCHOLOGICAL PROBLEMS WITH BREAST-FEEDING

Some women just aren't comfortable with either the idea or physical reality of breast-feeding. There can be a vast number of reasons for this. For example, a woman who can't stand the idea of breast-feeding may have been rejected as a child and is now afraid of warm, close relationships. Some women cannot nurse because unconsciously they identify with their own mother who was cold and rejecting. One learns to be a good mother from having had one.

If you are unhappy or tense breast-feeding you shouldn't bang your head against a wall. You will probably be able to relax, cuddle, and enjoy your baby more with a bottle. There are many people who believe that *how* a baby is fed is as important as *what* he is fed. A baby gets two things in his mother's arms: he gets food and love (and develops the capacity to love). If you can give that to your baby more freely and easily by *not* breast-feeding, then a bottle will be better for you both.

### DIABETES AND BREAST-FEEDING

Breast-feeding is usually advised against for diabetic mothers. Initially, breast-feeding may be associated with hypoglycemic episodes; milk production is often deficient and nursing is rarely successful. However, breast-feeding can help offset the high-risk atmosphere associated with diabetic pregnancy, as well as giving a diabetic mother the pleasure of nursing and of knowing her body can do it. Here are some possible complications:

*Hypoglycemia* can be expected between 5 and 7 hours postpartum. Immediately after delivery there is an increased risk of hypoglycemia while your body makes diet/insulin/exercise adjustments, whether you are breast-feeding or not. The loss of human placental lactogen is accompanied by an increased insulin sensitivity. I.V. glucose and insulin are monitored until stabilization is reached at about 18 to 24 hours postpartum. Then you can take daily insulin again by injection.

Your daily insulin requirement will probably be only 60 percent of the dose you were taking before you became pregnant. The requirement will gradually increase for 4 to 6 weeks postpartum. Breast-feeding may reduce your insulin requirement beyond this 4- to 6-week period. Nursing may reduce it due to a prolonged attenuation of growth hormone secretion. Insulin need declines in women who rigidly control their diets and increase their activity postpartum, independent of the effect of breast-feeding.

Hypoglycemic reactions (insulin reactions) are associated with rapid falls in your glucose levels. The symptoms are: visual disturbances, headache, sweating, shaking, loss of coordination, and finally loss of consciousness. Hypoglycemia triggers the release of epinephrine, which inhibits oxytocin, the hormone that mediates the let-down reflex. Thus high levels of epinephrine can inhibit your let-down reflex and interfere with breast-feeding. Trace amounts of insulin and epinephrine reach the breast milk but the infant's digestive enzymes deactivate the hormones.

*Hyperglycemia:* occasional high blood sugar may occur as diet/insulin/exercise adjustments are being made throughout the breast-feeding period. Any infection, illness, or even emotional upset can cause an increase in your blood glucose and glycosuria. You can test your urine 3 or 4 times daily for sugar, and periodic fasting and random blood sugar tests can be made to assess diabetic control.

*Acetonuria* may accompany high blood sugar. Acetones are detected in your urine by Ketodiastix or Acetest tablets. The usual treatment for ketosis is increased insulin, increased carbohydrates, and bed rest. If you are breast-feeding you have to be particularly concerned about avoiding acetonuria. Ketones can enter the breast milk but are not harmful. They are ingested by the infant and utilized along with other dietary substances.

*Lactose* may be found in your urine during late pregnancy and lactation. You will have to use urine-testing materials which will not react positively to lactose but are specific for glucose. TesTape, unlike most others, is specific for glucose.

*Infections* must be treated aggressively with a nursing diabetic mother. If you develop infection, antibiotics are usually prescribed, but many of them are detrimental to the nursing baby and enter your breast milk in high concentrations (see pages 683–687). *Antibiotics to avoid are:* erythromycin, Estolate, Symmetrel, tetracycline, streptomycin, and Doxycycline, to name a few. Alternatives can usually be prescribed and many antibiotics (including erythromycin) do not necessitate weaning, just a temporary interruption.

*Treat plugged milk ducts promptly* because they can quickly develop into an infection. Clogged ducts often result from wearing a too-tight bra or wearing a nursing bra while you sleep. If an infection does develop, keep the breast emptied, apply heat and stay in bed. Allowing milk to stay in your breast will result in painful engorgement and further obstruction of an already plugged duct.

*Abrupt weaning* should be avoided: it may cause an emotional upset for you and the baby and will make diabetic control difficult.

*Monilial infections* of the vagina: a diabetic woman is susceptible to them, especially if her glucose control is poor. When you are breast-feeding, monilia can infect the nipple. The prevention is to keep nipples dry between feedings or the infection will return despite treatment. The doctor may prescribe Lotrimin cream or suppositories or Monistat ointment. Mycostatin was popular at one time but it only has a 3- to 4-week shelf life. Be sure to wash these ointments off the breast before nursing.

*Weaning:* Infant teething or illness in you or the baby may mean you have to decrease nursing for a while and then nurse more frequently. This may cause mysteriously high urine or blood sugar, followed by unexpectedly low test values. You can usually compensate for this by eating less, exercising more, or adjusting your insulin.

## WORKING AND BREAST-FEEDING

There are two contemporary trends at odds with each other which meet head-on when a working woman decides to breast-feed. On the one hand there is increased employment and more substantial careers for women, but this conflicts with a trend toward increased breast-feeding and what is referred to as "natural mothering." This is a philosophy that a mother should have constant contact with her child, including breast-feeding on demand, for the first one or two years of his life—a belief system that is incompatible with employment outside the home.

A working mother also has a twofold problem in juggling her commitment to her job and her child. At work she must almost pretend that her child does not exist, yet she has to arrange her life as much as she can to take the child into consideration. She faces criticism from both sides: if she works she is considered a selfish, "bad" mother by those who favor "natural mothering" and because of her commitment to her child she may be reprimanded by those in the workplace if she rearranges her time on the child's behalf.

The reality is that there are increasing numbers of women who want to have a life outside their home. Many of the women having babies today are doing so after they have firmly established themselves in a career they do not want to relinquish. On top of that, there are women who may wind up forced to work to support their children. Statistics show that one-quarter of the children in America do not live with both their natural parents—and the vast majority stay with their mother. A full one-half of black children do not live with both their parents. By the age of eighteen, 35 to 45 percent of all children in the United States will spend five years or more in a single-parent home. Since most men do not meet child-support payments, the mother usually seeks employment.

Breast-feeding and working outside the home not only are possible but have great benefits if you are willing to make the effort. Working and raising children at the same time can produce a destructive guilt—you feel torn between the two, as if you are cheating the children, have to make it up to them, and so on. Breast-feeding provides an important source of confidence in your mothering ability. The practical aspect is that breast-fed babies are usually healthier. Preventing sickness in your baby is important to your psychological well-being. As hard as it may be to leave a baby to go to work, it creates that much more guilt to leave a sick baby. Breast-feeding itself is not a common choice among American women, and working and breast-feeding is even more unusual. It may be difficult, but the rewards are worth the investment of your time and energy if you are interested in pursuing the combination.

*Certain character traits* may hamper you. For instance, independence and a motivation to succeed, which help in a career, can hinder you with breast-feeding. Nursing is not a rational, predictable process: it cannot be controlled and organized in the way that many jobs can. Breast-feeding is emotional, intuitive, sensual, and enjoyable. Your expectation of accomplishing too much during early breast-feeding—and pride in your independence—may keep you from asking for help. You are going to have to overcome the antidependency sentiments which our society applauds, particularly for people with careers, so that you can reach out for help with breast-feeding if you need it.

*The La Leche League group* may not be the place to go for advice and support. La Leche members are often unemployed and many of them believe in "natural" or "total" mothering and may frown on mothers who work. Criticism is the last thing you need—it is a stress and can inhibit your let-down reflex during the initiation of lactation and undermine your efforts. Try to find other women who are in your position and even organize a support group among yourselves. You can share mutual problems and solutions—just knowing other women sharing your situation can be a great comfort.

*The initiation of breast-feeding* is the foundation for success when you return to work. It is absolutely essential that you have encouragement from everyone close to you. This is vital for breast-feeding success even for women who are not simultaneously pursuing careers. Especially if you are a first-time mother, you should optimally take off a minimum of 4 weeks from work and preferably 6 weeks. It is rare to be able to establish a good nursing relationship— with a well-conditioned let-down reflex and an adequate milk supply—in less than a month.

*Hand-expression of milk* will be necessary to maintain a milk supply once you are separated from your child. It will also be necessary so you can deal with breast engorgement. Practice the hand-expression of colostrum before the baby is born. If you aren't comfortable using your hands then try a breast pump because you have to be able to hand-express your milk.

*In the hospital you should realistically expect little or no help* with breast-feeding. Find women who have breast-fed before your baby is born so that you have someone to call if you need help. Breast-feeding will go much smoother if you have minimal medication during the birth— that way the baby will be alert and will suck more enthusiastically. An early start to breast-feeding—preferably on the delivery table—will also help establish your relationship with the baby. Be sure to have rooming-in, if possible, and make certain that your baby is given *no bottle supplements,* which sabotage breast-feeding.

*The day a woman comes home* from the hospital is considered the most critical time for lactation failure. Your let-down reflex is affected by *fatigue, anxiety, insensitive remarks,* and other stressful factors. If these occur in the early days, their impact can interfere with your milk supply.

You should literally come home and go right to bed, taking the baby with you. Take along your favorite food and drink; wine and beer in moderation are traditional aids to relaxation. Remove yourself from the responsibilities of the house and arrange for help in the beginning. Household help that contributes to good nursing—by freeing you to relax with your new baby—is a well-deserved indulgence.

***Returning to work*** and how you handle breast-feeding is a personal choice. However, it is vital that you maintain a flexible attitude. *There is no absolute definition of success in breast-feeding for a working mother.* There is no measurement of success as gauged by a number of weeks or any other absolute scale. Remember this: if your nursing relationship brings satisfaction to you and your baby, then you have succeeded.

Every drop of breast milk you give your baby helps him. The longer you nurse, the more protection against disease and allergy you've offered the baby. If you find you go back to work and cannot sustain breast-feeding, you have not failed. If you nurse for six weeks and then discontinue nursing, you can be pleased that you've given your baby the best possible nutrition in the important early weeks.

***You have several options*** about how to handle breast-feeding and your return to work. You can take the baby to work or you can work at home. A sitter can bring the baby to you at lunch or during coffee breaks, although there is no guarantee that the baby will nurse on your schedule. And then there is substitute feeding, which is probably the most practical.

***Substitute feeding is best if your milk is used,*** although formula can be substituted. You can begin to collect your milk before you return to work. Express the milk into a container that is cold and sterile: putting it through the dishwasher is sufficient sterilization. Cover it securely and label it with the date. It will last up to 2 years in a deep-freeze and up to 6 months in a refrigerator freezer. The antibodies in the milk are stable when frozen, but some other anti-infective properties are not. But having frozen milk gives you security: you won't have to worry about manual expression on a daily basis for the first few weeks and if you have days when you can't produce fresh milk, the baby will still have some.

It is best to express the next day's milk at work and refrigerate it until use, saving the frozen milk for when fresh is not available. If you express milk at work do it at the same time and place each day. This conditions your milk to let down to a stimulus other than sucking. You can also collect the leakage from your breasts by wearing a Netsy Milk Cup, which is a plastic dome-shaped cover (from the Netsy Co., 34 Sunrise Avenue, Mill Valley, California 94941).

*You have to refrigerate the collected milk right away, as it will spoil rapidly, especially when the weather is warm.*

**Introduce the baby to the person who will be giving the substitute feedings** before you return to work. The person should stay for increasingly long periods of time but with *no attempts to feed the child* the first few times. With older babies—past 6 or 7 months—they may already be experiencing separation anxiety, so the introduction should be more gradual for them.

At first you should go out for 1 to 2 hours, staying within reach. The substitute should try to feed the baby about half an hour *before* the baby's usual feeding time. Feeding before the baby gets really hungry gives her time to deal with the bottle before acute hunger sets in. This prevents the escalating panic in the infant who has to cope with an unfamiliar way of eating *and* extreme hunger.

The substitute should gently insert the nipple in a back-and-forth manner . . . and stop if the baby gets too upset. The sitter should try again 15 to 20 minutes later. Using Nuk nipples is a good idea as they are closest to human nipples. If the baby gets really upset you should return and try again the following day. Don't worry—some babies just take longer to adjust to substitute feeding.

**Rejecting the bottle or breast** is not uncommon. Some babies 6 months and over who are receiving solid foods may choose to wait as long as 6 to 7 hours for you to return. This is okay. Bottle rejection may indicate a loss of the *mothering person:* it is important for the substitute to "mother" the baby, not just feed her. If the baby refuses the bottle, the substitute should cuddle the baby, coo and talk to her, and then attempt the feeding again.

Refusing your breast may mean the baby is refusing you. You have to make an extra attempt at prolonged and continuous tactile contact: stroking, cuddling, holding, and maintaining eye contact. The danger here is that you may withdraw because the baby has rejected you for leaving. A rejection cycle can be established: the infant is suffering most from feelings of separation and loss, yet you withdraw. Signs of your withdrawal are: wanting to avoid the infant, not wanting to nurse, the failure of your let-down reflex, and the expectation that the nursing relationship is going to fail. If not stopped in time, this cycle can terminate the breast-feeding relationship.

*Maintaining milk supply* does not just happen by itself, as is the case with breast-feeding mothers who do not work. Hand-expression of milk stimulates about one-third as much milk as sucking does. You *must* allow the baby to nurse when you are home—roughly 4 feedings a day is usually right.

*Starting the morning right* is important: your breasts are fullest after a night's rest. Each day you should try to get up half an hour early so you can have a relaxed feeding and avoid feeling guilty because you had to rush.

*Coming home at the end of the day* is also very important because you and the baby have mutual emotional and physiological needs at that time. Your breasts are full and the baby is hungry. You must plan to set aside this homecoming time for the baby. Arrange with your mate and other children that all family business has to be postponed until one hour after you get home and that their needs will be met at that time. Try to get help with the dinner—either paid help/your mate/children or convenience foods—so that there is one less demand on you.

***Nighttime feedings help*** to maintain your milk supply. Most infants will continue to nurse at night—the easiest way is to take the baby to bed with you so that you can roll over and nurse without fully waking up. This gives you extra closeness to the baby and the extra energy you save by not having to get up is especially important since you have to go to work in the morning.

***The main problem*** you will encounter is that some days your milk supply will be low. You should expect this to happen. Some minimal curtailment of activity usually solves the problem. *Stress is the biggest offender.* When signs of stress approach the danger stage, you should try to reduce pressure and demands both at home and in your business life. Some signs are: the it's-too-much-trouble syndrome, excessive concern about the baby having enough to eat, worry about expressing milk, and a significantly reduced milk supply. *Stress tolerance is reached* when you are no longer able to nurse the baby when he's hungry. Take the day off, go to bed with the baby, drink plenty of fluids, and you should be back on course by the following day.

## DRUGS AND BREAST-FEEDING

Almost any drug you take will appear quickly in your breast milk, in approximately the same concentration as in your blood. The amount of drug in your milk and its effect on the baby varies; consult your doctor as well as the chart that follows because many drugs will not have an adverse effect. However, there should be a *careful and continuous observation* of a nursing infant for possible unwanted effects from drugs in breast milk.

Although only trace amounts of a drug may be found in breast milk, the cumulative effect over a 24-hour period of nursing may equal a full dose for an infant. Within the first postpartum days certain enzyme systems which are normally required to metabolize or detoxify some drugs may not be fully developed in the newborn. Some drugs, such as insulin and corticotropin, are destroyed in the infant's gastrointestinal tract and are therefore unimportant constituents of breast milk.

Some sulfa drugs prescribed for postpartum urinary tract infections in the mother will pass into her breast milk, remain active after withstanding the acidity of the infant's stomach, and may cause kernicterus or Gray's syndrome (jaundice).

Several anti-infective agents will cause vomiting and skin rash; some of the penicillin compounds may cause sensitization of the infant. Tetracycline may discolor the infant's teeth. Atropine can cause drowsiness, urinary retention, tachycardia, and respiratory symptoms in the baby. Anticoagulants and aspirin taken just before nursing may delay the infant's clotting time. Laxatives, excluding senna derivatives, may cause diarrhea in the baby. Bromides, which are found in Bromo-Seltzer and many over-the-counter sleeping aids, have caused rash and drowsiness in the nursing baby.

A number of psychotropic drugs cause lethargy and weight loss in the baby, including Valium, Lithium, Meprobamate, and Primidone. The effects of barbiturates are controversial but they probably should be avoided due to their action on the infant's liver enzymes. Ergot preparations for migraine headaches can cause vomiting, diarrhea, weak pulse, and unstable blood pressure in the infant. Some drugs are toxic to the nursing baby if taken over a long period of time and require close monitoring of the infant and determining whether the benefit of taking the drug outweighs the risk. Steroids, diuretics, and oral contraceptives are among these medications.

Iodides affect the infant's thyroid gland. Radioactive iodine, sodium, and gallium should be avoided if possible; even mothers who are not breast-feeding should have no contact with the baby for 48 hours afterward.

It is said that if a nursing mother does have to take medication of any kind that it is best to take it right before breast-feeding. If she takes the drug as she is beginning to nurse, by the end of the breast-feeding session the drug will have reached peak serum concentration at a point when there will be very little breast milk left for the drug to pass into. This strategy is not always workable when the infant is nursing 7 or 8 times a day, but as a general rule, try to take medication right when you start to nurse.

***Marijuana is stored in mammalian milk,*** and there have been no studies to suggest that it is acceptable for mothers to smoke marijuana while they are nursing. Because the effects on the infant of chronic exposure to THC and its products are unknown, nursing mothers should abstain from using it. Mother's milk (both animal and human) is very high in fat and is therefore a prime place for the deposit and accumulation of the by-products of marijuana. Furthermore, milk is one of the routes through which the female body excretes, or gets rid of, THC, the chemical component of marijuana.

Animal tests have shown cannabinoid present in all organs of suckling infant rats whose mothers were exposed to THC. When female mice took the drug either just before or just after birth, their male offspring had long-range sexual alterations. This included hormonal imbalances that decreased the size of the testes, as a result of exposure through the placenta and/or breast milk. In addition, when these animals went through puberty there were changes in their sexual behavior and hormone levels that were apparently due to their early exposure to marijuana.

***Cocaine can reach a baby through breast milk,*** as confirmed by recent research. Studies have demonstrated that cocaine not only crosses into breast milk, but remains there for over 36 hours. Researchers found that there can be severe damage, even death, if a baby gets a high enough dose of cocaine through the breast milk. In one study, the mother was snorting cocaine while breast-feeding: within 3 hours of using half a gram of cocaine her child had become irritable, had vomited, and had developed diarrhea. It took two and a half days for the cocaine to clear from the child's urinary tract, after which the child did well. In another case, a child died and the autopsy showed high levels of cocaine in his blood. The mother admitted to using crack before breast-feeding. It shouldn't be necessary to say anything more: breast-feeding mothers should get the message loud and clear.

---

**CHART 44. DIRECTORY OF DRUGS TO AVOID WHEN BREAST-FEEDING**

| DRUG | EFFECT |
|---|---|
| **ANALGESICS** | |
| *Aspirin, Phenacetin &* *combinations* (Alka-Seltzer, Bufferin, Cope, Excedrin, Rhinex, Vanquish) | possible bleeding |
| Ergotamine (antimigraine) *(Cafergot, Ergomar, Gynergan, Migral) | vomiting, diarrhea, weak pulse, unstable blood pressure, shock in 90 percent of infants |
| **ANTACIDS** | |
| (Alka-Seltzer, Gelusil, Maalox) | possible bleeding |
| **ANTIBIOTICS** | |
| *Chloromycetin | anemia, shock, death |
| *Erythromycin | sensitization, allergy to drug |
| Erythromycin Estolate (Ilosone) | hepatoxic |
| Symmetrel | vomiting, rash |
| Tetracycline | bone-growth retardation |
| Streptomycin | nephrotoxicity |
| *Penicillin | possible sensitization, allergy |
| *Antituberculosis (Isoniazid) | mental retardation |
| **ANTICOAGULANTS** | |
| *Dicumarol | prothrombin time less, or |
| *Heparin | hemorrhage in infant |

*Especially harmful*

---

**CHART 44. DIRECTORY OF DRUGS TO AVOID
WHEN BREAST-FEEDING *(continued)***

| DRUG | EFFECT |
| --- | --- |

**ANTICONVULSANTS**

| | |
| --- | --- |
| Primidone | mother should not nurse |
| Mysoline | drowsiness |

*Dilantin* has no acute side effects, occurs in only small amounts in milk; *Mysoline* appears in milk but causes only drowsiness

**ANTINEOPLASTICS**

| | |
| --- | --- |
| MAO inhibitors (an antihypertensive drug) | nursing should stop |

**ANTISPASMODICS**

| | |
| --- | --- |
| *Atropine combinations* *(Artane, Arlidin) | diminish milk secretion; heart irregularities in infant |

**BARBITURATES**

| | |
| --- | --- |
| (Amytal, Luminal, Seconal, Tuinal) | may have inducing effect on baby's liver enzymes; avoid |
| Nembutal | may sedate infant |
| *Hypnotics* (Doriden) | drowsiness |
| *Chloral hydrate and combinations* | drowsiness |
| *Bromides and others* (Bromural, Equanil, Phenergan, Bromo-Seltzer) | drowsiness, rash |

**CARDIOVASCULAR PREPARATIONS**

| | |
| --- | --- |
| *Hypotensives* & *combinations with diuretics* | |
| Ismelin | is hazard to infant |

***Especially harmful***

## CHART 44. DIRECTORY OF DRUGS TO AVOID WHEN BREAST-FEEDING *(continued)*

| DRUG | EFFECT |
|---|---|
| **CARDIOVASCULAR PREPARATIONS** *(cont.)* | |
| *Reserpine | increased respiratory-tract secretions, cyanosis, and anorexia in infant, galactorrhea in mother |
| **COCAINE** | mother should not nurse: can lead to infant death |
| **COUGH PREPARATIONS** | |
| Potassium Iodide | possible thyrotropic effect in infant, skin rash |
| **DIURETICS** | |
| *Thiazides & combinations* (Diuril, Enduron) | dehydration possible; may be harmless if taken under supervision (but manufacturer says to avoid if nursing) |
| **HORMONES** | |
| *Androgen-Estrogen combinations* (Deladumone, Premarin w/ Methyltestosterone) | all estrogens cause gynecomastia and lower milk production |
| *Estrogens* (DES, TACE) | see above |
| *Corticoids and analgesic combinations* | all corticosteroids may cause poor growth and development |
| *Glucocorticoid anti-inflammatory combinations* (Aristocort, Cetacort lotion) | poor growth of infant |

*Especially harmful*

## CHART 44. DIRECTORY OF DRUGS TO AVOID WHEN BREAST-FEEDING (continued)

| DRUG | EFFECT |
|---|---|
| **HORMONES** (cont.) | |
| *Progestins* (Depo-Provera, Gynorest, Nortulate) | lower milk production |
| *\*Progestins and estrogens in combination* (Demulen, Enovid, Ortho-Novum, Ovulen) | lower milk production |
| *\*Parathryoid-Dihydrotachysterol Thyroid inhibitors* *(Tapazole)* | osteoporosis, bone dysgenesis, reduced thyroid activity, goiter anemia |
| **LAXATIVES** | |
| Senokot | loose stool |
| *Dorbantyl, Dorbane | diarrhea |
| **MARIJUANA** | is hazard to infant |
| **MUSCLE RELAXANTS** | |
| Carosoprodol | manufacturer suggests avoiding nursing |
| Valium—see PSYCHOTROPICS | |
| **PSYCHOTROPICS** | |
| *Butyrophenones and combinations* (Haldol) | causes rash, diarrhea, vomiting in infant |
| *Hydroxyzines* (Vistaril, Atarax) | nursing discouraged: effect unknown |
| *Lithium Carbonate* | effects unknown; breast-feeding discouraged |

*Especially harmful*

## CHART 44. DIRECTORY OF DRUGS TO AVOID
## WHEN BREAST-FEEDING *(continued)*

| DRUG | EFFECT |
|---|---|
| **PSYCHOTROPICS** *(cont.)* | |
| *Meprobamate and combinations* | |
| *(Equanil, Miltown) | alternate drug advised |
| Librium | effects not known |
| *Valium | effects unknown; nursing not recommended |
| **RADIOISOTOPES** | |
| $I^{131}$ | suppress thyroid gland; all mothers, breast-feeding or not, should not have contact with baby for 48 hours |
| **URINARY ANTI-INFECTIVES** | |
| (Bactrim, Septra) | sulfanilamides contraindicated if infant less than 2 months old |
| (Thiosulfil, Nalidixic Acid) | may be noxious if taken continuously |
| Mandelic Acid | photosensitivity, rashes |
| **VAGINALS** | |
| *AVC cream and other sulfanilamides | |
| *Flagyl vaginal insert | jaundice of newborn (Gray's syndrome or kernicterus) |
| *Vaginal douches and gels containing povidone-iodine | possible thyroid problems from high iodine levels |

***Especially harmful**

## ENVIRONMENTAL CONTAMINATION OF BREAST MILK

We are all exposed daily to chemicals through food, air, and water. Some of these environmental contaminants are soluble primarily in water and others are soluble primarily in fat. When we ingest or inhale water-soluble chemicals, our bodies generally metabolize and excrete them. Fat-soluble chemicals are not excreted: they are stored in body fat for many years. As fat-soluble chemicals are accumulated they reach a steady-state level after which further chemical residues are no longer stored but are directly excreted. There are two ways of mobilizing (getting rid of) these fat stores and the chemicals they contain: weight loss and lactation. Otherwise the fat stores remain relatively immobile.

The fat-soluble chemicals which affect breast-feeding are called chlorinated hydrocarbons. Human breast milk can be contaminated with this type of chemical from agricultural and industrial sources. These chemicals increase the risk of cancer to the nursing infant and pose a threat of other physiological responses. The average amount of these chemicals in breast milk in the United States exceeds the safety standards proposed by the World Health Organization and the Food and Drug Administration (FDA). The information herein on the dangers of breast milk has been drawn from the excellent report *Birthright Denied* by the Environmental Defense Fund.

Chlorinated hydrocarbons fall into two categories, agricultural and industrial:

### AGRICULTURAL CHEMICALS

The chief ones are pesticides—DDT, aldrin, dieldrin, chlordane, heptachlor, toxaphene, benzene hexachloride (BHC), etc. They all have similar characteristics—they concentrate in the fat of organisms leading to *bioaccumulation*—for example, the residues of DDT in a fish can be thousands of times greater than the residues of DDT in the water it lives in) and *biomagnification;* persistence in the environment for many years; carcinogenicity and other chronic and acute toxic effects.

There is global contamination from these long-lived

pesticides. They concentrate in the fat of animals. Of all foods tested by the FDA the categories with the highest residues are meat, fish, and dairy products.

The Environmental Protection Agency (EPA) establishes tolerance levels of pesticide residues in food, allowing low levels which they believe are safe for human consumption. These tolerances are often based more on the expected level of the chemical rather than on a current evaluation of toxological data—therefore we cannot assume that foods will not harm us just because the government says they are safe.

Pesticide residues occur more frequently and in higher concentration in human milk than in cow's milk or infant formula. DDE (the form in which DDT is stored in the body) is the most frequently found pesticide in human milk, with dieldrin the second most common. The FDA has not done conclusive testing of formula. Theoretically the pesticide residues should be much lower in formula than in cow's milk because in processing cow's milk which could be contaminated with pesticides, the fat is removed; in most formulas it is replaced with vegetable fat, which is usually less contaminated.

## INDUSTRIAL CHEMICALS

There are many of these but only two have been officially reported as appearing in breast milk: PCBs (polychlorinated biphenyls) and their chemical cousins, PBBs (polybrominated biphenyls).

*PCBs:* PCB contamination of food is essentially limited to fish that spend part or all of their lives in fresh water. PCBs have had a widespread and uncontrolled industrial application for the past several decades. Industrial chemicals are discharged by factories into the air and water. They find their way into the food chain where they can be concentrated and bioaccumulated. Fish reflect the pollution of water that receives industrial discharges. Because fish can concentrate PCBs in their bodies up to 9 million-fold, the levels of PCBs in the flesh of many fish far exceed the established FDA tolerance level. Fishing has been restricted in several areas of the country—this is not a localized problem but one with national significance. See page 153 for more information.

**PBBs:** In Michigan this chemical (used as a flame retardant) accidentally got mixed into livestock feed in 1973 and 1974, causing illness and death to thousands of exposed animals. By now the contaminated food has mostly disappeared from grocery shelves, but it has not disappeared from mother's milk. So far the Public Health Department in Michigan has advised only women from contaminated farms to discontinue nursing, although urban consumers of milk and meat were also exposed.

Currently, PBB contamination is limited to Michigan. However, millions of pounds of this chemical have been manufactured and distributed throughout the United States in commerce. When these products are disposed of in landfills and dumps and thereby enter the environment, this problem can become more widespread.

## WAYS TO MINIMIZE CONTAMINANTS IN YOUR DIET

No one knows how long it takes to cleanse the fat stores of all chemical residues. Some scientists are optimistic and say that being on a chemical-free diet for a few years would assure a woman of minimal residues in her milk; others contend that a woman should start a chemical-free diet as soon as she reaches puberty to prepare for her later childbearing years.

**Fish** that have lived in fresh water for part or all of their lives are the major dietary source of PCBs. *This is one food that should be eliminated from your diet.* In particular, the fish to avoid are bottom-feeding estuarine fish (catfish, flounder, sole), Great Lakes fish (salmon, carp), fatty fish (buffalofish, eel), and fish from the Hudson River. Ocean fish (cod, haddock, halibut) are usually free from PCB residues so you should eat these if you include fish in your diet. See page 153.

***Animal origin*** foods are the major dietary source of chlorinated hydrocarbon pesticides. In these foods—meat, fish and dairy products—the pesticide residues are bioaccumulated in the fat over the lifetime of the animals and fish.

***Meat*** was monitored by the U.S. Department of Agriculture. The types of meat in which pesticide residues were most frequently found were: *beef, veal, chicken, and turkey,* with grass-fed beef having a much lower residue level than the usual grain-fed beef. The meat in which pesticides were least frequently found were: *sheep, goats, swine.*

If you eat meat you should remove the fat and discard the drippings. In general, the better cooked the meat, the lower its fat content. And the fat is where the pesticide residues are stored.

***Dairy products*** should be only *lowfat:* yogurt, skim milk, buttermilk, ice milk, and uncreamed cottage cheese. *Avoid high-fat dairy products:* butter cream, high-fat cheese. Again: the fat contains the residues.

***Eggs*** have a surprisingly low residue of most pesticides (with the exception of DDE) and so can be eaten with relatively low risk.

***Margarine*** made of corn oil is least likely to contain pesticide residues, including DDT. Look at labels carefully: many margarines are made with DDT-containing cottonseed oil.

***A lowfat, semivegetarian diet*** would seem to be the most residue-free. Such a diet also lowers dietary fats and cholesterol, which is recommended to prevent heart disease and cancer.

***A totally vegetarian diet*** may be an excellent way to reduce pesticide residues in your system if you start it well enough in advance of breast-feeding. A French study published in 1974 sampled the milk of women who were primarily vegetarians. The results showed that if 70 percent or more of the diet contained organic food, i.e., grown without synthetic chemical pesticides or fertilizers, that the pesticide residues in the breast milk were less than one-half of those in the median French human milk samples. All of the women who had significantly lower pesticide residues in their milk had been on the diet for 6 or more years while those women whose pesticide residues were higher were generally on the diet for 3 years or less.

The Environmental Defense Fund is doing a study to determine whether a vegetarian diet can reduce chemical contaminants in a woman's breast milk. Preliminary results show that the pesticide and PCB levels in vegetarian women are one-half to one-third the levels found in the 1976 EPA survey. This supports the findings of the 1974 French study.

*Your drinking water* can be a source of problems. See page 142.

# 12

# Taking care of baby

Most pregnancy and childbirth books end right at the birth of the baby—which is sort of like leading you down a road and stopping at the edge of a cliff! Although this chapter is by no means a complete guide to newborn baby care, it is an attempt to present some aspects which may involve consumer decisions on your part: choosing a pediatrician, circumcision, buying baby things, diet after weaning, etc. There is also a section on "what to expect"—bringing a newborn home is a thrilling, exhausting, and sometimes overwhelming experience. Many new parents in America have never been around little babies until they have their own: this chapter lets you know which "strange" aspects are actually normal and also how to recognize symptoms that require a doctor's care.

## CHOOSING A PEDIATRICIAN

This is something you should do before the baby is born. Some pediatricians will meet with you and your mate without charge when you are pregnant. If you have chosen a doctor beforehand, it can be a relief not to have to scramble around for professional advice if questions or problems arise in the early postpartum weeks.

Also, if there are nonroutine procedures that you want in the hospital you can ask your pediatrician to make requests before the birth. If you want to nurse on the delivery table, want your baby with you in the recovery area or released from the stabilization nursery quickly, or if you don't want the baby to receive any artificial nipples, you have a better chance of a positive reaction from the hospital staff if arrangements have been made through a medical channel. If you choose a pediatrician ahead of time, the hospital notifies him as soon as the baby is born and he will come to do the first examination rather than a hospital staff pediatrician. He may submit a separate bill for this or it may be part of his total fee for first-year baby-care visits.

*The office location* can be important if transportation is a problem. It helps not to have to go a far distance if you have to bring a sick child to the doctor.

*What is the waiting room like?* Is it cozy? Is it geared to children, with small chairs and toys and books? Just as you can tell quite a bit about people from their living rooms, you can tell something about a pediatrician from his waiting room. If the waiting room has a formal adult-oriented decor, this can tell you about the pediatrician's attitude toward children.

*House calls* are a fast-disappearing luxury, but pediatricians are just about the only doctors who will sometimes make them. If you have a feverish baby and it is wintertime, it is preferable not to have to take her outdoors. Ask whether the doctor will make house calls and, if so, under what circumstances.

*How busy is his practice?* You shouldn't have to call too far ahead for an appointment and you should be able to come in quickly in an emergency.

*Does he have a group practice?* If the pediatrician shares his practice with one or more doctors, will your child see a different doctor each time? A child feels more secure with continuity and stability, and it is preferable for you and the child to develop a relationship with the pediatrician you choose—rather than having to try to relate to the doctor(s) *he* has chosen to practice with. It is understandable if his colleagues handle telephone calls or emergencies in the evenings or on weekends, for example, but you should find out ahead of time.

*Personality* is the first important criterion in choosing a pediatrician. Does he have a sense of humor and seem warm toward children? Do you and your mate feel at ease with him, comfortable asking questions, and satisfied with his replies? Does he treat you as equals or is he patronizing?

*His style of child rearing* will affect you even if you imagine that a pediatrician is there only for medical problems. In the areas of health and nutrition, for example, a doctor's attitudes about how to raise a child are tied up with decisions about when and what to feed. Does the doctor prefer a rigid style of raising children? For instance, does he have an automatic date for the introduction of solid foods—as opposed to introducing them when the baby is ready? There is no "right" way—whatever makes you more comfortable is best. Precise instructions make some parents feel more secure; they make some parents, who might prefer things more loose and unstructured, feel hemmed in.

*Breast-feeding* is an area in which there will be problems if you don't share the same views as a pediatrician. If you choose *not* to breast-feed and a doctor strongly recommends nursing for all his patients, then you may feel pressured and judged if you bottle-feed. And if you *want* to breast-feed you may have a tough time unless a pediatrician is actively supportive. It is not enough for a doctor's attitude to be, "Sure, breast-feeding is fine with me." Especially if you are a first-time mother, you are going to need encouragement and help from everyone around you. For example, a doctor is *not* supportive if his response to problems you may have is to suggest supplementing breast-feeding with formula. And a doctor who recommends the early introduction of solids is not actively supporting breast-feeding. Discuss nursing with a pediatrician ahead of time and make sure that your beliefs are compatible.

*A good attitude toward a working mother* is essential in a pediatrician. If you are going to work when your baby is small, you're going to have to contend with a negative response from various people—there's no sense in adding to your burden by paying a professional to add to the negativism! A doctor's disapproval can undermine your confidence in your mothering. His attitude may come out in subtle ways—small comments about you being gone all day when the baby is sick, for instance—and can make you uncomfortable. The problems will only be greater if you are breast-feeding and working. It is important to find a pediatrician who respects your personal goals independent of your child. The baby is his patient, so the child's welfare will be his primary concern—so if he feels that a mother who works is cheating her child then he isn't the doctor for you.

*Circumcision* is a decision you should make before the baby is born and discuss with a pediatrician. A doctor can give you his opinion about the pros and cons but the decision ultimately rests with you: the section on circumcision that follows should help you decide. If you have a strong opinion either way you should find a pediatrician who is either noncommittal or agrees with you.

*Be sure to contact any doctors* you meet if you decide not to choose them. This is an important courtesy, especially if they did not charge you for the interview.

*Once you have chosen a pediatrician* it's good to know when you should call him. Many new parents worry about calling a doctor too much for seemingly unimportant matters that nevertheless concern them. On the other hand, there are times a doctor should be contacted because the baby's symptom *may* be a signal of a problem.

---

**CHART 45. CALL PEDIATRICIAN IF BABY
HAS THESE SYMPTOMS**

---

- EXCESSIVE CRYING and unusual irritability
- EXCESSIVE DROWSINESS; sleeping at times when he/she usually plays
- POOR SLEEP with frequent waking, restlessness, and crying
- FEVER with a rectal thermometer; flushed face, hot and dry skin
- SEVERE LOSS OF APPETITE; refusal to take familiar foods
- REPEATED VOMITING; throwing up most of a feeding more than once
- BOWEL MOVEMENTS WITH BLOOD or pus, mucus, a green color, or unusually loose or frequent
- COUGH OR SEVERE RUNNY NOSE
- INFLAMMATION OR DISCHARGE FROM EYES
- RASH that covers a large portion of the body or persists after changing laundry habits
- TWITCHING, CONVULSIONS, INABILITY TO MOVE
- PAIN

---

# CIRCUMCISION

Circumcision has been practically a routine procedure in this country for many years—until recently. It is now being aggressively questioned by both health professionals and parents. Many of the supposed medical advantages to circumcision have now been disproven, and people have begun to worry about the pain and trauma to newborn babies from this surgical procedure.

The practice of circumcision came from ancient Semitic cultures, when there were months of traveling across deserts without water to bathe in. This is obviously not applicable to life in modern society, although Jewish parents may want to continue to have their baby boys circumcised for reasons of religious tradition. However, other parents should weigh this decision carefully before submitting to what has become a routine hospital procedure.

It is significant to know that a committee from the American Academy of Pediatrics concluded that circumcision is a "nonessential surgical procedure" and that the health benefits previously ascribed to it can be as easily obtained with good hygiene. In 1989 there was a study done by military physicians which concluded that circumcision protects against kidney and urinary system infections. This might have rekindled the debate about circumcision except that the American Academy of Pediatrics had independent experts review the military study: they found there were flaws in how the study was conducted. Therefore the 37,000-member academy did *not* recommend routine circumcision.

However, the American Academy of Pediatrics, in contradiction to its earlier noncircumcision position, now suggests that newborn circumcision has potential medical benefits and advantages, which it recommends discussing between parents and pediatricians, along with the disadvantages and risks.

Recent evidence has shown that uncircumsized newborn males are 10 to 15 times more likely to have a urinary tract infection (UTI) than circumcised infants. Retrospective studies show that circumcising a newborn can have at least one medical benefit: it can reduce the frequency of early infantile urinary tract infection (UTI) by about 90 percent. Because of these findings, the AAP formed a new task force on circumcision and released a report in April of 1989, modifying its firm stance opposing routine neonatal circumcision. The report further stated that "circumcision may result in a decreased incidence of urinary tract infections" and that "evidence concerning the association of sexually transmitted disease and circumcision is conflicting." Further studies are needed about this controversial subject before the final word is written.

There is a growing trend against infant circumcision. It goes hand in hand with current desires for natural childbirth and breast-feeding. People now seem to accept the logical concept that the human body is well designed as it normally comes into the world. Parents are rebelling against surgically altering this natural design, particularly when it means causing their babies unnecessary pain.

In America, 60 percent of babies are still circumcised. Many parents who have attended a circumcision have been shocked to see what the baby undergoes and have suffered anguish and guilt over having allowed it to be done to their infant. Many are crusading to educate other people about circumcision in hopes of sparing other parents and babies. Although expectant couples usually try to learn everything they can about pregnancy, birth, and infant care, it is rare for them to question circumcision. Couples learn about nutrition, drugs, prepared-childbirth techniques, and breast-feeding, but often the only thing they know about circumcision is that it's done because "that's the way a penis is supposed to look and it's cleaner."

Parents who have had their babies circumcised and regret it recommend that a couple attend a circumcision before deciding to have it done to their son. They believe that few parents would consent if they had to be present at their baby's circumcision and saw what is done to him. They say that most parents would not permit it if they even saw pictures of what is actually involved.

*A description of circumcision:* The baby is placed on his back in a "circumstraint," a plastic tray in which his arms and legs are strapped down. Sterile drapes are placed over him with a hole through which his penis is exposed. A hemostat is applied to the tip of the foreskin to crush it and a slit is made to enlarge the tip. A small instrument is then used to reach inside the tip of the penis to separate the foreskin from the glans, tearing away the two layers of skin which normally adhere to each other.

There are several different methods of circumcision. In one method a metal clamp is placed over the foreskin for about five minutes to control postoperative bleeding. Then the foreskin is cut off and the clamp removed. Alternatively, a small protective bell is placed over the glans and under the foreskin. In this method a string is tied tightly over the foreskin and the plastic bell. Some of the foreskin in front of the string is trimmed away and then a plastic ring is left around the end of the penis. The remaining foreskin atrophies (dries up) in about a week and the plastic ring then falls off. Yet another method is for the foreskin to be cut off with a knife or scissors; then stitches are put in to control the bleeding. Sometimes a cauterizing needle is used to stop bleeding, although this procedure has been known to cause problems like hemorrhage, infection, and damage to the penis from electrical burns, but this is unusual.

*No anesthetic is used.* This is tied to a belief that newborns' nervous systems are not yet fully developed: the conclusion is drawn that therefore they do not feel as much pain as later on. Many parents report the anguished screams of their babies when they are circumcised, although some studies have shown that many babies do not cry out. However, other experts believe that the babies who do not react outwardly are having a stress-withdrawal reaction, in which they lapse into a deep, abnormal sleep pattern rather than crying out. The truth is that the degree to which the baby suffers is not known, although there has never been a scientific study which could support the theory that babies have little or no feelings. But when a circumcision is performed on an older child or man, it is considered painful enough to use anesthesia.

The American Academy of Pediatrics notes that circumcision has "inherent disadvantages and risks"; the academy acknowledges that the baby experiences pain in the procedure and for a few hours afterwards. There is a new local anesthesia technique called a dorsal penile block that can eliminate the newborn's pain and reduce his distress during circumcision. However, the academy cautions that there is only limited experience with the technique. Instead of generally recommending local anesthesia for newborn circumcision, the academy has recommended waiting for the results of large, scientific studies on the possible risks of this procedure.

*Hemorrhage and infection* are fairly uncommon complications of circumcision. There have also been mild distortions of the penis because of scarring, and in some cases plastic surgery has been necessary because of accidental damage. A common complication is called "meatal ulceration": the exposed glans, without the protective foreskin, develops painful urine burns from contact with wet diapers.

*Misinformation about circumcision* is rampant. Despite what was believed at one time, circumcision does not reduce the occurrence of cancers. It was previously thought that there was less penile and prostate cancer and less cervical cancer in women who had intercourse with circumcised men. It has been found that venereal disease and a lack of good hygiene in uncircumcised men was the cause of the higher cancer rate—not the lack of circumcision itself.

It has never been proven that circumcised men can hold an erection for longer. It has also never been proven that uncircumcised men have greater sexual pleasure.

*Good hygiene* is a viable alternative to circumcision, but many people seem to be misinformed about it. They are concerned when they are told that smegma collects under the foreskin and must be washed away. However, smegma is the same substance that collects on female genitals and is regularly washed away. Children are taught to wash behind their ears and to brush their teeth, so there is no reason why a boy cannot be taught to wash his penis.

Many people, doctors included, do not understand the normal development and correct care of the infant's foreskin. The general belief is that circumcision is "cleaner" and that care of a child's intact penis is difficult. Frequently a doctor will forcibly retract the infant's foreskin in the hospital or when the baby comes into the office for a visit. Sometimes parents are instructed to retract and clean under the baby's foreskin every day. Manipulating the foreskin forcefully is not a good idea. It can be more traumatic for the baby than circumcision, since that happens only one time. People have to be educated to leave the normally tight and nonretractable foreskin of the infant alone until it gradually loosens on its own, which can take up to 3 or 4 years. Ninety-six percent of infants have a nonretractable foreskin at birth. Eighty-five percent are nonretractable at 6 months, and 50 percent remain so at one year of age. This is the norm. The foreskin is not expected to retract easily until 2 years or older. In some boys the foreskin is not fully retractable until late puberty.

### Recommendations for hygienic care of uncircumcised infants:

- The newborn's foreskin should not be manipulated in the first days of life.
- Parents should not retract the foreskin for cleaning. Some doctors may recommend doing this, but it can cause unnecessary problems.
- A mother should show her son how to retract his foreskin and wash his penis when he is 4. She should supervise for a while and then expect him to care for himself.

**Sex identification with the father,** male siblings, and other boys later on in school is often given as a reason for circumcision. Some psychologists believe that a boy has an easier time making a sex identification with his father and other close male figures if his penis looks the same as theirs. Also, a boy who has a foreskin may suffer some social stigma when he goes to school and most of the other boys have been circumcised. However, with 40 percent of American boys now intact (uncircumcised), chances of being the "only one" are unlikely. The locker rooms of the 1990s will have boys with both kinds of penises.

As for a boy's identification with his father, there are other significant differences between the adult and child penis, besides the foreskin or lack of it. A young boy rarely notices circumcision status; when and if he does, you can offer him a simple explanation. For instance, you might say, "Doctors used to think circumcision was a good thing, but now we know it's important to keep your body whole."

Those who favor leaving boys intact also suggest that parents can help children feel good about their own bodies.

Children can learn to respect differences with other people, whether it's the other person's penis, nose, or other personal aspects. These advocates point out that education is the answer, not circumcision. The fact that other boys had unnecessary surgery is the worse possible reason to recommend that another child undergo the procedure!

*If you decide to circumcise your child,* there are several pointers to keep in mind:

• The procedure should not be performed postnatally in the delivery room. At some hospitals this is done for the doctor's convenience. It is unfair to the newborn baby, who is coping with the difficult adjustment to life outside the womb. Leaving aside the issue of how much pain the baby does or does not feel at this stage, there should be some respect for his need and right to have as gentle a beginning in life as possible.

• Circumcision should be delayed at least until 12 to 24 hours after birth.

• The baby's weight must be considered. If he weighs less than 6 pounds, the doctor may want to delay the operation until the baby is larger.

• The mother or father may want to hold the baby for the procedure, as this might lessen the trauma for the infant.

• Care of the penis after circumcision involves applying petroleum jelly to help protect it until it has healed.

## PKU TEST

This is done to screen all babies after birth. Some hospitals administer this screening test between the 2nd and 4th day of life, others wait until the 6th or 14th day. PKU is a rare metabolic disorder (occurring 1 in 10,000 births) that causes mental retardation. There is no cure, but the disease can be controlled through diet, which is why all babies are tested. If both parents have PKU, then all offspring will inherit it. If another family member already has PKU, then a baby with a negative PKU test should be retested at 1, 2, and 6 weeks of life to be absolutely sure. A small blood sample is obtained by pricking the baby's heel.

If a baby has PKU she lacks the ability to metabolize an amino acid called phenylalanine. All natural proteins contain an average of 5 percent of this amino acid. Excessive amounts of phenylalanine build up in the bloodstream and cause severe mental retardation and/or brain damage. The untreated symptoms of PKU are: irritability, hyperactivity, vomiting, convulsions, skin rashes or severe eczema, a musty barnlike odor with urine or sweat. Treatment involves excluding milk, meat, eggs, and cheese from the diet and substituting Lofenalac milk for as long as the major portion of brain growth occurs, or several years.

## NAMING THE BABY

This may pose a problem for couples who are not married or who are married but each use their own last names.

*It is only custom which dictates that a baby take his father's surname.* If parents, married or not, use different surnames, a child can be given either one's surname on a birth certificate.

*State laws differ* and can be challenged in court. Find out the laws in your state. Do not accept what is told you by a clerk. People who stand behind counters and work for the government have an unpleasant way of "laying down the law." They may not know any better, but they accept "common practice" (i.e., what most people do) as law—which it is not. Do not allow an officious clerk to intimidate you.

*In Massachusetts, Virginia, and other states,* married couples have given the mother's birth-given surname to their children.

*In common law,* a child born to a married couple does not automatically assume the father's surname. In common law, a child born to an unmarried couple does not automatically assume the mother's surname. This is also true for marriage: although the custom is for women to give up their surnames and take their husbands', common law does not automatically dictate this.

*The law may clearly allow you* to name your children as you please, but custom is so entrenched and prejudiced against the concept of children from a marriage being given the mother's surname that you may have to take legal action to enforce your rights. By the same token, the social expectation is that the children from an unmarried couple will be given the mother's surname, and there may be resistance if you want to give the baby the father's surname.

## PREPARATION AND SUPPLIES FOR THE BABY

*The baby's room should be painted* with nontoxic, nonyellowing paint. You should not repaint over old paint because babies can get lead poisoning from flakes of old paint, and as they get older, babies put *everything* in their mouths.

*A bassinet or cradle* is cute, but the baby will outgrow it immediately. Therefore don't buy one, but if someone gives or lends you a cradle, you can use it until the baby gets bigger.

*A crib should meet these requirements,* and you should only borrow a crib if it meets these important safety factors.

- bars no farther apart than 2⅜ inches, or the baby's head can get stuck between
- a railing 26 inches higher than the lowest level of the mattress support, so the baby can't climb over easily
- a mattress that fits snugly, or a baby can get her head stuck between the mattress and crib
- smooth surfaces, safe and sturdy hardware, and a secure teething rail all the way around
- A crib with one side-drop is more stable and less expensive than one in which both rails can be lowered.

• Crib guards make it safer and softer for the baby. *Never use pillows for this purpose:* they can smother the baby and are bad for posture.

WARNING: Mesh-sided cribs and playpens can be dangerous if the sides are left down. Children have suffocated when they rolled into the space between the mat and the loose mesh siding, when the sides were down. The government has sued nine manufacturers that make mesh-sided cribs and playpens; as a result there are now warning labels on the products. However, there are an estimated 6.5 million people with unlabeled products whose babies are in danger. When buying, look for a product with no gap at all between the mattress and sides. A child can become caught in a gap of as little as two inches. *Never, ever* leave a child in one of these cribs with the side down—always lock the hinges.

***Basic bedding needs:*** a waterproof mattress; 2 to 3 waterproof mattress pads; 2 quilted crib pads; 4 to 6 crib sheets; crib bumpers; 2 crib blankets or bag-type sleepers

***Basic supplies*** you'll need are:

• a rectal thermometer
• blunt baby nail scissors, which are easiest to use when the baby is asleep
• premoistened wipe cloths if there is no water nearby
• rubbing alcohol to dab on the umbilical cord until it falls off
• baby soap and mild, "no tears" shampoo
• diaper rash ointment (Desitin, Diaparene, Peri-anal; more economical is a 1-pound plastic jar of zinc oxide from a pharmacy)
• CONTROVERSIAL: Some people say that oils and powders are bad for a baby's skin, but you'll have to judge for yourself. Talcum powder is ground rock; brands like Johnson's do not contain asbestos. Alternatively you can use cornstarch; put it in a large salt shaker for convenience.

- DO NOT USE: *Cotton swabs* in either ears or nose—they can cause damage—or *mineral oil,* which absorbs all the oil-soluble vitamins through the skin
- a strap on the changing table is essential—even if you're going to use a bureau top for changing, be sure to make a secure strap; babies can fall off easily in the time it takes you to turn around
- a pacifier can be useful at times when the baby won't quiet down, or has the need to suck but you are not able to feed him right then, or has been fed but his sucking needs are not satisfied. Even parents with an adamant prejudice against pacifiers are usually won over by their usefulness. NUK brand—or another orthodontic model—is the most humanlike nipple; it is curved so that it doesn't harm the developing palate.

**Diapers** are a decision you have to make for yourself, although it seems most parents choose disposable diapers. Disposables are more expensive and add a lot of waste ecologically, but they are less trouble. Some brands fit newborns best, while others are better afterward. Since most everyone leans toward using disposable diapers, here is some information about cloth diapers to balance out the scales. This is not an endorsement of one kind over the other, just an attempt to let you see both sides before you decide. You might consider trying a diaper service for a few weeks and comparing the two.

- EVEN WITH A DIAPER SERVICE, cloth diapers are less costly. With a service, you'll need 80 to 100 diapers a week.
- IF YOU'RE GOING TO WASH THEM YOURSELF every day, you need 2 dozen. If you're going to wash them every other day, you need 3 to 4 dozen. This staggering amount is an indication of why mothers have turned to disposables. It does seem as though cloth diapers would add an enormous burden unless you could arrange for a diaper service.
- YOU'LL NEED 3 TO 6 PAIR OF WATERPROOF PANTS to go over cloth diapers. You can also use diaper liners once the child has a schedule of bowel movements. That way you can lift the liner out and flush it away.

- CLOTH DIAPERS WITH RUBBER PANTS OVER DO NOT LEAK through the leg openings the way disposable diapers can. With disposables it is not uncommon for this to happen.
- IF YOU USE CLOTH DIAPERS you will still want to use disposables when you travel. You can also use a disposable diaper opened up underneath the baby so that you don't make a mess if you're changing the baby at someone's house.

## BABY CLOTHES

*Hand-me-downs are sometimes softer* than newly purchased clothes because they are often made of 100 percent cotton instead of the fire-retardant synthetics used now. Don't be bashful about accepting other people's baby clothes—the child will grow out of them so quickly and it's wasteful to spend and accumulate your own basic clothing if there's someone willing to give (lend) you theirs.

*The fire-retardant chemical TRIS* has been banned from use in sleepwear. Government tests showed that it can cause cancer and was absorbed through the baby's skin or ingested orally by sucking on pajama sleeves. Many of these products were on the market but not labeled as containing TRIS. Be very careful about sleepwear you buy.

*Get the 6-month size* in any clothes for a newborn.

*You will need 6 to 10 T-shirts.* Some mothers favor the over-the-head style of T-shirts, while others find it hard to push and pull the baby's head and arms through the small openings. Those mothers prefer the snap-across or other wraparound styles. Try one of each kind for yourself before deciding.

*Other basic needs are:* 4 to 6 stretch coveralls, 2 to 4 gowns (kimonos or sacques), and 4 to 6 receiving blankets. If you aren't using cloth diapers, you'll want to have a dozen around for general nursery use: wiping up, over your shoulder for burping, etc. "Onesies," or one-piece underwear that snaps between the baby's legs, are very convenient.

***If the baby develops a rash,*** it may be from clothes washed with detergent containing phosphate or from fabric softener. If the rash is on the baby's face it may be from sheets and blankets laundered that way. Change your washing habits to eliminate this possible cause of rash.

### EXERCISE EQUIPMENT FOR BABY

***Jumpers*** are not recommended by some doctors, who contend that they force physical development ahead of natural timing.

***Bouncers and walkers*** can be very hazardous if the "X" part of the supporting frame does not have a plastic cover. Babies' fingers have been amputated when the design of the bouncer did not provide for the "X" being covered. Springs should stretch no more than ⅛ inch apart for the same reason—a baby's fingers could get caught and chopped off. Walkers should not tip if the child bumps into another object.

***These devices should not be used too much*** or they may impair development of reflexes when the child learns to fall naturally.

### TRAVEL EQUIPMENT

***The stroller*** should be tested with the baby in it—it should not tip if the child reaches out. It should have no sharp edges and no scissor-type action parts, which can harm fingers. Umbrella-type strollers can be rickety, but they are popular because they fold up for getting in and out of buses and cars and are no storage problem. Strollers can also be used inside the house as a chair for the baby.

***Infant car seats*** are an absolute must if you own a car. Nearly 1,000 children under 5 years of age die every year in car accidents and there are significant injuries yearly to another 60,000. If you always use a car seat you can prevent such a tragedy. You have to develop the strict habit of *always* using the car seat for *any* length trip. Even if a baby gets active or vocal you should not remove him from the carrier while the car is moving—instead, take a rest stop. Car seats for small babies are designed so that the infant rides backward with his entire head and body cushioned by impact-absorbing materials. A built-in harness holds the baby firmly in place. *Always use a car seat exactly as the instructions read.* Some brands convert to a forward-riding seat.

- CHECK THE LENGTH OF YOUR CAR'S SEAT BELTS. Infant car seats are attached with the car's seat belt—some car dealers can supply a belt extender if yours are too short to accommodate the infant seat. Also, measure the space where you are going to put the seat to be sure it will fit.
- SOME MODELS REQUIRE A TOP ANCHOR STRAP which has to be bolted to the rear window-ledge of the car. If you have a sedan-type car this will work, but installation may be difficult in the cargo area of a station wagon or with a fast-back car, so make sure you are able to install this style of seat.
- THE NATIONAL CHILD PASSENGER SAFETY ASSOCIATION issued a shopping guide to child car seats. *The following convertible safety seats can be used from birth to approximately 43 pounds*, and were deemed the easiest to use correctly. Therefore potentially the safest seats are: the Century 200 and Century 400XL (made by Century), the One Step (by Evenflo/Questor), the Quick Click Booster 605 (by Strollee), and the Quickstep (by Kolcraft). Of these, the One Step has a 5-point harness/shield that spreads the crash force over the widest area of the child's body and is thus safer.
- THERE ARE OTHER CARRIERS WHICH WERE FOUND SAFE in tests that were sanctioned by the group Action for Child Transportation Safety. If you want more information you can contact this organization at 400 Central Park West, #15P, New York, NY 10025.

- INFANT CAR SEATS CAN BE QUITE COSTLY, so watch want ads and garage sales for used models.
- THE PETERSON SAFETY SHELL #75 converts from an infant seat to a toddler seat with an optional insert that is sold separately.
- IF A CHILD CAN SEE OUT THE WINDOW from a car seat she will not fuss as much. The Strollee model designed for 6 months to 3 years is one carrier that raises the child up enough so that she can see out the window.

---

CHART 46. DIRECTORY OF RULES ABOUT CAR SEATS

---

- FASTEN THE HARNESS OR ANCHOR STRAPS *TIGHTLY*. This allows the child to sustain a very severe jolt during a collision because harness webbing is not stretched to absorb impact.
- ALWAYS PLACE THE BABY FACING *BACKWARD*. No child should be placed sitting forward until he weighs 17–20 pounds and can sit up well.
- CHECK INSTRUCTIONS FOR SAFE DEGREE OF TILT. Some infant seats can be reclined with an adjustable tilt feature. Never set the seat farther down than the instructions indicate; doing so could permit the child to be forced out head-first in an accident. And do not recline a forward-facing car seat. Child car seats are safer when used in the upright position. Children learn easily how to sleep sitting up.
- ALWAYS SECURE THE SEAT WITH THE AUTO SEAT BELT. If the lap belt does not fit around the car seat or through its frame, try another seating position in the car or get a seat-belt extender.
- ALWAYS USE THE HARNESS. If you don't do up the harness, the child can be thrown out of the car seat.
- DO NOT MISTAKE THE PADDED ARMREST FOR PROTECTION. Always use the harness in any car seat. The armrest on pre-1981 models is a cosmetic feature and will not protect the child in any way. In fact, it is a hazardous object for an unharnessed child to be thrown against.

---

CHART 46. DIRECTORY OF RULES ABOUT CAR SEATS *(continued)*

---

- DO NOT BUNDLE THE INFANT IN BLANKETS. The shoulder harness can't be correctly positioned if the infant is heavily bundled before being placed in the seat. In cold weather you can cut holes in one blanket you'll use only for the car: pull the straps through the holes, buckle the harness, then fold the blanket over.
- FOR THE BABY'S COMFORT use clothing with legs for a snug fit of the harness between his legs. Do not use papoose bunting or a sack sleeper.
- THE BABY'S POSITION IN THE SEAT should be with her back flat against the back of the seat, not curved. You should support a small infant's head and body with rolled diapers or thin blankets placed in the small of her back and on either side of her body.
- ALWAYS FASTEN THE TOP ANCHOR STRAP. If you forget to do this, the car seat can pivot forward in a frontal crash.
- BE SURE TO DOUBLE STRAPS BACK THROUGH BUCKLES. If strap buckles of the harness and anchor straps are incompletely threaded, they can pull out unnoticed. This defeats the entire safety system.
- NEVER LET CHILDREN RIDE LOOSE. If you allow your child to ride without the car seat a few times, it will only make buckling-up more difficult the next time. Do not give in, even if the child complains or manages to climb out of the car seat. You can keep your restless passenger happy with frequent stops, music, or games; don't make any exceptions to the rule about using a car seat.

---

## BATHING THE BABY

A daily bath is not necessary for a baby, although some grandmothers may disagree! Every 2 or 3 days is plenty for a full bath, since the only part of the baby that gets dirty is washed with every diaper change. Also, soap and shampoo are not necessary on newborn skin—and some people say should *not* be used at all in the early period of a baby's life.

You can bathe a baby in the kitchen sink, which saves you from having to bend over.

*Sponge-bathe a baby* until the umbilical cord falls off about a week after birth. You can dab the stump with cotton dipped in alcohol or just leave it alone. After that you can get the baby wet all over.

*The temperature of the water* should not be too hot; it should feel just warm to *your elbow,* not to your hands. Also, be careful that the baby does not get chilled because a newborn's temperature-regulating mechanism is not yet efficient. Be sure the room where you bathe him is not chilly or drafty and dry the baby off right away.

*Most babies love the water* and enjoy moving around in it. Some children, however, scream when they are bathed— if yours does this, don't worry: she will soon learn to enjoy the water.

*Basic supplies* for bathing are 3 to 4 towels and 3 to 4 washcloths made of soft terrycloth. *Do not use cotton swabs in the nose or ears*—they can easily hurt the baby.

*Try going into the bathtub* with the baby. Hold him securely (it's slippery!) and you'll find the baby will play, move his muscles, and make swimming motions. You can also breast-feed in the tub, which is relaxing and enjoyable for both of you.

## WHAT TO EXPECT IN A NEWBORN

Most parents have never even seen a newborn baby before. There are certain "oddities" you should be prepared for so that they don't surprise or concern you. Most newborns do not look like cherubs; some parents are so disappointed by this that they have a hard time accepting their baby's looks. Try to see some pictures of newborns so that your expectations are realistic. The parent-child bond can be hindered if you are displeased with how your baby looks.

*All new babies* sound like they have a cold—they sniffle and sneeze. This is because their breathing organs are new and have to adjust.

*The "startle reflex"* is normal and something a baby grows out of. A newborn tends to jump at noises and may tremble. You may worry that the baby is nervous, but this is just a sign of her system adjusting.

*The rooting reflex* causes the baby to turn her head toward anything that touches her cheek. This is an instinctive mechanism that helps the baby find food. You need only touch the baby's cheek with the nipple. Do not touch both the baby's cheeks at the same time or hold her by both cheeks to guide her head toward the nipple—this will just confuse her.

*A wobbly head* occurs because a baby's head is large and her neck muscles are not developed. The head always needs support in the first few months.

*Hearing* is impaired during the first few days after birth because the middle part of the baby's ear behind the eardrum is still full of amniotic fluid. Gradually it gets absorbed and evaporates, but until then, sounds reaching the baby's ears are muffled.

*Smells and textures* all interest the newborn. You can wear different fabrics when holding the baby to give him varying sensory stimulation. The baby may be excited by crinkly, colorful paper that makes a noise when the infant touches it.

*The umbilical cord* should be kept dry. You can cleanse it with alcohol on a piece of cotton or just leave it alone. Keep the cord stump protected and above the diaper. Notify the doctor if it bleeds, gets red, or has an unusual odor, all signs of infection. Most stumps take about 6 or 7 days to drop off and there may be a slight amount of bloody drainage when this happens.

*The external genitals* are often swollen at birth. The maternal hormones of pregnancy have passed to the baby; this swelling recedes gradually. The girl's clitoris may be swollen so that it looks like a little penis and she may have vaginal bleeding. This is from the estrogenic hormones that were in the mother's system: it will disappear in a short time.

*Milk in the baby's breasts* is fairly common for both males and females. The same hormones that prepare your breasts to lactate affect the baby, who can have milk in her breasts for a few days after birth.

*The nails* may be long at birth. They will be soft and are easiest to trim when the baby is asleep. If you are nervous at first using even blunt baby scissors, you can just make a small cut on the side of the nail and peel off the rest.

*The baby's temperature* is something you should be aware of because a newborn has an inefficient heating system. If a baby has cool hands and feet but a warm body, that means he is at a good temperature. Feel with your finger along his neck or legs to determine if the body is warm.

THE BABY'S SKIN

*The skin of a newborn is very sensitive.* It is susceptible to infection so all nursery linens and clothes should be sterilized by washing in hot water in a machine and all attendants should wash their hands carefully.

*Skin color at birth* may be a blotchy red or grayish blue regardless of the baby's race. Some babies start to develop racial color when born and others remain a very light color for at least the first few hours.

*The skin may peel* a few days after birth, like a peeling sunburn. Do not use lotions or pull off the skin—it will come off naturally.

*Lanugo:* the downy hair covering the baby's skin at birth can be quite heavy and noticeable, especially if it's dark. Lanugo is most abundant over the back, shoulders, forehead, and cheeks. It usually falls out and is rubbed away during the first weeks of life. This does not mean the child will have hairy skin later on—there is no relation between that and lanugo.

*Mottling,* or marbleized spots on the skin, is normal when you are undressing the baby.

*Mongolian spots* are irregular, greenish-blue pigmentation over the lower back that occurs in Negro, Mediterranean, and Asian races. These spots will disappear by school age.

*Prickly heat* is clusters of minute pink pimples surrounded by areas of pink skin. It is due to the overactivity of sweat glands. It can be cured by ventilating the skin using a weak solution of bicarbonate of soda and a bland powder, but be sure the baby cannot touch the mixture and then put his fingers to his mouth. Most important, put lighter clothes and covers on the baby.

*Milia* look like whiteheads. They are concentrated on the baby's nose, chin, and forehead. These are immature oil glands and will disappear by themselves. Leave them alone—squeezing them can cause infection.

*Diaper rash* can be caused by too-strong soap used on diapers or diapers that haven't been boiled long enough to kill the bacteria. Change your laundry habits and use zinc oxide or a commercial preparation like Desitin, which contains zinc oxide, on the affected area.

### THE BABY'S EYES

The baby's eyes are usually blue or slate-gray. The permanent color comes in between 6 months and 1 year. The iris flecks with brown about the 3rd month if the eyes are going to be hazel or brown. A blue-eyed child retains the blue shade.

*A newborn's eyes are crossed* because the muscles that keep both eyes pointing in the same direction aren't working yet. In a few weeks they will correct themselves as they develop.

*Seeing:* It has only recently been realized that little babies can see at all. However, they do have a fairly rigid distance of focus—around 9 inches away from their eyes. If you want the baby to look at something, it is best to show it at this distance. An amazing natural phenomenon is that during breast-feeding this is just about the distance from your face to the baby's. It is evidently a built-in part of the mothering system that a baby's focal distance is correlated to where her mother holds her for nursing.

*Tears* usually don't arrive until around the 3rd month. The tear glands don't function at all for the first weeks, so crying is tearless until then.

*The baby may have a red spot or two* in his eye postpartum. This is caused by a blood vessel that broke during delivery and will clear up by itself.

## BOWEL MOVEMENTS

*The first elimination* will be meconium, the greenish, tarlike substance that is in the baby's intestines at birth. If you are in the hospital and don't have rooming-in you may never even see this dark material which is eliminated for the first few days. If you are breast-feeding, after your milk comes in, the baby's bowel movements become loose and yellow. At first the meconium is streaked with yellow from the colostrum, and then when your milk comes in, the baby's bowel movements are yellow, watery curds. As the baby gets older, the stools are more the consistency of wet toothpaste.

*A newborn may seem constipated* because he strains when he has his first bowel movements. This is because his organs are new and have to adjust to this new task.

*A breast-feeding baby may not urinate much* for the first day or so because he isn't getting many fluids at first. Eventually he will soak 8 to 10 diapers a day once your milk is in.

*If a baby's urine is dark,* he may be dehydrated. Call your doctor, who may suggest giving some water.

## JAUNDICE

*Jaundice* has three forms: normal (or physiologic) jaundice, abnormal jaundice, and breast-milk jaundice, which is very rare.

*Physiologic jaundice* is normal and has no complicating factors. Babies show signs of it around 3 to 4 days postpartum, but before one to two weeks of age. A baby is born pink, regardless of race; with jaundice a baby will show a slight yellowing of the skin—a tinge of yellow almost like a tan. The other characteristics are a whiteness of the eyes, mucous membranes, and body fluids due to excess bilirubin in the blood.

*The cause of jaundice* is that in utero the baby has more red blood cells than she needs after birth. During the first week of life the baby must break down the excess red blood cells and discard them through the feces, urine, skin, and lungs. The liver picks up one of these unnecessary substances, bilirubin, an orange or yellow substance in the bile, and converts it to a conjugated bilirubin—a form that can be easily excreted. Sometimes it takes a newborn's liver a week or so to catch up on converting the bilirubin to a nontoxic substance that her body can excrete. This is why jaundice happens, accounting for the yellowish cast to the skin.

---

**CHART 47. FACTORS THAT MAY CONTRIBUTE TO JAUNDICE**

---

- The possibility of an ABO blood group incompatability: if you are O and your baby is A or B, you may have antibodies that will destroy some of the baby's cells
- The baby is dehydrated: has not had enough fluids, the weather is hot, and/or the baby is not receiving enough colostrum or milk, which is why some doctors recommend giving a newborn water during early feedings
- The baby is too cool
- The baby experienced a lot of bruising during birth, which means an excess number of red blood cells must be broken down quickly
- While pregnant you took aspirin, caffeine, sulfa, Valium, or other drugs which can interfere with the baby's ability to convert bilirubin
- The baby's liver is immature
- The baby is premature, making her more susceptible to becoming jaundiced because premies' livers are almost always immature
- You're an RH negative mother with an RH positive baby: occasionally this combination results in the destruction of some of the baby's red blood cells

---

***You should do something*** if the baby is obviously jaundiced—if the yellow color is medium to strong. This may be hard for you to judge, since you probably don't have any experience in gauging a newborn's jaundice! The best way to determine whether the baby has normal or abnormal jaundice is to take him to the pediatrician, who will determine whether he needs a blood test.

***Treatment of abnormal jaundice*** is especially important if it occurs in conjunction with fever, lack of meconium passage, cold, oxygen deprivation in labor, or a diabetic mother. The dangerous causes of jaundice are a hemolytic disease or an infection because of the rapid destruction of red blood cells. Some doctors will leave the jaundice alone to correct itself, but standard treatment is to admit the baby to a hospital, put him in an incubator with his eyes covered, and turn on fluorescent lights ("bili lights"). The baby's blood is tested every 12 hours to 24 hours if the level is rising significantly by heel prickings.

*The disadvantages of hospitalization* are that you and the baby are separated, breast-feeding is limited or often discouraged and skin-to-skin contact is limited. In some hospitals it is standard procedure *not* to remove the protective eye coverings even when the baby is not under the bili lights. You must guard against this lack of photic (light) stimulation in the first days of life. If your baby is put in the hospital or kept there be sure to read page 575 about the importance of spending time feeding and holding with a baby kept in the nursery.

*Alternative treatment* should be discussed with your pediatrician. Do not attempt these alternatives to hospitalization without your doctor's support. Give the baby a 2- to 3-minute sunbath in the early morning and late afternoon, protecting the infant's eyes. The vitamin D—which the sunlight contains—is known to help jaundice. Extra fluids help "flush out" the system, so you can give plain boiled water in an eye dropper after breast-feeding or in a bottle if you're bottle-feeding. You will still have to take the baby twice daily to the hospital for a blood test to determine the bilirubin count and whether it is rising, falling, or stable.

*Home photo-therapy* is offered by many pediatricians who understand the drawbacks of hospitalizing a newborn. Home therapy for jaundice consists of a nurse who comes out to your home, sets up the photo-therapy unit, and explains the simple use of it, including putting patches on the baby's eyes. Then the nurse will return every 24 hours to obtain follow-up bilirubin tests. This takes place under the supervision of your pediatrician, who continues to manage the situation with the help of the visiting nurse.

Ask your pediatrician whether home photo-therapy is available and if he's comfortable with this alternative to hospitalization. A great deal will depend upon you, and whether you are too anxious or uncomfortable to take on the responsibility of the extra care involved.

*The dangers of jaundice* are that high levels of unconjugated (unconverted) bilirubin in the blood can directly damage the baby's nervous system and brain cells. This is particularly true if the infant is immature or under stress. If the jaundice continues to be increasingly severe the most effective and rapid way to remove dangerous concentrations of bilirubin in the blood is to give the baby an exchange transfusion.

*Breast-milk jaundice* is most unusual. It sometimes occurs 4 days or more postpartum, mostly at the beginning of the second week of life. It is probably caused by a hormone related to progesterone called pregnendiol that is secreted in the milk. You can continue breast-feeding unless bilirubin levels approach 20 mg/100 ml during the first week of life. If that happens, you have to discontinue nursing temporarily. You can hand-express your milk for 2 to 3 days to allow the bilirubin level to go down. Breast-milk jaundice *does not* cause any harm to the baby.

## CRYING

Crying is a baby's way of expressing discomfort or hunger, but it may also be a way of "letting off steam." If the baby cries you should check his diaper for wetness and determine how long ago he last ate. Once you've eliminated those two reasons and the baby still cries when you put him back down, you have a couple of options. Some people set a 15-minute limit on crying—they let the baby cry that long before picking him up again. Although it may jangle your nerves, a baby will usually not continue crying that long: 15 minutes can feel like *hours* to you! It may just be that the baby needs to cry as a way of releasing tension.

However, the important thing to remember is that a tiny baby does not cry as a manipulative way of getting your attention. At such an early stage a baby's mind doesn't work that way. Years ago it was said that you'd "spoil" a baby by picking him up. *You cannot "spoil" a tiny baby.* By picking up a crying baby you are setting up a communication system: you're letting the baby know that his cries are heard and that somebody out there cares. *You can be as responsive and indulgent as you want.* Responding to a crying baby gives him a sense of security early on—and this can help a baby develop into a person with more independence later in life.

It is now known that a lack of nurturing as a child can cause unusual behavior and even violence later. If you reply to a baby's only way of communicating with you—by tending to him when he cries—you are laying the foundation for a child's ability to reach out and trust that his needs will be met. A baby who has not had good nurturing may grow up to be a person who is unable to relate one-to-one with another person. The way that you treat a small baby has a lot to do with what kind of person he becomes. For example, if you pick up the baby when he cries and he stops crying, you can view the baby either as "socially responsive" (he made a demand and was satisfied when it was answered) or you can see him as "exploitative and spoiled." There is a tendency to construct a fantasy about a baby's personality from the way that you perceive the crying and then to handle the baby accordingly. If you have the first attitude toward crying, you will give the baby attention; if you choose the second way to look at it, you will leave the baby to cry. In each case your response or lack of it will contribute to the way the child comes to perceive himself and others.

It is possible that overhandling of a baby can tire him out and *cause* crying and fussiness. This can also happen if there are many people around or the baby is going along with you on extended outings, for instance. A baby needs time to sleep peacefully and be left alone. One way to comfort and quiet an overstimulated baby is to swaddle him. Most hospitals swaddle babies in the nursery: they wrap the baby securely in a receiving blanket so that he is snug and cozy. If your baby gets fussy from too much sensory input, you can swaddle him so he calms down and sleeps.

## SLEEP PROBLEMS

*Sleeping through the night* is not something that some babies do "naturally" and others "refuse" to do. The way that you organize your baby's environment has a profound effect on whether the child can sleep through the night. Solid sleeping habits should be developed early on. From a very young age, many children resist sleep. As a parent, this can become a test of whether you have the self-confidence to impose limits on your baby's behavior.

The most important thing for new parents to realize is that they should be in control of the baby's sleep and feeding schedule—and not the other way around. Several of the couples interviewed for this book went through hellish months of sleeplessness—needlessly. They did not understand the part they played in having a baby that would not sleep. The loss of sleep for the parents—as a couple and individually—is a heavy burden. A situation like this can also cause you to resent the baby, and the baby to suffer a diminished sense of self-esteem and independence if he continues to depend on you throughout the night.

If you feel that a problem is developing with your baby's sleep habits, nip it in the bud. There is an excellent paperback book that covers the subject with intelligence, humor, and compassion. *Helping Your Baby Sleep Through the Night* is written by Joanne Cuthbertson and Susie Schevill, both of whom are married to pediatricians.

## A TEMPERAMENTALLY DIFFICULT BABY

*A very alert, sensitive baby can be difficult.* One way she may show fatigue from too much attention is to have intestinal cramps and gas. You should try to make this kind of baby's environment as placid as possible. Don't have the baby around when there are adult arguments going on; even the raised voices of a heated discussion can upset her. Give the baby enough privacy. This kind of baby needs solitude and a chance to explore her quiet room before catapulting into a house full of people. When you go out with an alert baby who is very sensitive to sensory input and new experiences carry her wrapped in your arms or in a front carrier. Holding her close to your body helps her feel secure in new situations.

## LOVE AND KISSES

Loving a baby—in the way you feed and play with him— teaches him the capacity to love. It appears that a child who fails to make the vital human connections in infancy will have varying degrees of difficulty in making them later in childhood. The formation of the love bond takes place during infancy. Later on, his ability to regulate the aggressive drive is largely dependent upon the quality and durability of these bonds. The absence of human bonds or the rupture of them early in life can have permanent effects on the later capacity for human attachment and for the regulation of aggression.

The baby is an active participant in attachment: the baby elicits nurturing and protective behaviors in you, stimulating your maternal instinct. Do not worry, however, if you don't feel this instinct right away. For many women it is a gradual process and takes time. You may feel like a partner in an arranged marriage, expected to instantly love and cherish someone you've never met before. You should not feel there is something wrong with you if you aren't overcome by a wave of emotion for your baby right at the start—give yourself a chance to ease into it. Try to spend as much time with the baby as feels comfortable, so that you get to know each other.

Regardless of what you are feeling, you should know that the baby becomes attached to you very early in his life and with increasing intensity. A baby in the 3rd and 4th weeks of life, for example, will smile selectively in response to his mother's voice. Experiments have demonstrated that no other sounds in the same frequency will elicit the baby's smile. At about 8 months a baby demonstrates through smiling a clear discrimination of your face. By the time your baby is 8 to 12 months old you are discriminated from all other people: the baby will demonstrate his needs and attachment to you by showing distress when you leave and by having grief reactions if the absence is prolonged beyond the baby's endurance. Studies have shown that accidental or experimental separations of baby and mother lead to panic states in both of them. Infant monkeys, during prolonged separations from their mothers, suffer grief and mourning states that cannot be distinguished from those seen in human infants. Pathological behaviors will occur as the infant settles into a stuporous state. One hears of the babies in orphanages who receive food but become seriously ill and even die because they do not receive sufficient emotional nourishment. This is called "failure to thrive." Never underestimate the importance of your expressions of love to your baby.

***Let the baby adjust to your life-style.*** A big mistake new parents make is to readjust their lives and schedules to accommodate a newborn. It will be much better for you and the baby won't know the difference if you just incorporate the child into *your* life-style. Let a baby get used to normal household noises—voices, music, machines—and she will accommodate. If you tiptoe around and whisper when the baby is asleep she will become accustomed to that kind of quiet and will have trouble getting used to normal sounds. There are many ways in which a baby will change your life, over which you *cannot* exercise any control—so let your lives continue as normally as possible and the baby will fit in.

Another example is that a baby doesn't have to be put to sleep at any magic hour. A baby's bedtime can be whatever is good for you. If you like to get up late and go to bed late the baby can fit into that pattern as comfortably as if you "get up with the chickens and go to sleep with the cows." There also does not have to be any strict regularity—if you can be flexible, so can the baby. She will be perfectly fine and happy just as long as she gets sleep, has clean diapers, a full tummy, and plenty of hugging.

***Immunization*** of the baby is usually begun at 2 months of age. Most pediatricians believe that the medications should be begun at this early age because they prevent diseases which can take a child's life. However, some doctors

are questioning whether exposure to these powerful medications could be safely delayed until the child is a bit older.
If you have questions about the timing of immunization, take
it up with your doctor, although most doctors do adhere to
the immunization schedule on the chart below.

Free immunization is available through many health
departments. Contact your local County Health Department for information.

---

**CHART 48. IMMUNIZATION CALENDAR**

---

| | |
|---|---|
| 2 months: | DTP 3-in-1 shot (Diphtheria, Tetanus, Pertussis) |
| | Sabin Oral live polio vaccine |
| 4 months: | DTP booster |
| | Polio booster |
| 6 months: | DTP booster |
| 1 year: | Tuberculin test |
| 15 months: | Measles/rubella vaccine |
| | Mumps vaccine |
| 18 months: | DTP booster |
| 2 years: | Polio booster |
| | HIB vaccine (hemophilus influenza type B) |
| 4 to 6 years: | DTP booster |
| | Polio booster |

---

*Colic* can be agonizing for you and the baby. A baby with
colic has abdominal cramps and her knees draw up from
the gas and pain—inevitably she cries a lot. Breast-fed babies tend to have colic less frequently because breast milk
is more easily digested. Colic occurs mostly in the evening;
walking and rocking a baby can help. You can try tummy
massage or placing the baby on her stomach over your warm
hand or knee. A towel or receiving blanket warmed in the
dryer and folded under the baby's painful stomach may help
soothe her to sleep.

Although colic usually disappears around 3 months

of age it can be very hard on new parents. The frequent crying and wakefulness can stretch your physical and mental tolerance to the limit. Perhaps worse of all is that you know your baby is suffering and you are impotent—your sense of helplessness can frustrate and make you angry. One solution is to have other people around to hold and comfort the baby so that you can at least get out of the house for part of each day to restore your sanity!

## FEEDING THE BABY

Breast-feeding was covered in the preceding chapter because it has as much to do with your body as the baby's. What follows here is some basic information about feeding a baby, a discussion of bottle-feeding and a comparison of infant formulas, and a section on baby's diet after weaning.

### SOME POINTERS ABOUT FEEDING

*Begin a feeding in a calm,* relaxed atmosphere. If the baby is hungry and crying do not let yourself get upset so you rush and get tense. The baby isn't going to starve. All babies cry sometimes—it's nothing to get anxious about. Quiet the baby down before you feed him; sometimes just putting him into a nursing position can do this. But if the baby is tense his stomach will be tight, his breathing will be out of rhythm and he won't nurse or digest as well.

*When you nurse, hold the baby firmly* so that he knows you are there and feels secure. Hold his foot or bottom with a firm touch and keep his back fairly straight—he can't digest well if he's all hunched over. If you are bottle-feeding there are certain important aspects of nursing you should know that are covered in the following section.

*When you give the baby a night feeding,* change his diaper before you feed him. This way he will be clean and dry and will wake up, which means he will nurse well rather than dozing and reawakening.

*Burping* a baby is important after feeding, depending on the individual. You will learn your baby's patterns: whether he is a quick or slow burper, or whether he needs to burp at all, and which position works best. You can burp a baby over your shoulder or with his face downward on your lap, patting his back in either case. Another position is with the baby sitting up: you support his back and head with one hand, gently moving the baby back and forward as if he was bowing. He is less likely to spit up in this position.

*Choking* can happen because there is a delicate balance between a baby's breathing and swallowing. If the baby spits up, chokes, and gags *sit him up immediately*. This should be an automatic reflex on your part—you should not worry about the baby making a mess or anything like that. Sit the baby up instantly if he chokes.

*Lay the baby on his side or stomach to sleep.* That way mucus or milk cannot go down the wrong passageway.

*If you are bottle-feeding* it's important to offer the bottle on both sides. If you always hold the baby on your left side and the bottle in your right hand, the baby's eye coordination can suffer. Breast-feeding mothers automatically have to alternate sides so the baby can get both breasts.

### BOTTLE-FEEDING

*There are a number of advantages to bottle-feeding over breast-feeding:*

- You have more freedom of movement: you are not the only person who can supply the baby's food and therefore you aren't restricted by a feeding schedule, since other people can give a bottle. If you have a job, you may be able to return to it sooner.
- You can get more rest because your mate and others can feed the baby.
- The gratification and closeness associated with feeding can be shared by all—the father, mother, and grandpar-

ents. However, this should be a secondary consideration. Other people can share the care of the baby in many ways: by changing and dressing, bathing, or taking her for a walk.

- You escape the potential discomforts of breast-feeding (leaky breasts, sore nipples), and not nursing may preserve the shape of your breasts better. Although it is pregnancy itself which softens a firm breast regardless of whether you nurse, breast sagging is more common in those who breast-feed. However, it doesn't occur in all or even most of those who do breast-feed.
- Formula feeding may fill the baby up more so she will go longer between feedings.
- There is more certainty for you because you know exactly how much the baby is getting. This visible evidence is gratifying to some women who would not know the exact quantity a breast-feeding baby was receiving. This seems a weak rationale that caters to some people's compulsive need to measure and time things strictly. A breast-feeding baby gets just as much as she needs because of the natural supply-and-demand system.
- Your condition does not affect the milk, so if you were ill or taking drugs it would not affect your supply or pass the medication on to the baby.

**There are two disadvantages to bottle-feeding** in addition to the loss of all the *advantages* of breast-feeding:

1. THE INJECTION GIVEN IN THE HOSPITAL to dry up your milk supply is potentially dangerous. Your milk production will stop by itself if you don't nurse the baby, so why intervene when nature will take care of it? Some hospitals give an injection of testosterone (a male hormone) to prevent lactation. *Many hospitals use the hormone DES (diethylstilbesterol), a known human carcinogen* which could increase your chances of cancer in later years. There is also evidence that the risk of thromboembolism is increased tenfold if DES is used to suppress lactation. One option you should consider is to nurse for the first week and then gradually dry up your milk supply. You will be

giving your baby all the benefits of colostrum and you will be avoiding the use of these potentially dangerous drugs.

2. OBESITY IN MOTHER AND CHILD can be greater with bottle-feeding. The 30 percent increase in your weight during pregnancy prepares your body for the greater nutritional stress of lactation. You lose the opportunity to shed that body fat accumulated during pregnancy, specifically to support breast-feeding. Also, a bottle-fed child gains and grows more rapidly than one that breast-feeds. This creates more fat cells, which may lead to obesity later in life.

*Bottles and nipples require sterilization*—some people say that careful washing or putting them in the dishwasher is sufficient. Ask your doctor his opinion.

*Plastic bottles* are safer than glass.

*Nursers* (with a disposable plastic inner lining) are more expensive but it means less washing. The liner collapses during drinking so the baby takes in less air.

*Nipples should be discarded* when they become flabby. If the flow is not fast enough you can enlarge the opening with a heated needle; if you make the hole too big you can close it by boiling the nipple for 5 minutes. The Nuk nipple is the most like a human nipple and is orthodontic, enabling the palate to develop more naturally. However, the nipple has an "up" and a "down" side, so you have to explain this to anyone giving the baby the bottle and to the child later on.

## THE EMOTIONAL RISK OF BOTTLE-FEEDING

*The psychological aspects of nursing may be lost in bottle-feeding unless you understand them.* It is essential to know what takes place naturally during breast-feeding so that you can re-create it in bottle-feeding. Breast-feeding creates a biological synchrony of suckling, tactile intimacy, cradling, comforting, sensory arousal, and communication through signs. These are all somewhat technical ways of saying that the baby has many needs besides just nourishment that are met during nursing. A breast-feeding mother does not have to premeditate meeting any of these needs: If you bottle-feed, you have to make sure you are meeting these needs. There is the risk that many of these aspects can be sacrificed if you do not know about them. If the bottle is substituted for the breast, the biological necessity for the baby to experience intimacy in a close grasp has to be compensated for by your intelligent knowledge that *the baby receives both food and love in your arms.*

Most mothers *do* approximate the breast-feeding position when they give a bottle. However, there are many who feed their baby by means of a propped bottle in the crib or who give the bottle while the baby reclines in a plastic seat. *Body intimacy in an embrace is essential for the psychological and physiological growth of the baby.* There are many solitary babies who do not know—or are intermittently deprived of—the sensual delights and comforts of their mother's embrace. The baby of an unknowing mother can be deprived of essential conditions of attachment if she isn't nursed close to her mother's body in a close grasp.

The breast automatically binds the baby to a specific person—the bottle does not guarantee this union. The mother who doesn't know any better can easily adopt the attitude that *anyone* can give the baby a bottle. The section on Love and Kisses, pages 724–727, makes it clear that a baby needs to make a strong attachment to one person for her development. The minimum guarantee for the evolution of the human bond is for an infant to have prolonged intimacy with a nurturing person, a condition which is biologically insured by breast-feeding. With bottle-feeding the continuity of the nurturing experience becomes dependent on your personality. You may want mobility and freedom and perceive that your baby—and particularly the need for you to be the primary person nurturing that baby—as something that ties you down. This is a frequently cited reason for bottle-feeding—thus a woman who does not recognize the biological necessity for her baby to receive both food and love in her arms may be absent for many feedings.

The breast was "intended" to bind a baby and her mother for the first year or two of life. Breast-feeding insures the continuity of mothering as part of the formation of human bonds. The point here is not that everyone "should" breast-feed or that you are cheating your baby emotionally by bottle-feeding; what is at stake is *how* a baby is fed and by whom. It is in your arms that a baby's ability to relate and to communicate with other people is initiated. A baby who is fed by a variety of care-givers while she sits in a hard plastic seat, a baby who is congratulated for holding her own bottle as soon as possible, is a baby who is deprived of the pleasure and security of her mother's arms, which may have ramifications in later relationships. If you feed your baby with a bottle, it places a responsibility on you that you would not have if you breast-fed. It is now your conscious effort, rather than an automatic corollary, that insures the integrity of the human bond between you and your baby.

### INFANT FORMULA

The alternative to breast-feeding is artificial formula; in order to decide between these two methods of feeding you need full information about formulas. Although they may not be contaminated with residues of chlorinated hydrocarbons as frequently as human milk, formulas may contain different contaminants. If you decide to bottle-feed your baby or to supplement breast milk, you should know which formulas pose the fewest health problems and are the most balanced nutritionally.

Infant formulas try to approximate the natural composition of human milk; although there is no formula that is identical in composition, some come closer than others. The aspects to consider in comparing a formula to breast-milk are its protein-to-fat ratio, the amino-acid content, the type of carbohydrate used, and the levels of minerals present. The directory on pages 735–737 is a comparison between human milk, cow's milk, evaporated cow's milk, and milk-base formula and soy-base formula. Cow's milk in fluid and evaporated form is significantly different in its protein-to-fat ratio than human milk. Therefore you should not consider feeding these to your baby instead of formula—they are less expensive substitutes for breast milk but are not good for a growing infant.

The formulas which most closely approximate human milk in their content of protein, fat, amino acids, carbohydrates, and minerals are: PM 60/40, SMA, and Optimil. PM 60/40 is manufactured specifically for infants whose kidneys cannot handle a high concentration and is the only formula to contain lactalbumin, the same type of protein found in human milk.

If you have a family history of allergies and are not going to breast-feed you should probably avoid milk-base formulas. You can use either a soy-base formula like Neo-Mull-Soy or Isomil or a predigested cow's milk formula like Nutramigen. Although these alternative formulas do not resemble human milk as closely as milk-based ones (there are differences in carbohydrates, protein and nutrient levels), they can prevent an allergenic response in the baby.

Corn is also a common allergen. Therefore, parents concerned about allergies should find a milk-free *and* corn-free formula, one that has no corn syrup, corn oil, etc. Consult the directory that follows in making your decision, but double-check the ingredients listed on any formula before purchasing it.

***Soy milk is not a substitute*** for mother's milk or formula. The Food and Drug Administration has warned parents not to use Edensoy or similar soy drinks instead of breast milk or infant formula. Soy drinks, sometimes sold as soy milk, are not the same as soy protein infant formulas. Some health-food stores and literature from Eden Foods, Inc., may give the false impression that soy drinks are nutritionally comparable to cow's milk. The FDA has stated that this is not true; Eden Foods voluntarily recalled their misleading pamphlets.

***Protein-to-fat ratio:*** Human milk has a high-fat, low-protein content. This is believed necessary to provide enough calories and to aid in the absorption of small quantities of iron. Infant formulas approximate this ratio and several come close: SMA, PM 60/40, and Enfamil. However, even when the ratio is similar, the composition of the protein and fat is usually different, except in the cases of SMA and PM 60/40. The protein in human milk is primarily lactalbumin which is easily digested by infants. The protein in formula is primarily casein, which is not as easily digested.

***Sugar:*** Sugar is added to formulas to simulate the natural sweetness of breast milk. Most cow's milk formulas add lactose, the natural sugar present in human milk, but all milk-substitute formulas (soy milk) add sucrose. Sucrose is refined white sugar—and some formulas contain as much as 40 to 50 percent sucrose by weight.

***Cholesterol:*** The level of cholesterol in human milk is higher than that in formula. Human milk has 20 mg cholesterol per 100 mg while most formulas have between 1.5 and 3.3 mg per 100 mg. The effects of this are not fully known, but it is speculated that exposure to high cholesterol in early life may be necessary to stimulate the metabolic systems which break down cholesterol later on. The amount of cholesterol needed by infants has not been determined but animal studies show that *low* cholesterol in infancy led to *higher* serum cholesterol levels when the animals got older, compared to those that had moderate amounts of cholesterol in their infant diets. The implication is that low-cholesterol formulas may contribute to atherosclerosis in later life, a big national health problem in the United States.

***Mineral content:*** Human milk contains lower levels of minerals, which minimizes the load on the baby's kidneys. Only PM 60/40, SMA, and Optimil have a low-soluble load similar to that in breast milk. There is also a higher level of sodium (salt) in cow's milk and formula, which can cause water loss from the kidneys. In cases of dehydration from diarrhea or overheating this can lead to hypernatraemia, a condition in which the abnormally high sodium level in the blood may result in brain damage and later intellectual re-

## CHART 49. DIRECTORY OF COMPARISON OF COMMONLY USED INFANT FORMULAS AND HUMAN AND COW'S MILK

| STANDARD FORMULAS | Normal Dilution | Cal./ Oz. | Percentage Fat | Protein | CHO | Units A | Units D | mg C | mg Iron | Fat Composition | Carbohydrate Composition |
|---|---|---|---|---|---|---|---|---|---|---|---|
| Human milk* | — | 20 | 3.8 | 1.25 | 7.0 | 1419 | 95 | 40 | Trace | butterfat (human) | lactose |
| Cow's milk* (undiluted) | — | 20 | 4.1 | 3.5 | 5.0 | 946 | 38 | 17 | Trace | butterfat (cow) | lactose |
| Evaporated 1:2* | 1:2 | 15 | 2.7 | 2.4 | 3.4 | 800 | 265 | — | Trace | butterfat (cow) | lactose |
| Bremil | 1:1 | 20 | 3.5 | 1.5 | 7.0 | 2500 | 400 | 50 | Trace | coconut, corn, peanut oil | lactose |
| Carnalac | 1:1 | 20 | 2.7 | 2.4 | 8.2 | 1035 | 400 | 80 | Trace | butterfat | lactose |
| Enfamil | 1:1 | 20 | 3.7 | 1.5 | 7.0 | 1500 | 400 | 50 | 1.4 | coconut, corn, oleo | lactose |
| Lactum | 1:1 | 20 | 2.8 | 2.7 | 7.8 | 400 | 400 | 2 | Trace | butterfat | lactose, maltose, dextrins |
| Modilac | 1:1 | 20 | 2.7 | 2.15 | 7.7 | 1500 | 400 | 45 | 10 | corn oil | lactose, maltose, dextrose, dextrins |
| Optimil | 1:1 | 20 | 3.8 | 1.47 | 7.2 | 2500 | 400 | 80 | 8 | corn, coconut, olive oil | lactose |

*Information and statistics concerning cow's milk, evaporated milk, and human milk present many variables: seasonal and breed variations in cow's milk, different manufacturing formulations and processing techniques of evaporated milk, varying degrees of maturity and other factors in human milk.

(From *Handbook of Infant Formulas*, J.B. Roerig Div., Chas. Pfizer & Co., Inc., N.Y. 1967)

## CHART 49. DIRECTORY OF COMPARISON OF COMMONLY USED INFANT FORMULAS AND HUMAN AND COW'S MILK (continued)

| STANDARD FORMULAS | Normal Dilution | Cal./Oz. | Percentage | | | Per qt. @ Normal dilution | | | | Fat Composition | Carbohydrate Composition |
|---|---|---|---|---|---|---|---|---|---|---|---|
| | | | Fat | Protein | CHO | Units A | Units D | mg C | mg Iron | | |
| Purevap | 1:2 | 20 | 2.6 | 2.3 | 8.0 | 800 | 400 | — | Trace | butterfat | lactose, maltose, dextrose, dextrins |
| Similac | 1:1 | 20 | 3.4 | 1.7 | 6.6 | 2500 | 400 | 50 | Trace | corn, coconut oil | lactose |
| SMA S-26 | 1:1 | 20 | 3.6 | 1.5 | 7.2 | 2500 | 400 | 50 | 7.5 | corn, coconut, soy, oleo | lactose |
| **SOY FORMULAS** | | | | | | | | | | | |
| Isomil | 1:1 | 20 | 3.6 | 2.0 | 6.8 | 1419 | 378 | 47 | 11.4 | corn, coconut oil | sucrose, maltodextrins |
| Mull-Soy | 1:1 | 20 | 3.6 | 3.1 | 5.2 | 2000 | 400 | 40 | 5 | soy oil | sucrose |
| Neo-Mull-Soy | 1:1 | 20 | 3.5 | 1.8 | 6.4 | 2000 | 400 | 50 | 8 | soy oil | sucrose |
| ProSobee | 1:1 | 20 | 3.4 | 2.5 | 6.8 | 1500 | 400 | 50 | 8 | soy oil | sucrose, maltose, dextrose, dextrins |
| Sobee | 1:1 | 20 | 2.6 | 3.2 | 7.7 | 1500 | 400 | 50 | 8 | coconut, soy oil | sucrose, maltose, dextrins |
| Soyaloc | 1:1 | 20 | 4.0 | 2.1 | 5.9 | 1500 | 400 | 30 | 10 | soy oil | sucrose, maltose, dextrose, dextrins |

## SPECIAL FORMULAS

| | | | | | | | | | | Fat | Carbohydrate |
|---|---|---|---|---|---|---|---|---|---|---|---|
| Alacta (powder only) | — | — | 1.2 | 3.4 | 10.8 | — | — | — | Trace | butterfat | lactose, maltose, dextrins |
| Dryco (powder only) | 1:2 | 16 | 1.5 | 4.0 | 5.7 | 2500 | 400 | — | Trace | butterfat | lactose |
| Lofenalac (powder only) | 1:2 | 20 | 2.7 | 2.2 | 8.5 | 1500 | 400 | 50 | 15 | corn oil | arrowroot starch, maltose, sucrose, dextrins |
| Nursette Premature | Premixed | 24 | 3.7 | 2.84 | 9.1 | 1500 | 400 | 50 | Trace | corn oil | lactose, corn starch, sucrose |
| Nutramigen (powder only) | 1:2 | 20 | 2.6 | 2.2 | 8.5 | 1500 | 400 | 30 | 9.5 | corn oil | sucrose, arrow-root starch |
| Olac (powder only) | 1:1 | 20 | 2.7 | 3.4 | 7.5 | 2500 | 400 | — | Trace | corn oil | lactose, maltose, dextrins |
| PM 60/40 (powder only) | 1:2 | 20 | 3.4 | 1.5 | 7.2 | 2500 | 400 | 50 | 2 | corn, coconut oil | lactose |
| Similac with Iron | Premixed | 24 | 4.2 | 2.12 | 8.0 | 3000 | 480 | 60 | 15 | corn, coconut oil | lactose |

tardation. There are also higher levels of phosphate in cow's milk and formulas—in certain circumstances this can prevent adequate absorption of calcium. This can lead to hypocalcaemia or neonatal tetany, newborn diseases caused by a deficiency of calcium in the blood, which causes convulsions. These diseases are not a problem for most formula-fed infants—but they do occur and therefore must be mentioned.

## CONTAMINANTS IN FORMULA

Lead has been a serious problem in liquid formulas, where it has been found in a variety of studies over the years. Unfortunately, the results of these studies are contradictory in terms of how much lead was detected and whether there was more in canned or bottled formula. However, just the possible presence of lead is a cause for concern. It can cause neurological disorders ranging from learning disabilities, mental retardation, and hyperactivity to paralysis, convulsions, and coma. The blood system and kidneys can also be adversely affected.

It is not known what minimal amount of lead will *not* cause toxological effects in children. The FDA has a standard for lead intake by infants, but the Environmental Defense Fund, a private organization, states that it is too lenient. Evidently the FDA acceptable levels of lead are based on inaccurate measurements and do not take into account the reported fiftyfold increase in absorption of lead from milk compared to lead in other foods. There is no doubt that infants are particularly susceptible to lead poisoning. Also, children absorb substantially higher amounts of lead from dietary sources than adults do; infants may absorb even higher amounts.

Experts cannot agree on where the lead in formulas is coming from, but there is no doubt that it is present in many liquid formulas. Some say that the lead derives from the solder used on the seams of the cans—which does not explain why bottled formula sometimes contains lead. Others speculate that lead could be associated with the food additive carageenan which is added to stabilize formula.

There have been two studies of liquid formula: one indicates that glass-bottled formula is preferable but the other study contradicts this. Powdered formula was not tested and although lead levels might be lower, the tap water added to prepare it has contaminants of its own. This lack of conclusive data makes it even more difficult for you to decide how and what to feed your baby. Although it is necessary to include this information about lead contamination of formula, it is not sufficiently definitive to be used in choosing one formula over another.

***The tap water used to dilute formula can contain contaminants.*** The Environmental Protection Agency made a survey to test the amount of pollution in water supplies in 113 cities of more than 75,000 people in the United States. The report was released in early 1978 and the accompanying chart on pages 741–742 shows the levels of a group of chemicals called trihalomethanes (THMs). Thirty-one of these cities had more than the now-acceptable standard set by the EPA of 100 parts per billion (ppb). This means 100 drops of THMs per billion drops of water. Since this study was done, some of the cities with concentrations of THMs higher than 100 ppb may have taken action to reduce this pollution. Under proposed regulations, cities with high levels will be *required* to use filtering systems to reduce the THMs.

THMs are formed during the chlorination of water, which kills the bacteria that cause infectious diseases. The chlorine reacts with the organic matter in the water supply to form THMs. Chlorination cannot be stopped because it is the most effective disinfectant method available and the EPA states that it is necessary for public health safety. The irony is that THMs have been shown to cause cancer in test animals and the EPA says that they *may* pose the same risk to humans. According to the EPA, studies in areas of high cancer rates have suggested a link between cancer and chemical contaminants in drinking water.

A granulated activated carbon (GAC) filtering system in a community can safeguard its water. The EPA report showed that *industrial chemicals* discharged into surface waters are not usually removed by current drinking water treatment facilities. Many organic chemicals, some mutagens and suspected carcinogens are present in drinking water samples from all over the country. These chemicals *could* be removed at the treatment plants by filtration with activated carbon, but this is still rare in most communities. The EPA estimates that a GAC filtering system would cost a community from $6 to $10 per family per year.

If a formula manufacturer does not properly treat the water used in preparing formula, then these organic chemicals will be present. If you use concentrated or powdered formula and dilute it with tap water it will introduce these chemicals. You can find out if your community is one of the few in the country that does filter its drinking water supply with activated carbon, which removes these impurities. Otherwise you can purchase a carbon filter system for your home or buy distilled water. You might consider using such water for yourself and the rest of your family as well.

Another problem with tap water in certain parts of the country is *high nitrate levels.* Approximately 5 percent of communities in the United States have high levels in the drinking water, and public health officials recommend that it not be used for infants. Nitrate, when reduced to nitrite in the stomach, can combine with hemoglobin in the blood and prevent oxygen from being adequately distributed throughout the body, causing the baby to turn blue, a disease known as methemoglobinemia. High-nitrate-containing water is a serious health hazard to infants if it is added to their formula.

In certain parts of the country lead pipes have been corroded by water and the *lead level* is high—Boston is one such area. If this water is used to dilute concentrated formula or frozen orange juice, or in the preparation of cereals, it poses a health hazard to the baby. Prenatal exposure can also be a problem because lead exposure can cause birth defects in the fetus.

**CHART 50. EPA RATING OF 113 U.S. CITIES'
WATER POLLUTION IN 1978**

(The ratings are listed in parts per billion of the chemical
pollution in the water supply. Under 100 ppb is considered
safe.)

| | | |
|---|---|---|
| 1. Albuquerque, NM | 15ppb | |
| 2. Amarillo, TX | 130 | |
| 3. Annandale, VA | 200 | |
| 4. Atlanta, GA | 75 | |
| 5. Baltimore, MD | 65 | |
| 6. Baton Rouge, LA | 1.6 | |
| 7. Billings, MT | 13 | |
| 8. Birmingham, AL | 75 | |
| 9. Bismarck, ND | 100 | |
| 10. Boise, ID | 16 | |
| 11. Boston, MA | 5 | |
| 12. Brownsville, TX | 450 | |
| 13. Buffalo, NY | 23 | |
| 14. Burlington, VT | 91 | |
| 15. California Aqueduct, CA | 110 | |
| 16. Camden, AZ | 120 | |
| 17. Cape Girardeau, MO | 140 | |
| 18. Casper, WY | 41 | |
| 19. Charleston, SC | 200 | |
| 20. Charlotte, NC | 71 | |
| 21. Chattanooga, TN | 98 | |
| 22. Cheyenne, WY | 130 | |
| 23. Chicago, IL | 50 | |
| 24. Cleveland, OH | 49 | |
| 25. Columbus, OH | 210 | |
| 26. Concord, CA | 110 | |
| 27. Corvallis, OR | 57 | |
| 28. Dallas, TX | 79 | |
| 29. Davenport, IA | 100 | |
| 30. Dayton, OH | 40 | |
| 31. Denver, CO | 39 | |
| 32. Des Moines, IA | 15 | |

| | |
|---|---|
| 33. Detroit, MI | 34 |
| 34. Duluth, MN | 12 |
| 35. Elizabeth, NJ | 86 |
| 36. Erie, PA | 31 |
| 37. Eugene, OR | 25 |
| 38. Fort Worth, TX | 61 |
| 39. Fort Wayne, IN | 59 |
| 40. Fresno, CA | 37 |
| 41. Grand Rapids, MI | 69 |
| 42. Greenville, MS | 2.4 |
| 43. Hackensack, NJ | 110 |
| 44. Hagerstown, MD | 100 |
| 45. Hartford, CT | 36 |
| 46. Houston, TX | 250 |
| 47. Huntington, WV | 110 |
| 48. Huron, SD | 300 |
| 49. Ilwaco, WA | 250 |
| 50. Indianapolis, IN | 82 |
| 51. Jackson, MS | 240 |
| 52. Jacksonville, FL | 8.7 |
| 53. Jersey City, NJ | 64 |
| 54. Kansas City, MO | 34 |
| 55. Lincoln, NE | 28 |
| 56. Little Rock, AR | 42 |
| 57. Los Angeles, CA | 49 |
| 58. Las Vegas, NV | 76 |
| 59. Louisville, KY | 150 |
| 60. Madison, WI | .02 |
| 61. Manchester, NH | 60 |
| 62. Melbourne, FL | 550 |
| 63. Memphis, TN | 17 |
| 64. Milwaukee, WI | 16 |
| 65. Monroe, MI | 58 |
| 66. Montgomery, AL | 110 |

---

### CHART 50. EPA RATING OF 113 U.S. CITIES' WATER POLLUTION IN 1978 *(continued)*

---

(The ratings are listed in parts per billion of the chemical pollution in the water supply. Under 100 ppb is considered safe.)

| | | | | |
|---|---|---|---|---|
| 67. | Mount Clemens, MI | 48 | 92. San Diego, CA | 97 |
| 68. | Nashville, TN | 24 | 93. San Francisco, CA | 78 |
| 69. | New Haven, CT | 49 | 94. Santa Fe, NM | 180 |
| 70. | Newport, RI | 160 | 95. Sioux Falls, SD | 79 |
| 71. | Norfolk, VA | 150 | 96. So. Pittsburgh, PA | 43 |
| 72. | Oakland, CA | 45 | 97. Spokane, WA | 1.9 |
| 73. | Oklahoma City, OK | 200 | 98. Springfield, MA | 20 |
| | | | 99. Syracuse, NY | 18 |
| 74. | Omaha, NE | 120 | 100. Tacoma, WA | 8.9 |
| 75. | Passaic Vly., NJ | 130 | 101. Tampa, FL | 230 |
| 76. | Phoenix, AZ | 130 | 102. Terrebonne Parish, LA | 140 |
| 77. | Portland, ME | 7.4 | | |
| 78. | Portland, OR | 20 | 103. Toledo, OH | 38 |
| 79. | Poughkeepsie, NY | 78 | 104. Topeka, KS | 180 |
| 80. | Providence, RI | 8 | 105. Tulsa, OK | 50 |
| 81. | Provo, UT | 12 | 106. Washington, DC | 110 |
| 82. | Pueblo, CO | 9.6 | 107. Waterbury, CT | 110 |
| 83. | Richmond, VA | 34 | 108. Waterford Township, NY | 83 |
| 84. | Rockford, IL | 7.9 | | |
| 85. | Rome, GA | 79 | 109. Wheeling, WV | 160 |
| 86. | Sacramento, CA | 29 | 110. Whiting, IN | 3.6 |
| 87. | St. Croix, VI | 23 | 111. Wichita, KS | 27 |
| 88. | St. Louis City, MO | 51 | 112. Wilmington/ Stanton, DE | 64 |
| 89. | St. Paul, MN | 90 | | |
| 90. | Salt Lake City, UT | 43 | 113. Yuma, AZ | 86 |
| 91. | San Antonio, TX | 13 | | |

***Improper handling of formula*** can lead to bacterial contamination. If there are unsanitary conditions—which often occurs in poor areas—bottles and formulas can be contaminated with bacteria and cause gastrointestinal illness. This can be a life-threatening problem to a baby, who can easily become dehydrated from vomiting and diarrhea.

The other problem in poor areas is that formula can be overdiluted to cut costs.

### INTRODUCING SOLID FOODS

***The age to introduce solids*** should be governed in part by the baby's physical capabilities. The voluntary transfer of food from the front to the back of the mouth is not evident until 3 to 4 months of age.

***Appetite*** appears to be regulated by the hypothalmic portion of the brain. Normally, the desire to eat is suppressed when an adequate number of calories has been consumed. It is not known when this appetite-regulating mechanism begins in infants. The use of solid foods in higher caloric density than breast milk or formula during the period when an infant cannot yet regulate her intake by calories may result in excessive energy (calorie) intake. Human milk or formulas have 67 to 77 calories per 100 grams. For an equivalent 100 grams of meat there are 103 calories, for desserts, 96 calories, and for dry cereals with milk, there are 107 calories.

***Parents can overestimate a baby's caloric*** need and encourage the baby to finish all the food in the jar or on the plate. To make this potential problem even worse, some companies are now marketing jars that are 11 percent larger in order to capture a bigger share of customers. This will further encourage overfeeding.

***Some doctors say*** that the early introduction of solids predisposes an infant to allergy. They say that delaying the use of the more allergenic foods (egg white, citrus fruit, wheat) until 12 months of age will minimize the likelihood of allergy.

***The early introduction of home-prepared foods*** is equally undesirable.

***The early introduction of solids*** is not only physiologically unsound, it is also a bad idea economically. Commercially prepared baby foods are more expensive per unit calorie than most milks or formulas.

**There are some doctors who urge de-emphasizing** the role of milk in a baby's diet. They feel that lean meat and vegetables provide all the calcium and protein of milk without the saturated fats and cholesterol in milk. These doctors recommend that after 3 months of age you should discontinue formula or breast-feeding and use a maximum of 14 to 18 ounces of lowfat (2 percent fat) milk daily. This is only one theory—you can discuss it with your pediatrician.

### DIET AFTER WEANING

**Human milk or a substitute** supports the normal growth of most infants from 4 to 6 months of age with some vitamin and iron supplementation. Some mothers—particularly those who bottle-feed—are unaware that the American Academy of Pediatrics has urged against the *unnecessary early introduction of solid foods* into a baby's diet. One reason that parents rush to start a baby on solid foods is because it is considered a mark of accomplishment. "My child is already eating cereal," you may hear a woman say with pride. Another reason that solids are introduced quickly is because some people believe it causes the infant to sleep through the night—but this claim has not been substantiated. There is no data to support linking solid foods and better sleeping. And then there is the pressure from advertisements that induce women to start solids.

According to one study, bottle-feeding mothers are more likely to introduce solids at a much earlier age than those who breast-feed; those who begin solids before the baby is 3 months old are more likely to use commercially prepared foods rather than home-processed ones. The International Pediatric Association disfavors the early introduction of solids and found that many mothers who did this were using the free samples of commercial baby food that were distributed in the hospital. The group called for a ban on this "dissemination of propaganda" by companies that manufacture formula and baby food.

*Skim milk* (nonfat) does not provide enough energy to sustain an infant's growth during the first year. It doesn't contain enough calories, which are the gauge used to express the fuel or energy value of food. Skim milk is deficient in iron, ascorbic acid, and essential fatty acids. It is also too high in salt and protein (protein provides 40 percent of the calories in skim milk), which put too much pressure on a baby's kidneys. A baby needs some fat because he has to build up a fat storage in case of serious illness when his food intake might be temporarily interrupted.

*If your family has a history of high cholesterol levels* or premature coronary deaths you should have your child checked. People with this tendency can be singled out before age 3 with a series of blood tests.

*Nitrate-rich foods* can cause methemoglobinemia. This is a disease which causes a baby to turn blue because oxygen is not adequately distributed throughout the body. Nitrate in the diet can convert to nitrite in the intestines, which then combines with hemoglobin in the blood and prevents oxygen distribution. There is a very small risk of this happening, but *spinach, carrots, and beets* should not be given to a child under 3 months because of susceptibility to methemoglobinemia. Ideally, these vegetables should be served only after 5 to 7 months of age. They are best served fresh; mashed, boiled, or steamed rather than kept in the refrigerator several days.

*Home-prepared foods should not be salted.* The drawbacks to salt in commercial baby foods are discussed below. There are several good books available on home-preparation with recipes. Basically you should feed your baby appropriate family foods minus the seasonings.

*Commercially prepared baby foods* have drawbacks in the areas of salt, starch, and sugar. Several manufacturers now offer certain items minus the salt or sugar that was once routinely added—read labels carefully. You should also not be misled by certain kinds of advertising: for example, Gerber claims that it adds no preservatives, artificial flavors, or colors to its foods. This may be true, but Gerber *does* add sugar to 55 percent of its products, and the other major companies add even more. So read this section and then consider making all or some of your baby's food at home.

NEVER STORE opened commercial baby food in the refrigerator for more than 3 days. Take out only the portion your baby will eat.

DO NOT FEED THE BABY DIRECTLY FROM THE JAR until an age when the baby can eat the entire contents. The enzymes in saliva start breaking down food in the jar and cause the uneaten portion to be "watery" because of this process.

YOU SHOULD KNOW WHAT YOU'RE PAYING FOR and what you're actually giving your baby: vegetable/meat dinners contain an average of only 9 percent meat. So-called "high meat" dinners have around 30 percent meat.

SALT has been added to baby foods for a long time. Manufacturers used to claim that salt helped maintain the sodium/potassium balance, aided in kidney function, and that the iodine in it helped prevent thyroid problems like a simple goiter. The National Academy of Sciences Committee recommends a limit of 0.25 percent salt, but some pediatric nutritionists consider even this an excessive amount.

As of 1977, Beech-Nut and Heinz removed all salt from their products. Gerber still uses it at the $\frac{1}{4}$ of 1 percent "recommended" level except in specially marked foods. There is a possible relation of salt to hypertension and experts tend to agree that salt has no benefit to the infant, who cannot tell the difference between salted and unsalted food. Human milk can be used as the appropriate standard by which to measure: per 100 calories of human milk there is 0.9 mEq of sodium. In baby foods with salt the average per 100 calories is 7.0 for meats, 11.3 for plain vegetables, and 10.8 for soups and combination dinners. If you accept that human milk is the appropriate yardstick then these differences in salt content are worrisome.

STARCH in baby food is defended by the manufacturers. They claim that modified starches derived from corn or tapioca act as stabilizers, are an energy source, and that they are never more than 6 percent of the total product. However, modified starch may comprise as much as one-fourth of the total solids. It adds only calories and replaces more expensive, nutritious ingredients that have protein, minerals, and vitamins. Few single-ingredient foods contain modified starch. Combination-foods give a manufacturer increased shelf-space in stores, but it is the consumer who pays: larger volumes of few choices would cost the companies less to produce and this saving *could* be passed on to you.

SUGAR is a real problem in commercial foods. Studies show that infants can differentiate and will generally eat more of a sweet food. Companies put sugar in more than half their foods, which accustoms children to sweetness and teaches them to expect it. Gerber adds sugar to 55 percent, Heinz to 65 percent, and Beech-Nut to 66 percent of their products. It is often added to foods that do not naturally contain much sugar. Cereals, especially those in jars, often have sugar added. In desserts, sugar is often the principal ingredient.

Sugar adds only extra calories: no vitamins, minerals, or protein. Some studies relate sugar to atherosclerosis, diabetes, and hyperactivity in childhood. The regular eating of sweet foods in infancy may stimulate a preference for sweet foods in childhood and adulthood. *Every possible step should be taken to reduce a baby's intake of and taste for sugar.*

HONEY should not be fed to children under 12 months of age. This recommendation is made by the Centers for Disease Control and by the world's largest honey producer, the Sioux Honey Association of Sioux City, Iowa. Honey poses a threat of botulism if fed to infants. There is a significant link between honey exposure and type-B infant botulism, and many samples of honey were tested and found to be contaminated.

SODIUM NITRITE OR NITRATE is in some baby foods. Gerber adds it to ham-containing "toddler meals" as a coloring and flavoring. It is not needed as a preservative: all baby food is heat-sterilized, killing all microorganisms and spores. Nitrite may react with other chemicals in the body to form nitrosamines, small amounts of which cause cancer in animals. Infants are the most sensitive segment of the population and should not be exposed to even the tiniest amounts of potential carcinogens.

## MISCELLANEOUS DANGERS TO THE BABY

*Infant swim classes* have become popular for babies only a few months old, but they present some dangers. The California Medical Association has issued strong warnings, especially about the dangers of forced infant submersion. Instructors often use this technique to get a child used to getting her face wet: *parents don't know that children have died or been permanently harmed by water intoxication.* This is a condition which occurs when a child ingests too much water: the victim may have convulsions, seizures, go into shock, or even become comatose. *This condition can happen hours or days after the swim class, even if the child did not seem affected at the time of the lesson.*

The most dangerous classes are those aimed at the youngest children, the classes which promise to "waterproof" or "drownproof" children under age 3. Although they can learn to propel themselves, children that age don't understand water safety—and it is the age at which a child is most vulnerable to drowning.

An additional hazard of kiddie swim classes is that there can be bacterial infections in the water from other children which can result in ear infections, sinus conditions, and ingestion of bacteria into the lungs. The California Medical Association recommends that you avoid submerging any child until she has developed immunities to bacteria, and until other physiological and psychological growth have also taken place.

***The use of vitamins for infants*** is an area of controversy. Although vitamin supplements are sometimes routinely prescribed as "nutritional insurance," many knowledgeable pediatricians are opposed. The consensus is that a healthy, full-term baby has no need for vitamin supplementation. A breast-fed baby gets everything he needs from mother's milk, while infant formula already contains vitamins to approximate breast milk.

***Waterbeds are dangerous*** for babies less than 2 years old: they cannot turn over on a waterbed and can smother. *Do not leave a young child of any age unattended on a waterbed: if the child is under two, do not even turn your back on the child.*

***Bath support rings*** can be lethal for babies. Never leave a small child alone in one of these "support ring" bathing devices, which usually are constructed with 3 or 4 legs with suction cups. The suction cups can suddenly release from the bottom of the bathtub, allowing the device and the baby to tip over. A baby can also slip between the legs of the device and become entrapped under the ring. *An adult should always be present when a bath ring is used.*

***Certain crib toys are hazardous*** for babies, some of whom have hung themselves on these devices. Numerous babies, most over 5 months old, have strangled, suffered brain damage, or been narrowly rescued from strangulation due to these playthings. Though some of the stuffed animals, dolls, mirrors, etc., that are strung from mobiles or stretched across the crib are more dangerous than others, the hazard exists with all of them once a baby is able to reach the toys. *Remove all crib toys strung across the crib or playpen when your child is beginning to push up on hands and knees or is 5 months of age, whichever occurs first. These toys can cause strangulation.*

## HOUSEHOLD PETS

Household pets may have had a central part in your life before the birth of your baby. In some ways pets may even have been surrogate children and received a great deal of loving from you. It is inevitable that when you bring a newborn home it will change the kind of attention your pets now receive. This can create jealousy in the animal and set up a rivalry between it and the new baby. Make an effort to include your pet as much as you can when the baby joins the household. New parents have a tendency to push the pet away—both because they haven't got as much time for it and because they want to protect the baby. This will only increase the animal's feeling of rivalry. Make a careful observation of the animal when it is around the baby—some dogs become protective and nurturant of a baby, others may feel antagonistic. When you aren't there, it may be a good idea to close the nursery door, at least in the early postpartum period. There is an old wive's tale (untrue) that a cat can jump into a crib and smother a baby. However, household pets do pick up dirt and germs and it's best not to have them in nose-to-nose contact with a newborn.

*Structured exercise programs for infants* are not recommended by the American Academy of Pediatrics, in a policy statement released in October of 1988. These programs, most of which involve massage and passive exercise, have become increasingly popular in the United States. Some of these programs involve purchasing equipment and instructional materials for enhancing a baby's quiet alert states and "learning." Promoters claim that this will improve a baby's physical prowess or intelligence. However, the AAP feels there should not be pressure on parents and infants to accelerate the child's normal development, especially because "the possibility exists that adults may inadvertently exceed the infant's limitations."

The American Academy of Pediatrics emphasized in the policy statement that although it is important to provide a stimulating environment for infants, parents do not need special skills or equipment to do this. "An infant should be provided with opportunities for touching, holding, face-to-face contact, and minimally structured playing with safe toys. If these opportunities occur, an infant's intrinsic motivation will guide his or her individual development. . . ." The point here is to avoid getting caught up in the Super Baby Syndrome and allow your child to blossom naturally.

## SOME FINAL THOUGHTS

I'm glad to say that I am still passionate about childbirth even after ten years of being immersed in the subject. If anything, the health-care, social, and personal issues surrounding pregnancy and birth seem more important than ever. Women have told me that because of this book they came to view me as a friend during their childbearing experience. I am honored. And I don't take that trust lightly: I want to do everything possible to make pregnancy and childbirth safe and beautiful for parents and babies. So if you have questions this book doesn't answer, or you can't get what you want from your health-care providers, or you just need some reassurance, get in touch with me. I learn something from everyone who contacts me, and I can pass it on to others.

I still get crazy when I hear bad hospital stories; I still get frustrated when I meet couples who complain about The System and are doing nothing to take responsibility for their own health care; I am still in awe of the miracles of medicine; I still get all choked up when I see a baby coming into this world. It seems as though the world has another chance every time a baby is born; we all have to make sure that birth is the very best it can be.

I still have an urge to stop pregnant women in the street and ask if they're okay. "Is everything all right?" I want to ask. "Are you satisfied with your doctor? Are you eating enough protein? How about breast-feeding? How's your relationship doing?"

I also still weep inside when I learn of couples with tiny children whose marriages are suffering—sometimes to the point of separation or divorce. It is vital that you find your strength together as a couple during pregnancy so that childbirth and raising a family together can be a powerfully positive time in your lives.

In fact, I was so concerned about the effect of a new baby on a couple's relationship that I wrote a whole book about it! I wrote *Childbirth & Marriage* for parents-to-be and new parents because I could see that new parents need all the help they can get if they're going to have a mutually satisfying marriage while raising a child. Until *Childbirth & Marriage* there was nowhere to turn for support and information about that transition to parenthood and the effect it has on your relationship. I hope that the two books together will help you get the full measure of joy and fulfillment from giving birth and raising a child together.

# Bibliography

(This listing is of books and periodicals consulted for research purposes. It is not intended as a recommendation that you read these publications. Alphabetical by title.)

AMERICAN JOURNAL OF NURSE MIDWIFERY 1975–1982
AMERICAN BABY MAGAZINE 1976–1978
BIRTH, Caterine Milinaire (Harmony, 1974)
BIRTH BOOK, Raven Lang (Genesis Press, 1972)
BIRTH AND THE FAMILY JOURNAL 1974–1989
THE BIRTH PRIMER, Rebecca Rowe Parfitt (Running Press, 1977)
BIRTH WITHOUT VIOLENCE, Frederick Leboyer, M.D. (Knopf, 1975)
BIRTHRIGHT DENIED: *The Risks of Breast-feeding,* Harris and Highland (Environmental Defense Fund, 1977)
BRIEFS (FOOTNOTES ON MATERNITY CARE) (Maternity Center Association, 1975–1983)
THE CHILDBEARING YEAR, Peg Beals (ICEA, 1975)
CHILDBIRTH AT HOME, Marion Sousa (Bantam, 1976)
CHILDBIRTH WITHOUT PAIN, EDUCATION LEAGUE STUDENT MANUAL, compiled by Maryann Roulier (1972, 1975)
CHOICES IN CHILDBIRTH, Silvia Feldman, M.D. (Grosset & Dunlap, 1978)
COMMONSENSE CHILDBIRTH, Lester Dessez Hazell (Berkeley Windhover, 1969–1976)
COMPLETE BOOK OF MIDWIFERY, Barbara Brennan & Joan Rattner Heilman (Dutton, 1977)
DIET FOR A SMALL PLANET, Frances Moore Lappé (Ballantine, 1971)
EMERGENCY CHILDBIRTH, Gregory White, M.D. (Police Training Foundation, Franklin Park, Illinois, 1958, 1976)
EVERY CHILD'S BIRTHRIGHT: IN DEFENSE OF MOTHERING, Selma Fraiberg (Basic Books, 1977)

EVERYWOMAN: *A Gynaecological Guide for Life,* Derek Llewellyn-Jones (Faber & Faber, 1973)

THE FIRST NINE MONTHS OF LIFE, Geraldine Lux Flanagan (Simon & Schuster, 1962)

HAVE IT YOUR WAY, Vicki Walton (Henry Philips Publishing Co., 1976)

HAVING A CESAREAN BABY, Hausknecht & Heilman (Dutton, 1978)

HELPING YOUR CHILD SLEEP THROUGH THE NIGHT, Joanne Cuthbertson and Susie Schevill (Doubleday, 1985)

HOME BIRTH, Alice Gilgoff (Coward, McCann, Geoghegan, 1978)

THE HOME BIRTH BOOK, Charlotte & Fred Ward (Inscape, 1976)

HOME ORIENTED MATERNITY EXPERIENCE: *A Comprehensive Guide to Homebirth* (H.O.M.E., Inc., 1976)

HUSBAND-COACHED CHILDBIRTH, Robert Bradley, M.D. (Harper & Row, 1965)

IMMACULATE DECEPTION, Suzanne Arms (Houghton Mifflin, 1975)

THE LAMAZE EXPERIENCE (3 records and workbook), Elizabeth Bing and Ferris B. Urbanowski (Tratec, Inc., 1972)

LET'S HAVE HEALTHY CHILDREN, Adelle Davis (Signet, 1951, 1972)

METHODS OF CHILDBIRTH, Constance Bean (Doubleday, 1972)

MAKING LOVE DURING PREGNANCY, Elizabeth Bing and Libby Colman (Bantam, 1974)

MATERNAL INFANT BONDING, Marshall Klaus and John Kennell (C.V. Mosby Co., 1976)

NATUREBIRTH: *You, Your Body and Your Baby,* Danae Brook (Pantheon, 1976)

NINE MONTHS: *A Practical Guide for the Expectant Mother,* Alice Fleming (Barnes & Noble, 1974)

9 MONTHS 1 DAY 1 YEAR, Jean Marzollo (Harper, 1976)

NINE MONTHS' READING, Robert Hall (Bantam, 1973)

NOURISHING YOUR UNBORN CHILD, Phyllis S. Williams (Avon, 1975)

OUR BODIES, OURSELVES (Boston Women's Health Book Collective, 1971, 1976)

THE PEOPLE'S PHARMACY, Joe Graedon (Avon, 1977)

PREGNANCY: *The Psychological Experience,* Arthur and Libby Colman (Seabury Press, 1971; Bantam, 1977)

PREGNANCY, BIRTH AND FAMILY PLANNING, Alan F. Guttmacher, M.D. (Signet, 1937, 1973)

THE PSYCHOLOGY OF CHILDBIRTH, Aidan MacFarlane (Harvard University Press, 1977)

THE RIGHTS OF THE PREGNANT PARENT, Valmai Howe Elkins (2 Continents Publishing Group, 1976)

SAFE ALTERNATIVES IN CHILDBIRTH, David and Lee Stewart, editors (NAPSAC, 1976)

A SEASON TO BE BORN, Suzanne Arms (Harper & Row, 1973)

SIX PRACTICAL LESSONS FOR AN EASIER CHILDBIRTH, Elizabeth Bing (Bantam, 1967)

SPIRITUAL MIDWIFERY, Ina May Gaskin (The Book Publishing Co., 1978)

21ST CENTURY OBSTETRICS NOW!, Vols. 1 & 2, David Stewart and Lee Stewart, editors (NAPSAC, 1977)

WHAT EVERY PREGNANT WOMAN SHOULD KNOW: *The Truth about Diet and Drugs in Pregnancy,* Gail Sforza Brewer (Random House, 1977)

THE WOMANLY ART OF BREASTFEEDING, La Leche League, 1963

YOU'RE NOT TOO OLD TO HAVE A BABY, Jane Price (Farrar, Straus & Giroux, 1977)

# BOOKS ON INFERTILITY

THE INFERTILITY BOOK: *A Comprehensive Medical and Emotional Guide,* Carla Harkness (Volcano Press, 1987)

INFERTILITY: *A Guide for the Childless Couple,* Barbara Eck Menning (Prentice-Hall, 1977)

IN SEARCH OF PARENTHOOD: *Coping with Infertility and High-Tech Conception,* Judith N. Lasker and Susan Borg (Beacon Press, 1982)

THE MIRACLE SEEKERS: *An Anthology of Infertility,* Mary Martin Mason (Perspectives Press, 1987)

NEW CONCEPTIONS: *A Consumer's Guide to the Newest Infertility Treatments,* Lori B. Andrews (St. Martin's Press, 1984)

NEW MIRACLES OF CHILDBIRTH, Elliott H. McCleary (Dell, 1974)

YOU CAN HAVE A BABY: *Everything You Need to Know About Fertility,* Joseph H. Bellina, M.D., and Josleen Wilson (Crown Publishers, 1985)

WHAT WE KNOW ABOUT INFERTILITY: *Diagnosis and Treatment Alternatives,* Robert Winston, M.D. (Free Press, 1986)

# The Appendices

There are five appendices which may be useful to you:

**APPENDIX I** is a state-by-state listing of the organizations dedicated to pregnancy, childbirth, and parenting. By contacting these groups you will be able to find out what birth options are available in your area—whether you are seeking a home-birth attendant, a childbirth educator, support for breast-feeding, recommendations about hospitals, supportive physicians, etc.

    This listing is not an endorsement of the organizations or individuals. You will have to decide for yourself whether particular groups or people meet your needs; this appendix simply lets you know who is part of the "birth movement" in your state.

    Groups called CEA are members of the International Childbirth Education Association (ICEA)—as are a number of other listed organizations which do not use those letters as part of their name. C/SEC is the abbreviation used by groups dedicated to information and support for women who have had cesareans.

**APPENDIX II** is a listing of national organizations. By contacting these groups you can get information about nationwide programs and organizations relating to childbearing, as well as references for groups in your part of the country.

**APPENDIX III** is "Help for Grieving Parents," with support groups listed by state. By contacting these organizations you will find invaluable help and comfort if you have lost your baby through miscarriage, stillbirth, neonatal death or SIDS.

**APPENDIX IV** is a listing of "Infertility and Genetics Organizations" which can provide information and counseling for couples with infertility problems.

APPENDIX V is a listing of "Lactation Consultants," from which breast-feeding families can get advice and support for beginning breast-feeding or if problems arise.

# APPENDIX I

## CHILDBIRTH GROUPS BY STATE

**ALABAMA**
CEA of Greater Birmingham
441 Shenandoah Dr.
Birmingham 35226

CEA of West Alabama
P O Box 3003
Tuscaloosa 35401

Decatur CEA
P O Box 411
Decatur 35602

**ALASKA**
CEA of Greater
    Anchorage Area
P O Box 8-484
Anchorage 99508

Childbirth & Parent Assoc. of
    Sitka
Box 1941
Sitka 99835

Parent & Child Inc. of Juneau
P O Box 2926
Juneau 99803

**ARIZONA**
Childbirth Education Assoc.
P O Box 26393
Tucson 85726

CEA of Greater Phoenix
6308 N. 13th Place
Phoenix 85014

Committee for Arizona
    Midwifery
114 E. Mohave Rd.
Tucson 85705

**ARKANSAS**
Arkansas Valley Parent
    Education Assoc.
22 Ridgewood
Russelleville 72801

Better Births
Fayetteville Women's Center
207 Razorback Rd.
Fayetteville 72701

Prepared Childbirth
P O Box 5821
Little Rock 72205

**CALIFORNIA**
Adelphian Childbirth
    Educators
1920 E. Katella, Suite G
Orange 92667

American Academy of
  Husband-Coached Childbirth
Box 5224
Sherman Oaks 91413

American Institute of Family
  Relations
5287 Sunset Blvd.
Los Angeles 90027

Assoc. for Childbirth at Home
  International
Box 1219
Cerritos 90701

B.I.R.T.H.
6052 Ethel Ave.
Van Nuys 91401

CEA of Los Angeles
3309 Big Cloud Circle
Thousand Oaks 91360

CEA of the Peninsula
308 Iris St.
Redwood City 94062

CEA of San Diego
4138 30th St.
San Diego 92104

CEA of San Jose
1722 Sweetbriar Dr.
San Jose 95125

Center for Family Growth
555 Highland Ave.
Penngrove 94951

Central Valley Prepared Ch.B.
  Educators
6434 Savannah
Stockton 95209

Childbirth Education League
  of the Monterey Peninsula
P O Box 6628
Carmel 93921

Childbirth Education League
  of Salinas
P O Box 1423
Salinas 93901

Childbirth w/o Pain League of
  Sonoma County
638 Acacia Lane
Santa Rosa 95405

Childbirth w/o Pain Parent
  Leagues
22271 McClaren Rd.
Colton 92324

Childbirth w/o Pain Parent
  Leagues
P O Box 233
Dana Point 92629

Childbirth w/o Pain Education
  League
3940 11th St.
Riverside 92501

Clovis Adult School Prepared
  Childbirth Education
914 4th St.
Clovis 93612

Community Child Care
  Council
1030 2nd St.
Santa Rosa 95404

Conference of Practicing
  Midwives
7351 Covey Rd.
Forestville 95436

Discovery Institute
1020 Corporation Way
Palo Alto 94303

East Bay Birth Center
2908 Ellsworth
Berkeley 94705

Entrepoint Foundation
P O Box 38
San Geronimo 94963

Holistic Childbirth Institute
1627 10th Ave.
San Francisco 94122

International Scientific Lay
  Midwives for Natural
  Homebirth
315 Sampson
San Diego 92113

Life After Birth
34334 Calle Naranja
Capistrano Beach 92624

Los Angeles C/SEC
812 17th St.
Santa Monica 90403

Midpeninsula CEA
Box 242
Menlo Park 94025

Mother (Mary Ann Bennett)
P O Box 718
Inverness 94937

Organization for Safe
  Alternatives in Childbirth
  (OSAC)
1072 Pinehurst Place
Camarillo 93010

Preparing Expectant Parents
P O Box 838
Pomona 91769

Read Natural Childbirth
  Foundation
1300 S. Eliseo Dr., Suite 102
Greenbrae 94904

Safe Birthing Information
  Network
4146 51st St., Suite 2
San Diego 92105

Santa Cruz Women's Health
  Center
250 Locust St.
Santa Cruz 94060

Society for Humanized Birth
P O Box 255502
Sacramento 95825

Turlock CEA
1690 Lantana
Turlock 95380

Womencare Inc. Childbearing
  Clinic
1050 Garnet
San Diego 92109

**COLORADO**
CEA of the Pikes Peak Region
P O Box 4641
Colorado Springs 80930

CEA of Pueblo
P O Box 3276
Pueblo 81005

Mesa County Parenthood
Education Assoc.
P O Box 516
Grand Junction 81501

Parents' League of Trinidad
P O Box 51
Trinidad 81082

Poudre Valley CEA
P O Box 1443
Ft. Collins 80522

CONNECTICUT
Calm-Childbirth Assoc.
35 Hawthorne Dr.
Norwalk 06851

Connecticut Midwives
84 High St.
Mystic 06355

Family Oriented Childbirth
Information Society
P O Box 748
Manchester 06040

Focis/Elaine Camposeo
22 Tunxis Trail
Bolton 06040

Monthly Extract New Moon
Communications
Box 3488, Ridgeway Station
Stamford 06905

Pace/Janet & Richard Miller
36 Shady Hill Lane
Glastonbury 06033

Palm/Barbara Behan
Woodland Hill Rd.
Southbury 06488

Parenthood & Childbirth
Education Assoc.
1680 Albany Ave.
Hartford 06105

Waterbury Area Parents'
Assoc. for the Lamaze
Method
c/o Pam Kreis
Old Waterbury Rd.
Southbury 06488

DELAWARE
Family Centered Parents
Box 142
Rockland 19732

DISTRICT OF COLUMBIA
DC Area Chapter of ASPO
4401 Cathedral Ave., N.W.
Washington 20016

FLORIDA
CEA of Alachua County
P O Box 12886
Gainesville 32604

CEA of Broward County
P O Box 6294
Ft. Lauderdale 33310

CEA of Jacksonville
P O Box 8224
Jacksonville 32211

CEA of Northwest Florida
P O Box 1901
Pensacola 32589

CEA of the Palm Beaches
P O Box 10042
Riviera Beach 33404

Childbirth Education League
of Brevard County
P O Box 174
Cape Canaveral 32920

Childbirth & Parent Education
Assoc.
P O Box 264
S. Miami 33143

Childbirth & Parent Education
Assoc. of Polk County
P O Box 655
Winter Haven 33880

Childbirth & Parent Education
League of Pinnellas County
P O Box 1281
Largo 33540

Education for a Gentle Birth
220 Toms Rd.
DeBary 32713

Feminist Women's Health
Center
1017 Thomasville Rd.
Tallahassee 32303

Parents & Childbirth
Education Assoc. of Collier
County
P O Box 7872
Naples 33940

Prepared Childbirth of Halifax
Area
P O Box 2522
Daytona Beach 32015

**GEORGIA**
Atlanta APSAC
533 Linwood Ave., N.E.
Atlanta 30306

CEA of Atlanta
201 Washington St., S.W.
Atlanta 30303

CEA of Augusta
3406 Wentwood Place
Augusta 30906

Childbirth & Parent Education
Assoc.
P O Box 696
Waycross 31501

Childbirth & Parent Education
Assoc. of Macon
2597 Hyde Park Rd.
Macon 31201

Feminist Women's Health
Center
580 14th St., N.W.
Atlanta 30318

Griffin CEA
c/o Pam Pinson
Rt. 6, Box 549
Griffin 30223

**HAWAII**
Ahahui Kumu Hanau-Assoc. of
Childbirth Educators
818 Keolu Dr.
Lailua 96734

Maui CEA
P O Box 974
Paia 96779

**IDAHO**
Family Centered Education
    Assoc. of Pocatello
P O Box 462
Pocatello 83201

Prepared Childbirth Assoc.
c/o Millie Andrus
Rt. #2
Rexburg 83440

**ILLINOIS**
American College of Home
    Obstetrics
664 N. Michigan, Suite 600
Chicago 60611

Assoc. for Childbirth
    Preparation & Family Life
P O Box 345
Macomb 61455

CEA of Northwestern Illinois
1707 21st St.
Rock Island 61201

Childbirth & Parent Education
    Assoc. of Peoria
P O Box 24
Peoria 61601

Home Opportunity for the
    Pregnancy Experience
P O Box 78
Wauconda 60084

The Life Center
Richard Talsky, DC
5613 W. Cermak Rd.
Cicero 60650

Midwest Parentcraft Center
627 Beaver Rd.
Glenview 60025

Parent & Childbirth Education
    Society
P O Box 213
Western Springs 60558

Parents for Prepared
    Childbirth & Family
    Centered Maternity Care
152 S. Highland
Aurora 60506

Successful Childbirth &
    Organized Parent Education
P O Box 175
Crystal Lake 60014

**INDIANA**
Childbirth Educator Training
    Assoc.
4029 Roland Rd.
Indianapolis 46208

Childbirth & Parenting
P O Box 13
Richmond 47374

Evansville CEA
c/o Judy Leahy
RR #3 Box 735
Newburgh 47630

H.O.M.E.
c/o Mary Douglas
RR #1
Box 101
Coatesville 46121

Home of Muncie
1353 E. Jackson
Muncie 47305

Maternity Family League
  Foundation
P O Box 50183
Indianapolis 46250

**IOWA**
CEA of Cedar Rapids
340 Jacolyn Dr.
Cedar Rapids 52405

CEA of Southeastern Iowa
P O Box 281
Fort Madison 52627

CEA of Waterloo-Cedar Falls
802 Eldora Rd.
Hudson 50643

Dubuque Childbirth & Parent
  Education Assoc.
P O Box 54
Dubuque 52001

Family Centered CEA
2531 Euclid
Des Moines 50310

Siouxland CEA
5501 Broken Kettle Rd.
Sioux City 51108

**KANSAS**
Birth at Home League
4010 W. 90th St.
Prairie Village 66207

CEA of Greater Kansas City
P O Box 1284
Mission 66202

CEA of Wichita
345 N. Hillside
Wichita 67214

**KENTUCKY**
Lexington Assoc. for Parent
  Education
P O Box 5544
Lexington 40505

Owensboro CEA
207 E. 23rd St.
Owensboro 42301

**LOUISIANA**
Baton Rouge Parent-Child
  Assoc.
12367 Brookshire Ave.
Baton Rouge 70815

Greater New Orleans CEA
10120 Deerfield Dr.
New Orleans 70127

Lamaze Assoc. for Childbirth
  Education
P O Box 1575
Morgan City 70380

**MAINE**
CEA of Greater Portland
P O Box 984
Portland 04101

Maternal & Child Health
   Council
611 Hammond St.
Bangor 04401

Midcoast Maine Assoc. of
   Parents & Professionals for
   Safe Alternatives in
   Childbirth
c/o Kitty Pfeiffer
R.F.D.
Jefferson 04348

Parenthood Education Assoc.
1 Summer St.
Hallowell 04347

Waterville CEA
6 Middle St.
Waterville 04901

Wellborn
188 Main St.
Eliot 03903

**MARYLAND**
Birth
5304 Ludlow Dr.
Temple Hills 20031

CEA of Baltimore
2530 N. Calvert St.
Baltimore 21218

Family Life & Maternity
   Education
10113 Parkwood Terrace
Bethesda 20014

Homebirth
2113 Kentucky Ave.
Baltimore 21218

Home Oriented Maternity
   Experience (HOME)
511 New York Ave.
Takoma Park 20012

Maternity Center Associates
Janet Epstein, CNM
5415 Cedar Lane, Suite 107-B
Bethesda 20014

Parent & Child
420 University Blvd. East
Silver Spring 20901

**MASSACHUSETTS**
Assoc. for Childbirth at Home
47 Ronald Rd.
Arlington 02174

Berkshire-Bennington
   Parenthood Education
   Assoc.
c/o Sharon Bray Clark
Hancock Rd.
Williamstown 01267

Birthday
Box 388
Cambridge 02138

Birthday
128 Lowell Ave.
Newtonville 02160

Boston Assoc. for Childbirth
   Education
Box 29
Newtonville 02160

Cesareans/Support, Education,
   Concern
181 High St.
North Billerica 01862

CEA of Central Massachusetts
Box 193, West Side Station
Worcester 01602

CEA of Greater Springfield
210 Elm St.
Holyoke 01040

C/SEC
23 Cedar St.
Cambridge 02140

C/SEC
22 Forest Rd.
Framingham 01701

Homebirth
Box 162
Norton 02766

Homebirth, Inc.
89 Franklin St., Suite 200
Boston 02111

Pioneer Valley CEA
P O Box 699
Amherst 01002

Women's Community
  Health Center
137 Hampshire St.
Cambridge 02139

**MICHIGAN**
Assoc. for Shared Childbirth
4361 Keller Rd.
Holt 48842

Birth Information Services
Rt. #1, Box 73A
Suttons Bay 49682

Cadillac Childbirth Assoc.
P O Box 341
Cadillac 49601

CEA of Manistee
P O Box 72
Manistee 49660

CEA of Marquette County
806 W. College Ave.
Marquette 49855

Childbirth Information Service
Box 36451
Grosse Pointe 48236

Childbirth Preparation Assoc.
P O Box 73
Lincoln Park 48146

Childbirth Preparation Service
  of Jackson
P O Box 742
Jackson 49201

Childbirth w/o Pain Education
  Assoc.
20134 Snowden
Detroit 48235

Delta CEA
Rt. 1, Box 232A
Bark River 49878

Expectant Parents
  Organization
2022 Cooper Ave.
Lansing 48910

Family Life Forum
P O Box 2083
Ann Arbor 48106

Joys of Parenthood
Rt. 5, Box 149A
Dowagiac 49047

Kalamazoo Assoc. for
  Prepared Childbirth
154 Fairview
Kalamazoo 49001

Lamaze Childbirth Assoc. of
  Greater Detroit
c/o Jim Spaulding
5617 Cliffside
Troy 48098

Lamaze CEA of Livonia
P O Box 2811
Livonia 48151

Lamaze Childbirth Education
  of Grand Rapids
P O Box 284
Jenison 49428

Lamaze Childbirth Preparation
  Assoc. of Ann Arbor
P O Box 1812
Ann Arbor 48106

Lenawee County Prepared
  Childbirth Service
Box 632
Adrian 49221

M&M Prepared Childbirth
  Assoc.
2116 11th Ave.
Menominee 49858

Mt. Pleasant Assoc. for
  Prepared Childbirth
1101 Watson Rd.
Mt. Pleasant 48858

Parent Education Program
3296 Christopher Court
Bay City 48706

Parents Inc. of Albion
P O Box 584
Albion 49224

Plymouth CEA
P O Box 311
Plymouth 48170

Saginaw Valley CEA
P O Box 821
Bay City 48706

**MINNESOTA**
Austin CEA
2305 16th Ave.
Austin 55912

CEA of Fairmont
520 E. First
Fairmont 56031

CEA of Greater Minneapolis-
  St. Paul
P O Box 20091
Minneapolis 55420

CEA of Kanabec County
c/o Marcia Scheiber
Rt. 2
Mora 55051

CEA of Northeastern
  Minnesota
P O Box 312
Duluth 55801

CEA of Queen of Peace
c/o Joan Goggins
Rt. 2
Box 287
New Prague 56071

CEA of Renville County
c/o Mary Fahey Rozycki
202 Primrose Lane
Olivia 56277

CEA of Southeastern
  Minnesota
P O Box 6522
Rochester 55901

Genesis
5101 Queen Ave. S.
Minneapolis 55410

New School of Family Birthing
993 Portland Ave.
St. Paul 55104

Scott-Carver CEA
409 E. 1st St.
Chaska 55318

Women's Counselling Service
621 West Lake St.
Minneapolis 55458

**MISSISSIPPI**
CEA of Metro Jackson
Box 5124
Jackson 39216

The Childbirth Preparation
  Assoc. of Greenville
2453 Hummingbird Dr.
Greenville 38701

Coast Assoc. for Parent
  Education
3903 Washington Ave.
Pascagoula 39567

**MISSOURI**
Assoc. for Childbirth At Home
  (A.C.A.H.)
1520 Manor Place
Blue Springs 64015

Childbirth & Parent Education
  of Kansas City
P O Box 17725
Kansas City 64134

Childbirth Preparation Classes
P O Box 1164
Cape Girardeau 63701

Childbirth Preparation Seminar
  of Greater Kansas City
c/o Lynn Talley
1600 Country Club Dr.
Pleasant Hill 64080

Expectant Parents Classes
1614 W. 18th
Sedalia 65301

H.O.M.E.
c/o Debra Alstott
6221 Harrison
Kansas City 64110

Northeast Missouri Childbirth
  Assoc.
Box 31
LaBelle 63447

Parent & Child/St. Louis
P O Box 9985
Kirkwood 63122

St. Joseph CEA
1103 Dewey Ave.
St. Joseph 64501

**MONTANA**
Family Centered Education
   Assoc. of Great Falls
502 53rd St.
Great Falls 59405

**NEBRASKA**
CEA of Lincoln
3401 "R"
Lincoln 68503

CEA Mid-Plains, No. Platte
5002 Cedarberry Lane
No. Platte 69101

CEA of Western Nebraska
P O Box 937
Scottsbluff 69361

Central Nebraska Childbirth &
   Parent Assoc.
P O Box 864
Grand Island 68801

**NEVADA**
CEA of Clark County
P O Box 42235
Huntridge Station
Las Vegas 89104

Help Educate Learning Parents
c/o Marcella Posthuma
656 Ave. G.
Boulder City 89005

**NEW HAMPSHIRE**
La Famille Inc.
56 High St.
Claremont 03743

Maternal & Child Health Dept.
Dartmouth Medical School
Hanover 03755

New Hampshire CEA
29 Woodknoll Dr.
North Hampton 03862

**NEW JERSEY**
Birth Alternatives
43 Clover Lane
Princeton 08540

Cape-Atlantic CEA
Box 156
Linwood 08221

CEA of South Jersey
P O Box 462
Toms River 08753

Childbirth & Parent Education
   Assoc.
RD 1, Box 189
Cape May 08204

Childbirth & Parent Education
   Assoc. of Northern New
   Jersey
Box 381
Dover 07801

Lamaze Childbirth Preparation
   Assoc.
P O Box 223
Moorestown 08057

Metropolitan Medical Assoc.
Lonnie Holtzman, CNM
464 Hudson Terrace
Englewood Cliffs 07670 (BC)

Northern New Jersey Chapter
of ASPO
Box 562
Ridgewood 07450

**NEW MEXICO**
Albuquerque CEA
P O Box 26173
Albuquerque 87125

Dona Ana County CEA
P O Box 3293
Las Cruces 88003

Santa Fe CEA
1702 Callejon Cordelia
Santa Fe 87501

**NEW YORK**
Assoc. for Childbirth at Home
John & Sue Crockett
69 Moseman Ave.
Catonah 10536

Assoc. of Mothers for
Educated Childbirth
Box 720 Far Rockaway
New York 11691

Cesarean Birth Assoc.
133-29 122nd St.
So. Ozone Park
Queens 11420

CEA of Albany
P O Box 3
Albany 12204

CEA of Cayuga County
P O Box 444
Auburn 13021

CEA of Greater Syracuse
P O Box 15
Syracuse 13201

CEA of the Hunsbruck OB
Clinic, c/o Joyce Mullins
USAF Hospital
Hahn AFB
APO New York 09109

CEA of Rochester
Box 9612, Midtown Plaza
Rochester 14604

CEA of Tompkins County
15 Lake St.
Dryden 13053

CEA of Watertown
Box 175
Cape Vincent 13618

International Scientific Lay
Midwives for Natural
Homebirth
1364 E. 7th St.
Brooklyn 11230

Long Island Chapter ASPO
165 Ithaca St.
Bayshore 11706

Maternity Center Assoc.
48 E. 92nd St.
New York 10128

Metropolitan New York CEA
30 Beekman Place
New York 10022

New York Fertility Research
  Foundation
123 E. 89th St.
New York 10028

Oswego Co. CEA
234 E. 7th St.
Oswego 13126

Project: Child Growth
30 Stillman Rd.
Glen Cove 11542

Shoshana
1122 Beach 12th St.
Far Rockaway 11690

Women's Action Alliance
370 Lexington Ave.
New York 10017

Women's Counselling Project
East Hall, Columbia University
117th St. & Broadway
New York 10027

Women's Health Forum/
  Healthright
175 5th Ave.
New York 10010

**NORTH CAROLINA**
Childbirth & Parenthood
  Education Assoc. of Chapel
  Hill
310 Umstead Dr.
Chapel Hill 27514

National Assoc. for Parents &
  Professionals for Safe
  Alternatives in Childbirth
Box 1307
Chapel Hill 27514

Tri-County Health Services
P O Box 266
Aurora 27806

**OHIO**
Action for Newborns
Rt. 4, Box 72
Galion 44833

Alliance CEA
984 Mill Circle #95
Alliance 44601

Bluffton CEA
253 Grove St.
Bluffton 45817

CACE/LaMaze
P O Box 1062
Columbus 43216

Canton CEA
P O Box 8654
Canton 44709

CEA of Akron
P O Box 1061
Akron 44309

CEA of Cleveland
P O Box 21272
Cleveland 44121

Center for Humane Options in
  the Childbirth Experience
  (CHOICE)
P O Box 02003
Columbus 43202

Childbirth Education Assoc.
P O Box 5051
Cincinnati 45205

Childbirth Education Classes
of Hamilton
1601 Peck Blvd.
Hamilton 45011

Childbirth & Parenting
Education Assoc.
146 Water St., Suite 2
Kent 44240

Cloverleaf Organization for
Parent Education
P O Box 852
Cambridge 43725

Clyde CEA
3315 Linerick Rd.
Clyde 43410

Dayton CEA
P O Box 2108
Dayton 45429

Educated Childbirth
P O Box 2613
Lakewood 44107

Family Centered Assoc. for
Childbirth Education
P O Box 2826
Mansfield 44906

Fremont CEA
523 S. Clover St.
Fremont 43420

Husband-Coached Natural
Childbirth Assoc.
P O Box 11258
Cincinnati 45211

Lamaze Childbirth Assoc.
3590 Milton Ave.
Columbus 43214

Parents for Prepared
Childbirth
P O Box 591
Marietta 45750

Prepared Childbirth of Lorain
County
P O Box 591
Elyria 44035

Sisters & Others United for
Responsible Childbirth
Education (SOURCE)
2456 Glenwood
Toledo 43610

Tiffin CEA
2964 W. State St. 18
Tiffin 44883

Total Parent Education of
Greater Cincinnati
P O Box 39382
Cincinnati 45239

Trained Childbirth Assoc. of
Lancaster & Fairfield County
P O Box 1033
Lancaster 43130

Tri-County Trained Childbirth
Assoc.
8283 Troy Rd.
Springfield 45502

Wayne County CEA
P O Box 568
Wooster 44691

**OKLAHOMA**
Central Oklahoma CEA
P O Box 25606
Oklahoma City 73125

CEA of Stillwater
1522 Hanson Circle
Stillwater 74074

Childbirth & Family Life
2802 E. 48th St.
Tulsa 74105

Oklahoma Parent Education
  League
216 Overton Dr.
Norman 73071

**OREGON**
Birthcenter/Irene Nielsen,
  CNM
514-516 Adams, P O Box 797
Cottage Grove 97424

CEA of Southern Oregon
P O Box 1394
Medford 97501

Childbirth Educators of Bess
  Kaiser Hospital
2889 N.E. Edgehill Place
Portland 97212

Hermiston CEA
c/o Shari Ford
Rt. 3, Box 3302
Hermiston 97838

Home Oriented Maternity
  Experience (HOME)
Dorothy Fitzgerald
1920 N.W. 29th Place
Corvallis 97330

Josephine County CEA
P O Box 5
Murphy 97533

Prepared Childbirth Assoc.
6446 S.W. Capitol Highway
Portland 97201

Salem CEA
840 Jefferson
Salem 97303

**PENNSYLVANIA**
Berks County Assoc. for
  Childbirth Education
P O Box 374
Reading 19610

CEA of Greater Monongahela
  Valley
RD #2, Box 437
Charleroi 15022

CEA of Greater Philadelphia
814 Fayette St.
Conshohocken 19428

CEA of Luzerne County
61 Corlear St.
Wilkes-Barre 18702

CEA of State College
P O Box 1074
State College 16801

Clearfield Area Prepared
  Childbirth Assoc.
216 S. Front St.
Clearfield 16830

Dubois Area Prepared
  Childbirth Assoc.
P O Box 62
Dubois 15801

Fathers & Mothers Learning
  Through Education &
  Experience
Box 15
Telford 18969

Lebanon Valley CEA
RD 1, Box 65
Lebanon 17042

OTH Maternity Center
51 Overbrook Ave.
Philadelphia 19131

Parents' Assoc. for Childbirth
  Education
P O Box 14429
Philadelphia 19115

Pittsburgh Organization for
  Childbirth Education
P O Box 143
Murrysville 15668

Wayne County CEA
355 Ridge St.
Honesdale 18431

**RHODE ISLAND**
Assoc. for a Better Childbirth
  & Developmental
  Experience
Box 20
Warwick 02886

Greater Providence CEA
P O Box 2477
Providence 02906

**SOUTH CAROLINA**
Childbirth & Parent Education
  Assoc. of Greenville
16 Lakeview Circle
Greenville 29611

**SOUTH DAKOTA**
South Dakota Educated
  Childbirth Assoc.
Rt. 3, Box 77
Aberdeen 57401

**TENNESSEE**
CEA of Oak Ridge
P O Box 551
Oak Ridge 37830

Childbirth Information Assoc.
2113 Ashwood Ave.
Nashville 37212

Organization for the Art of
  Parenthood
330 Peterson Lane
Clarkeville 37040

**TEXAS**
Arlington Organization for
  Parent Education
P O Box 1261
Arlington 76010

CEA of Victoria
P O Box 3852
Victoria 77901

Conference of Practicing
  Midwives
P O Box 13063
El Paso 79912

Dallas Assoc. for Parent
  Education
5531 Dyer St., Room 203
Dallas 75206

Family Life Educational Assoc.
P O Box 1191
Abilene 79604

Houston Organization for
   Parent Education
3521 Richmond, Suite 330
Houston 77098

The Maternity Center
1119 E. San Antonio Ave.
El Paso 79901

Nacogdoches Parents Assoc.
3309 Tyler Rd. #54
Nacogdoches 75961

Orange CEA
P O Box 644
Orange 77630

Parents' Assoc. for Childbirth
   Education
P O Box 2286
Freeport 77541

Prepared Childbirth Education
   League
1017 S. Alabama
Amarillo 79102

Southeast Assoc. for Childbirth
   Education
P O Box 57124
Webster 77598

**UTAH**
Cache Valley CEA
P O Box 581
Logan 84321

Cameron, Joyce/
College of Nursing
University of Utah
Salt Lake City 87112

Tooele CEA
173 S. First St.
Tooele 84074

**VERMONT**
Matthews, Kay
Thetford Academy
Thetford Center 05075

**VIRGINIA**
CEA of the New River Valley
Box 801
Blacksburg 24060

Childbirth Education Assoc.
Box 5078
Alexandria 22305

Roanoke Childbirth Educators
P O Box 13123
Roanoke 24031

Tidewater Childbirth
   Educators Assoc.
P O Box 62125
Virginia Beach 23462

**WASHINGTON**
Assoc. for Childbirth at Home
   (ACAH)
Virginia Day
5821 S. Fletcher
Seattle 98118

CEA of Snohomish County
P O Box 2407
Everett 98203

CEA of Tacoma
1509 S. 7th
Tacoma 98405

Childbirth & Parent Education
  Assoc. of the Tri-Cities
6710 W. Arrowhead
Kennewick 99336

Fremont Women's Clinic
6817 Greenwood Ave. N.
Seattle 98103

Parent Assoc. for Learning
P O Box 767
Aberdeen 98520

Spokane's Assoc. for Family
  Education-Parents Helping
  Parents
P O Box 9016
Spokane 99209

**WEST VIRGINIA**
CEA of Huntington
817 2nd St.
Huntington 25701

CEA of the Mid-Ohio Valley
P O Box 856
Parkersburg 26101

Childbirth & Parent Education
  Assoc. of Morgantown
P O Box 1106
Morgantown 26505

Parent & Childbirth Education
  Assoc.
Central District Mental
Health Center
#6 Hospital Plaza
Clarksburg 26301

**WISCONSIN**
Childbirth Assoc./Lamaze
  Method of Janesville
P O Box 1041
Janesville 53545

CEA of Green Bay
P O Box 54
Green Bay 54305

CEA of Hudson River Falls
P O Box 345
Hudson 54016

CEA of Milwaukee
11040 W. Bluemound Rd.
Milwaukee 53226

Childbirth Education Services
P O Box 109
Racine 53401

Childbirth & Parent Assoc. of
  Madison
P O Box 565
Madison 53701

Hayward Area CEA
c/o Linda Anderson
Rt. 6
Box 287
Hayward 54843

Health Writers
306 N. Brooks St.
Madison 53715

Institute for Childbirth &
  Family Research
P O Box 129
Cottage Grove 53527

Madison Birth Education
1043 Hebbufer St.
Madison 53703

Northland CEA
422 Abner St.
Rhinelander 54501

Parentcraft Teachers Assoc.
1614 Meadowcrest Lane
Middleton 53562

Sheboygan CEA
818 Swift Ave.
Sheboygan 53081

Stevens Point Area CEA
2522 North Reserve Dr.
Stevens Point 54481

WYOMING
Casper Family Centered
  League
2918 Saratoga Rd.
Casper 82601

Cheyenne CEA
4709 Maple Way
Cheyenne 82001

# APPENDIX II

## NATIONAL BIRTH ORGANIZATIONS

American Academy of
  Husband-Coached Childbirth
Box 5224
Sherman Oaks, CA 91413

American College of Nurse-
  Midwives
1522 K St., N.W.
Suite 1120
Washington, DC 20005

The American Fertility Society
1801 Ninth Ave. South #101
Birmingham, AL 35205

American Public Health Assoc.
Maternal-Child Health Section
1015 Eighteenth St., N.W.
Washington, DC 20036

American Society for
  Psychoprophylaxis in
  Obstetrics (ASPO)
1523 L. St., N.W.
Washington, DC 20005
(this is the official name of
  Lamaze childbirth training)

Down's Syndrome Congress
16470 Ronnies Dr.
Mishawaka, IN 46544

H.O.M.E. c/o Esther Herman
5 New York Ave.
Takoma Park
Washington, DC 20012

International Childbirth
  Education Assoc. (ICEA)
P O Box 20852
Milwaukee, WI 53220

International Council for
  Infant Survival
1515 Reisterstown Rd. #300
Baltimore, MD 21208

La Leche League International
9616 Minneapolis Ave.
Franklin Park, IL 60131

Lamaze
See American Society for
  Psychoprophylaxis in
  Obstetrics (ASPO), above

National Assoc. for Parents &
  Professionals for Safe
  Alternatives in Childbirth
  (NAPSAC)
Box 1307
Chapel Hill, NC 27514

National Association of
  Childbearing Centers
RD 1, Box 1
Perkiomenville, PA 18074

National Sudden Infant Death
  Syndrome Foundation
310 S. Michigan Ave.
Chicago, IL 60604

National Women's Health
  Network
1302 18th St., N.W., Suite 203
Washington, DC 20036

The National Midwives Assoc.
P O Box 163
Princeton, NJ 08540

Non-Circumcision Information
  Center
P O Box 404
Ipswich, MA 01938

Society for the Protection of
  the Unborn Through
  Nutrition (SPUN)
17 N. Wabash Ave. #603
Chicago, IL 60602

# APPENDIX III

## HELP FOR GRIEVING PARENTS
### (Listed by State)

If you have lost your baby through miscarriage, stillbirth, neo-natal death or SIDS, the following groups can help support you during your grieving. If your town or city is not listed, contact your local hospital, childbirth educators, or Family Health Association to obtain information about groups in your area.

## CALIFORNIA

**AMEND** (Aiding a Mother Experiencing Neonatal Death), Los Angeles Chapter, 4032 Towhee Drive, Calabassas, CA 91302. Local Groups in Tampa, FL; Carbondale, IL; Alton, IL; St. Louis, MO; and Tulsa, OK.

**HAND** (Helping After Neonatal Death), c/o Barbara Jones, P.O. Box 62, San Anselmo, CA 94960, (415) 459-1770. Outreach and group support for parents after stillbirth or neonatal death; information for hospital staffs.

**SHARE** (A Source of Help in Airing and Resolving Experiences), Diane Bremesth, 5854 East Lansing, Fresno, CA 93727, (209) 291-3275; or Joan Christman and Mary Amacher, Social Services, St. Agnes Hospital, 1313 E. Herndon, Fresno, CA 93710.

## COLORADO

**Newborn and Fetal Loss Support Group,** c/o Mary Krugman, Coordinator, Parent Education, Rose Medical Center, 4567 East Ninth Avenue, Denver, CO 80200, (303) 320-2121. Counseling and group meetings for parents; information for hospital staffs.

## CONNECTICUT

**AID** (Aid in Infant Death), c/o Nancy Baranowski, 28 Wesley Drive, Huntington, CT 06484.

# FLORIDA

**AMEND** (Aiding a Mother Experiencing Neonatal Death), Tampa Chapter, c/o Dottie Cannon, 5104 - 127th Avenue, Tampa, FL 33617, (813) 961-3662; or Karen Frazier, (813) 988-7996. Support for mothers after neonatal death.

**HOPES** (Helping Other Parents Experiencing Sorrow), P.O. Box 1143, Lutz, FL 33549.

# ILLINOIS

**AMEND** (Aiding a Mother Experiencing Neonatal Death), Madison County Chapter, c/o Jane Borman, 2209 Gillis, Alton, IL 62002, (618) 466-7129.

**AMEND,** Memorial Hospital, 404 West Main Street, Carbondale, IL 62901, (618) 549-4415; or Malinda Sawyer, Rt. #5, Box 353, Marion, IL 62959.

**Bereaved Parents,** P.A.C.E.S. (Parent and Child Education Society), c/o Cathy McNeilly, 619 S. Humphrey, Oak Park, IL 60304.

**The Compassionate Friends, Inc.,** National Headquarters, P.O. Box 1347, Oak Brook, IL 60521, (312) 323-5010. A self-help organization of bereaved parents helping each other: local chapters exist throughout the world. Newsletter for $5/year.

**SHARE,** St. Elizabeth Hospital, 220 West Lincoln Street, Belleville, IL 62220, (618) 234-2415.

# INDIANA

**Bereaved Parents Group,** Parents and Friends of Children, Inc. (ICEA), c/o Linda Runden, 101 South Capitol Avenue, Corydon, IN 47112, (812) 738-3277.

**Project Comfort,** c/o Gerald C. Machgan, Chaplain, Parkview Hospital, 2200 Randalia Drive, Ft. Wayne, IN 46805, (219) 484-6636. Counseling and group meetings for parents of dying infants and after newborn death.

# IOWA

**Support for Parents with Empty Arms,** c/o Dr. Russell Striffler, St. Luke's Methodist Hospital, 1026 Avenue A., N.E., Cedar Rapids, IA 52402, (319) 398-7347. Individual and group support for parents after miscarriage, stillbirth, neonatal death, and crib death.

# KENTUCKY

**Norton-Children's Hospital,** c/o Chaplain Wayne Willis, P.O. Box 25070, Louisville, KY 40232, (502) 589-8176.

# MARYLAND

**National Sudden Infant Death Foundation** (SIDS), 2 Metro Plaza, Suite 205, 8240 Professional Place, Landover, MD 20785, (301) 459-3388.

# MASSACHUSETTS

**Boston Stillbirth Study Group,** c/o Ann Ross, Jean Stringham, and Judith Riley, 53 Country Corners Road, Wayland, MA 01778. Counseling and referral of parents; training and consultation with professionals.

**COPE** (Coping with the Overall Pregnancy/Parenting Experience), 37 Clarendon Street, Boston, MA 02116, (617) 357-5588. Counseling after miscarriage, ectopic pregnancy, and therapeutic abortion.

**Grief Support Group,** Childbirth Education Association of Central Massachusetts, c/o Linda Brink and Merilyn Bambauer, P.O. Box 193, West Side Station, Worcester, MA 01602. Group for parents after miscarriage, abortion or stillbirth.

**HOPE** (Helping Other Parents Endure), c/o Susan Harrington, South Shore Hospital, 55 Fogg Road, South Weymouth, MA 02190, (617) 337-7011, ext. 332. Group for parents after miscarriage, stillbirth, or infant death.

**Resolve,** 5 Water Street, Arlington, MA 02174, (617) 643-2442.

**Support Group for Bereaved Parents,** c/o Patricia Berman and Laura Simons, Department of Social Services, Brigham and Women's Hospital (Lying-In Division), 221 Longwood Avenue, Boston, MA 02115, (617) 732-4060. Group for parents after miscarriage, stillbirth, or infant death.

## MICHIGAN

**Bereaved Parents Group,** c/o Sister Mary Ruth, Providence Hospital, Southfield, MI 48075.

**Hoping,** The Edward Sparrow Hospital, 1215 E. Michigan Avenue, Lansing, MI 48901, (517) 483-3873.

**PEND** (Parents Experiencing Neonatal Death), c/o Neonatal I.C.U., Marcia Eager, Butterworth Hospital, Grand Rapids, MI 49503, (616) 774-1774. Group providing information and support for parents after neonatal death.

**Survivors—Up from Grief,** 17125 Fordline Avenue, Riverview, MI 48192.

## MINNESOTA

**Loving Arms** (Pregnancy and Infant Loss Center), 1415 E. Wayzata Boulevard, Suite 22, Wayzata, MN 55391. An organization providing resources and educational materials on pregnancy loss.

**Parents' Grief Support Group,** c/o Kathy Peterson, St. Mary's Hospital, Duluth, MN, (218) 727-4551, ext. 384; or Barbara Elliott, 4340 London Road, Duluth, MN 55804, (218) 525-7268.

## MISSOURI

**AMEND** (Aiding a Mother Experiencing Neonatal Death), c/o Maureen Connelly, 4324 Berrywick Terrace, St. Louis, MO 63128, (314) 487-7582; or Mary Wyss, 9161 Rusticwood Trail, St. Louis, MO 63126, (314) 843-3681. Individual counseling and group meetings for parents.

**HOPE** (Helping Other Parents Endure), P.O. Box 153, Florissant, MO 63032.

**Mothers-in-Crisis,** c/o Terry Weston, Social Service Department, Freeman Hospital, Joplin, MO 64801, (417) 623-2801. Individual and group support for mothers after miscarriage, stillbirth, and infant death (including Sudden Infant Death Syndrome).

## NEW JERSEY

**Compassionate Friends,** c/o Pat Turoczy, P.O. Box 63, Verona, NJ 07044, (201) 857-2464.

**HELP,** c/o Eileen Thompson, 607 North Oxford Avenue, Ventnor, NJ 08706, (609) 822-5265.

## NEW YORK

**Bereavement Clinic,** Nancy O'Donohue, Kings County Hospital, 451 Clarkson Avenue, Brooklyn, NY 11203; or c/o Joanne Middleton, Downstate Medical Center, 450 Clarkson Avenue, Brooklyn, NY 11203, (212) 270-1885. Individual and group support for parents after stillbirth and neonatal death.

**Bronx Bereaved Parents,** Holy Rosary Church, Eastchester and Gunhill Roads, Bronx, NY 10469, (212) 881-3852.

**Infant Bereavement Group,** 52 Davis Avenue, White Plains, NY 10605, (914) 472-5766 and (914) 472-9477.

**Miscarriage and Stillbirth Support Group,** c/o Dorothy Hai, 209 York Street, Olean, NY 14760, (716) 375-2111, 372-7021.

**National Self-Help Clearing House,** 33 W. 42nd Street, Room 1227, New York, NY 10036. A newsletter is available.

**Perinatal Bereavement Hotline,** Mary and John Wasacz, Scarsdale, NY, (914) 472-5766.

**SHARE** (Source of Help in Airing and Resolving Experiences), Lois Sugarman, 6726 Gleason Place, Fayetteville, NY 13066, (315) 446-1262. Group meetings for parents after miscarriage, stillbirth, and infant death; inservice for professionals.

## NORTH CAROLINA

**Kinder-Mourn,** 605 East Boulevard, Charlotte, NC 28203, (704) 376-2580. Group and individual counseling for families whose children died at any age (pregnancy to age thirty).

**Parent Care, Inc.,** P.O. Box 125, Cary, NC 27511.

## OHIO

**Bereaved Parents Group,** Denny and Janie Churchill, 3136 Ellet Avenue, Akron, OH 44312, (216) 628-8335.

**CARE,** The Toledo Hospital, 2142 North Cove Boulevard, Toledo, OH 43606.

**Compassionate Friends,** c/o Ann Arpasi, 27075 Sleepy Hollow Drive, Westlake, OH 44145, (216) 871-5077. Self-help group for parents, grandparents, and siblings of children who have died.

**HOPE** (Helping Other Parents Emotionally), Cleveland Metropolitan General Hospital/Highland View Hospital, 3395 Scranton Road, Cleveland, OH 44109, (216) 459-5918. Information and support for grieving parents.

**Parent Support Group,** Childbirth Education Association of Akron, c/o Linda Baily, 2183 Larchdale, Cuyohoga Falls, OH 44221.

**PEND** (Parents Experiencing Neonatal Death), Nancy Bartell, Rainbow Babies and Children's Hospital, 2101 Adelbert Road, Cleveland, OH 44106, (216) 831-1171.

## OKLAHOMA

**AMEND** (Aiding a Mother Experiencing Neonatal Death), Tulsa Group, 1344 East 26th Place, Tulsa, OK 74100.

# PENNSYLVANIA

**Booth Maternity Center,** c/o Nancy Johns and Laurie Rendall, 6051 Overbook Avenue, Philadelphia, PA 19131, (215) 878-7800. Group for parents after miscarriage and infant death.

**Grieving Clinic,** c/o Dr. Susan Jasin, Temple University Health Sciences Center, 3401 North Broad Rd., Philadelphia, PA 19140.

**Medical Social Work Department,** Magee Women's Hospital, Forbes Avenue and Halket Street, Pittsburgh, PA 15213, (412) 647-4255. Individual and group support for parents after miscarriage and infant death.

**UNITE** (Understanding Newborns in Traumatic Experiences), c/o Bernadette Foley, Social Services Department, Jeanes Hospital, 7600 Central Avenue, Philadelphia, PA 19111, (215) 728-2082. Support for parents after miscarriage or infant death.

# TENNESSEE

**PEPR** (Parents Experiencing Perinatal Death), P.O. Box 38455, Germantown, TN 38138, (901) 767-8727. Outreach, group and public education.

# TEXAS

**HAND** (H.O.P.E.'s Aid in Neonatal Death), c/o Karen Riley, Houston Organization for Parent Education, 3311 Richmond Avenue, Suite 330, Houston, TX 77098, (713) 524-3089. Group for parents after neonatal death.

# UTAH

**Sharing Heart,** c/o Thomas D. Coleman, University of Utah Medical Center, Department of Pediatrics, Room 2B425, 50 North Medical Drive, Salt Lake City, UT 84132, (801) 581-7052.

# WASHINGTON

**Parents of Prematures,** c/o Lauri Lowen, 13616 Northeast 26th Place, Bellevue, WA 98005, (206) 883-6040. Outreach and groups for parents of premature babies.

**P.S.** (Parents of Stillborns), c/o Bill and Doreen Dolleman, 6210 South 120th Street, Seattle, WA 98178, (206) 772-5338. Individual and group support for parents; educational programs for professionals.

**Parents of Stillborns,** c/o Judy Campbell, Group Health Cooperative—East Side, Redmond, WA, (206) 883-5761.

**Parents of Stillborn Newsletter,** 3509 N.E. 33rd Street, Tacoma, WA 98422.

# WASHINGTON, D.C.

**The Candlelighters Foundation,** National Headquarters, Suite 1011, 2025 Eye Street, N.W., Washington, DC 20006, (202) 659-5136. Support group for parents who have lost children or whose children are under treatment for cancer.

# WISCONSIN

**AID** (Aid in Infant Death), Childbirth Education Association of Milwaukee, c/o Katie Walker, 5636 W. Burleigh, Milwaukee, WI 53210, (414) 445-7470. Group for parents after miscarriage, stillbirth or infant death.

**Bereaved Parents Support Group,** Childbirth Education Association of Madison, c/o Carol Gowler, 1016 Van Buren, Madison, WI 53711, (608) 257-6352.

**Parents Supporting Parents,** c/o Mary Berg, Rice Clinic, 2501 Main Street, Stevens Point, WI 54481.

**Resolve Through Sharing,** La Crosse Lutheran Hospital, 1910 South Avenue, La Crosse, WI 54601, (608) 785-0530, ext. 3696.

**SHARE** (Source of Help in Airing and Resolving Experiences), St. Vincent Hospital, 835 South Van Buren Street, Green Bay, WI 54305, (414) 432-8621. Local groups in Sheboygan and LaCrosse.

# APPENDIX IV

## INFERTILITY AND GENETICS ORGANIZATIONS

The Barren Foundation
60 East Monroe Street
Chicago, IL 60603

Center for Communications in
Infertility, Inc.
P.O. Box 516
Yorktown Heights, NY 10598

March of Dimes Birth Defects
Foundation
1275 Mamaroneck Avenue
White Plains, NY 10605
Provides information on
genetic counseling and
testing and referrals to
physicians and genetics
centers; has local chapters
across the country.

National Genetics Foundation
555 West 57th Street
New York, NY 10019

Resolve
Box 474
Belmont, MA 02178
Provides information and
support to infertile couples;
has local chapters
nationwide.

United Infertility Organization
P.O. Box 23
Scarsdale, NY 10583

# APPENDIX V

## LACTATION CONSULTANTS

Breastfeeding and Human Milk
Study Center
University of Rochester
Medical Center
601 Elmwood Avenue
Rochester, NY 14642
(716) 275-0088

International Board of
Lactation Consultant
Examiners, Inc.
Nancy Clark
3400 Charleston Street
Annadale, VA 22003

International Lactation
Consultant Association
P.O. Box 4031 University of
Virginia Station
Charlottesville, VA 22903

Lactation Associates
Marsha Walker
254 Conant Road
Weston, MA 02193-1756
(617) 893-3553

The Lactation Institute and
  Breast-feeding Clinic
16161 Ventura Boulevard,
  Suite 223
Encino, CA 91436
(818) 995-1913

National Capital Lactation
  Center
Community Human Milk Bank
Georgetown University
  Hospital
3800 Reservoir Road, N.W.
Washington, DC 20007
(202) 784-MILK

The San Diego Lactation
  Program
4062 First Avenue
San Diego, CA 92103
Breast-feeding Helpline: (619)
  295-5193

# Index

KAREN BLANCHARD received her medical training at Johns Hopkins Medical School. She went on to a Fellowship in Maternal–Fetal Medicine at UCLA Medical Center in Los Angeles and continued her specialization in obstetrics and gynecology with an additional year of research at UCLA as a Walter C. Teagle scholar. Although Dr. Blanchard is a subspecialist in high-risk pregnancies, she has also been an advisor to a home-birth clinic and was a pioneer in the movement allowing couples to stay together for cesarean births.